MICROBIOLOGY
FOR
MEDICAL LABORATORY
TECHNOLOGY STUDENTS

Other Books by Dr. D.R. Arora

- Textbook of Microbiology, 5/e
- Textbook of Microbiology for Dental Students, 4/e
- Medical Parasitology, 5/e
- Medical Mycology, 2/e
- Essentials of Microbiology for B.Sc. Nursing Students
- Practical Microbiology
- Practical Microbiology for Dental Students
- Exam-Oriented Microbiology (Questions & Answers)
- Microbiology for Nursing and Allied Sciences, 2/e

MICROBIOLOGY FOR MEDICAL LABORATORY TECHNOLOGY STUDENTS

Dr. D.R. Arora M.D., Ph.D., M.N.A.M.S.

Ex-Professor & Head, Department of Microbiology,
Postgraduate Institute of Medical Sciences, Rohtak, Haryana (India), and
Maharaja Agarsen Medical College, Agroha, Haryana (India)

Ex-Professor & Head, Department of Microbiology,
Medical Superintendent, and Dean Faculty of Allied Health Sciences,
SGT University, Gurugram, Haryana (India)

Ex-W.H.O. Fellow; and Visiting Professor, University of Mauritius

Lead Assessor and Member, Accreditation Committee,
National Accreditation Board for Testing and Calibration Laboratories (NABL),
Gurugram, Haryana (India)

Principal Assessor, National Accreditation Board for Hospitals &
Healthcare Providers (NABH), New Delhi (India)

Assessor, National Accreditation Board for
Education and Training (NABET), New Delhi (India)

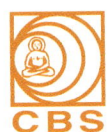

CBS

CBS Publishers & Distributors Pvt. Ltd.

New Delhi • Bengaluru • Chennai • Kochi • Kolkata • Mumbai
Hyderabad • Nagpur • Patna • Pune • Jharkhand • Uttarakhand

ISBN: 978-93-86827-57-9

First Edition: 2018

Published by **Satish Kumar Jain** and produced by **Varun Jain** for
CBS Publishers & Distributors Pvt. Ltd.,
4819/XI Prahlad Street, 24 Ansari Road, Daryaganj, New Delhi - 110002
delhi@cbspd.com, cbspubs@airtelmail.in • www.cbspd.com
Ph.: 23289259, 23266861, 23266867 • Fax: 011-23243014

Corporate Office: 204 FIE, Industrial Area, Patparganj, Delhi - 110 092
Ph: 49344934 • Fax: 011-49344935
E-mail: publishing@cbspd.com • publicity@cbspd.com

Branches:
• *Bengaluru:* 2975, 17th Cross, K.R. Road, Bansankari 2nd Stage,
  Bengaluru - 70 • Ph: +91-80-26771678/79 • Fax: +91-80-26771680
  E-mail: cbsbng@gmail.com, bangalore@cbspd.com
• *Chennai:* No. 7, Subbaraya Street, Shenoy Nagar, Chennai - 600030
  Ph: +91-44-26681266, 26680620 • Fax: +91-44-42032115
  E-mail: chennai@cbspd.com
• *Kochi:* Ashana House, 39/1904, A.M. Thomas Road, Valanjambalam,
  Ernakulum, Kochi • Ph: +91-484-4059061-65
  Fax: +91-484-4059065 • E-mail: cochin@cbspd.com
• *Kolkata:* 6-B, Ground Floor, Rameshwar Shaw Road, Kolkata - 700014
  Ph: +91-33-22891126/7/8 • E-mail: kolkata@cbspd.com
• *Mumbai:* 83-C, Dr. E. Moses Road, Worli, Mumbai - 400018
  Ph: +91-9833017933, 022-24902340/41 • E-mail: mumbai@cbspd.com

Representatives:

• Hyderabad: 0-9885175004	• Nagpur: 0-9021734563
• Patna: 0-9334159340	• Pune: 0-9623451994
• Jharkhand: 0-9811541605	• Uttarakhand: 0-9716462459

Printed at:
Neekunj Print Process

Dedicated to the
sweet memories of

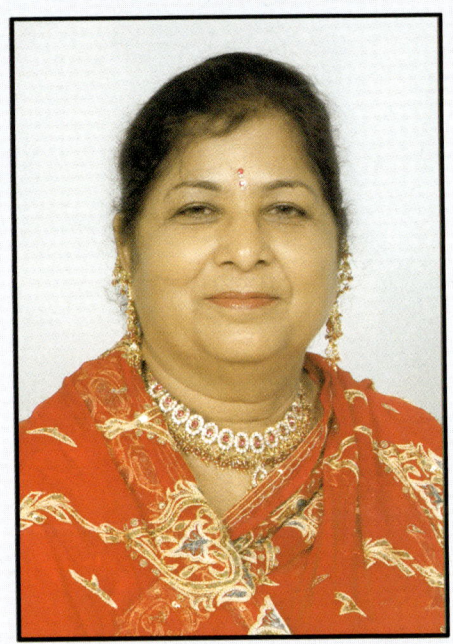

Dr. Brij Bala Arora
(04.03.1947 – 21.11.2014)

Preface

Microbiology is a valuable and useful discipline that offers an exhaustive view of an invisible world around us. Infectious diseases account for 26% of the total deaths in the world and this percentage is much higher in the developing world including India. A sound knowledge of microbial infections particularly methods of laboratory diagnosis is vital for medical laboratory technologists. A few books on medical laboratory technology are available. All these books cover mainly the practical part. They are lacking in theory part of the microorganisms and parasites. For the diagnosis of microbial infections the theoretical knowledge of microorganisms is essential because "what mind does not know eyes cannot see". Moreover, for getting through the examination, the medical laboratory technology students have to pass both in theory and practical examinations. This book covers both theory and practical aspects of microbiology and parasitology.

Traditionally, the identification of bacteria and fungi has been based on conventional procedures which often yield poor results because of low microbial load and increased chances of contamination. The conventional methods for identification (ID) and antimicrobial susceptibility testing (AST) are labour-intensive, have long turnaround time, poor reliability and reproducibility, and are prone to higher chances of cross-contamination. Due to the need for simpler and faster methods with better outcomes, automated systems have been introduced. In this book, automated systems for the ID and AST have been described in one of the chapters.

Text has been presented in a lucid manner for the students to help them imbibe the basics of the subject. It is illustrated with coloured figures, clinical photographs and microphotographs. Diagrams of the life cycle of the parasites are computer-drawn with simple line sketches. This makes the book colourful and the readers can have better understanding of the biology of the microorganisms. The book has been divided into five sections. These are General Bacteriology, Systemic Bacteriology, Virology, Mycology, and Parasitology.

I express my sincere thanks to Dr. Ashima Katyal, Senior Resident; Dr. Deepinder Singh, Resident; and Dr. Paramjit Singh Gill, Professor, Department of Microbiology, Postgraduate Institute of Medical Sciences, Rohtak, for contributing a chapter on "Automation in Microbiology".

I am grateful to Mr. B.M. Singh for meticulous proof-reading and valuable professional help and support. I am also grateful to Mr. Anurag Trivedi for designing the book. I honestly acknowledge the most sincere and dedicated support and advice of Mr. Dharmvir.

The readers are requested to send suggestions for the improvement of the book which will be incorporated in the subsequent editions. Shortcomings, if any, may please be communicated at *draroradr@rediffmail.com*.

D.R. Arora

Contents

Preface vii
General Instructions to Medical Laboratory Technologists xi

SECTION 1
GENERAL BACTERIOLOGY — 1

Chapter 1   Introduction 3
Chapter 2   Morphology of Bacteria 5
Chapter 3   Growth and Nutrition of Bacteria 11
Chapter 4   Collection of Specimens, Identification of Bacteria and Taxonomy 23
Chapter 5   Sterilization, Disinfection, and Disposal of Biomedical Waste 33
Chapter 6   Bacterial Genetics 42
Chapter 7   Bacteria in Health and Disease 49
Chapter 8   Immunity 54
Chapter 9   Antigens 60
Chapter 10   Antibodies 63
Chapter 11   The Complement System 69
Chapter 12   Antigen-Antibody Reactions 73
Chapter 13   Architecture of the Immune System 83
Chapter 14   Immune Response 89
Chapter 15   Hypersensitivity 95
Chapter 16   Autoimmunity 101
Chapter 17   Transplantation Immunology 103

SECTION 2
SYSTEMIC BACTERIOLOGY — 107

Chapter 18   Staphylococcus 109
Chapter 19   Streptococcus and Enterococcus 114
Chapter 20   Streptococcus Pneumoniae (Pneumococcus) 120
Chapter 21   Neisseria, Moraxella and Acinetobacter 123
Chapter 22   Corynebacterium Diphtheriae 127
Chapter 23   Bacillus Anthracis 131
Chapter 24   Clostridium 134
Chapter 25   Mycobacterium tuberculosis 139
Chapter 26   Nontuberculous Mycobacteria 144

Chapter 27   Mycobacterium Leprae 147
Chapter 28   Spirochaetes 152
Chapter 29   Bacteroides, Propionibacterium and Fusobacterium 161
Chapter 30   Escherichia, Klebsiella, Enterobacter, Serratia, Proteus and Morganella 162
Chapter 31   Shigella and Salmonella 167
Chapter 32   Yersinia Pestis 173
Chapter 33   Vibrio, Pseudomonas and Burkholderia 175
Chapter 34   Campylobacter and Helicobacter 181
Chapter 35   Legionella Pneumophila 184
Chapter 36   Haemophilus and Bordetella 186
Chapter 37   Brucella 191
Chapter 38   Mycoplasma and Ureaplasma 194
Chapter 39   Rickettsia and Orientia 198
Chapter 40   Chlamydia and Chlamydophila 202
Chapter 41   Actinomyces and Nocardia 207
Chapter 42   Gardnerella, Erysipelothrix and Streptobacillus 210
Chapter 43   Antimicrobial Sensitivity Testing 212
Chapter 44   Bacteriology of Water, Milk and Air 215
Chapter 45   Automation in Microbiology 220

SECTION 3
VIROLOGY
227

Chapter 46   General Properties of Viruses 229
Chapter 47   Bacteriophage 237
Chapter 48   Poxviruses and Herpesviruses 239
Chapter 49   Adenoviruses, Papillomaviruses and Rotaviruses 244
Chapter 50   Polioviruses and Rabies Virus 247
Chapter 51   Influenza, Parainfluenza, Mumps, and Measles Viruses 251
Chapter 52   Chikungunya, Rubella, Dengue, Japanese Encephalitis and Kyasanur Forest Disease 257
Chapter 53   Human Immunodeficiency Viruses: AIDS 260
Chapter 54   Hepatitis Viruses 262

SECTION 4
MYCOLOGY
267

Chapter 55   Mycology 269

SECTION 5
PARASITOLOGY
291

Chapter 56   Parasitology 293
Chapter 57   Parasitic Diagnostic Procedures 346

Index 357

General Instructions to Medical Laboratory Technologists

- Protect your clothings in the laboratory by wearing an overall. This should not be worn outside the laboratory.
- All microorganisms should be regarded as capable of causing disease.
- Long hair should be tied back to avoid risks from fire and accidental contamination.
- Mouth-pipetting is not allowed.
- Always flame the bacteriological loop before and after use.
- Do not try to smell any bacterial culture.
- Do not expose microbiological cultures longer than necessary.
- Do not shake liquid cultures.
- Do not place cotton-wool plugs or other stoppers on the bench.
- Do not place contaminated pipettes on the bench top.
- Do not sit on the bench top.
- Do not lick labels with tongue.
- Do not put pencils, fingers and other objects in your mouth.
- Do not eat or drink in the laboratory.
- Discard the used and contaminated slides and other materials in disinfectant jar.
- Do not wander about in the laboratory.
- Do not forcibly expel material from a pipette.
- Always wash your hands thoroughly at the end of your work.
- Bench tops should be disinfected immediately after experiment is over.
- All accidents like cuts and burns in the laboratory should be reported to your teacher.
- Accidental spillage of bacterial growth or other contaminated material should be reported to your teacher or laboratory incharge.

SECTION 1

GENERAL BACTERIOLOGY

Chapter 1   Introduction
Chapter 2   Morphology of Bacteria
Chapter 3   Growth and Nutrition of Bacteria
Chapter 4   Collection of Specimens, Identification of Bacteria and Taxonomy
Chapter 5   Sterilization, Disinfection and Disposal of Biomedical Waste
Chapter 6   Bacterial Genetics
Chapter 7   Bacteria in Health and Disease
Chapter 8   Immunity
Chapter 9   Antigens
Chapter 10   Antibodies
Chapter 11   The Complement System
Chapter 12   Antigen-Antibody Reactions
Chapter 13   Architecture of the Immune System
Chapter 14   Immune Response
Chapter 15   Hypersensitivity
Chapter 16   Autoimmunity
Chapter 17   Transplantation Immunology

Introduction

Microbiology is the study of living organisms of microscopic size. This term was introduced by French chemist Louis Pasteur, who demonstrated that fermentation was caused by the growth of bacteria and yeasts. **Medical microbiology** is the study of microbes that infect humans, the disease they cause, and their diagnosis, prevention and treatment. It also deals with the response of the human host to microbial infection. The term **microbe** was first used by Sedillot in 1878, but it has now been replaced by **microorganism**.

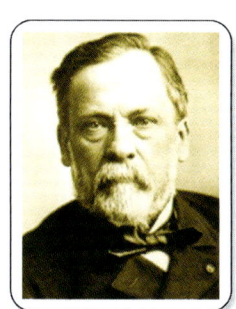

Louis Pasteur
(1822–1895)

The construction and use of the compound microscope (*micro*, small; and *skop*, to see) was an essential prerequisite to study the microbial forms. To **Antonie van Leeuwenhoek** (1632–1723) must be ascribed the credit of placing the science of microbiology on the firm basis of direct observation. This Dutch maker of lenses from Holland devised an

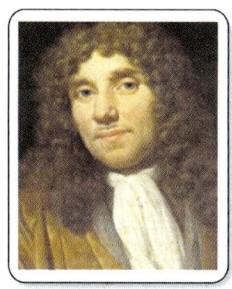

Antonie van
Leeuwenhoek
(1632–1723)

apparatus and technique which enabled him to observe and describe various microbial forms with accuracy and care.

THE DEVELOPING SCIENCE OF MICROBIOLOGY

In the course of studies, Pasteur introduced the techniques of sterilization and developed steam sterilizer, hot air oven and autoclave. **Robert Koch** (1843–1910), a German physician, perfected the bacteriological techniques, staining procedures and methods of obtaining bacteria in pure culture using solid media during his studies on the culture and characters of anthrax bacillus.

KOCH'S POSTULATES

A microorganism can be accepted as the causative agent of an infectious disease only if following postulates, known as Koch's postulates, are satisfied (Fig. 1.1):

1. The microorganism must be present in the lesions in every case of the infectious disease.
2. It should be possible to isolate the microorganism in pure culture from the lesions.
3. Inoculation of the pure culture by a suitable route into a suitable laboratory animal should produce a similar disease.
4. It should again be possible to re-isolate the microorganism in pure culture from the lesions produced in the experimental animals.

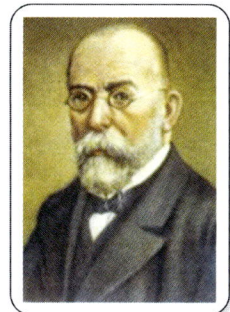

Robert Koch
(1843–1910)

A fifth criterion introduced subsequently states that specific antibodies to the organism should be demonstrable in the serum of the patient suffering from the disease. These postulates have proved extremely useful in confirming the authenticity of doubtful claims made regarding the causative agents of infectious diseases.

THE BEGINNING OF VIROLOGY

For many years the term virus was used to describe any poison or microbial agent capable of causing an infection. In a large number of diseases such as smallpox, chickenpox, measles, influenza, poliomyelitis and the common cold, no bacterial cause could be established. Pasteur had suspected that rabies in dogs could be caused by a microbe too small to be seen under the microscope.

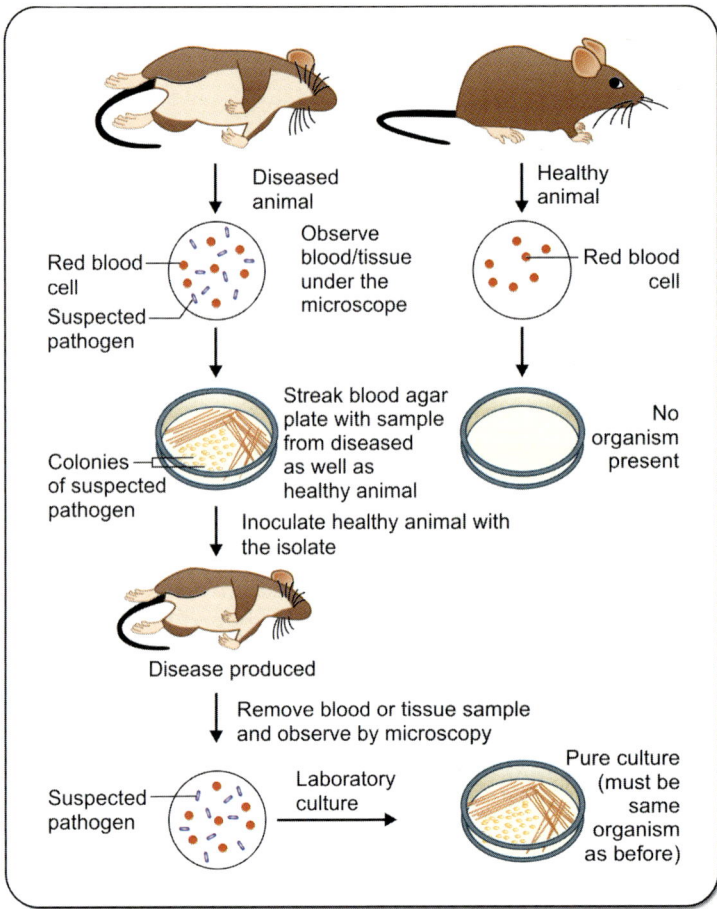

Fig. 1.1. Koch's postulates.

Morphology of Bacteria

Bacteria are free-living, microscopic, unicellular organisms capable of performing all the essential functions of life, e.g., growth, metabolism and reproduction. They possess both deoxyribonucleic acid (DNA) and ribonucleic acid (RNA) and lack chlorophyll. Bacteria have been placed in a kingdom separate from the animal and plant kingdoms, **Monera**.

Cells that have a well-defined nucleus are called **eukaryotes** (*eu*, true; and *karyon*, nucleus), whereas cells that lack a well-defined nucleus are called **prokaryotes** (*pro*, primitive; and *karyon*, nucleus). Bacteria and blue-green algae are prokaryotes, while fungi, other algae, slime molds and protozoa are eukaryotes.

Bacteria do not contain a membrane-bound nucleus. Their DNA consists of a single circular chromosome, which is attached to a mesosome, a saclike structure in the cell membrane. Bacterial ribosomes are found free in the cytoplasm and attached to the cytoplasmic membrane. The cell envelope, in bacteria, consists of cytoplasmic (cell) membrane and cell wall. Some species also produce capsules and slime layers.

SIZE OF BACTERIA

Bacteria are very small in size. The unit of measurement of bacteria is called micrometre (μm). One μm is a millionth part of a metre or a thousandth part of a millimetre (mm). One nanometre (nm) is a thousandth part of a μm, and one Angstrom unit (Å) is one tenth of a nanometre. The diameter of the smallest body that can be resolved and seen clearly with naked eye is about 100 μm.

Medically important bacteria, generally, measure 0.2–1.5 μm in diameter and 3–5 μm in length. Therefore, to visualize most bacteria one must use the higher powers of magnification of a good light microscope and enlarge them about 1000 times. To visualize their surfaces distinctly, it is usually necessary to stain them. Electron microscopy is essential for clear visualization of internal structures of the bacteria.

Microscopy

The study of the morphology of bacteria requires the use of microscopes. Following types of microscopes are used for examination of bacteria:

Light microscope

Bacteria may be examined under light microscope, either in the living state or after fixation and staining. The arrangement, motility and approximate size of the organisms can be observed by the examination of wet films or 'hanging drops'. But, due to lack of contrast, details cannot be appreciated.

Phase-contrast microscope

The phase-contrast microscope takes advantage of the fact that light waves passing through transparent objects such as cells, emerge in different phases depending on the properties of the materials through which they pass. A special optical system converts difference in phase into difference in intensity, so that some structures appear darker than others. It can be used to reveal some details of the internal structures in living cells.

Dark-ground (Dark-field) microscope

This microscope renders visible delicate organisms such as *Treponema pallidum*. Dark-field microscopy is frequently performed on the same microscope on which bright field microscopy is performed. By means of a special condenser with a circular central stop, the specimen is illuminated by oblique light only. The rays do not enter the tube of the microscope, and in consequence, do not reach the eye of the observer unless they are scattered by objects (e.g., bacteria) of different refractive index from the medium in which they are suspended. As a result, the organisms appear brightly illuminated against a dark background.

The advantage of this method is that the resolving power of the dark-field microscopy is significantly improved compared with that of bright-field microscopy. The disadvantage of this method is light passes around rather than through the organisms, making it difficult to study their internal structure.

Fluorescence microscope

When ultraviolet or short-wavelength or invisible light falls on a fluorescent substance, the wavelength of the invisible light increases, so that it becomes luminous and is said to fluoresce. If tissues, cells or bacteria are stained with a fluorescent dye and are examined under the microscope with ultraviolet light instead of ordinary visible light, they become luminous and are seen as bright objects against a dark background.

Electron microscope

The greatly increased resolving power of the electron microscope (EM) has enabled scientists to observe the detailed structures of prokaryotic and eukaryotic cells. The superior resolution of the EM is due to the fact that electrons have a much shorter wavelength than the photons of white light. In EM, a beam of electrons is employed instead of the beam of light used in the optical microscope.

The resolution that can be obtained with EM is hundred times more than that of the light microscope.

SHAPE OF BACTERIA

Bacteria exist in different shapes as under (Fig. 2.1):

1. **Cocci** (from *kokkos* meaning berry) are round or oval cells.
2. **Bacilli** (from *baculus* meaning rod) are rod or stick-shaped. The ends may be square or rounded. The bacilli with tapered, pointed ends are termed fusiform. In some of the bacilli the length of the cells may be equal to width. Such bacillary forms are known as **coccobacilli**. The latter have to be carefully differentiated from cocci.
3. **Vibrios** are curved or comma-shaped rods.
4. **Spirilla** are non-flexuous spiral forms with one to three fixed curves in their rigid bodies.
5. **Spirochaetes** (from *spira* meaning coil and *chaite* meaning hair) are slender and flexuous spiral forms.
6. **Mycoplasmas** are cell wall deficient organisms. Therefore, they do not possess stable morphology. They occur as round or oval bodies or as interlacing filaments.

GROUP PATTERNS

The most frequent method of reproduction among bacteria is asexual binary fission, that is, each cell splits in half, forming two new cells. As they increase in number they form distinct groups. Cocci that split along one plane only tend to arrange themselves in pairs (**diplococci**) or in chains (**streptococci**). When the division occurs alternatively in each of two planes, groups of four (**tetrads**) or eight (**octads**) are formed. Haphazard splitting in several planes results in the formation of clusters of cocci (Fig. 2.1).

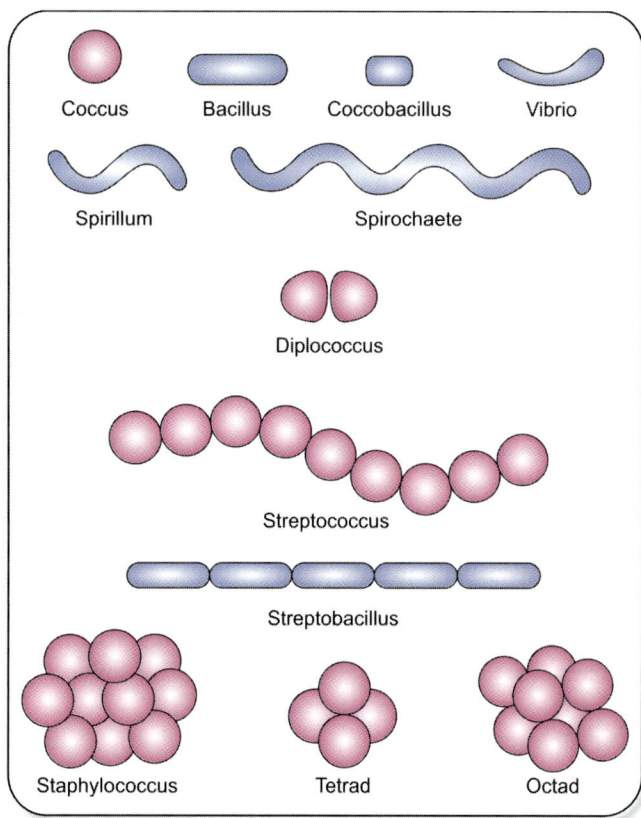

Fig. 2.1. Shapes and group patterns of bacteria.

Bacilli split only across their short axes, therefore, the patterns formed by them are limited. They may appear as end to end pairs (**diplobacilli**), or chains (**streptobacilli**) (Fig. 2.1). In some instances, there occurs incomplete separation of the daughter cells after binary fission. The bacilli remain attached to each other at various angles, resembling the letters V or L. This is called **Chinese letter arrangement** and is characteristic of *Corynebacterium diphtheriae*.

ANATOMY OF A BACTERIAL CELL

The principal structure of a bacterial cell is shown in Fig. 2.2. The interior of the cell, the protoplast, is differentiated into cytoplasm and nuclear material. Cytoplasm is bounded by a thin, elastic and semipermeable cytoplasmic membrane. Outside this lies cell wall, which gives the bacterium its shape and rigidity. Cell wall, in many bacteria, is enclosed by a protective gelatinous covering layer called capsule. Many bacteria also possess flagella which are the organelles of motility and some species have fimbriae (pili) too.

Bacterial cell wall

- It is a complex rigid structure which gives bacteria their definite shape.
- It is permeable to passage of liquid nutrient material into the cell, and to outward passage of substances produced within the cell.

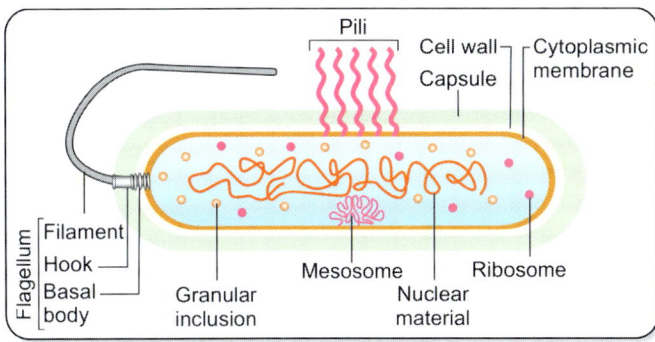

Fig. 2.2. Anatomy of a bacterial cell.

- It is about 10–20 nm in thickness and constitutes 20–30% of dry weight of the cell.
- The cell walls of Gram-positive bacteria are generally thicker than those of Gram-negative bacteria.
- The strength of the bacterial cell wall is due to the presence in it of a substance referred to as **peptidoglycan**, muco-peptide or murein.

Gram-positive bacterial cell wall

- The Gram-positive bacterial cell wall is 16–80 nm thick and is composed mostly of several layers of **peptidoglycan**.
- It constitutes **50–90%** of the dry weight of the wall.
- In addition to peptidoglycan, Gram-positive cell wall also contains teichoic acids and polysaccharides. There are two types of teichoic acids – cell wall teichoic acid, covalently linked to peptidoglycan; and membrane teichoic acid, covalently linked to cytoplasmic membrane.

Gram-negative bacterial cell wall

- The cell wall of Gram-negative bacteria is thinner (2 nm) than that of Gram-positive bacteria but is structurally more complex. It consists of peptidoglycan, lipoprotein, outer membrane, and lipopolysaccharide.

Acid-fast cell wall

Certain genera (*Mycobacterium* and *Nocardia*) have a Gram-positive cell wall structure but, in addition, contain a waxy layer of glycolipids and fatty acids (**mycolic acid**) bound to the exterior of the cell wall. This makes *Mycobacterium* species difficult to stain with the Gram stain. The mycobacteria and nocardiae can be stained with an acid-fast stain, in which the bacteria are stained with carbol fuchsin, followed by treatment with sulphuric acid or acid alcohol as decolourizer. Other bacteria are decolourized, whereas mycobacteria and nocardiae retain the stain. They are, therefore, known as **acid-fast bacteria**.

Cytoplasmic membrane

Bacterial cytoplasmic membrane, also called cell membrane, limits the bacterial protoplast externally. It is thin (5–10 nm), elastic and consists of a phospholipid bilayer, in which various constituent proteins are embedded. **It acts as a semi-permeable membrane controlling the inflow and outflow of metabolites to and from the protoplasm.** It permits the passive diffusion inward and outward of water and other small molecular substances, but it actively effects the selective transport of specific nutrients into the cell and that of waste products out of it.

Cytoplasm

Cytoplasm of the bacterial cell is a viscous watery solution of soft gel, containing a variety of organic and inorganic solutes. It contains all biosynthetic components required by the bacterium for the growth and cell division, together with genetic material.

It contains ribosomes which are composed of ribosomal RNA (rRNA) and ribosomal proteins. They measure 10–20 nm in diameter and have a sedimentation coefficient of 70S. Each 70S particle is composed of a 30S and a 50S subparticle. Each cell contains thousands of ribosomes strung together on strands of messenger RNA (mRNA) to form polysomes and it is at this site that code of mRNA is translated into peptide sequences.

Bacterial nucleus

The genetic information of a bacterial cell is contained in a single, circular, double-stranded molecule of DNA. It is often accompanied by a smaller extrachromosomal DNA known as **plasmid**. It is 1000 μm or more in length, about 1000 times the length of the cell. Therefore, it occurs tightly coiled like a skein of woollen thread.

Capsule and slime layer

Cell wall in many bacteria is enclosed by a protective gelatinous covering layer. If it is easily washed off and does not appear to be associated with the cell in any definite fashion it is referred to as a **slime layer**, on the other hand, if it appears as discrete, thickened gel around each cell, it is called a **capsule** (Fig. 2.3). If capsule is too thin to be seen with light microscope, it is called **microcapsule**. In most species it is made-up of a complex polysaccharide (e.g., pneumococcus), though in some species its main constituent is polypeptide (e.g., anthrax bacillus). When slime forming bacteria are grown on a solid culture medium, the slime remains around the bacteria as a matrix in which they are embedded and its presence confers on growth a **mucoid** character.

Functions

- Capsules protect the bacteria from antibacterial agents such as lytic enzymes found in nature.
- They inhibit phagocytosis, thus contributing to the virulence of the bacteria.
- The capsular antigen is specific for bacteria, therefore, it can be used for identification and typing of bacteria.

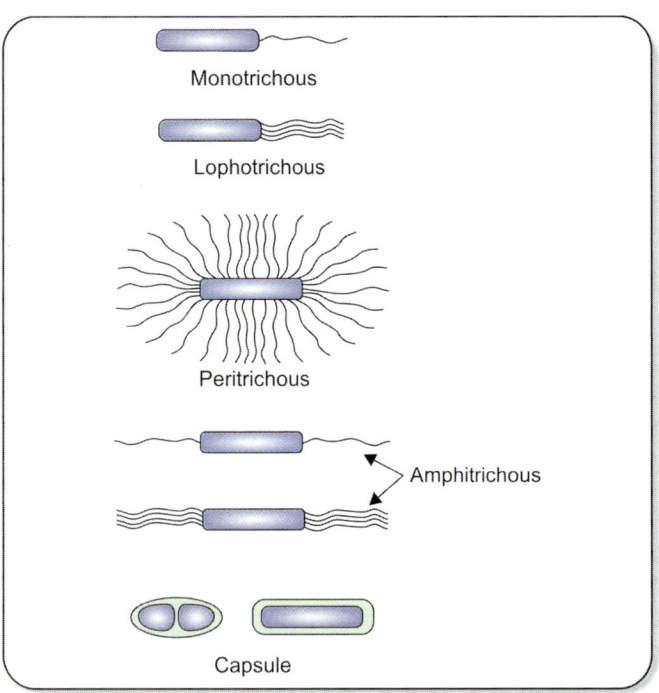

Fig. 2.3. Arrangement of flagella and capsule.

Demonstration of capsule

- Capsule cannot be stained with ordinary stains like Gram staining.
- It can be visualized by suspending the organisms in India ink and observing microscopically the exclusion of the colloidal ink particles from the area around the cell that is occupied by the capsule.
- It may also be visualized by reaction with specific antibody, which causes a characteristic swelling of the capsule. It is known as **Quellung reaction**. This phenomenon is seen in and allows rapid identification of capsular serotypes of *Streptococcus pneumoniae*, *Neisseria meningitidis*, several groups of streptococci, *Klebsiella* and *Haemophilus influenzae*.

For demonstration of polypeptide capsule of *Bacillus anthracis* (McFadyean's reaction) refer to Chapter 23.

Flagella

A large number of bacteria are motile by means of flagella. Flagella are long, hollow, helical filaments, usually several times the length of the cell. They are 10–20 nm in diameter, 3–20 μm in length and are found on both Gram-positive and Gram-negative bacteria. Their number varies from 1 to 20 flagella per bacterial cell.

Arrangement

There are four types of arrangement of flagella (Fig. 2.3).
1. **Monotrichous:** These organisms have a single polar flagellum.

2. **Lophotrichous:** They have a tuft of flagella at one pole.
3. **Amphitrichous:** They have single polar flagellum or tuft of flagella at both poles.
4. **Peritrichous:** Flagella are distributed all round the cell.

Demonstration of flagella

- Flagella can be demonstrated by:
  - Ordinary light microscope by special staining techniques in which their thickness is increased by mordanting.
  - Dark-ground microscopy.
  - Electron microscopy.
  - Occurrence of spreading growth in semisolid agar medium.

Indirect methods by which motility of bacteria can be demonstrated

- On microscopic examination of wet films, motile bacteria are seen swimming in different directions across the field with darting (*V. cholerae*), very active (*Proteus* spp.), active (*Escherichia coli*), sluggish and tumbling (*Listeria monocytogenes*) motility. True motility should be differentiated from Brownian movement which is a rapid oscillation of the bacterium within a very limited area due to bombardment by the water molecules.

Structure of flagellum

The flagellum consists of three parts – the **filament**, the **hook** and the **basal body**. The basal body, anchored in the cytoplasmic membrane, comprises a rod and two or more sets of encircling rings. In Gram-negative bacteria four types of rings (M, S, P and L) are seen. Through ring M it attaches to the cytoplasmic membrane, ring S is located just above cytoplasmic membrane and through rings P and L it is attached to peptidoglycan and outer lipopolysaccharide membrane respectively (Fig. 2.4). Rings P and L are absent in Gram-positive bacteria.

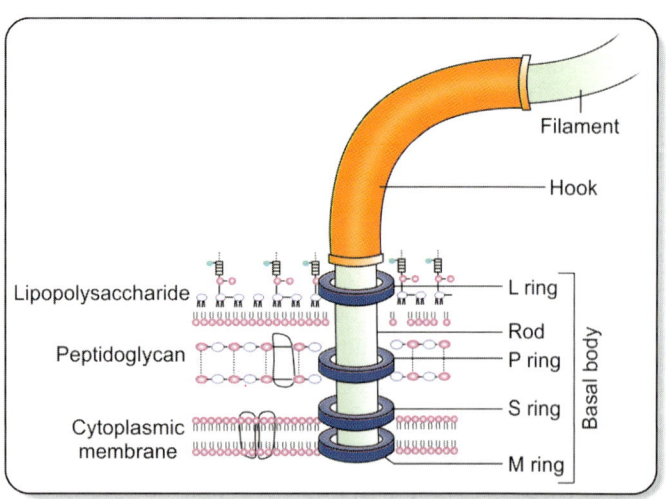

Fig. 2.4. Structure of flagellum.

Fimbriae or pili

They are hair-like microfibrils 1–1.5 μm in length and 4–8 nm in diameter. They are straighter, thinner and shorter than flagella (Fig. 2.2). They are present on many Gram-negative cells and provide a means for adherence to other cells, either bacterial or animal. Each bacterium possesses 100–500 peritrichously-borne fimbriae. They can be seen by electron microscopy. They originate in the cytoplasmic membrane and are composed of self-aggregating protein monomers.

In stagnant liquid medium, the fimbriate bacteria grow attached together in the form of a pellicle that floats on the surface of the medium where the growth is greatly enhanced by the free supply of oxygen.

Certain bacteria possess specialized fimbriae or pili which are longer and thinner than the common type. These appear to be hollow and constitute conjugation tubes through which DNA is transferred from one organism to another during conjugation. They are determined by sex factors and are referred to as **sex pili**.

Spore

Some species of bacteria (Gram-positive only), particularly those of the genera *Bacillus* and *Clostridium*, are capable of forming spores inside original cell. These spores can be released from original cell as free spores. Each bacterium forms one spore which on germination forms a single vegetative cell. Sporulation in bacteria, therefore, is a method of preservation and not of reproduction. Spores are small, highly resistant, metabolically dormant structures which develop as a response to starvation.

Sporulation

It develops from a portion of protoplasm near one end of the cell. This part of the bacterial cell is known as **forespore** and the remaining part as **sporangium** (Fig. 2.5). Bacterial DNA replicates and partitions into two halves and one of them, which is equivalent to one genome of the cell, is incorporated into forespore. A transverse septum derived from the cytoplasmic membrane is then formed by a process of invagination which divides forespore and sporangium. The forespore is, subsequently, completely encircled by dividing septum as a double layered membrane.

The two spore membranes now engage in active synthesis of various layers of the spore. The inner layer becomes the **inner membrane**. Between the two layers is laid **spore cortex** and outer layer is transformed into **spore coat** which consists of several layers. In some species from outer layer also develops **exosporium**, which bears ridges and folds. Finally, exosporium disintegrates and the spore is freed. Mesosomes

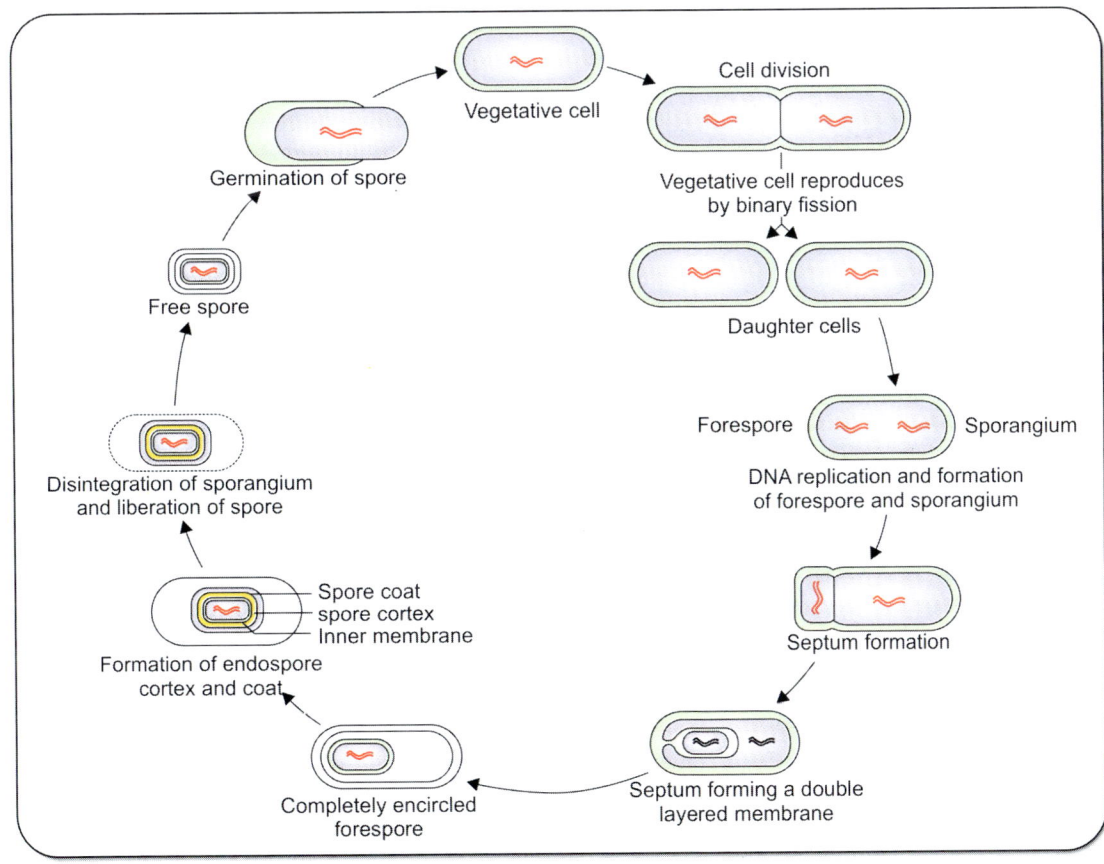

Fig. 2.5. Morphological events in sporulation.

appear to play a role in the development of spore and may be involved in the compartmentation of the spore's share of the nuclear material.

Shape and position

The spores may be round, oval or elongated occupying a terminal, subterminal or central position. They may be narrower than the width of the bacilli or broader and bulging (Fig. 2.6).

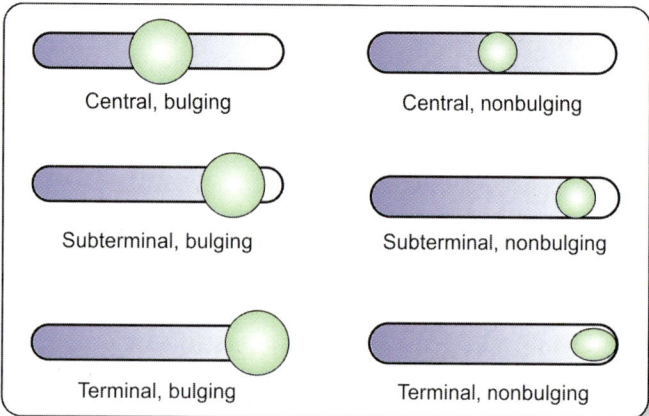

Central, bulging **Central, nonbulging**

Subterminal, bulging **Subterminal, nonbulging**

Terminal, bulging **Terminal, nonbulging**

Fig. 2.6. Types of spores.

Resistance

Spores can remain dormant for many years. They are extremely resistant to chemical and physical agents. Their killing requires moist heat at 100–120°C for 10 minutes while vegetative cells can be killed by heating at 60°C for 10 minutes.

Germination

Spores are able to **germinate** when the external conditions become favourable to growth by access to moisture and nutrients particularly trigger nutrients such as a particular amino acid, pyrimidine or sugar in a suitable aqueous environment. Within a short period of time spore loses its heat resistance, refractility, dipicolinic acid and calcium. It then swells and absorbs water, after which the spore coat ruptures, and a new vegetative cell grows out.

Demonstration

- In unstained preparations, the spore is recognized within the parent cell by its greater refractility. In simple stains like Gram it remains unstained and appears as a clear space within the stained cell protoplasm.
- They are slightly acid-fast and may be demonstrated by modified Ziehl-Neelsen staining.

L-forms of bacteria

L-forms (after Lister Institute, London) of bacteria are cell wall deficient bacteria derived by variation, usually in the laboratory, from bacteria of normal morphology. They are stable in the sense that special conditions of culture, such as presence of penicillin, are not required to prevent their reversion to the parental bacterial forms. They lack regular size and shape. They may be spherical or disc-like and measure 0.1–20 μm in diameter.

Cultural characteristics

L-forms are difficult to grow and usually require a medium that is solidified with agar as well as having the right osmotic strength. L-forms are produced more readily with penicillin than with lysozyme.

Colonies of L-forms of bacteria on agar medium show a characteristic **'fried-egg'** appearance with a dark thick centre, where many of the organisms embed themselves and grow within the agar, and a lighter periphery consisting of organisms lying on the surface of the agar. In liquid medium they grow in the form of clumps. Some L-forms are capable of reverting to normal bacillary forms upon removal of the inducing stimulus. Other L-forms are, however, stable and never revert. Presence of residual peptidoglycan is essential for reversion. It acts as a primer in its own biosynthesis.

3

Growth and Nutrition of Bacteria

Bacteria reproduce by a process called binary fission, in which a parent cell divides to form a progeny of two cells. This results in a logarithmic growth rate – one bacterium will produce 16 bacteria after four generations.

Generation time

The time required for a bacterium to give rise to two daughter cells is known as **generation time**. Under constant conditions, the generation time for any organism is quite reproducible, but differs greatly among different bacteria. The fastest growing bacteria have generation time of 15–20 minutes under optimum growth conditions. Many bacteria, however, have generation times of hours or even days. In *Escherichia coli* it is 20 minutes, in tubercle bacilli it is 20 hours and in lepra bacilli it is 20 days.

1. Total count

This is total number of bacteria present in a specimen irrespective of whether they are living or dead. This is done by counting the bacteria under microscope using counting chamber and by comparing the growth with standard opacity tubes.

2. Viable count

This measures only viable (living) cells which are capable of growing and producing a colony on a suitable medium.

BACTERIAL GROWTH CURVE

When a bacterium is inoculated into a suitable culture medium and incubated, its growth follows a characteristic course. If both total and viable counts are made at different intervals and plotted in relation to time, then a characteristic growth curve is obtained. A typical growth curve contains four major phases (Fig. 3.1).

1. Lag phase

When bacteria are seeded into fresh medium, multiplication usually does not begin immediately. The period between

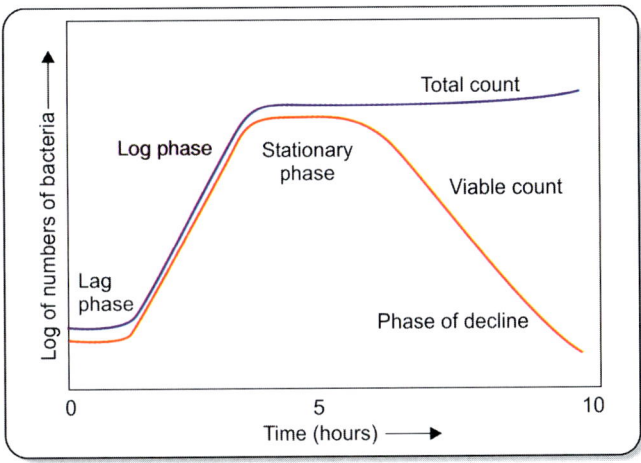

Fig. 3.1. Bacterial growth curve.

inoculation and beginning of multiplication is known as lag phase. **During this period the organisms adapt themselves to growth in fresh medium and increase in size and metabolic activity. Therefore, lag phase is regarded as a period not of rest but of intense metabolic activity.**

2. Log or exponential growth phase

During this phase the bacteria are multiplying at their maximum rate and their number increases exponentially or by geometric progression with time. If logarithm of bacterial count is plotted against time a straight line is obtained. **In the log phase, the bacterial cells are smaller and stain uniformly.** Exponential phase is of limited duration because of:

- exhaustion of nutrients,
- accumulation of toxic metabolic cnd products,
- rise in cell density,
- change in pH, and
- decrease in oxygen tension (in case of aerobic organisms).

3. Stationary phase

Due to above reasons exponential growth slows down and the bacterial population enters the stationary phase, in which the number of viable cells remains constant. There is almost a balance between the bacterial reproduction and bacterial death. **During this phase, bacteria become Gram-variable, show irregular staining and spores start forming in spore-forming bacteria.**

4. Phase of decline

Stationary phase is followed eventually by the phase of decline because rate of death exceeds the rate of reproduction and the number of viable cells declines. **Finally, after a variable period, all the cells die and culture becomes sterile.**

Bacterial nutrition

The growth of microorganisms depends upon an adequate supply of suitable nutrients, pH, oxygen and temperature. They require the elements present in their chemical composition. Nutrients must provide these elements in a metabolically accessible form. All bacteria have three major nutritional needs for growth:

1. A source of carbon for making cellular constituents.
2. A source of nitrogen for making proteins.
3. A source of energy (ATP) in order to synthesize macromolecules and maintain essential chemical gradients across their membranes.

Smaller amounts of molecules such as phosphate for nucleic acids and a variety of metals and ions for enzymatic activity must also be present. Although, the basic building blocks required for growth are the same for all cells, bacteria vary widely in their ability to use different sources of these molecules.

Nutritional requirements for growth

Bacteria are divided into two basic groups according to how they meet their nutritional needs:

1. Autotrophs

Some organisms possess considerable synthetic power, therefore, they can utilize very simple inorganic compounds, such as carbon dioxide as carbon source and ammonium salts as nitrogen source. These are known as autotrophs or lithotrophs.

2. Heterotrophs

Bacteria that are unable to synthesize their own metabolites and depend on preformed organic compounds are known as heterotrophs. They require an organic source of carbon, such as glucose, and obtain energy by oxidizing or fermenting organic substances. Often, the same substance (for example, glucose) is used as both the carbon source and energy source. Some bacteria require certain organic compounds in minute quantities. These are known as growth factors or bacterial vitamins. All bacteria that inhabit the human body fall into the heterotrophic group.

CULTURE MEDIA

Numerous culture media have been devised. The original media used by Louis Pasteur were liquids such as urine or meat broth. Liquid media have many disadvantages. Bacteria growing in these media may not exhibit specific characteristics for their identification. With liquid media it is difficult to isolate different types of bacteria from mixed populations. However, liquid media are used for obtaining bacterial growth from blood or water when large volumes have to be used as inoculum, for preparing bulk cultures for antigens and vaccines, and for preparation of inoculum for biochemical reactions and antibiotic susceptibility testing.

In 1881, Robert Koch described means of cultivating bacteria on solid media. First he used as his growth medium pieces of potato, then 2.5–5.0% gelatin to prepare solid media fortifying them with 1% meat extract as an essential ingredient. But gelatin is not satisfactory as liquefies at 24°C (incubation temperature for most pathogenic bacteria is 37°C). At the suggestion of Anglina Hesse, the American wife of his assistant, he substituted agar-agar in place of gelatin as solidifying agent for the media. She had used it to solidify broths in her kitchen.

Agar-agar or '**agar**' for short is prepared from a variety of seaweeds; the product is clarified, dried and supplied as a powder. The chief component of agar is a long-chain polysaccharide, mainly composed of D-galactopyranose units. It also contains a variety of impurities including inorganic salts, a small amount of protein like material and sometimes traces of long-chain fatty acids which are inhibitory to growth.

Agar does not add to the nutritive properties of medium and is not affected by the growth of bacteria. The exact concentration to be used may require some adjustment according to the batch of agar. A concentration of 1–2% usually yields a suitable gel. In preparing agar media, the appropriate amount of agar powder is added to the liquid medium and dissolved by placing the mixture in a steamer at 100°C for 1 hour or longer. Most agars dissolve to give a clear solution but sometimes it is necessary to filter off particulate impurities.

The melting and solidifying points of agar solutions are not the same. At the concentrations normally used, most bacteriological agars melt at about 95°C and solidify only when cooled to about 42°C. Agar can be added to any nutrient liquid medium if the advantages of a solid medium are desired. Most of the culture media are sterilized by autoclaving at 121°C for 15 minutes. Nutrients that are damaged by autoclaving are sterilized separately by filtration, etc. The sterilized agar base is then melted in the steamer and cooled to about 45–50°C followed by addition of heat-labile ingredients, but once these are added the medium must at once be poured into petri dishes because it cannot be remelted without damaging the heat-sensitive ingredients.

If heated at a low pH, agar is hydrolysed to products that do not solidify on cooling. Agar usually does not alter the pH of the medium, to which it is added, but if it contains free acid this must be neutralized before it is autoclaved.

Another important ingredient of common media is **peptone**. It consists of water-soluble products obtained from lean meat or other protein material such as heart muscle, casein, fibrin or soya flour, usually by digestion with the proteolytic enzymes pepsin, trypsin or papain. Its constituents are peptones, proteoses, amino acids, a variety of inorganic salts including phosphates, potassium and magnesium, and certain accessory growth factors such as nicotinic acid and riboflavin. Special brands of peptone such as neopeptone and proteose peptone are available for special use.

Other common ingredients of the culture media include casein hydrolysate, meat extract, yeast extract, malt extract, blood and serum.

While bacteria grow diffusely in liquid media, they produce discrete visible growth on solid media in petri dishes. If a mixed culture is inoculated in suitable dilution on solid medium, different bacteria form well-separated colonies, which are clones of cells originating from a single bacterial cell. On solid media, bacteria have distinct colony morphology and exhibit many other characteristic features such as pigment production or haemolysis.

Types of culture media

Culture media have been classified in many ways:

1. Solid, semisolid and liquid.
2. Simple (basal), complex, synthetic, defined, semidefined and special media. Special media are further divided into enriched, selective, enrichment, indicator or differential, storage media, sugar media and transport media.
3. Aerobic media and anaerobic media.

Basal media

These include peptone water and nutrient broths which form the basis of most media used in the study of the common pathogenic bacteria.

Enriched media

These are prepared to meet the nutritional requirements of fastidious organisms by addition of substances such as blood, serum and egg to a basal medium. Important examples of enriched media are blood agar for isolation of *Streptococcus*, chocolate agar for isolation of *Neisseria* and *Haemophilus*, and Loeffler's serum slope for the isolation of *Corynebacterium diphtheriae*.

Selective media

When a substance is added to a solid medium which inhibits the growth of unwanted bacteria but permits the growth of wanted bacteria in the form of colonies, it is known as selective medium. Important examples of this type of media are MacConkey agar for *E. coli*, deoxycholate citrate agar (DCA) for *Salmonella* and *Shigella*, Wilson and Blair's medium for *Salmonella*, Lowenstein-Jensen medium for *Mycobacterium tuberculosis*, and blood tellurite agar medium for isolation of *Corynebacterium diphtheriae*.

Enrichment media

When a substance is added to a liquid medium which inhibits the growth of unwanted bacteria and favours the growth of wanted bacteria it is known as enrichment medium. Important examples of this type of media are tetrathionate and selenite broth for *Salmonella* and *Shigella*, and alkaline peptone water for *Vibrio cholerae*.

Indicator media or differential media

When a substance is added into a medium which would produce a visible change in the medium following the growth of a particular organism, it is designated as indicator or differential medium. For example, MacConkey medium contains lactose and neutral red. Lactose-fermenting organisms after growth on this medium produce acid and in acidic pH neutral red becomes red in colour. Thus *E. coli* which is lactose fermenter produces red or pink colonies on this medium.

Christensen's medium contains urea and phenol red. When urease producing organisms like *Proteus* and *Klebsiella* grow on this medium, urea is split-up into ammonia and carbon dioxide. Ammonia makes the medium alkaline and in alkaline pH the medium becomes pink in colour (in alkaline pH phenol red is pink in colour). Enriched media can also be differential on the basis of certain growth characteristics evident on the medium. Blood agar is considered both an enriched and differential medium because it differentiates organisms based on whether they are α-haemolytic, β-haemolytic or non-haemolytic.

Transport or holding media

When the clinical sample is being transported from the hospital to the laboratory, delicate organisms like *Neisseria gonorrhoeae* may not survive or the normal flora (*E. coli*) may overgrow pathogenic flora (*Salmonella*, *Shigella* and *V. cholerae*). Transport media maintain the viability of micro-organisms present in a specimen without supporting the growth of any organism. These maintain the organisms in a state of suspended animation, so that no organism overgrows another or dies out. These media typically contain only buffers and salts. They lack carbon, nitrogen and organic growth factors, hence do not facilitate microbial multiplication. Stuart's transport medium and Amies transport medium are examples of transport media.

Storage media

Bacteria are best preserved and stored by lyophilization. But for preservation and storage for a few months or so, they can be stab inoculated on semisolid agar or on Dorset egg medium followed by incubation. When growth appears they can be stored in refrigerator.

Sugar media

For the identification of most of the organisms, sugar fermentation reactions are carried out. Glucose, lactose, sucrose and mannitol are widely used sugars. For the preparation of sugar media, 1% of the concerned sugar is added to peptone water with a suitable indicator. Durham's tube (a small tube) is kept inverted in the tube containing this medium to detect gas production. For fastidious organisms like *C. diphtheriae* and pneumococci, Hiss's serum sugar is used.

Anaerobic media

For the growth of anaerobes, the media used contain reducing substances. These include thioglycollate broth and cooked meat broth. The sterile muscle tissue, in cooked meat broth, contains reducing substances, particularly glutathione, which permit the growth of many strict anaerobes. In addition to its reducing effect, the meat provides a variety of nutritional substances for bacterial growth. In this medium, saccharolytic clostridia rapidly produce acid and gas but do not digest the meat. The cultures may have slight sour smell and the meat is often reddened. The proteolytic clostridia produce blackening of the meat, decomposing it and reducing it in volume with the formation of foul-smelling products.

Preparation of commonly used culture media

Peptone water

This medium is used chiefly as the basis for carbohydrate fermentation media, and for subculture of bacteria for anti-microbial susceptibility testing. It is also used to test for the formation of indole.

Peptone	10 g
Sodium chloride	5 g
Water	1 litre

Dissolve the ingredients in warm water, adjust the pH to 7.4–7.5 and filter. Distribute as required and autoclave it at 121°C for 15 minutes.

Alkaline peptone water

It is prepared in the same manner as above. However, pH is adjusted to 8.6.

Sugar fermentation media (peptone water sugars)

Peptone water is prepared as above, pH is adjusted to 7.8, and 1% Andrade's indicator is added. Steam for 20 minutes at 100°C. Filter and add 1% of different sugars (but in case of dulcitol, 0.5%). Sugars commonly tested are glucose, mannitol, sucrose, lactose and maltose. Add 5 ml each of sugar media in test tubes containing inverted Durham's tubes completely filled with liquid and containing no air bubble.

Steam for three successive days at 100°C for 20 minutes. Production of acid is indicated by change in the colour of the medium to red or pink, and gas, if produced, collects in Durham's tube.

Andrade's indicator is prepared from 0.5% aqueous acid fuchsin to which sufficient 1 M sodium hydroxide has been added to turn the colour of the solution yellow.

Hiss's serum sugar media

These media are used to test the fermentation reactions of nutritionally exacting bacteria such as diphtheria bacilli and streptococci. One part of serum (sheep or ox serum) is mixed with three parts of distilled water. The reaction of the medium is adjusted to pH 7.5, and 5 ml of 0.2% solution of phenol red per 100 ml of the medium is added prior to sterilization. The various sugars are incorporated in the proportion of 1%. Sterilization is done by intermittent steaming at 100°C for 20 minutes each day on three successive days and distribute it aseptically in 2.5 ml amounts in screw-capped 6 ml bottles. Fermentation is indicated by the production of acid, which alters the indicator and causes coagulation of the medium.

Selenite F broth

The selenite in this enrichment medium inhibits coliform bacilli while permitting salmonellae and many shigellae to grow.

Sodium hydrogen selenite, $NaHSeO_3$	4 g
Peptone	5 g
Lactose	4 g
Disodium hydrogen phosphate, $Na_2HPO_4.2H_2O$	9.5 g
Sodium dihydrogen phosphate, $NaH_2PO_4.2H_2O$	0.5 g
Sterile water	1 litre

Dissolve the ingredients with sterile precautions and distribute the yellowish solution in about 10 ml amounts in screw-capped containers. Steam at 100°C for 20 minutes (once only). Do not autoclave, because excessive heating spoils the medium. A slight red precipitate may form but it is of no consequence. The pH of the medium should be 7.1.

Care must be taken in the preparation and use of the medium, because selenium salts are toxic and teratogenic, and volatile derivatives, including hydrogen selenide, are toxic when inhaled.

Tetrathionate broth

The tetrathionate formed by the chemical action of sodium thiosulphate and iodine is inhibitory to coliform organisms and permits the growth of salmonellae.

Thiosulphate solution

Sodium thiosulphate	24.8 g
Sterile water	100 ml

Mix the salt and water and steam for 30 minutes at 100°C.

Iodine solution

Potassium iodide	20 g
Iodine	12.7 g
Sterile water	100 ml

Dissolve potassium iodide in about 50 ml warm water, add iodine and make-up the volume to 100 ml.

Complete medium

Calcium carbonate	2.5 g
Nutrient broth	78 ml
Thiosulphate solution	15 ml
Iodine solution	4 ml
Phenol red, 0.02% in 20% ethanol	3 ml

Calcium carbonate is added to nutrient broth and sterilized at 121°C for 15 minutes by autoclaving. When cool, thiosulphate, iodine and phenol red solutions are added with sterile precautions. Distribute 10 ml amounts in sterile screw-capped bottles or test tubes. Even in the refrigerator, the completed medium does not keep for more than about 1 week. It is convenient to keep the stock solutions and prepare the complete medium as required. Ideally, the medium should be used within a few hours of adding the iodine solution to the other reagents.

Cooked meat broth

This medium is suitable for growing anaerobes in air and also for the preservation of stock cultures of aerobic organisms. The inoculum is introduced deep in the medium in contact with the meat. Fresh sheep/goat heart is minced after removing all fat.

Cooked meat particles

Minced meat	500 g
Water	500 ml
Sodium hydroxide (1 N NaOH)	1.5 ml

Boil for 20 minutes. Sodium hydroxide will neutralize lactic acid present in the meat. Filter off the liquid while still hot through the lint. Dry the meat particles by spreading on a filter paper at 37°C.

Peptone infusion broth

Liquid filtered from cooked meat	500 ml
Peptone	2.5 g
Sodium chloride	1.25 g

Steam at 100°C for 20 minutes, add 1 ml pure hydrochloric acid and filter. Bring the reaction of the filtrate to pH 8.2. Steam at 100°C for 30 minutes and adjust reaction to pH 7.8.

Preparation of complete medium

Place meat in 30 ml bottles to a depth of 2.5 cm and cover with about 15 ml nutrient broth. Autoclave at 121°C for 20 minutes.

Thioglycollate broth

This medium is used to grow anaerobic organisms.

Yeast extract, water-soluble	5 g
Casein hydrolysate, pancreatic digest	15 g
Glucose	5.5 g
L-cystine	0.5 g
Agar	0.75 g
Sodium chloride	2.5 g
Sodium thioglycollate	0.5 g
Resazurin sodium solution, 1 in 1000, freshly prepared	1 ml
Water	1 litre

Dissolve ingredients except thioglycollate and resazurin by steaming at 100°C. Add thioglycollate and adjust the pH to 7.3. Filter while hot and add methylene blue solution. Add resazurin solution, mix thoroughly, distribute and sterilize at 121°C for 15 minutes. After autoclaving, cool it at once to 25°C and store in the dark preferably between 20°C and 30°C. Before use, if it is seen that more than the upper third is pink in colour, anaerobic conditions may be restored by steaming at 100°C for a few minutes.

Glycerol saline transport medium for enteric bacilli

If there is likely to be delay of some hours before specimens of faeces for culture of enteric bacilli reach the laboratory, this transport medium prevents other intestinal organisms from overgrowing the enteric bacteria.

Glycerol	300 ml
Sodium chloride	4.2 g
Disodium hydrogen phosphate, Na_2HPO_4, anhydrous	10 g
Phenol red, 0.02%, aqueous	15 ml
Water	700 ml

Dissolve sodium chloride in water. Add glycerol and shake well. Add phosphate and place it for 15 minutes in steamer to dissolve. Then add enough phenol red to give a purple pink colour. Distribute in 6 ml amounts in screw-capped bottles. Sterilize by autoclaving at 115°C for 15 minutes. When the colour of the medium changes from pink to yellow (indicating acidity), it should not be used.

Stuart's transport medium

This soft agar medium is used to maintain the viability of gonococci on swabs during their transportation to the laboratory.

Sodium thioglycollate	1 g
Sodium glycerophosphate	10 g
Calcium chloride	0.1 g
Agar	6 g
Methylene blue, 0.1%, aqueous	4 ml
Distilled water	1 litre

Dissolve all the solids in distilled water at 100°C. Adjust pH to 7.3–7.4. Add methylene blue solution and distribute in bijou bottles, filling nearly full. Sterilize at 121°C for 15 minutes and immediately tighten caps. When cool, the medium should be colourless.

Nutrient (meat extract) broth

Peptone	10 g
Meat extract	10 g
Sodium chloride	5 g
Water	1 litre

Mix the ingredients and dissolve them by heating briefly in the steamer. When cool, adjust pH to 7.5–7.6. A precipitate of phosphates may appear and this may be removed by filtration through filter paper. Distribute in tubes or bottles and sterilize by autoclaving at 121°C for 15 minutes.

Nutrient agar

Nutrient agar is nutrient broth solidified by addition of 1–2% agar. If the concentration of agar is lowered to 0.2–0.5%, it is called semisolid agar. If its concentration is raised to 6%, it is called hard agar. In semisolid agar, the motile organisms show growth in entire medium, and on surface of hard agar, swarming of *Proteus* is inhibited.

Blood agar

Blood agar is prepared by adding sterile 10% sheep blood to sterile nutrient agar that has been melted and cooled to 50°C. It is then poured in petri dishes. It is an enriched medium. It is also an indicator medium showing the haemolytic properties of bacteria such as *Streptococcus pyogenes*.

Heated blood agar ('chocolate agar')

It is prepared by heating 10% of sterile blood in sterile nutrient agar. Melt the agar, cool it in a water bath at 75°C, add the blood and allow the medium to remain at 75°C, mixing the blood and agar by gentle agitation from time to time until the blood becomes chocolate-brown in colour, within about 10 minutes. Then pour as slopes or plates.

An alternative method of preparing plates of heated blood agar involves the heating of already poured and set plates of ordinary blood agar. The blood agar plates are held in an incubator or hot air oven at 55°C for 1–2 hours.

This medium is used for isolation of *Haemophilus influenzae* and other fastidious organisms such as neisseriae and the pneumococci.

MacConkey agar

Peptone	20 g
Sodium taurocholate	5 g
Water	1 litre
Agar	20 g
Neutral red solution, 2% in 50% ethanol	about 3.5 ml
Lactose, 10% aqueous solution	100 ml

Dissolve peptone and sodium taurocholate in water by heating. Add agar and dissolve it in the steamer or autoclave. If necessary, clear by filtration. Adjust the pH to 7.5. Add lactose and neutral red, which should be well shaken before use, and mix. Heat in the autoclave or free steam (100°C) for 1 hour, then at 115°C for 15 minutes. Pour plates.

Deoxycholate citrate agar (DCA)

This medium is used for isolation of *Shigella* and *Salmonella* from faeces.

Neutral red lactose agar

Meat extract	5 g
Peptone	5 g
Agar	22.5 g
Neutral red, 2% in 50% ethanol	1.25 ml
Lactose	10 g
Water	1 litre

Dissolve meat extract in 50 ml of water over a flame. Make just alkaline to phenolphthalein by addition of sodium hydroxide, boil at 100°C and filter through filter paper. Adjust pH to 7.4, make up the volume to 50 ml and add peptone. Dissolve the agar in 950 ml of water by steaming for 1 hour at 100°C. Filter, if necessary, to clarify. Add meat extract and peptone solution to the agar solution and mix well. Add neutral red and lactose, mixing again. Bottle in 100 ml lots and sterilize by steaming at 100°C for 20 minutes on three successive days.

Solution A

Sodium citrate	17 g
Sodium thiosulphate	17 g
Ferric ammonium citrate	4 g
Sterile water	100 ml

Solution B

Sodium deoxycholate	10 g
Sterile water	100 ml

These two solutions are prepared separately and heated at 60°C for 1 hour.

Complete medium

Neutral red lactose agar	100 ml
Solution A	5 ml
Solution B	5 ml

Melt agar and add solutions A and B with separate pipettes, in that order. Mix and pour plates.

Mueller Hinton agar

Beef infusion	300 ml
Casein hydrolysate	17.5 g
Starch	1.5 g
Agar	10 g
Distilled water	1 litre

Emulsify the starch in a small amount of cold water, pour into the beef infusion and add the casein hydrolysate and agar. Make up the volume to 1 L with distilled water. Dissolve the constituents by heating gently at 100°C with agitation. Filter, if necessary. Adjust pH to 7.4. Dispense in screw-capped bottles and sterilize by autoclaving at 121°C for 20 minutes. Pour plates.

Culture media for isolation of fungi

Media for isolation of pathogenic fungi are designed to be inhibitory to bacteria and in certain cases selective against other fungi as well. Following culture media are commonly used in the mycology laboratory.

For primary isolation of fungi

1. Sabouraud dextrose agar (SDA)

Original formula:

Dextrose	40 g
Peptone	10 g
Agar	15 g
Distilled water	1000 ml

Dissolve the ingredients by boiling and adjust pH at 5.6. Dispense in tubes, and autoclave at 121°C for 10 minutes. Allow tubes to cool in slanted position. Store in refrigerator.

2. Emmons' modification of Sabouraud dextrose agar

Dextrose	20 g
Peptone	10 g
Agar	20 g
Distilled water	1000 ml

Dissolve the ingredients by boiling and adjust pH at 6.8–7.0. Dispense in tubes, and autoclave at 121°C for 10 minutes. Allow tubes to cool in slanted position. Store in refrigerator.

3. Sabouraud-cycloheximide-chloramphenicol agar

Dextrose	20 g
Peptone	10 g
Agar	20 g
Chloramphenicol	40 mg
Cycloheximide	500 mg
Distilled water	1000 ml

After dextrose, peptone and agar are dissolved, heat to boiling, add 40 mg of chloramphenicol which has been suspended in 10 ml of 95% alcohol and quickly remove from heat. Add 500 mg cycloheximide, which has been dissolved in 10 ml of acetone. Dispense in tubes, and autoclave at 121°C for 10 minutes. Allow tubes to cool in slanted position. Store in refrigerator.

This medium is useful for isolation of fungi from contaminated specimens. **Chloramphenicol** inhibits bacterial contaminants. **However, it partially inhibits *Nocardia* and actinomycetes.**

Cycloheximide reduces the rate of growth of many saprophytic fungi. It is toxic for *Cryptococcus neoformans*, *Candida* spp. and other yeasts. It also inhibits growth of the yeast forms of some dimorphic fungi when they are incubated at 37°C.

Nutritionally deficient media

1. Cornmeal agar

Cornmeal	40 g
Agar	20 g
Tween 80 (polysorbate 80)	10 ml
Distilled water	1000 ml

Mix cornmeal well with 500 ml of water; heat to 65°C for 1 hour. Filter through gauze and then paper until clear; restore to original volume. Adjust to pH 6.6–6.8; add agar dissolved in 500 ml of water. Add Tween 80, autoclave at 121°C for 15 minutes. Dispense into petri plates.

Cornmeal agar is low in nutrients. It suppresses vegetative growth while stimulating sporulation of many fungi. It is used in distinguishing the different genera of yeasts and various species of *Candida*. It is also useful in slide culture. If 10 g of dextrose is added to the medium in place of the Tween 80, the medium can be used to differentiate *Trichophyton mentagrophytes* from *T. rubrum* on the basis of pigment production. On this medium the latter produces red pigment while the former is negative.

2. Rice-Tween 80 agar

Cream of rice	10 g
Tween 80	10 ml
Agar	10 g
Distilled water	1000 ml

To 1 litre of boiling distilled water add 10 g cream of rice and continue boiling for 30 seconds. Filter through cotton and restore volume. Add 10 g agar and dissolve with heat. Add 10 ml Tween 80. Autoclave at 121°C for 15 minutes. Pour into a cylinder and leave overnight in a water bath at 60°C. Decant clear portion, refilter through cotton, dispense in flasks and autoclave at 121°C for 15 minutes. Pour in petri plates.

Rice-Tween 80 agar is used for the production of chlamydoconidia by *Candida albicans* faster as compared to cornmeal agar.

Enriched media

Brain heart infusion (BHI) agar

Brain heart infusion	8 g
Peptic digest of animal tissue	5 g
Pancreatic digest of casein	16 g
Sodium chloride	5 g
Dextrose	2 g
Disodium phosphate	2.5 g
Agar	13.5 g
Distilled water	1000 ml

Dissolve ingredients by boiling and dispense into screw-cap tubes and autoclave at 121°C for 15 minutes. Chloramphenicol 40 mg is often added to inhibit bacteria, and sheep blood is added to further enrich the medium and enhance the growth of fastidious pathogenic fungi. BHI agar is recommended for the cultivation of fastidious pathogenic fungi, such as *Histoplasma capsulatum* and *Blastomyces dermatitidis*.

Selective and differential media

1. Bird seed agar or niger seed agar

Bird seed agar is a selective and differential medium used for primary isolation of *Cryptococcus* spp. The colonies of *Cryptococcus* spp. on this medium are dark brown to black in colour because phenoloxidase produced by these organisms breaks down the substrate (*Guizotia abyssinica* seeds or niger seed) to melanin, which is deposited in the yeast cell wall. This imparts a dark brown to black pigmentation of the colonies.

Guizotia abyssinica	
(niger seed or bird seed)	50 g
Distilled water	1000 ml

Boil for 30 minutes. Filter through gauze and add the following:

KH_2PO_4	1 g
Creatinine	1 g
Agar	15 g

(Glucose, 1 g is added in the formulation for identification of *Candida dubliniensis*, but it inhibits pigment production by *Cryptococcus neoformans*. Chloramphenicol, 1 g may be added in the formulation for pigment production by *C. neoformans*.)

Mix well. Autoclave at 121°C for 15 minutes. Pour into tubes and cool in slanted position.

Test procedure

A. For pigment production by C. neoformans

Inoculate with suspected *Cryptococcus* spp. and incubate at 25–30°C for 7 days. Only *C. neoformans* varieties *neoformans* and *gattii* produce phenoloxidase which break down the substrate resulting in the production of melanin and the development of dark brown to black colonies. Colonies of other yeasts are cream in colour.

B. For differentiation of C. dubliniensis vs. C. albicans

Inoculate a plate of this medium with a 48-hour-old colony. Incubate at 30°C for 3–5 days. Examine macroscopic morphology of colonies. Colonies of *C. dubliniensis* are rough and may have hyphal fringe. On the other hand, colonies of *C. albicans* are smooth.

2. Dermatophyte test medium (DTM)

Phyton	10 g
Dextrose	10 g
Agar	20 g
Phenol red solution	40 ml
0.8 M HCl	6 ml
Cycloheximide	0.5 g
Gentamicin sulphate	0.1 g
Chlortetracycline HCl	0.1 g
Distilled water	1000 ml

Dissolve phyton, dextrose, and agar by boiling them in water. While stirring, add 40 ml of phenol red solution (0.5 g of phenol red dissolved in 15 ml of 0.1 N NaOH made up to 100 ml with distilled water). While stirring, add 0.8 M HCl. Dissolve cycloheximide in 2 ml of acetone, and add to hot medium while stirring. Dissolve gentamicin sulphate in 2 ml of distilled water, and add to the medium while stirring. Autoclave at 12 lb/in^2 for 10 minutes and cool to approximately 47°C. Dissolve chlortetracycline in 25 ml of sterile distilled water in sterile container, and add to medium while stirring. Dispense into sterile 30-ml screw-cap tubes; slant and cool. The final pH of the medium is 5.4–5.6, and the medium should be yellow in colour. Store in refrigerator at 4°C.

The dermatophyte test medium is used for presumptive diagnosis of dermatophytes. They change the colour of the medium from yellow to red due to liberation of alkaline metabolites within 14 days. Care must be taken in specimen collection and interpretation of results, as many contaminants and other fungi increase the number of false-positive changes in colour. DTM cannot be used to study pigment production because of the intense red colour of the indicator.

3. Urea agar (Christensen medium)

Peptone	1 g
Dipotassium hydrogen phosphate (K_2HPO_4)	2 g
Sodium chloride (NaCl)	5 g
Phenol red	
(1 in 500 aqueous solution)	6 ml
Agar	20 g
Distilled water	1 litre
Glucose, 10% solution, sterile	10 ml
Urea, 20% solution, sterile	100 ml

Sterilize the glucose and urea solutions by filtration. Prepare the basal medium without glucose and urea. Adjust to pH 6.8–6.9 and sterilize by autoclaving in a flask at 121°C for 30 minutes. Cool to about 50°C, add glucose and urea and tube the medium as deep slopes.

This medium detects the ability of an organism to produce urease enzyme. In the presence of suitable substrates, urease splits urea producing ammonia. It raises pH of the medium and phenol red indicator changes amber colour to pinkish red.

Urease-positive fungi are *Trichophyton mentagrophytes*, *Trichosporon* spp., *Cryptococcus neoformans* and *Rhodotorula*. Urease-negative fungi are *Trichophyton rubrum*, *Geotrichum candidum*, *Candida* and *Saccharomyces*.

Assimilation media for yeasts

Assimilation is the utilization of carbon (or nitrogen) source by a microorganism in the presence of oxygen. A positive reaction is indicated by the presence of growth or a pH shift in the medium. **Since all yeasts assimilate glucose, it acts as a positive control.**

1. Carbon assimilation medium

Yeast nitrogen base	6.7 g
Appropriate pure carbohydrate	5 g
Distilled water	100 ml

Heat to dissolve. Sterilize by Seitz or membrane filtration. Add 0.5 ml of the solution to 4.5 ml of sterile distilled water in screw cap tubes. Store in refrigerator. These may be used for one month.

2. Nitrate assimilation medium

Yeast carbon base	11.7 g
Potassium nitrate	0.78 g
Distilled water	100 ml

Warm gently to dissolve. Sterilize by Seitz or membrane filtration. Add 0.5 ml of medium to 4.5 ml of sterile distilled water in screw-cap tubes. Store in refrigerator. These may be used for one month.

Test procedure

Make a suspension of the yeast in sterile distilled water. This suspension should not exceed the turbidity of McFarland No. 1 standard. Add 0.1–0.2 ml of the yeast suspension to each tube of medium. Include a tube of yeast nitrogen base without any carbon source, and a tube of yeast carbon base without potassium nitrate, as controls for carryover. Incubate tubes at the yeast's optimal temperature. Examine cultures over a period of 7–14 days for dense turbidity caused by growth. The negative-control tubes without a carbon or nitrogen source should show no growth.

Auxanographic plate method

1. Carbon assimilation tests

Yeast nitrogen base	0.67 g
Noble or washed agar	20 g
Distilled water	1000 ml

Dispense in 20-ml quantities into 18 × 150 mm screw-cap tubes. Autoclave at 121°C for 15 minutes. Allow to harden as butts. Store in refrigerator.

Test procedure

- Melt a tube of nitrogen base medium in a boiling-water bath. Allow to cool to 47–48°C.
- With a sterile cotton-tipped applicator, make a heavy suspension of a 24- to 72-hour yeast culture in 4 ml of sterile distilled water. The density of the suspension should be equal to that of a McFarland No. 4 or 5 standard.
- Pour the yeast suspension into the tube of molten yeast nitrogen base agar. Mix thoroughly by inverting tube several times.
- Pour the yeast-agar mixture into a sterile 15 × 150 mm petri plate. Allow to solidify at room temperature.
- Place carbohydrate-containing disks, evenly spaced, on the plate.
- Incubate at 30°C for 18–24 hours and then examine for growth around each disk. Growth around a disk indicates that the yeast assimilates that sugar.

2. Nitrate assimilation tests

Medium

Yeast carbon base	12 g
Noble or washed agar	20 g
Distilled water	1000 ml

Tube in 20-ml aliquots and autoclave at 121°C for 15 minutes. Store in refrigerator.

Peptone solution for positive control

Peptone	10 g
Distilled water	100 ml

Sterilize by filtration and store in refrigerator

Test procedure

- Melt a tube of yeast carbon base medium in a boiling-water bath. Allow to cool to 47–48°C.
- Make an aqueous solution suspension of the yeast to a density equal to a McFarland No. 1 standard.
- Add 0.1 ml of yeast suspension to the tube of medium. Mix thoroughly.
- Pour the yeast-agar mixture into a sterile petri plate. Allow to solidify at room temperature.
- Place approximately 1 mg of potassium nitrate crystals on agar surface away from the centre of the plate.
- Place about 0.1 ml of peptone solution (positive control) on agar surface opposite potassium nitrate site.
- Incubate at 30°C for 48–96 hours.

For test to be valid growth must occur in the peptone area. If growth is seen in the "peptone area", examine for growth in the potassium nitrate area (growth indicates assimilation of potassium nitrate).

ENVIRONMENTAL FACTORS INFLUENCING GROWTH

Oxidation-reduction (Redox) potential

On the basis of the influence of oxygen on growth and viability, the bacteria are divided into two categories – aerobes and anaerobes:

- **Aerobes** require oxygen for their growth. They may be obligate aerobes like *Pseudomonas aeruginosa* which can grow only in the presence of oxygen, and facultative anaerobes. The latter are ordinarily aerobes, but they can also grow in the absence of oxygen though less abundantly.

- **Anaerobes**, on the other hand, are organisms that do not require oxygen for life and reproduction. In addition, oxygen's direct toxic effect may prohibit the growth of these organisms in environments, in which oxygen is present. They may be obligate anaerobes such as *Clostridium tetani*, which cannot grow even in the presence of traces of oxygen, and **microaerophilic** such as *C. perfringens* which can grow under microaerophilic conditions.

Carbon dioxide

Some organisms such as *Brucella abortus* require extra CO_2 in the air in which they are grown and others such as pneumococci and gonococci grow better in air supplemented with 5–10% CO_2 (**capnophilic**).

Temperature

Each bacterium multiplies best within a restricted temperature range. For most of the pathogenic bacteria optimum temperature for growth is 37°C (our body temperature) with upper and lower temperature limits of 40–50°C and 15–20°C respectively. The organisms with optimum temperatures of 37°C, less than 20°C and 55–80°C are known as mesophiles, psychrophiles and thermophiles respectively.

Moisture and desiccation

Moisture is very essential for the growth of bacteria because 80% of their body weight is made up of water.

pH

Like other living organisms, microorganisms are very susceptible to changes in the acidity or alkalinity of the surrounding medium. Most of the medically important bacteria can grow at neutral or slightly alkaline pH (7.2–7.6). Some bacteria like lactobacilli and cholera vibrio grow at acidic and alkaline pH respectively.

CULTURE METHODS

The methods of bacterial culture used in the clinical laboratory include streak culture, lawn culture, stroke culture, stab culture, pour-plate culture and liquid culture.

Streak culture

This method is routinely employed for the isolation of bacteria in pure culture from clinical specimens. A platinum or nichrome wire loop 2–4 mm in diameter is used. The loop is first sterilized in the Bunsen flame by making it red hot and cooled by touching an uninoculated part of the medium. Then a loopful of the specimen is smeared thoroughly over area A (Fig. 3.2), on the surface of a well dried plate, to give a well-inoculum or 'well'. The loop is re-sterilized and drawn from

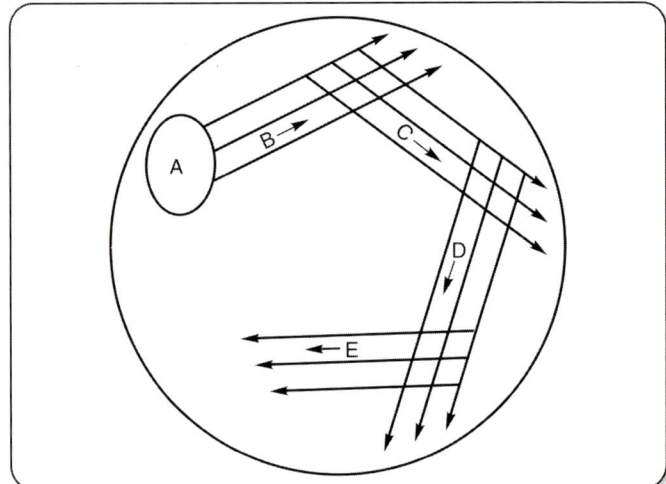

Fig. 3.2. Streak culture.

the well in 2 or 3 parallel lines onto the fresh surface of the medium (B). This process is repeated as shown (C, D, E), care being taken to sterilize the loop, and cool it on unseeded medium, between each sequence. On incubation, growth may be confluent at the site 'well', but becomes progressively thinner, and well separated colonies are obtained over the final series of streaks.

Lawn culture

Lawn cultures are prepared by flooding the surface of the plate with a liquid culture or suspension of bacteria and pipetting off the excess inoculum or by applying a swab soaked in the bacterial culture or suspension. After incubation, lawn culture provides a uniform surface growth. It is useful for antibiotic susceptibility testing by disc diffusion method and bacteriophage typing.

Stroke culture

Stroke culture is made in tubes containing agar slope or slant. Slopes are seeded by lightly smearing the surface of agar with loop in a zig-zag pattern taking care not to cut the agar. It is used for obtaining pure growth for slide agglutination and other diagnostic tests.

Stab culture

Stab cultures in solid media (nutrient gelatin or glucose agar) are inoculated by plunging the charged wire into the centre of the medium and withdrawing it in the same line to avoid splitting the medium. These are employed mainly for demonstration of gelatin liquefaction and for the maintenance of stock cultures.

Pour-plate culture

This method is used for counting the number of living bacteria or groups of bacteria in a liquid culture or suspension. Prepare serial 10-fold dilutions of the bacterial suspension over a range (6–9 tubes) ensuring that one dilution will contain between 50–500 viable bacteria/ml (number which can be accurately counted). Starting with the greatest dilution, pipette 1 ml amounts of each dilution into each of three 9 cm petri dishes. Then pour into each dish about 10 ml of clear nutrient agar, melted, and cooled at 45–50°C. Mix well by rapidly moving the plate for about 10 seconds. Allow the agar to set and incubate at 37°C for 48 hours. After incubation, colonies will be seen well distributed throughout the depth of the medium and can be enumerated using colony counters. Count the colonies in three plates containing 50–500 colonies/plate. Multiply the average number/plate by the dilution factor to obtain the viable count/ml in the original suspension.

Liquid culture

Liquid cultures in tubes, bottles or flasks may be inoculated by touching with a charged loop or by adding the inoculum with pipettes or syringes. Large inocula can be employed in liquid cultures and hence this method is adopted for blood culture and for sterility tests, where the concentration of bacteria in inocula are expected to be small. Liquid cultures are also preferred when large yields are desired.

AEROBIC CULTURE

For cultivation of aerobes the incubation is done in an incubator under normal atmospheric condition. The temperature of incubation for most of the human pathogenic bacteria is 37°C. To prevent drying of the medium when prolonged incubation is necessary, as in the cultivation of the tubercle bacilli, screw-capped bottles should be used instead of test tubes or plates.

CULTURE IN AN ATMOSPHERE WITH ADDED CARBON DIOXIDE

Some organisms such as *Brucella abortus* and capnophilic streptococci, require extra CO_2 in the air in which they are grown and others, such as the pneumococcus and gonococcus grow better in air supplemented with 5–10% CO_2. For this CO_2 jars are used. The required amount of air is withdrawn with a vacuum pump and replaced with CO_2 from a cylinder. CO_2 incubators which provide a predetermined and regulated amount of CO_2 in a suitably humid atmosphere are commercially available. Screw caps on containers of liquid media must not be tight and should preferably be replaced by a closure that allows entry of CO_2.

CULTURE IN MICROAEROPHILIC ATMOSPHERE

Microorganisms like *Campylobacter*, *Helicobacter pylori* and *Actinomyces israelii* are microaerophilic. Culture of such organisms is done by an evacuation replacement method with 5% O_2, 10% CO_2 and 85% N_2.

ANAEROBIC CULTURE

Anaerobic culture methods

A variety of methods are available for the culture of anaerobic organisms in the clinical laboratory. Exclusion of oxygen from the medium is the simplest method, and is effected by growing the organisms within the culture medium such as freshly steamed liquid media containing reducing agent such as glucose, ascorbic acid, cysteine, sodium thioglycollate and cooked meat pieces.

Cooked meat broth, **CMB** (original medium known as 'Robertson's bullock-heart medium') has a special place in anaerobic bacteriology; and **thioglycollate broth** and its modifications are also very useful. CMB is suitable for growing anaerobes in air and also for the preservation of stock cultures of aerobic organisms. The inoculum is introduced deep in the medium in contact with the meat. Cooked meat pieces are placed in 30 ml bottles to a depth of about 2.5 cm and covered with about 15 ml broth.

Anaerobic jars

When an oxygen-free or anaerobic atmosphere is required for obtaining surface growths of anaerobes, anaerobic jars provide the method of choice. The most reliable and widely used anaerobic jar is the **McIntosh-Fildes' anaerobic jar**. It is a cylindrical vessel made of glass or metal with a metal lid which is held firmly in place by a clamp (Fig. 3.3). The lid has two tubes with taps, one acting as gas inlet and the other as the outlet. On its undersurface it carries a gauze sachet carrying alumina pellets coated with palladium. It acts as a room temperature catalyst for the conversion of hydrogen and oxygen into water. It acts as a catalyst, as long as the sachet is kept dry.

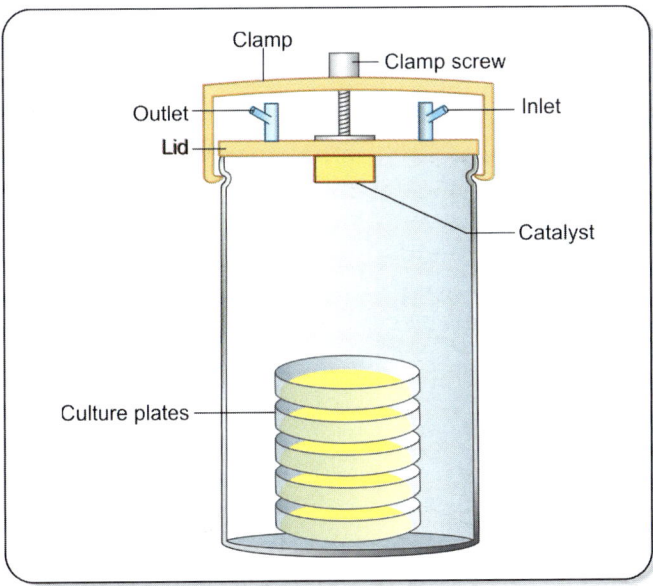

Fig. 3.3. Anaerobic jar.

Inoculated culture plates are placed inside the jar and the lid clamped tight. The outlet tube is connected to a vacuum pump and the air inside is evacuated. The outlet tap is then closed and the inlet tube connected to a hydrogen supply. Hydrogen is drawn in rapidly. As soon as this inrush of gas has ceased the inlet tap is also closed. After about 5 minutes inlet tap is again opened. There occurs again an immediate inrush of hydrogen since the catalyst creates a reduced pressure within the jar due to the conversion of hydrogen and left over oxygen into water. If there is no inrush of hydrogen, it means the catalyst is inactive and must be replaced. The jar is left connected to the hydrogen supply for about 5 minutes, then the inlet tap is closed and the jar is placed in the incubator, catalysis will continue until all the oxygen in the jar has been used up.

The **GasPak** is now the method of choice for preparing anaerobic jar. The GasPak is commercially available as a disposable envelope containing chemicals which generate hydrogen and carbon dioxide on the addition of water. After the inoculated plates are kept in the jar, the GasPak envelope with water added, is placed inside and the lid screwed tight. Hydrogen and carbon dioxide are liberated and the presence of a cold catalyst in the envelope permits the combination of hydrogen and oxygen to produce an anaerobic environment.

The outstanding feature of the GasPak system is the disposable gas generator envelope, which does away with the need for a vacuum pump and cylinders of compressed gas; the operation of the jar is consequently very quick and simple. As the standard GasPak jar is not evacuated before use a relatively large volume of water is formed during catalysis.

An **indicator** should be used for verifying the anaerobic condition in the jar. Methylene blue is generally used for this purpose. When it is placed in an anaerobic environment it is reduced from its coloured oxidized form to a colourless reduced leuco compound.

In addition to, or instead of, using a chemical indicator, some workers include in the jar a plate inoculated with a known strict anaerobe such as *Clostridium tetani* or *Bacteroides fragilis*, and a strict aerobe, such as *Pseudomonas aeruginosa*. This method is quite reliable if the indicator anaerobe grows and the aerobe does not.

Incubation

Inoculated plates should be incubated at 37°C for at least 48 hours, and reincubated for another 2–4 days to allow slow-growing organisms (certain species of *Actinomyces* and *Eubacterium*) to form colonies.

4

Collection of Specimens, Identification of Bacteria and Taxonomy

The laboratory diagnosis of an infectious disease begins with the collection of a clinical specimen. Proper collection of an appropriate clinical specimen is the first step in obtaining an accurate laboratory diagnosis of an infectious disease. A poorly collected specimen not only may result in failure to recover important microorganisms, but may also lead to incorrect or even harmful therapy if treatment is directed towards a commensal or contaminant.

The quality of a clinical microbiological report is directly related to the quality of the specimen on which it is based. Care in obtaining a proper specimen and its prompt submission to the laboratory are essential. In general, specimens of frank pus, wound exudate or excised tissue sent in sterile containers are preferable to swab which is relatively inefficient sampling device.

General rules for collection and transportation of specimen

- Apply strict aseptic techniques throughout the procedure.
- Wash hands before and after the collection.
- Collect the specimen before the administration of anti-microbial agents.
- Prevent contamination of the specimen with externally present organisms or normal flora of the body.
- Collect the specimen at the appropriate phase of disease.
- Collect the specimen from the actual infection site.
- Collect adequate quantity for the desired tests.
- Collect the specimen aseptically in a sterile and appropriate container.
- Close the container tightly so that its contents do not leak during transportation.
- Ensure that the outside of the specimen container is clean and uncontaminated.
- Label the container appropriately and complete the requisition form.
- Immediately transport the specimen to the laboratory.

Criteria for rejection of specimens

- Missing or inadequate identifications.
- Incomplete forms.
- Leaking container or blood stained containers.
- Specimens collected in an inappropriate container.
- Haemolysed blood sample.
- Insufficient quantity.
- Dried-up specimen.
- Contamination suspected.
- Specimen collected in formalin.
- Inappropriate transport or storage.

Collection and transportation of specimens

Blood for culture

- Using a pressure cuff, locate a suitable vein in the arm.
- Wearing sterile gloves thoroughly disinfect the vene-puncture site as follows:
  - Using 70% ethanol (spirit), cleanse an area about 50 mm in diameter. Allow to air-dry.
  - Using 2% tincture of iodine and a circular action, swab the area beginning at the point where the needle will enter the vein. Allow the iodine to dry on skin for at least 1 minute.
- Lift the tape or remove the protective cover from the top of culture bottle. Wipe the top of the bottle using an ethanol swab.
- Using a sterile syringe and needle withdraw 5 ml of blood from an adult and 1 ml from a young child.
- Insert the needle through a hole in the cap and through rubber or plastic liner of the bottle cap, and dispense 5 ml of blood from an adult and 1 ml from a young child into the culture medium bottles (Fig. 4.1a) respectively. Cap must not be removed for introduction of the blood. In adults large quantity (5 ml) of blood is required since the number

of organisms in the blood particularly in mild and recovering cases may be quite small, even as few as one per ml. As blood's natural bactericidal or bacteriostatic action may interfere with the growth of any bacteria present, this effect is annulled by diluting (inoculating) 5 ml of blood in an adult and 1 ml of blood in a young child in 50 ml and 10 ml of the medium (10-fold dilution) respectively. **Organisms causing baceteraemia in young children are usually present in sufficient concentration to be detected in small volume (1 ml) of blood.**

- Using a fresh ethanol swab wipe the top of the culture bottle and replace the tape or protective cover. Without delay, mix the blood with the broth. Blood must not be allowed to clot in the culture medium because any bacteria will become trapped in the clot.
- Clearly label the bottle with the name and number of the patient, and the date and time of collection.
- As soon as possible, incubate the inoculated medium.
- Collect blood during early stage of disease since the number of bacteria is higher in acute and early stage of disease.
- Collect blood during paroxysm of fever since the number of bacteria is higher at high temperature in patients with fever.
- In the absence of antibiotic administration, 99% culture positivity can be seen with three blood cultures.
- Transport the specimen to the laboratory. If delay in transportation is expected keep in incubator or at room temperature. **Do not refrigerate.**

Anticoagulated blood sample

If anticoagulated blood specimen is required, use suitable anticoagulant, e.g., *EDTA for malaria parasites and trypanosomes, and sodium citrate for microfilaria. Mix blood well, but gently, with anticoagulant. The blood must be*

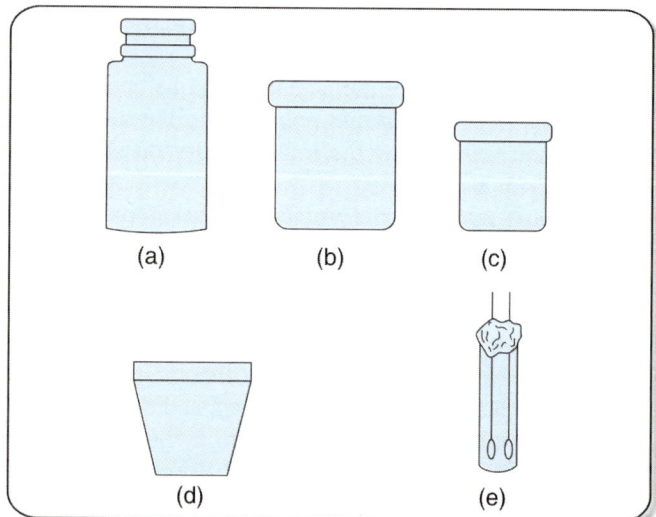

Fig. 4.1. (a) McCartney bottle, (b) Urine/stool container, (c) CSF container, (d) Sputum container, (e) Throat swabs.

examined within one hour of collection to avoid morphological changes in the appearance of parasites.

Blood for serological tests

For serological tests collect about 5 ml of blood to ensure there will be enough serum for all the tests that may be required. Immediately transfer the blood from the syringe into a dry stoppered sterile tube or bottle (without anticoagulant) and allow to clot. When the serum has separated, pipette it off into a sterile tube.

Urine

- Mid-stream urine sample is collected after giving proper instructions to the patient.
  - (a) Clean the genitalia properly. (In case of male, retract the prepuce, clean it with sterile normal saline. In case of female, wash perineum and periurethral area with soap and water. Separate apart labia with fingers of one hand).
  - (b) Collect a "clean-catch" mid-stream urine sample in a sterile container (Fig. 4.1b).
- Transport immediately to the laboratory. If a delay of more than 1–2 hours is unavoidable, refrigerate at 4°C.
- In catheterized patients, do not collect urine from collection bag or after opening the closed drainage. Clean the area over the collecting tubes and puncture with the help of a sterile needle and syringe and draw out the sample.
- Suprapubic aspiration under aseptic condition may be done in infants.

Cerebrospinal fluid (CSF)

Cerebrospinal fluid must be collected by an experienced physician. Rigorous aseptic precautions must be observed to prevent the introduction of infection into the central nervous system. The fluid is usually collected from the arachnoid space.

- A sterile wide-bore needle is inserted between fourth and fifth lumber vertebrae and the CSF is allowed to drip into a sterile dry container (Fig. 4.1c).
- Only 3–5 ml of fluid should be collected, because the removal of a larger volume may lead to headache.
- Immediately deliver the sample with a request form to the laboratory.
- CSF must be examined without delay and the results of the tests reported to the medical officer as soon as they become available. If delay in processing is inevitable then store it at 37° C. *Do not refrigerate.*
- The fluid should be handled with special care because a lumber puncture is required to collect the specimen.

Sputum

- Collect the sputum in a wide-mouthed container, which is preferably disposable, made up of transparent thin plastic, unbreakable and leak-proof (Fig. 4.1d).

- Ask the patient to rinse the mouth with plain water and then inhale deeply 2–3 times, cough-up deeply and spit in the sputum container by bringing it close to the mouth. If the patient has difficulty in coughing sputum, postural drainage, and appropriate physiotherapy often cause exudate to move in the bronchi and stimulate productive coughing.
- Make sure the sputum sample is of good quality and not just the saliva. A good sputum sample is thick, purulent and sufficient in amount (2–3 ml).
- Sputum sample may be refrigerated for up to 3–4 hours.

Throat swab

- Two swabs should be collected, one for smear and other for culture (Fig. 4.1e).
- Depress the tongue with a tongue blade.
- Swab the inflamed area of the throat, pharynx or tonsils with a sterile swab taking care to collect the pus or piece of membrane.
- Take care not to contaminate the swab with saliva.

Pus and other discharge

- Do not apply antiseptic before collection.
- Clean with normal saline.
- In case of discharge, 1–2 ml of sample is collected in a sterile vial.
- If swabs are to be collected then 2 swabs, in a sterile container, should be collected (one for direct microscopic examination and the other for culture).

Bone marrow

- Decontaminate the skin, overlying the site from where specimen is to be collected, with spirit and tincture of iodine.
- Aspirate 1 ml or more of bone marrow by sterile percutaneous aspiration with bone marrow aspiration needle.
- Collect in a sterile screw capped tube.
- Immediately transport to the laboratory.

Stool

- Should be collected in early stage of disease and prior to treatment with antimicrobials.
- Do not collect the specimen from bed pan.
- Should not be contaminated with urine.
- Collect about a spoonful of the specimen, especially that which contains mucus, pus or blood, into a clean, dry, leakproof container (Fig. 4.1b).
- If possible, submit more than one specimen on different days.
- The fresh stool specimen must be processed within 1–2 hours of passage.
- If delay is unavoidable then store it at 2–8°C.

Rectal swab

- Collect the swab only if stool collection is not possible.
- Insert swab at least 2.5 cm beyond the anal sphincter, so that it enters the rectum.
- Rotate it once before withdrawing.
- Transport in Cary-Blair or other transport medium.

IDENTIFICATION OF BACTERIA

Identification of the isolate is carried out by examination of stained and unstained smears of the morbid material, isolation in pure culture on appropriate culture media, study of macroscopic (colonial characters) and microscopic morphology of the isolate and biochemical characters. Finally, antibiotic susceptibility of the isolate is carried out and specific chemotherapy initiated.

Microscopic morphology of bacteria, appearance of bacterial colonies on solid media and appearance of bacterial growth in liquid media are given in Tables 4.1, 4.2 and 4.3, respectively.

Table 4.1. Microscopic morphology of bacteria

- **Shape:** Cocci, bacilli, coccobacilli, coma-shaped or filamentous.
- **Size:** Length and breadth, and diameter in μm.
- **Sides:** Parallel, convex, concave or irregular.
- **Ends:** Rounded, truncate, concave or pointed.
- **Arrangement:** Pairs, chains, groups of four or eight, clumps. Bacilli may be arranged at random, in short or long chains, in Chinese letter patterns, as palisades or in bundles. Vibrios may be single or in S forms.
- **Motility:** Non-motile, sluggishly motile, tumbling motility, actively motile, very actively motile or darting motility.
- **Flagella:** Without flagella (atrichate), monotrichate, lophotrichate, amphitrichate or peritrichate.
- **Spores:** These, when present, may be oval, spherical or ellipsoidal. These may be of the same width or wider than that of bacillary body. The spores may be equatorial, subterminal or terminal.
- **Capsules:** Present or absent.
- **Staining:** Even, irregular, bipolar, beaded, barred, presence of metachromatic granules, Gram-positive, Gram-negative, acid-fast, non-acid-fast.

Table 4.2. Appearance of bacterial colonies on solid media

- **Size:** In mm.
- **Shape:** Circular, irregular.
- **Elevation:** Flat, convex, concave, umbonate or umbilicate.
- **Edges:** Entire, undulate, crenated or fimbriate.
- **Colour:** White, buff, pink, etc.
- **Structure:** Translucent, transparent or opaque.
- **Consistency:** Membranous, friable, butyrous or viscid.
- **Emulsifiability:** Emulsifiable or autoagglutinable.
- **Degree of growth:** Scanty, moderate or profuse.
- **Haemolysis:** Type of haemolysis (α, β or nonhaemolytic) produced on blood agar.

Table 4.3. Appearance of bacterial growth in liquid media

- **Degree of growth:** Scanty, moderate or profuse.
- **Turbidity:** Present or absent. If present, uniform, granular or flocculent.
- **Deposit:** Present or absent. If present, powdery, granular or membranous.
- **Surface pellicle:** Present or absent.

Unstained wet film

An unstained wet film or **hanging drop preparation** is examined under light microscope for observation of motility, and an unstained wet film may be examined under **dark-ground microscope** for demonstration of motility of spirochaetes. Presence of *Treponema pallidum*, with characteristic spiral shape and motility, in exudate from a chancre is sufficient for presumptive diagnosis of syphilis.

Hanging drop preparation

Hanging drop preparations are frequently used for determination of bacterial motility.

- Take a glass slide having a circular concavity in the centre.
- By means of a matchstick dipped in petroleum jelly, a ring or square (according to the shape and size of the coverslip) is outlined round the concavity.
- With a wire loop place a drop of liquid culture or specimen such as stool on a coverslip laid on the bench.
- Invert the slide over the coverslip, allowing the glass to adhere to the jelly, and quickly turn round the slide so that the coverslip is uppermost. The drop should then be 'hanging' from the coverslip in the centre of the concavity.
- Place the slide on the microscope, rack down the condenser slightly and partially close the iris diaphragm.
- With low-power objective, focus the edge of the drop.
- Observe motility, shape and approximate size of the bacteria under high power.

It is essential to distinguish between true motility, where organism changes its position in the field, and Brownian movement, which is an oscillatory movement possessed by all small bodies (whether living or not) suspended in the fluid.

Staining techniques

A number of staining techniques for the identification of bacteria are available. Of these, Gram stain and Ziehl-Neelsen stain are most important. A Gram-stained smear shows the Gram reaction, size, shape and grouping pattern of bacteria, absence or presence of spores, their shape, size and intracellular position. Presence of Gram-negative diplococci inside the polymorphs in cerebrospinal fluid (CSF) and urethral discharge gives the provisional diagnosis of meningococcal meningitis and gonorrhoea respectively. With Ziehl-Neelsen staining, it is possible to identify tubercle bacilli and atypical mycobacteria, lepra bacilli, and *Nocardia*. They resist decolorization with 20%, 5% and 1% sulphuric acid respectively.

Gram stain

This staining method is most frequently used in diagnostic bacteriology.

Reagents

Ammonium oxalate crystal violet

Crystal violet	20 g
Methylated spirit	200 ml
Ammonium oxalate, 1% in water	800 ml

Gram's iodine

Iodine	10 g
Potassium iodide	20 g
Distilled water	1 litre

Dissolve 20 g potassium iodide in 250 ml of water and then add 10 g iodine. When iodine is dissolved, make up to 1 litre with water.

Decolorizer

Absolute alcohol or acetone.

Dilute carbol fuchsin

Basic fuchsin	0.5 g
Distilled water	1 litre

Method

- Prepare smear from clinical specimen, culture smear of colony or broth culture on a clean glass slide by spreading thinly on the slide.
- Allow it to dry in air and fix it by passing the dried slide, film downwards, three times slowly through the flame.
- Cover the smear with crystal violet (primary stain) for one minute. Other pararosaniline dyes such as methyl violet or gentian violet may also be used as primary stain.
- Pour Gram's iodine over the slide for two minutes.
- Decolorize with alcohol or acetone for 10–30 seconds.
- Counterstain with dilute carbol fuchsin or safranin for 30 seconds.
- Wash thoroughly with water; blot and dry in air.
- Examine under oil-immersion lens.

On the basis of their reaction to the Gram stain, bacteria can be divided into two groups, i.e., Gram-positive and Gram-negative. Both Gram-positive and Gram-negative bacteria take up violet colour with pararosaniline dyes. After treatment with decolourizing agent, Gram-positive bacteria retain this dye and violet colour while Gram-negative lose the dye and become colourless. They then take-up counterstain and appear red in colour.

The Gram stain is useful in two ways:

1. In the identification of many bacteria.
2. In influencing the choice of antibiotic.

Mechanism of Gram staining

The exact mechanism of Gram reaction is not known. It may, however, be attributed to:

- Gram-positive bacteria have a more acidic protoplasm, which may account for their retaining the basic primary dye more strongly than Gram-negative bacteria.
- The violet basic dye and the iodine form a dye-iodine complex inside both Gram-positive and Gram-negative bacteria but during alcohol or acetone wash, cell membranes (outer membrane of cell wall and cytoplasmic membrane) of Gram-negative bacteria are dissolved. However, dye-iodine complex is retained in Gram-positive cells by the thick peptidoglycan mesh, whereas it is readily washed out through the very thin peptidoglycan layer remaining in Gram-negative cells after both membranes have been dissolved.
- Gram-positive organisms that have lost cell wall integrity because of antibiotic treatment, old age, or action of auto-lytic enzymes may allow crystal violet to wash out with the decolorizing step and may appear Gram-variable, with some cells staining pink and others staining violet. However, for identification purposes these organisms are considered Gram-positive. On the other hand, Gram-negative bacteria rarely, if ever, retain crystal violet if staining procedure has been properly performed. Host cells, such as red and white blood cells, allow the crystal violet stain to wash out with decolourization and appear red. *If iodine solution is not added then Gram-negative bacteria stain violet than red, presumably because the organic solvent removes dye-iodine complex but not dye alone.*

Ziehl-Neelsen stain

Next to Gram stain, this is the method most frequently used in diagnostic bacteriology. It is of value in distinguishing a few bacterial species, e.g., tubercle bacilli, atypical myco-bacteria, lepra bacilli and *Nocardia* from all others. Tubercle bacilli, atypical mycobacteria and lepra bacilli are relatively impermeable to simple stains but when stained with hot concentrated carbol fuchsin, subsequently resist decolorization by 20%, 20% and 5% sulphuric acid respectively. Decolorized non-acid-fast organisms are counterstained with methylene blue. However, *Nocardia* which resists decolorization with 1% sulphuric acid, can be easily stained with Gram stain and is Gram-positive.

Modified Ziehl-Neelsen staining is used for detection of parasites such as *Cryptosporidium, Isospora, Cyclospora* and microsporidia.

Reagents

Carbol fuchsin

Basic fuchsin (powder)	5 g
Phenol (crystalline)	25 g
Absolute alcohol	50 ml
Distilled water	500 ml

Dissolve fuchsin in phenol by placing them in a 1 litre flask over a boiling water bath for about 5 minutes, shaking the contents from time to time. When solution is complete, add alcohol and mix thoroughly. Then add distilled water. Filter the mixture before use.

Sulphuric acid (20%) decolorizer

Concentrated sulphuric acid	250 ml
Distilled water	1 litre

Pour water into a large flask and place the flask in cold water in the sink. Add acid in 50 ml lots over 10 minutes, pouring slowly down the side of the flask into water. Mix gently. When cool, decant into a labelled bottle for use.

Methylene blue counterstain

Saturated solution of methylene blue in alcohol	300 ml
Potassium hydroxide, 0.01% in water	1 litre

Method

- Cover the slide with filtered carbol fuchsin and heat until steam rises. Allow the preparation to stain for 5 minutes, heat being applied at intervals to keep the stain hot. The stain must not be allowed to evaporate and dry on the slide. If necessary, pour more carbol fuchsin to keep the whole slide covered with carbol fuchsin.
- Wash with water.
- The stained smear is decolorized with 20% sulphuric acid and washed with water. This step is repeated till the film is only very faintly pink.
- Wash the slide well with water.
- Counterstain it with methylene blue for 15–20 seconds.
- Wash, blot, dry and examine under oil-immersion lens.

Result

Acid-fast bacilli stain bright red, while the tissue cells and other organisms are stained blue.

Principle of acid-fastness

Acid-fastness has been attributed to the high content of lipids, fatty acids and higher alcohols found in acid-fast bacteria. Of the lipids, mycolic acid, a high molecular weight hydroxy acid wax containing carboxyl groups, is most important because it is acid-fast even in free state.

Albert's stain

This method is useful for identification of *Corynebacterium diphtheriae*.

Reagents

Albert's stain

Toluidine blue	1.5 g
Malachite green	2 g
Glacial acetic acid	10 ml
Ethyl alcohol (95%)	20 ml
Distilled water	1 litre

Dissolve the dyes in alcohol and add to the water and acetic acid. Allow to stand for one day and then filter.

Albert's iodine

Iodine	6 g
Potassium iodide	9 g
Distilled water	900 ml

Method

- Prepare the film, dry in air, and fix by heat.
- Cover slide with Albert's stain and allow to act for 3–5 minutes.
- Wash in water and blot dry.
- Cover the slide with Albert's iodine, allow to act for one minute.
- Wash in water and blot dry.

Result

The granules and the protoplasm of *C. diphtheriae* are bluish-black and green respectively.

Other stains

A number of other staining procedures are available. They include:

- Simple stains such as methylene blue and basic fuchsin. They impart same colour to all organisms and are used only for colour contrast.
- Too thin bacteria may be rendered visible by light microscope by **silver impregnation method** which thickens the bacteria. This method is used for demonstration of spirochaetes and flagella.
- In case of **negative staining**, bacteria (spirochaetes) or fungi (*Cryptococcus*) are mixed with India ink or nigrosin that provide a uniform coloured background against which the unstained organisms can be seen. Bacterial capsules which do not take simple stains can be seen by negative staining.
- Special staining techniques for demonstration of spores, flagella, cell walls and capsules of bacteria are also available.

Differential identification characteristics

Accurate identification can be accomplished by isolation of bacteria in pure form followed by study of colonial morphology, examination of stained smear, biochemical reactions, antigenic structure, serotyping, biotyping, bacteriocin typing, phage typing, animal pathogenicity and antibiotic susceptibility determination. Clinical material is inoculated onto a solid medium (nutrient agar, blood agar or MacConkey agar) in such a way so as to ensure isolated discrete colonies. A colony represents a clone of descendants of a single bacterium, therefore, pure growth.

Enriched, enrichment, selective and differential media, depending upon the organism suspected, are employed. Selective growth conditions, i.e., presence or absence of oxygen and presence of CO_2, etc. are also employed keeping in view the organisms suspected. The culture plates are incubated at optimum temperature. Most of the pathogenic bacteria grow best at 37°C.

Biochemical reactions

A large number of biochemical tests can be employed for the identification of different bacteria. These include:

Indole production

Certain bacteria which possess enzyme **tryptophanase**, degrade amino acid tryptophan to indole, pyruvic acid and ammonia. Indole production is detected by inoculating the test organism into peptone water and incubating it at 37°C for 48–96 hours. Then add 0.5 ml of Kovac's reagent and shake gently. A **red colour** in the alcohol layer indicates a positive reaction. Kovac's reagent consists of:

Paradimethylaminobenzaldehyde	10 g
Amyl or isoamyl alcohol	150 ml
Concentrated hydrochloric acid	50 ml

Dissolve aldehyde in alcohol and slowly add the acid and store in refrigerator. Shake gently before use. Indole is extracted from the medium by amyl or isoamyl alcohol and forms red coloured ring by forming a red coloured complex with paradimethylaminobenzaldehyde. Negative test will show yellow coloured ring (colour of Kovac's reagent).

Methyl red (MR) test

This test detects the production of sufficient acid by fermentation of glucose, so that pH of the medium falls and it is maintained below 4.5. Inoculate the test organism in glucose phosphate broth and incubate at 37°C for 2–5 days. Then add five drops of 0.04% solution of methyl red, mix well and read the result immediately. Positive tests are bright red (indicating a low pH) and negative are yellow. If the test is negative after 2 days repeat it after 5 days.

Glucose phosphate broth

Medium

Peptone	5 g
Dipotassium hydrogen phosphate	5 g
Distilled water	1 litre
Glucose 10% solution (sterilized separately)	50 ml

Dissolve peptone and phosphate, adjust pH to 7.6, filter, dispense in 5 ml amounts and sterilize at 121°C for 15 minutes. Sterilize glucose solution by filtration and add 0.25 ml to each tube (final concentration 0.5%).

Voges-Proskauer (VP) test for acetoin production

Many bacteria ferment carbohydrates with the production of acetyl methyl carbinol (acetoin). In the presence of potassium hydroxide and atmospheric oxygen, acetoin is converted to diacetyl, and α-naphthol serves as a catalyst to form a red complex. This test is usually done in conjunction with the methyl red test. *An organism of the family Enterobacteriaceae is usually either methyl red positive and Voges-Proskauer negative or methyl red negative and Voges-Proskauer positive.*

Inoculate test organism in glucose phosphate broth and incubate at 37°C for 48 hours. Then add 1 ml potassium hydroxide and 3 ml of 5% solution of α-naphthol in absolute alcohol. A positive reaction is indicated by the development of **pink colour** in 2–5 minutes and crimson in 30 minutes.

Citrate utilization

This test is used to study the ability of an organism to utilize citrate as a sole source of carbon for the growth. Liquid (Koser's) and solid (Simmon's) media containing citrate as a sole source of carbon can be used. A part of colony is picked up with a straight wire and inoculated into either of these media. The ability of an organism to utilize citrate as a sole source of carbon is detected by the **production of turbidity** (due to growth) in liquid medium. Solid medium also contains bromothymol blue as indicator, therefore, on the solid medium the **appearance of growth and blue colour** is positive, and original green colour and no growth is negative.

The blue colour is due to the alkaline pH that results from utilization of citrate. It turns the indicator in the medium from **green to blue**. It is important to keep the inoculum light, since dead organisms can be a source of carbon, producing a false positive reaction.

Indole, MR, VP and citrate tests are done in routine for the classification of Gram-negative enteric bacteria. They are commonly referred to as **IMViC tests**.

Koser's medium

Sodium chloride	5 g
Magnesium sulphate	0.2 g
Ammonium dihydrogen phosphate	1 g
Potassium dihydrogen phosphate	1 g
Sodium citrate	5 g
Distilled water	1 litre

The pH of the medium should be 6.8. The medium is dispensed and sterilized by autoclaving at 121°C for 15 minutes.

Simmons' citrate medium

Koser's medium	1 litre
Agar	20 g
Bromothymol blue, 0.2%	40 ml

Dispense, autoclave at 121°C for 15 minutes and allow to set as slopes.

Sugar fermentation

The ability of an organism to ferment various sugars is tested by inoculation of the test organism in different sugar media containing Andrade's indicator. A small inverted tube (**Durham's tube**) completely filled with liquid and containing no air bubbles, is usually included in each culture tube. Production of acid is indicated by the change in the colour of the medium to red or pink, and gas, if produced, collects in Durham's tube (see sugar fermentation media in chapter 3).

Nitrate reduction

This test detects the production of enzyme nitrate reductase which reduces nitrate to nitrite. *All the organisms of the family Enterobacteriaceae are positive for this test.* Inoculate test organism in 5 ml medium containing potassium nitrate, peptone and distilled water. Incubate it at 37°C for 96 hours. Then add 0.1 ml test reagent which consists of equal volumes of 0.8% sulphanilic acid and 0.5% α-naphthylamine in 5 N acetic acid mixed just before use. A **red colour** developing within a few minutes indicates the presence of nitrite and hence the ability of test organism to reduce nitrate to nitrite.

If no colour develops, this may indicate that nitrate has not been reduced (a true negative reaction) or that nitrate has been reduced beyond nitrite to nitrogen gas (N_2), nitric oxide (NO), or nitrous oxide (N_2O). Because the test reagents detect only nitrites, the latter process would lead to a false negative reading. Thus, it is necessary to add a small quantity of zinc dust to all negative reactions. Zinc ions reduce nitrate to nitrite, and the development of a red colour after adding zinc dust indicates the presence of residual nitrates and confirms a true negative reaction.

Medium

Potassium nitrate (nitrite-free)	0.2 g
Peptone	5 g
Distilled water	1 litre

Tube in 5 ml amounts and autoclave at 121°C for 15 minutes.

Test reagents

- **Solution A:** Dissolve 8.0 g of sulphanilic acid in 1 litre of acetic acid 5 mol/litre.
- **Solution B:** Dissolve 5.0 g of α-naphthylamine in 1 litre of acetic acid 5 mol/litre.

Immediately before use, mix equal volumes of solutions A and B to give the test reagent.

Urease test

This test detects the ability of an organism to produce urease enzyme. The test organism is inoculated on the entire slope of Christensen's medium which contains urea and phenol red indicator in addition to other constituents including agar. It is incubated at 37°C and examined after 4 hours and after overnight incubation. Development of **purple-pink** colour indicates production of urease. The latter in the presence of water converts urea into ammonia and carbon dioxide. Ammonia makes the medium alkaline and phenol red indicator changes to purple-pink in colour.

Christensen's medium

Peptone	1 g
Sodium chloride	5 g
Dipotassium hydrogen phosphate	2 g
Phenol red (1 in 500 aqueous solution)	6 ml
Agar	20 g
Distilled water	1 litre
Glucose, 10% solution, sterile	10 ml
Urea, 20% solution, sterile	100 ml

Sterilize glucose and urea solutions by filtration. Prepare the basal medium without glucose and urea. Adjust pH to 6.8–6.9 and sterilize by autoclaving in a flask at 121°C for 30 minutes. Cool to about 50°C, and add glucose and urea and tube the medium as slopes.

Hydrogen sulphide production

Some organisms produce hydrogen sulphide from sulphur containing amino acids. It may be detected by suspending strips of filter paper impregnated with lead acetate between the cotton plug and the tube. Blackening of the paper indicates hydrogen sulphide production. It has variable sensitivity. When cultured in media containing lead acetate or ferric ammonium citrate or ferrous acetate they turn them black or brown. This method is more sensitive than lead acetate strip method.

Potassium cyanide test

This tests the ability of an organism to grow in the presence of potassium cyanide. Inoculate buffered peptone water medium, containing 1 in 13,000 concentration of potassium cyanide, with test organism. Incubate at 37°C for 24–48 hours. Development of **turbidity** in the medium indicates the ability of the organism to grow in the presence of potassium cyanide.

Catalase production

The enzyme catalase mediates the breakdown of hydrogen peroxide into oxygen and water. This principle is used for the detection of catalase enzyme in a bacterial isolate.

Put a loopful of 10% hydrogen peroxide on colonies of the test organism on nutrient agar. Alternatively, pick-up a few colonies of the test organism with platinum loop from nutrient agar plate and dip it in a drop of 10% hydrogen peroxide on a clean glass slide. The production of **gas bubbles** from the culture indicates a positive reaction. A false positive result may be obtained if the growth is picked-up from medium containing catalase, e.g., blood agar or if an iron wire loop is used.

Oxidase test

This test depends on the presence, in bacteria, of certain oxidases that catalyze the oxidation of reduced tetra-methyl-*p*-phenylenediamine dihydrochloride (oxidase reagent) by molecular oxygen. Put a drop of freshly prepared 1% solution of oxidase reagent on a piece of filter paper. Then rub a few colonies of test organism on it. If it is oxidase-positive, it will produce a **deep purple** colour within 10 seconds. Alternatively, pour oxidase reagent over the colonies of the test organism on the culture plate. The colonies of oxidase-positive organisms rapidly develop a deep purple colour.

Various species of *Neisseria, Pseudomonas, Aeromonas, Vibrio, Alcaligenes* and *Campylobacter* are oxidase-positive. All the members of the family Enterobacteriaceae are oxidase-negative.

Motility test

The motility test medium has agar concentration of 0.4% or less, to allow free spread of organisms. Inoculation is done by a single stab into the medium. After overnight incubation, movement away from the stab line or a hazy appearance throughout the medium indicates a motile organism.

Phenylalanine deaminase test

Phenylalanine deaminase determines whether the organism possesses the enzyme phenylalanine deaminase that deaminates phenylalanine to phenylpyruvic acid, which reacts with ferric salts to give a green colour. Agar slants of the medium containing DL-phenylalanine is inoculated with a single colony of the test organism. After incubation at 37°C for 18–24 hours, 4 or 5 drops of 10% solution of ferric chloride reagent are added directly to the surface of the agar. If the test is positive, a green colour will develop in the fluid and in the slope. This test is useful in initial differentiation of *Proteus, Morganella,* and *Providencia* from the rest of the Entero-bacteriaceae.

Medium

Yeast extract	3 g
DL-Phenylalanine	2 g
Disodium hydrogen phosphate	1 g
Sodium chloride	5 g
Agar	12 g
Distilled water	1 litre

Adjust the pH to 7.4, distribute and sterilize by autoclaving at 121°C for 15 minutes. Allow to solidify in tubes as long slopes.

Decarboxylase tests

Decarboxylase tests determine whether the bacterial species possess enzymes capable of decarboxylating specific acids in the test medium. The three amino acids commonly used to test for Enterobacteriaceae are lysine, ornithine, and arginine. Specific amine products and carbon dioxide are products of decarboxylation. The production of decarboxylases is induced by a low pH and, as a result of their action, the pH rises to neutrality or above. The lysine and ornithine reactions are truely decarboxylase tests, but the arginine reaction is more correctly recognized now as dihydrolase test.

Medium

Peptone	5 g
Meat extract	5 g
Glucose	0.5 g
Pyridoxal	5 mg
Bromocresol purple (1 in 500 solution)	5 ml
Cresol red (1 in 500 solution)	2.5 ml
Distilled water	1 litre

Dissolve the solids in water and adjust the pH to 6.0 before the addition of the indicators. This is the basal medium and to it is added the amino acid whose decarboxylation is to be tested. Divide the basal medium into four portions. To the first portion add 1% L-lysine hydrochloride, to the second 1% L-ornithine hydrochloride, to the third 1% arginine hydrochloride, and no addition to the fourth portion. Readjust pH to 6.0. Distribute 1 ml quantities in small tubes containing sterile liquid paraffin to provide a layer about 5 mm thick above the medium. Autoclave at 121°C for 15 minutes.

Method: Inoculate lightly through paraffin layer with a straight wire. Incubate and read daily for 4 days.

The medium first becomes yellow due to acid production during glucose fermentation; later, if decarboxylation occurs, the medium becomes violet. The control should remain yellow.

Bacteriocin, bacteriophage and serotyping

Each species of an organism contains a number of different strains. These epidemiological markers are useful for intraspecies differentiation of various strains.

Animal pathogenicity

Various experimental models used in diagnostic microbiology laboratory are mouse, rat, guinea-pig, rabbit, nine-banded armadillo and monkey. Various routes of inoculation are intradermal, subcutaneous, intramuscular, intraperitoneal, intracerebral and intravenous. Oral and nasal routes can also be used. The identification of the organism is carried out on the basis of clinical and postmortem findings, and cultural characteristics.

BACTERIAL TAXONOMY

The taxonomy of bacteria refers to three basic concepts – classification, nomenclature and identification.

Classification

It can be defined as the arrangement of organisms into taxonomic groups (taxa) on the basis of genotypic (genetic) and phenotypic (observable) similarities and differences. It allows the orderly grouping of microorganisms. For bacterial classification, three main approaches are usually followed. These include phylogenetic, Adansonian, genetic and intraspecies classification.

Phylogenetic classification

It is a hierarchial classification. It represents a branching tree-like arrangement, one characteristic being employed for division at each branch or level. This system is called phylogenetic because it denotes an evolutionary arrangement of species. Here some characteristics are given special weightage. For example, Gram staining, spore formation, lactose fermentation, etc. are used to differentiate major groups, whereas less important properties such as nutritional requirements for growth of bacteria, production of certain enzymes by bacteria, etc. are employed to distinguish minor groups such as genera and species.

The formal levels of classification, in successive smaller subsets, are kingdom, phylum or division, class, order, family, tribe, genus and species. At present no standard classification of bacteria is universally accepted and applied although **Bergey's Manual of Systematic Bacteriology** is widely used as authoritative source.

Adansonian classification

Adansonian classification makes no phylogenetic assumption but merely takes into account all the characteristics expressed at the time of study. It gives equal weight to all measurable features, and groups the organisms on the basis of similarities of several characteristics. The availability of computers has extended the scope of phonetic classification by permitting comparison of very large number of properties of several organisms at the same time. This is known as **numerical taxonomy**.

Genetic classification

This is based on homology of DNA base sequences of the microorganisms. DNA relatedness is determined by studying the nucleotide sequence of DNA by DNA hybridization or recombination methods. The study of messenger RNA and ribosomal RNA also provides useful information on genetic relatedness among bacteria. Genetic classification has been used more with viruses than with bacteria.

Intraspecies classification

Intraspecies classification is based on biochemical properties (biotypes), antigenic properties (serotypes), susceptibility to bacteriophages (phage types), resistance to various chemicals (resistotypes), or production of bacteriocins (colicin types).

Nomenclature

It refers to the naming of microorganisms. It is governed by the *International Committee on Systematic Bacteriology* and published as *Approved List of Bacterial Names* in the *International Journal of Systematic Bacteriology*. By accepted taxonomic convention, order names have the endings -ales (i.e., the order Eubacteriales), family names have the latinized ending -aceae (e.g., the family Enterobacteriaceae), and tribe names end in -eae (e.g., the tribe Proteae). The order, family and tribe names are capitalized. The genus name is also capitalized followed by species name which is not capitalized. If typed, the genus and species names should be italicized. If written, they should be underlined. Species should not be capitalized even when derived from the name of the person who discovered it. Often, the genus name is abbreviated by using the first letter of the genus followed by a period and the species epithet (name) (e.g., *E. coli*). The genus name followed by the word species (e.g., *Staphylococcus* species) may be used to refer to the genus as a whole. Species abbreviated sp. (singular) or spp. (plural) is used when the species is not specified. When the bacteria are referred to as a group, their names are neither capitalized nor underlined (e.g., staphylococci).

Identification

Suitable criteria for the purpose of identification include cell shape, Gram reaction and the presence or absence of specialized structures such as spores or flagella. Staining procedures such as Gram stain can provide reliable assessment of the nature of cell surfaces. Some bacteria produce characteristic pigments and others can be differentiated on the basis of their complement of extracellular enzymes (e.g., haemolysins). Tests such as oxidase test can be used to distinguish organisms on the basis of the presence of a respiratory enzyme, cytochrome C.

The traditional method of placing an organism into a particular genus and species is based on the similarity of all members in a number of phenotypic characteristics. This is accomplished by testing each bacterial culture for a variety of metabolic characteristics and comparing the results with those listed in established charts.

In rapid identification systems, a numerical taxonomy (also called computer taxonomy, phenetics, or taxometrics) is used. Numerical classification schemes use a large number (frequently 100 or more) of taxonomically useful characteristics. All these characteristics are assigned numerical value. The computer clusters different strains at selected levels of overall similarity (usually 80% at the species level) on the basis of the frequency with which they share traits.

5

Sterilization, Disinfection, and Disposal of Biomedical Waste

Sterilization

It is defined as the process by which an article, a surface or a medium is freed of all microorganisms including viruses, bacteria, their spores and fungi, both pathogenic and non-pathogenic.

Disinfection

It is a process of destruction or removal of organisms capable of giving rise to infection. Disinfectants are capable of killing vegetative bacteria, fungi, viruses and rarely bacterial spores. Therefore, disinfection must never be used when sterilization is possible.

Antisepsis

It is the destruction or inhibition of microorganisms in living tissues thereby limiting or preventing the harmful effects of infection. A disinfectant that is applied to living tissue, to kill microbes, is referred to as an **antiseptic**.

Various agents used in sterilization and disinfection may be divided into:

A. **Physical agents**
1. Sunlight
2. Drying
3. Heat
4. Filtration
5. Radiations

B. **Chemical agents**
1. Phenols
2. Halogens
3. Metallic salts
4. Aldehydes
5. Alcohols
6. Dyes
7. Vapour-phase disinfectants
8. Surface active disinfectants

A. PHYSICAL AGENTS

1. SUNLIGHT

Sunlight possesses ultraviolet rays which along with heat rays are responsible for appreciable germicidal activity.

2. DRYING

Water constitutes 80% of the weight of the bacteria and is also essential for the growth of bacteria. Therefore, drying has deleterious effect on many bacteria. However, spores are unaffected by drying.

3. HEAT

Heat is the most reliable, certain and rapid method of sterilization. It can be easily controlled and unlike chemical disinfection, leaves no potentially harmful residue. Unless the material to be sterilized is heat-sensitive, this method should be preferred.

Types of heat and principle

There are two types of heat – dry heat and wet heat.

Dry heat

It is believed to kill microorganisms by causing destructive oxidation of essential cell constituents. Dry heat at 100°C for 60 minutes and 115°C for 60 minutes can kill all vegetative bacteria and fungal spores respectively. Bacterial spores can be killed by dry heat at 160°C for one hour or 180°C for 20 minutes. On the whole dry heat is less efficient sterilization process than moist heat.

Moist heat

It causes denaturation and coagulation of proteins. When steam condenses on cooler surface, it releases its latent heat and raises the temperature of its surface. If spores are present, steam condenses on them and increases their water content leading to hydrolysis and breakdown of bacterial proteins. Most vegetative bacteria are killed by moist heat at 50–65°C in 10 minutes. Resistance of bacterial spores varies with different strains of the same species. For example, spores of most strains of *Clostridium tetani* are killed by boiling at 100°C for 10 minutes. However, some strains resist boiling for 1–3 hours. The spores of some strains of *C. botulinum* resist boiling at 100°C up to 8 hours. However, all spores are killed by autoclaving at 121°C for 10–30 minutes.

I. Sterilization by dry heat

(A) Red heat

Inoculating wires and loops, points of forceps and spatulas are sterilized by holding them almost vertical in a bunsen burner flame until red hot (Table 5.1).

(B) Flaming

Scalpel blades, needles, mouths of culture tubes, glass slides and cover slips are sterilized by passing the article through the bunsen flame without allowing them to become red hot.

(C) Incineration

This is an efficient method for rapidly destroying contaminated materials such as soiled dressings and pathological materials, etc.

(D) Hot air oven

It is a method of choice for sterilization of glassware such as assembled all glass syringes, test tubes, petri dishes, pipettes and flasks; metal instruments such as forceps, scissors and scalpels; sealed materials such as oils, jellies and powders which are impervious to steam; and swab sticks packed in test tubes. It is not suitable for materials like fabrics which may be damaged by heat.

Hot air oven is electrically heated and is fitted with a thermostat that maintains the chamber air at a chosen temperature and a fan that distributes hot air in the chamber (Fig. 5.1). It must not be overloaded and spaces must be left for circulation of air through the load. Holding time for sterilization in hot air oven is **one hour at 160°C or 20 minutes at 180°C**. It is timed as beginning when the thermometer first shows 160°C or 180°C respectively.

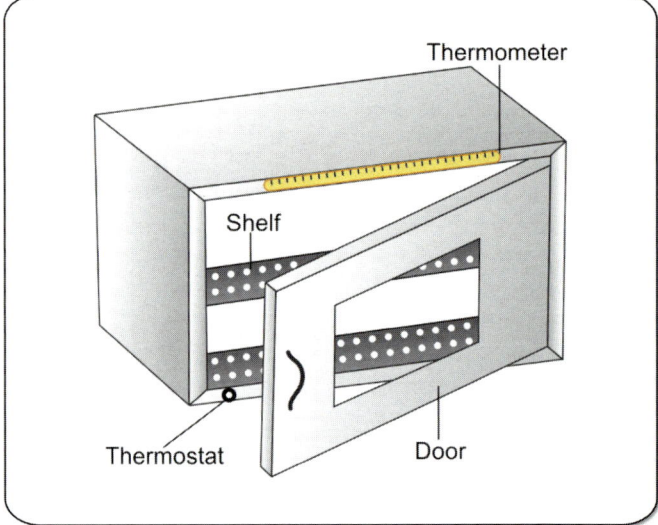

Fig. 5.1. Hot air oven.

Sterilization controls

Two types of controls are available:

1. Biological control

An envelope containing a filter paper strip impregnated with 10^6 spores of *Bacillus subtilis* subsp. *niger* (NCTC 10075 or ATCC 9372) is placed within the load (Table 5.2). After sterilization is over, the strip is removed and inoculated into tryptone soy broth and incubated anaerobically at 37°C for five days. No growth of *B. subtilis* subsp. *niger* indicates proper sterilization.

2. Chemical control

A Browne's tube containing red solution is placed within the load. A change of colour of the solution from **red to green** indicates proper sterilization.

II. Sterilization by moist heat

Sterilization by moist heat means killing of the micro-organisms with hot water or steam. Moist heat is divided into 3 forms (Table 5.3):

Table 5.1. Sterilization by dry heat

Mode of sterilization	Instrument	Temperature and time	Sterilization of	Advantages/disadvantages
Red heat	Bunsen burner	Till red hot	Inoculating wire loops, forceps and spatulas	Sterilization is rapid and thorough
Flaming	Bunsen burner	Waving through the flame	Scalpel blades, glass slides, mouth of culture tubes and bottles.	1. Surface sterilization is possible 2. Rapid method
Hot air	Hot air oven	160°C for 1 hour or 180°C for 20 minutes	Glassware, sealed materials like oils, greases, dry powder, etc.	Can be used for loads that cannot be penetrated by steam

Table 5.2. Biological controls of different sterilization methods

Method of sterilization	Biological control
Hot air oven	*Bacillus subtilis* subsp. *niger*
Autoclave	*Bacillus stearothermophilus*
Low temperature steam-formaldehyde	*Bacillus stearothermophilus*
Ethylene oxide	*Bacillus globigi* (a red-pigmented variant of *Bacillus subtilis*)
Ionizing radiations	*Bacillus pumilis*
Filtration	*Serratia marcescens*, *Pseudomonas diminuta*

A. At temperatures below 100°C.
B. At a temperature of 100°C.
  (a) Boiling water
  (b) Free steam
C. At temperature above 100°C.

(A) Moist heat at temperatures below 100°C

Heat-labile fluids may be disinfected (not sterilized) by heating at temperatures below 100°C. Such treatment is sufficient to kill mesophilic vegetative bacteria. This includes:

- **Pasteurization** of milk. The temperature employed is either **63°C for 30 minutes** (holder method) or **72°C for 20 seconds** (flash method) followed by rapid cooling to 13°C or lower.
- **Heat-labile fluids** such as serum may be disinfected by heating at 56°C for one hour. If temperature rises above 59°C it will coagulate.
- **Vaccines** prepared from non-sporing bacteria may be inactivated in a water bath at 60°C for one hour.
- **Household utensils** and **patient's clothing** may be disinfected by washing in water at 70–80°C for several minutes.
- Media such as Lowenstein-Jensen and Loeffler's serum slope are rendered sterile by heating at 80–85°C for half an hour on three successive days in an inspissator.

(B) Moist heat at a temperature of 100°C

(a) Boiling at 100°C: Boiling at 100°C for 10–30 minutes kills all vegetative bacteria and some bacterial spores. Therefore, it is not recommended for sterilization of instruments for surgical procedures.

(b) Free steam at 100°C: Steam at normal atmospheric pressure is at 100°C. But, in addition, it has latent heat which on condensing on the article to be sterilized releases its latent heat. A **Koch** or **Arnold steam sterilizer** consists of a vertical metal cylinder with a removable conical lid having a small opening for the escaping steam. Water is added on the bottom and there is a perforated shelf above water level (Fig. 5.2). On this shelf articles to be sterilized are placed.

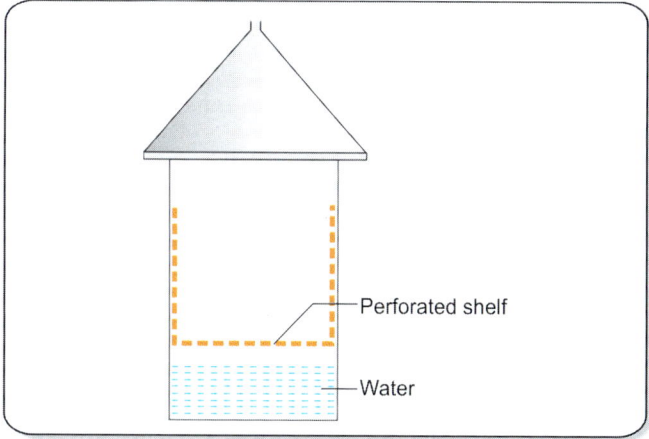

Fig. 5.2. Steam sterilizer.

One single exposure to steam for 90 minutes ensures complete sterilization but for media containing sugar and gelatin, which may get decomposed on long heating, an exposure of **100°C for 20 minutes on three consecutive days** is employed. This is known as **tyndallization** or **intermittent sterilization**. First exposure to steam kills all vegetative bacteria, and any spores present being in a favourable medium, will germinate and will be killed on the subsequent occasions. Therefore, non-nutrient media cannot be sterilized by this method.

Table 5.3. Sterilization by moist heat

Mode of sterilization	Instrument	Temperature and time	Sterilization of	Advantages/disadvantages
Below 100°C	Water bath	56°C for 1 hour	Serum	May be used for disinfection. Most vegetative mesophilic bacteria are killed.
At 100°C	Boiling water bath	100°C for 10–20 min.	Glass, metal and rubber items	Kills all vegetative bacteria and some spores.
Steaming at 100°C	Arnold steamer	100°C for 20 min. on 3 successive days	Culture media containing sugar and gelatin	Prevents decomposition of media. *Spores of thermophilic bacteria may escape killing.*
Above 100°C	Autoclave	121°C for 15–20 min.	Culture media and other aqueous solutions, dressing material, linen, gloves, etc.	Most reliable method of sterilization.

(C) Moist heat at temperature above 100°C

Steam above 100°C or saturated steam is a more efficient sterilizing agent than hot air because:

- it provides greater lethal action of moist heat,
- it is quicker in heating up the exposed articles, and
- it can penetrate easily porous material such as cotton wool stoppers, paper and cloth wrappers, bundles of surgical linen, and hollow apparatus.

Sterilization by **steam under pressure (autoclaving)** is suitable for culture media and aqueous solutions (since atmosphere of steam prevents evaporation during heating), dressing material, linen, gloves, etc. Satisfactory sterilization can be achieved at 15 pounds per square inch (psi) pressure equivalent to **121°C in 15–20 minutes**. In fact the only practical and dependable method of sterilization is steam under pressure using different types of autoclaves. *However, the autoclave is ineffective for sterilizing substances that repel moisture (oils, waxes or powders).*

All the air must be removed from the autoclave chamber and the articles to be sterilized, so that the latter are exposed to pure steam. There are three reasons for this:

- The admixture of air with steam results in lower temperature being achieved.
- Air hinders penetration of steam into the interstices of porous materials, surgical dressings, syringes, etc.
- The air being denser forms a separate and cooler layer in the lower part of the autoclave, so it prevents adequate heating of articles there.

Several types of steam sterilizers are available. The **laboratory autoclave** or **pressure cooker type autoclave** (Fig. 5.3) consists of a vertical or horizontal cylinder of gun metal or stainless steel in a supporting frame or case. The lid is fastened by screw clamps and rendered air tight by asbestos gasket. Lid bears a tap for discharge of air and steam, and a steam release valve or safety valve. The latter opens and closes when the steam pressure rises or falls the desired level respectively. On its upper part of the side, the autoclave has a discharge tap for air and steam, and an air and steam release knob. Heating is done by electricity. Water is added on the bottom of the autoclave. Above this is a perforated shelf on which articles to be sterilized are placed.

The lid is closed, discharge tap is opened and safety valve is adjusted to the required pressure. As heating continues, the steam and air mixture escapes. To know when all the air inside the autoclave has escaped the discharge tap is connected with one end of a rubber tube and the other end of it is placed in water. When the air bubbles stop coming it indicates that all the air from inside the autoclave has been removed. The discharge tap is now closed. Steam pressure rises inside and when it reaches the desired set level (15 psi) the safety valve opens and excess steam escapes. From this point the **holding time** (15 minutes) is counted.

When the holding time is over, the heating is stopped and autoclave allowed to cool till pressure gauze indicates that inside pressure has reached to the atmospheric pressure. The discharge tap is now opened and air is allowed to enter the autoclave. The lid is now opened and the sterilized articles removed. If the tap or lid is opened when the pressure inside is high, the liquid media boil violently and may explode. On the other hand, if the articles are not removed for a long time after the normal atmospheric pressure has reached inside the autoclave, an excessive amount of water will be evaporated and lost from the media.

Sterilization controls

Two types of controls are available:

1. Biological control

An envelope containing a filter paper strip impregnated with 10^6 spores of *Bacillus stearothermophilus* (NCTC 10003 or ATCC 7953) is placed with the load in the coolest and least accessible part of the autoclave chamber (Table 5.2). After sterilization is over the strip is removed and inoculated into tryptone soy broth and incubated at 56°C for 5 days. No growth of *B. stearothermophilus* indicates proper sterilization. Spores of this organism withstand 121°C for up to 12 minutes and this has made the organism ideal for testing autoclaves.

2. Chemical control

A Browne's tube containing red solution is placed within the load. A change of colour of the solution from **red to green** indicates proper sterilization.

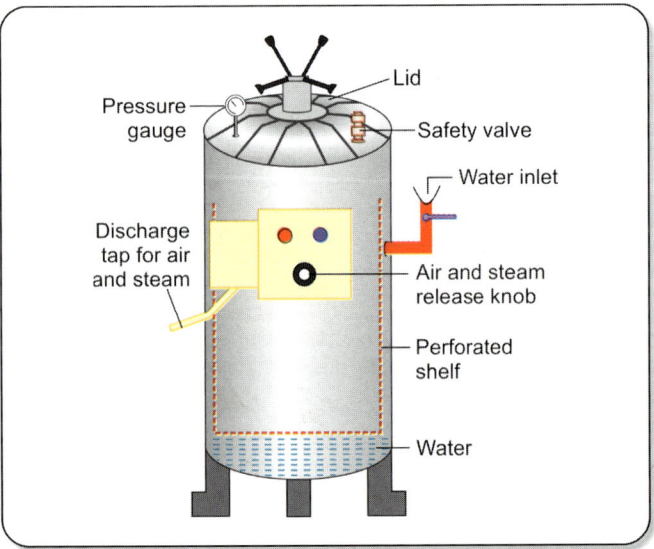

Fig. 5.3. Autoclave.

4. FILTRATION

Liquids such as sera and solutions of heat-labile substances such as sugars and urea, used for preparation of media, can be sterilized by filtration. Filtration does not kill microbes, it separates them out. This method is also useful for:

- sterilization of pharmaceutical substances,
- separation of bacteriophages and bacterial toxins from bacteria, and
- isolation of organisms which are scanty in fluids.

Most bacteria, yeasts and molds are retained by pore size of 0.45 μm; however, this pore size may allow passage of *Pseudomonas*-like organisms, and therefore a 0.22 μm size is available for critical sterilizing (e.g. parenteral solutions). Membranes with pore sizes of 0.01 μm are capable of retaining small viruses. Filtration of air is accomplished with the use of high-efficiency particulate air (HEPA) filters. HEPA filters are able to remove microorganisms larger than 0.3 μm and are used in laboratory hoods and in rooms of immuno-compromised individuals. *Serratia marcescens* and *Pseudomonas diminuta* have been used to test the efficacy of different filters (Table 5.2).

Types of filters

1. Earthenware filters

Important examples are earthenware filters made from kieselguhr (a fossil diatomaceous earth), and chamberland filters made of unglazed porcelain. They are made in the form of hollow candles with different grades of porosity. The fluid to be sterilized is passed through the candle. After use they can be sterilized by scrubbing with stiff brush followed by boiling and autoclaving.

2. Asbestos (Seitz) filters

They are made up of a disc of asbestos (magnesium trisilicate). It is supported on a perforated metal disc within a metal funnel. The latter with filter disc fitted is sterilized by autoclaving. It is then fitted onto a sterile flask through a silicone rubber bung. The fluid to be sterilized is put into the funnel and flask connected to the exhaust pump through its side tap. Sterilized fluid is collected from the flask and filter disc is discarded after use. These discs are available with different grades of porosity.

3. Sintered glass filters

These are made of finely ground glass fused together. These are available in different pore sizes. They are also available in the form of a disc fused into a glass funnel. After use they are washed with running tap water in reverse direction and cleaned with warm, strong sulphuric acid.

4. Membrane filters

These are made-up of cellulose esters and are widely used now-a-days for sterilization of heat-labile fluids. These are also known as millipore filters. They are available as discs of pore size varying from 0.015–12 μm. The 0.22 μm filter is the most commonly used because the pore size is smaller than that of bacteria. They can also be used for bacterial counts of water. A known amount of water is filtered through the membrane filter disc. The upper side of the disc is then placed on an appropriate moist culture medium and incubated. The colonies that develop can be counted and viable count calculated.

5. Syringe filters

Syringes fitted with membranes of 13 mm and 25 mm diameter are available. The fluid to be sterilized is forced through the disc by pressing the piston of the syringe.

6. Air filters

Large volumes of air may be rapidly freed from infectious agents by passage through high efficiency particulate air (HEPA) filters.

5. RADIATIONS

Two types of radiations (Table 5.4) are used:

- Non-ionizing.
- Ionizing.

Non-ionizing radiations

These include infrared and ultraviolet radiations:

Infrared rays

Infrared rays bring about sterilization by generation of heat. Articles to be sterilized are placed in a moving conveyor belt and passed through a tunnel that is heated by infrared radiators to a temperature of 180°C. The articles are exposed to that

Table 5.4. Sterilization by radiation

Type of radiation	Instrument	Dose	Application	Advantages/disadvantages
Ionizing	Cobalt 60	2.5 Mrad	Sterilization of antibiotics, hormones, sutures and prepacked disposable items such as plastic syringes, transfusion sets, catheters, cannulas, culture plates, etc.	Excellent sterilizing agent, penetrates deep into objects, produces less heat, can be used for heat sensitive items. But it is expensive.
Non-ionizing (UV radiation)	UV lamps, commercial UV units and mercury vapour lamps	250–260 nm wavelength for 30 min.	Disinfection of clear surfaces like inoculation hoods, laboratories, wards, operation theatres, etc.	Destroys microorganisms only on exposed surfaces. Hazardous for eyes and skin.

temperature for a period of 7.5 minutes. Articles sterilized include metallic instruments and glassware. It is mainly used in central sterile supply department. Efficiency can be checked by using Browne's tube No. 4 (blue spot).

Ultraviolet (UV) radiations

Ultraviolet (UV) radiations in the range of 250–260 nm wavelength are highly effective. Low pressure mercury vapour lamps emit over 95% of radiations with the wavelength of 253.7 nm. Most vegetative bacteria are susceptible to UV radiations. Spores are highly resistant and susceptibility of viruses is variable. **Human immunodeficiency virus is not inactivated by UV radiations.** Their use is best restricted to disinfection of clean surfaces like *inoculation hoods*, *laboratories*, *wards*, and *operation theatres*. Source of UV radiations must be shielded to prevent the radiations falling on eyes and skin because it may damage them.

Ionizing radiations

These include *X-rays*, *gamma rays* and *cosmic rays*. These have very high penetrative power and are highly lethal to all cells including bacteria. They damage DNA by various mechanisms. Spores are more resistant than vegetative bacteria. Large commercial plants use gamma radiations for sterilization of prepacked disposable items such as *plastic syringes, transfusion sets, catheters, cannulas, culture plates*, etc. that are unable to withstand heat because there is no appreciable increase in the temperature. Therefore, this method is known as **cold sterilization**. High cost of installation limits its use commercially. *Bacillus pumilis* has been used to test the efficacy of ionizing radiations (Table 5.2).

B. CHEMICAL AGENTS

Several chemical agents are used as antiseptics and disinfectants.

1. PHENOLS

These are obtained by distillation of coal tar and have a powerful microbicidal action. They cause cell membrane damage, thus releasing cell contents and causing cell lysis. They are resistant to inactivation by organic matter and are active against Gram-positive and Gram-negative bacteria, moderately active against mycobacteria, and have little activity against spores and viruses. They are used mainly for *discarded cultures, contaminated pipettes and other infected material*. Phenol is bactericidal at a concentration of 1%. At a concentration of 0.5% it is used for preservation of sera and vaccines. Certain phenol derivatives like cresols, chlorhexidine, chloroxylenol and hexachlorophene are commonly used as disinfectants.

2. HALOGENS

Halogens are oxidizing agents. They cause damage by oxidation of essential sulfhydryl groups of enzymes. Chlorine

and iodine are the halogens which are used as disinfectants. They are bactericidal and sporicidal. They are active in very high dilutions and their action is very rapid. In addition to chlorine itself there are three types of chlorine compounds, the hypochlorites, and the inorganic and organic chloramines. **The disinfectant action of all the chlorine compounds is due to release of free chlorine.** Hypochlorites have a wide spectrum of activity against viruses and very little activity against tubercle bacilli. They are available in liquid or powder form as salts of calcium, lithium and sodium. Iodine in alcoholic and aqueous solutions is used almost exclusively as a skin disinfectant (antiseptic).

3. METALLIC SALTS

All metallic salts have some degree of toxicity for bacteria. The most toxic are those of mercury and silver and the least toxic are those of sodium and potassium.

4. ALDEHYDES

Two aldehydes (formaldehyde and glutaraldehyde) are currently of considerable importance.

Formaldehyde

It is an irritant, water-soluble gas. It is highly lethal to bacteria and their spores, fungi and viruses. However, **it is not active against prions**. It is cheap and can be used for *sterilization of rooms, furniture* and a wide variety of articles liable to be damaged by heat, such as *clothing, woollen blankets, mattresses, respirators, heat-sensitive instruments*, etc.

Glutaraldehyde

It is more effective and less irritant than formaldehyde. It possesses high microbicidal activity against bacteria and their spores, mycelial and spore forms of fungi, and various types of viruses, including human immunodeficiency viruses and enteroviruses. Two per cent alkaline buffered solution is used for sterilization of heat-sensitive instruments like *cystoscopes, bronchoscopes, thermometers*, etc. *Glutaraldehyde is toxic and irritant to skin and mucous membranes, therefore, contact with it must be avoided. It must be used in a fume hood or in well ventilated area.*

5. ALCOHOLS

Several alcohols possess antimicrobial activity. The antimicrobial activity of alcohols can be attributed to their ability to denature proteins. Alcohol solutions containing 60–70% alcohol are most effective, and higher concentrations are less potent because proteins are not denatured easily in the absence of water. They are active against vegetative bacteria including tubercle bacilli, fungi and lipid-containing viruses but not against spores. Any solution of an alcohol that is used as an antiseptic or disinfectant should be filtered through a 0.22 μm filter to remove any spores that may be present.

- **Isopropyl alcohol** is preferred over ethyl alcohol as it is a better fat solvent, more bactericidal and less volatile. It is commonly used for *disinfection of clinical thermometers*.
- **Methyl alcohol** is effective against fungal spores.
- **Alcohol based hand rubs** are recommended for the decontamination of highly soiled hands in situations where proper hand washing is inconvenient or not possible. However, it must be remembered that alcohol is ineffective against spores and may not kill all types of non lipid viruses.

Alcohols are volatile and flammable and must not be used near open flames. Working solutions should be stored in proper containers to avoid evaporation of alcohol.

6. DYES

Two groups of dyes, the aniline dyes and the acridine dyes have been used extensively as skin and wound antiseptics. They are much more active against Gram-positive than Gram-negative bacteria.

7. VAPOUR-PHASE DISINFECTANTS

Two most important vapour-phase agents are ethylene oxide and formaldehyde.

Ethylene oxide

It is a colourless gas soluble in water. It is highly lethal to all kinds of microbes including spores and tubercle bacilli. It is useful for sterilization of articles liable to be damaged by heat, e.g., *plastic and rubber articles, blankets, pharmaceutical products (crude drugs and powders) and complex apparatus such as heart-lung machines.*

Formaldehyde gas

It is liberated by spraying or heating of formalin, by addition of formalin to potassium permanganate or by volatilization of paraformaldehyde. Its antimicrobial activity depends upon several factors. The atmosphere must have a high relative humidity (more than 60% and preferably 80 to 90%) and a temperature of at least 18°C. It is used for fumigation of operation theatres, wards and laboratories.

Hydrogen peroxide fogging

This is a better method replacing fumigation. It is done by fogging machine using hydrogen peroxide as disinfectant. It has the advantage of short cycle time and is non-toxic.

8. SURFACE ACTIVE DISINFECTANTS

Substances that alter the energy relationships at interfaces leading to reduction of surface or interfacial tension, are known as **surface active agents** or **surfactants**. They possess both hydrophobic (water-repelling) and hydrophilic (water-attracting) groups. On the basis of charge or the absence of ionization of the hydrophilic group, these surfactants are classified into anionic, cationic, non-ionic and amphoteric

compounds. Non-toxic surfactants do not have antimicrobial activity.

Cationic compounds such as quarternary ammonium compounds are the most important surfactants. **These act on phosphate groups of cell membrane phospholipids and also enter the cell.**

Anionic surfactants such as common soaps usually have strong detergent but weak antimicrobial properties.

Amphoteric agents such as tego compounds possess detergent properties of anionic and antimicrobial activity of cationic compounds.

Table 5.5 gives a list and the recommended concentrations of disinfectants commonly used in the hospitals.

Table 5.5. List and the recommended concentrations of disinfectants commonly used in the hospitals

Disinfectant	Recommended concentration
Ethanol	70%
Methylated spirit	70%
Glutaraldehyde	2% activated (available commercially as cidex)
Bleaching powder (calcium hypochlorite)	14 g/litre of water
Sodium hypochlorite	1%, 0.1%
Hydrogen peroxide	3%
Lysol	2.5%
Savlon®	2.0%, 5.0%
Dettol®	4.0%
Betadine	2.0%

Testing of disinfectants

The tests most commonly used for testing of disinfectants are as follows:

1. Minimum inhibitory concentration (MIC)

This test measures the lowest concentration of the disinfectant that inhibits the growth of *Salmonella* Typhi in a nutrient medium.

2. Phenol coefficient test

In this test similar quantities of organisms are added to rising dilutions of phenol and of the disinfectant to be tested. In the U.K. the organisms used are *S.* Typhi and in the U.S.A., *S.* Typhi, *Staphylococcus aureus* and *P. aeruginosa* are used. For testing, two methods, i.e., **Rideal-Walker** and **Chick-Martin** can be used. In the latter, but not the former, a source of organic matter (e.g., 2% killed yeast suspension or 20% inactivated horse serum or 3% dried human faeces) is used to simulate natural situations. The dilution of the disinfectant in question which kills the organisms in a given time is divided by the dilution of phenol which kills the organisms at the same time. This gives the phenol coefficient. A phenol coefficient of 1.0 means that the disinfectant in question has the same effectiveness as phenol and a coefficient of less than 1.0 means it is less effective and more than 1.0 means it is more effective.

3. Capacity test (Kelsey and Sykes test)

Capacity test is designed to simulate the natural conditions under which the disinfectants are used in hospitals. The main feature of the test is that instead of one addition of a large inoculum of the test organism, the additions are made in increments with or without organic matter. This gives a measure of the capacity of the disinfectant to cope with successive bacterial invasions. Test organisms (*S. aureus*, *Escherichia coli*, *P. aeruginosa* and *Proteus vulgaris*) in both clean (test bacteria in broth) and dirty (bacteria in 20% inactivated horse serum or 2% yeast suspension) conditions are added to the disinfectant in 3 successive lots at 0, 10 and 20 minutes. Each addition is in contact with the disinfectant for 8 minutes, therefore, samples are transferred at 8, 18 and 28 minutes respectively to a recovery medium. The disinfectant is judged on its overall performance, i.e., its ability to kill bacteria as judged by recovery on subculture and not by comparison with phenol.

DISPOSAL OF BIOMEDICAL WASTE

Biomedical waste (BMW)

It is a broader term applied to waste generated in the diagnosis, treatment or immunization of human beings or animals, in research or in the production or testing of biological products. It also includes waste coming out of medical treatment given at home.

Infectious waste

Medical waste which has the potential to transmit viral, bacterial or parasitic diseases. It includes both human and animal infectious waste and waste generated in laboratories, and veterinary practice. Infectious waste is hazardous in nature.

Hazardous waste

Waste which has a potential to pose a threat to human health and life. The persons most at risk are the staff of hospitals particularly nurses and waste handlers. In countries such as India, scavengers and ragpickers are at serious risk.

Waste segregation

The biomedical waste shall be segregated into containers or bags at the point of generation, since 80% of the waste is non-hazardous and can be disposed of easily into the municipal bin. It is important that hazardous waste component is separated from non-hazardous waste. Mixing of waste will render the entire waste potentially hazardous. Waste should be segregated in bags of different colours to facilitate appropriate treatment and disposal. Table 5.6 shows biomedical waste categories and their segregation, collection, treatment, processing and disposal options.

Table 5.6. Biomedical waste categories and their segregation, collection, treatment, processing and disposal options

Category	Type of waste	Type of bag or container to be used	Treatment and disposal options
Yellow	(a) **Human anatomical waste:** Human tissues, organs, body parts and foetus below the viability period (as per the Medical Termination of Pregnancy Act 1971, amended from time to time).	Yellow-coloured non-chlorinated plastic bags	Incineration or plasma pyrolysis or deep burial*.
	(b) **Animal anatomical waste:** Experimental animal carcasses, body parts, organs, tissues, including the waste generated from animals used in experiments or testing in veterinary hospitals or colleges or animal houses.		
	(c) **Soiled waste:** Items contaminated with blood, body fluids like dressings, plaster casts, cotton swabs and bags containing residual or discarded blood and blood components.		Incineration or plasma pyrolysis or deep burial*. In absence of above facilities, autoclaving or microwaving/hydroclaving followed by shredding or mutilation or combination of sterilization and shredding. Treated waste to be sent for energy recovery.
	(d) **Expired or discarded medicines:** Pharmaceutical waste like antibiotics, cytotoxic drugs including all items contaminated with cytotoxic drugs along with glass or plastic ampoules, vials, etc.	Yellow-coloured non-chlorinated plastic bags or containers	Expired cytotoxic drugs and items contaminated with cytotoxic drugs to be returned to the manufacturer or supplier for incineration at temperature > 1200°C or to common biomedical waste treatment facility or hazardous waste treatment, storage and disposal facility for incineration at > 1200°C or encapsulation or plasma pyrolysis at > 1200°C. All other discarded medicines shall be either sent back to manufacturer or disposed by incineration.

(Contd.)

Category	Type of waste	Type of bag or container to be used	Treatment and disposal options
	(e) **Chemical waste:** Chemicals used in production of biologicals and used or discarded disinfectants.	Yellow-coloured containers or non-chlorinated plastic bags	Disposed of by incineration or plasma pyrolysis or encapsulation in hazardous waste treatment, storage and disposal facility.
	(f) **Chemical liquid waste:** Liquid waste generated due to use of chemicals in production of biologicals and used or discarded disinfectants, silver X-ray film developing liquid, discarded formalin, infected secretions, aspirated body fluids, liquid from laboratories and floor washings, cleaning, housekeeping and disinfecting activities, etc.	Separate collection system leading to effluent treatment system	After resource recovery, the chemical liquid waste shall be pre-treated before mixing with other waste water.
	(g) Discarded linen, mattresses, beddings contaminated with blood or body fluid.	Non-chlorinated yellow plastic bags or suitable packing material	Non-chlorinated chemical disinfection followed by incineration or plasma pyrolysis or for energy recovery. In absence of above facilities, shredding or mutilation or combination of sterilization and shredding. Treated waste to be sent for energy recovery or incineration or plasma pyrolysis.
	(h) **Microbiology, biotechnology and other clinical laboratory waste:** Blood bags, laboratory cultures, stocks or specimens of microorganisms, live or attenuated vaccines, human and animal cell cultures used in research, industrial laboratories, production of biologicals, residual toxins, dishes and devices used for cultures.	Autoclave safe plastic bags or containers	Pre-treat to sterilize with non-chlorinated chemicals on-site as per National AIDS Control Organisation or World Health Organisation guidelines thereafter for incineration.
Red	**Contaminated waste (Recyclable):** Wastes generated from disposable items such as tubings, bottles, intra-venous tubes and sets, catheters, urine bags, syringes (without needles and fixed needle syringes) and vaccutainers with their needles cut) and gloves.	Red coloured non-chlorinated plastic bags or containers	Autoclaving or microwaving/hydroclaving followed by shredding or mutilation or combination of sterilization and shredding. Treated waste to be sent to registered or authorized recyclers or for energy recovery or plastics to diesel or fuel oil or for road making, whichever is possible. Plastic waste should not be sent to landfill sites.
White (Trans-lucent)	**Waste sharps including metals:** Needles, syringes with fixed needles, needles from needle tip cutter or burner, scalpels, blades, or any other contaminated sharp object that may cause puncture and cuts. This includes both used, discarded and contaminated metal sharps.	Puncture-proof, leak-proof, tamper-proof containers	Autoclaving or dry heat sterilization followed by shredding or mutilation or encapsulation in metal container or cement concrete; combination of shredding-cum-autoclaving; and sent for final disposal to iron foundries (having consent to operate from the State Pollution Control Boards or Pollution Control Committees) or sanitary landfill or designated concrete waste sharp pit.
Blue	(a) **Glassware:** Broken or discarded and contaminated glass including medicine vials and ampoules except those contaminated with cytotoxic wastes.	Cardboard boxes with blue-coloured marking	Disinfection (by soaking the washed glass waste after cleaning with detergent and sodium hypochlorite treatment) or through autoclaving or microwaving or hydroclaving and then sent for recycling.
	(b) **Metallic body implants.**	Cardboard boxes with blue-coloured marking	

* Disposal by deep burial is permitted only in rural or remote areas where there is no access to common biomedical waste treatment facility. This will be carried out with prior approval from the prescribed authority and as per the standards specified in Schedule-III. The deep burial facility shall be located as per the provisions and guidelines issued by Central Pollution Control Board from time to time.

Bacterial Genetics

6

Genetics is the study of genes, their structure and function, heredity and variation. Like other organisms, bacteria too obey the laws of genetics and breed true. However, a small proportion of their progeny exhibits variations in some properties. The genetic information in bacteria, as in other cells, is contained in the specific sequence of nucleotides in the cell's deoxyribonucleic acid (DNA). The DNA acts as a template for its own replication, so that at the time of cell division two copies are available. It also acts as a template (Fig. 6.1) for transcription of messenger RNA (mRNA) which is then translated, by ribosomes into particular polypeptide (DNA → RNA → polypeptide). This is the **central dogma of molecular biology**.

STRUCTURE OF DNA

DNA molecule is composed of two chains of nucleotides wound together in the form of double helix (Fig. 6.2). Each chain has a backbone of alternatively arranged molecules of deoxyribose sugar and phosphates. To each deoxyribose sugar is attached one of the four nitrogenous bases, i.e., pyrimidines (thymine and cytosine) and purines (guanine and adenine). Hydrogen (H) bond unites two nitrogenous bases of opposite strands, thus making it double-stranded. Adenine always binds to thymine and guanine to cytosine. Therefore, adenine is complementary to thymine and guanine to cytosine.

STRUCTURE OF RNA

Structure of RNA is similar to that of DNA with two differences:
1. It has sugar ribose instead of deoxyribose.
2. It has nitrogenous base uracil in place of thymine in DNA.

On the basis of structure and function RNA is of three types:

1. **Ribosomal RNA (rRNA):** This is RNA of ribosomes. It plays a basic role in the synthesis of proteins.

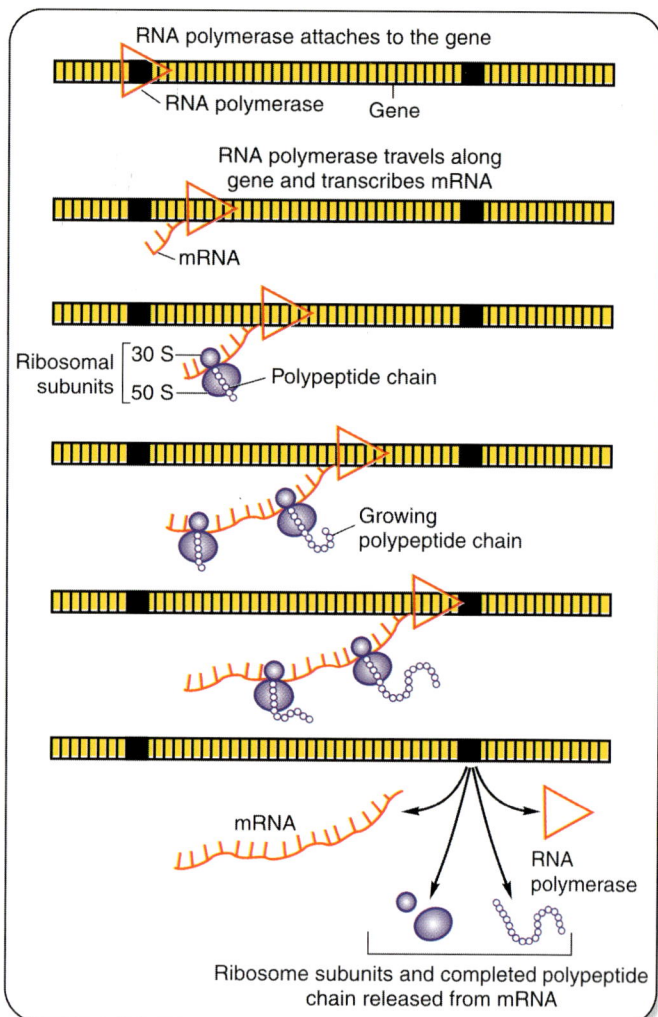

Fig. 6.1. Synthesis of polypeptide.

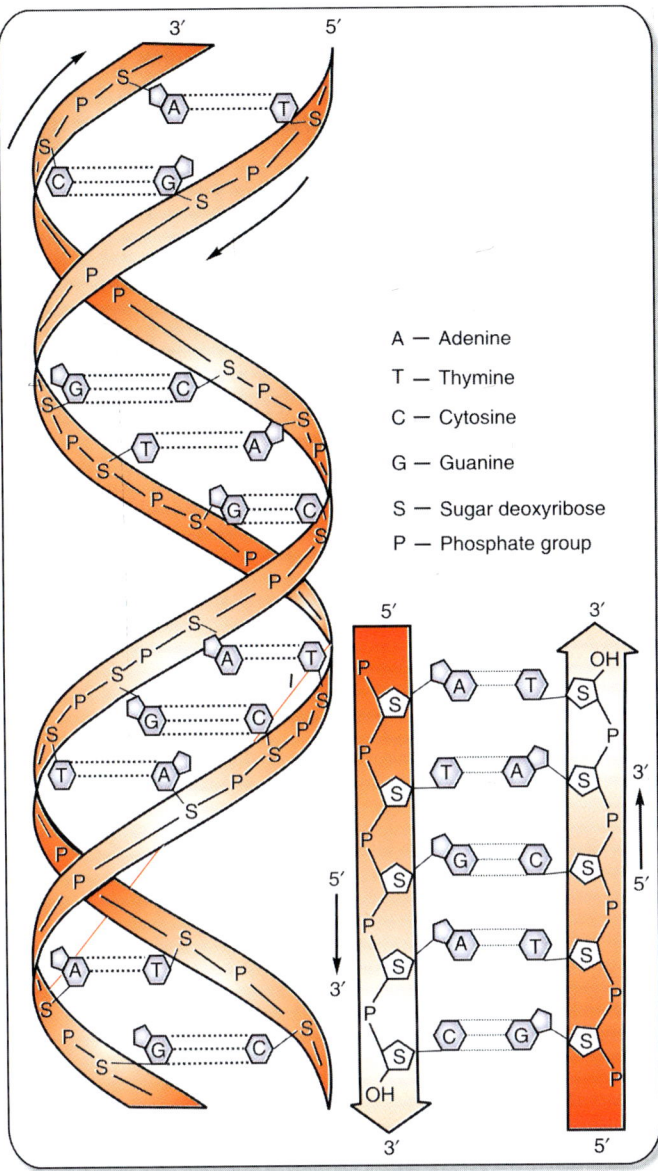

A — Adenine
T — Thymine
C — Cytosine
G — Guanine
S — Sugar deoxyribose
P — Phosphate group

Fig. 6.2. Watson and Crick model of DNA.

2. **Transfer RNA (tRNA):** This RNA has a specific terminal nucleotide sequence that enables it to accept a single molecule of an activated amino acid and transfer it to a ribosome.
3. **Messenger RNA (mRNA):** This RNA is formed by an enzyme RNA polymerase under the direct influence of DNA.

Codon

Genetic information is stored in DNA as a code. The unit of code is known as codon. It consists of a sequence of three bases.

A segment of DNA carrying a number of codons specifying for a particular polypeptide is known as **cistron** or **gene**. A large number of genes constitute a **locus** and a large number of loci constitute cell **genome**.

EXTRACHROMOSOMAL GENETIC ELEMENTS

Plasmid

In addition to chromosomal DNA, bacteria may also possess extrachromosomal genetic material known as plasmid. It may be defined as a small extrachromosomal piece of genetic material that can replicate autonomously and can maintain in the cytoplasm of a bacterium for many generations. It consists of a circular piece of double-stranded DNA. It may confer on the bacterium additional properties such as drug resistance, bacteriocin production, toxigenicity, etc.

GENOTYPIC AND PHENOTYPIC VARIATIONS

The characteristics expressed by a cell in a given environment are referred to as its **phenotype** (*pheno:* display) and the collection of genes encoding these characteristics, the **genotype**. Bacteria, in general, are very adaptable and may alter their phenotype in response to environmental change while the genotype remains unchanged. Not all the genes of the bacterial cell are expressed all the time. For example, typhoid bacillus is normally flagellated but when grown on phenol agar, the flagella are not synthesized, but when subcultured from phenol agar into nutrient broth flagellated cells appear.

Another example of environmental influence is the synthesis of an enzyme β-galactosidase, necessary for lactose fermentation to its constituent sugars – glucose and galactose, in *Escherichia coli*. This organism possesses genetic information for synthesis of the enzyme, but it is produced by the bacteria only when lactose is present in the growth medium. This enzyme is not synthesized if *E. coli* is grown in medium containing glucose only. Such enzymes, which are synthesized only when induced by substrate, are called **induced enzymes**, while those enzymes, which are synthesized both in the presence or absence of the substrate, are known as **constitutive enzymes**. Regulation of enzyme induction illustrates the economy of nature, the enzyme being produced only when appropriate substrates are present.

MUTATION

It is a random, undirected, heritable variation caused by an alteration in the nucleotide sequence at some point of the DNA of the cell, which may be due to addition, deletion or substitution of one or more bases. Mutations occur spontaneously at fairly constant rates, usually in the range of one per 10^2–10^{10} cell divisions.

ACQUISITION OF NEW GENES

Change in the genome of a bacterium may be due to mutation in the organism's own DNA or to acquisition of DNA from an external source. Transmission of genetic material may take place by:

1. Transformation
2. Transduction
3. Lysogenic conversion
4. Conjugation

1. Transformation

Acquisition of DNA by a bacterium from its environment and incorporation in its genome is known as transformation. It is perhaps the most important mechanism of genetic exchange for certain bacterial species, notably *Streptococcus pneumoniae*, *S. sanguis*, *Bacillus subtilis*, *Haemophilus influenzae* and *Neisseria gonorrhoeae*. For transformation to occur DNA must have been derived from a closely related strain, since a piece of DNA can undergo recombination with chromosome only when there is adequate nucleic acid homology. Transformation was first demonstrated by Griffith in 1928. *S. pneumoniae* in capsulated form is an extremely virulent organism for mice, whereas non-capsulated variants are avirulent. The virulence of the organism is due to polysaccharide capsule.

Mutant pneumococci that have lost their ability to synthesize this capsule arise spontaneously. These show rough (R) colonies on blood agar as compared to smooth (S) colonies of capsulated form of pneumococcus. Griffith mixed live non-capsulated cells that had originally produced a capsule of one antigenic type with heat-killed smooth cells of a different capsular type. Neither preparation alone caused disease in mice, but mixture of the two preparations was lethal and Griffith was able to isolate from blood of the mice live pneumococci having a capsule of the same antigenic type as that of heat-killed cells. It was later shown that **DNA was the transforming principle** that was released from the heat-killed bacteria and was able to confer upon a live recipient cell the ability to produce a new type of capsule. The DNA that was taken up by the rough cells supplied the genetic information needed to make the missing enzyme needed for capsule synthesis.

2. Transduction

Transfer of a portion of DNA from one bacterium to another by bacteriophages (phages) is known as transduction. It may be generalized when it involves any segment of donor DNA or it may be restricted when a specific bacteriophage transduces only a particular portion of DNA.

Generalized transduction

Phages are viruses that multiply in bacteria. They carry their genetic information inside a protein coat. During assembly each phage head is normally filled with a phage genome, but sometimes an occasional phage particle is formed at a frequency of 1 in 10^6 whose head has been accidentally filled with a similar length of host cell DNA. This is known as 'packing error'. When such a particle attaches to a second cell the DNA that enters the cell is not phage DNA capable of replicating and lysing the cell but a short segment of chromosome from first host, thus bacterial genes have been transduced by the phage into a second cell.

Since these phages pick up any portion of the host chromosome, they can transduce any gene. Each transducing phage can pick up a piece of bacterial DNA about the same size as its normal phage genome. Genes can be transduced only between fairly closely related strains because bacteriophage attacks a limited range of organisms with the same surface receptors. Transduction is not confined to transfer of chromosomal DNA. Plasmids may also be transduced. **The plasmid determining penicillin resistance in staphylococci is transferred from cell to cell by transduction.**

Restricted transduction

Bacteriophages that lyse the host cell are known as **virulent phages**, however, **temperate phage** may get incorporated into the host genome and divide with it. These cells are known as **lysogenic**. Molecular basis of lysogeny has been extensively studied in λ phage of *E. coli*. When infected with this phage majority of the cells go into lytic cycle while in a small proportion of them, they get incorporated into host cell genome (**lysogeny**). In some lysogenic cells lytic cycle is resumed. The **prophage** (integrated phage DNA) is excised and codes for viral proteins and DNA. In a small proportion of cells prophage is excised inaccurately so that a neighbouring portion of bacterial DNA is also removed.

Since phage head can contain only a standard amount of DNA, a transducing phage contains a few bacterial genes at one end of its DNA and lacks a few phage genes at the other end, i.e., **phage genome is defective**. When such a piece of DNA is transduced into a second cell the defective phage can still integrate into its normal site on the chromosome. The added bacterial genes are reproduced in the progeny of the recipient bacterium. Since the temperate phage has a specific insertion site it can pickup and transduce only a short length of DNA containing a few genes on either side of this site. This is known as restricted transduction. λ phage is always inserted between the genes for galactose utilization (*gal*) and biotin synthesis (*bio*) and thus can transduce either *gal* or *bio* genes.

3. Lysogenic conversion

In the lysogenic bacteria the prophage behaves as an additional segment of the bacterial chromosome, coding for new characters. This process by which prophage DNA confers additional genetic information to the host cell is known as **lysogenic or phage conversion**. An important example of lysogenic conversion is of *Corynebacterium diphtheriae* by β-phage. Only those organisms which are lysogenic produce diphtheria toxin because ***tox* gene** coding for the production of **diphtheria toxin** is present on the phage DNA. The cells that lose the phage, lose toxin production. Another example of lysogenic conversion is the production of **dick toxin** by *Streptococcus pyogenes*.

4. Conjugation

It is the transfer of DNA that occurs during contact between bacterial cells. This mechanism is much more efficient than transformation or transduction. Transfer of DNA by conjugation is very common among Gram-negative bacteria, but it is rare in Gram-positive bacteria. **It is a major mechanism of transfer of drug resistance and can occur among unrelated genera.**

Conjugation was first described by Lederberg and Tatum in 1946 in *E. coli* K12 strain and has been most extensively studied in this strain. The donor status of a bacterial cell is determined by the presence of a plasmid which codes for **sex pilus**. It is 1–2 μm in length. The tip of the pilus attaches to the surface of a recipient cell and holds the two cells together. The two strands of plasmid separate. One strand enters the recipient bacterium, probably along the sex pilus, while one strand remains in the donor. Each strand then makes a complementary copy (Fig. 6.3).

Fertility (F) factor or F plasmid

F factor or F plasmid is a transfer factor that contains the genetic information necessary for the synthesis of the sex pilus and for self transfer but it does not possess other identifiable genetic markers such as drug resistance. Cells that possess one or more copies of the F plasmid are called **F⁺** and the cells lacking the F plasmid are called **F⁻**. F⁺ cells have no distinguishing features other than their ability to mate with F⁻ cells and render them F⁺.

Certain *E. coli* strains contain an F plasmid that has become permanently integrated into the cell's chromosome. Such cells are able to transfer chromosomal genes to recipient cell with high frequency and are known as **Hfr (high frequency recombinant) cells**. F plasmid may revert from Hfr state to free state. Sometimes it may carry with it some chromosomal genes from near the site of its attachment leaving a part of its own DNA from other end in the donor chromosome (Fig. 6.4). Such F factor possessing chromosomal genes is known as **F′ (F prime) factor**. When an F′ cell mates with a recipient cell, it transfers, along with the F factor, the host genes incorporated with it. This process of transfer of host genes through F factor resembles transduction and is known as **sexduction**.

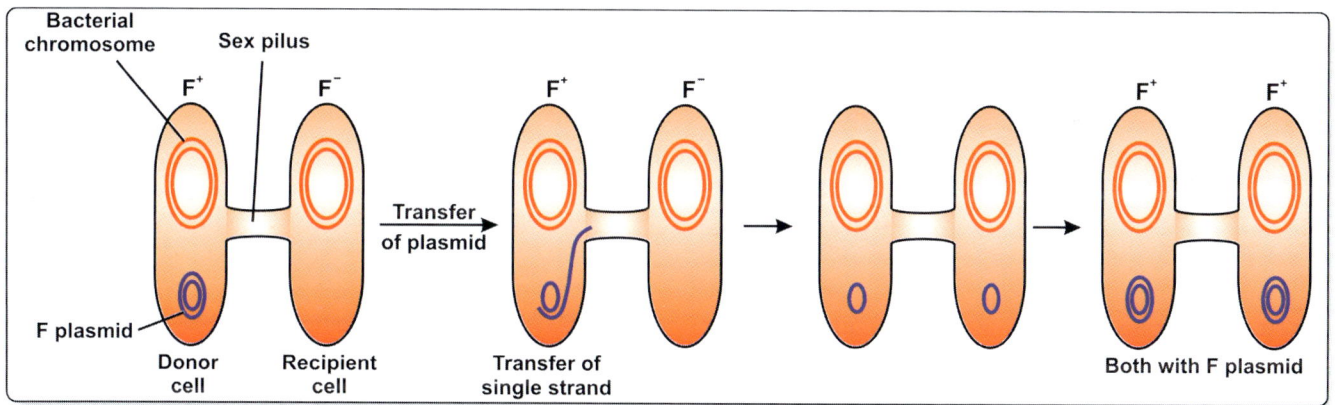

Fig. 6.3. Process of conjugation.

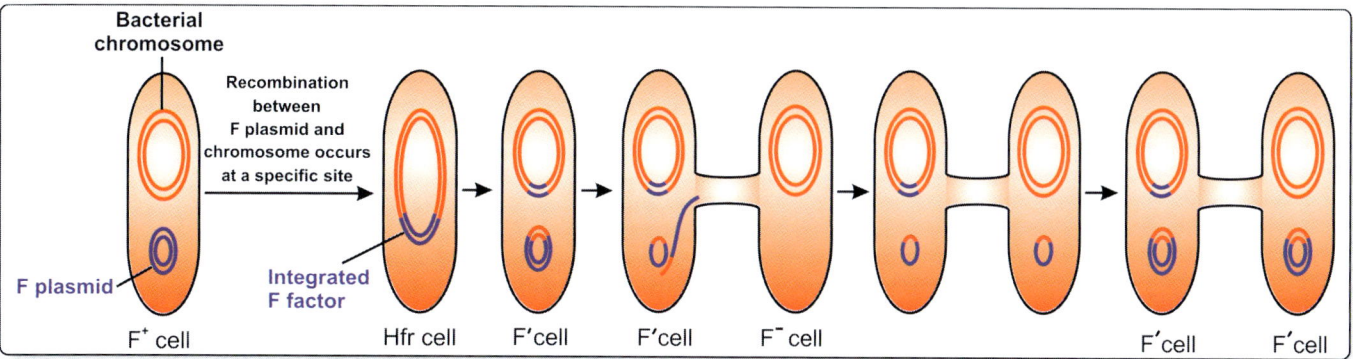

Fig. 6.4. Process of sexduction.

Resistance plasmid or R plasmid or R factor

It consists of two parts – resistance transfer factor and resistance determinants (RTF + r). RTF is responsible for conjugal transfer and r determinants code for resistance against various drugs. As many as eight or more r determinants may be carried on each plasmid. Therefore, resistance to eight or more drugs may be transferred simultaneously.

Colicinogenic (col) factor

Several strains of coliform bacteria produce colicins. These are antibiotic-like substances that are specifically and selectively lethal to other enterobacteria. Since similar substances are also produced by other than coliforms, e.g., pyocin by *Pseudomonas aeruginosa*, klebocin by *Klebsiella pneumoniae* and diphthericin by *Corynebacterium diphtheriae*, therefore, the name bacteriocin has been given to this group of substances. The specificity of action of bacteriocins enables intraspecies classification of certain bacteria, e.g., colicin typing (*Shigella sonnei*), klebocin typing (*Klebsiella* spp.), proticin typing (*Proteus* spp.), and pyocin typing (*Pseudomonas* spp.).

Colicin and klebocin production is known to be mediated by col and klebocin plasmids, respectively.

Transposon

In 1974, the discovery of a new type of transposable element that encoded a recognizable gene product (β-lactam antibiotic resistance) was reported. It was termed a **transposon (tn)**. Since then many others carrying a variety of resistance and other genes have been identified. Because of the ability of transposable elements to move from one plasmid to another or to a phage or to the bacterial chromosome they have assumed the popular name of **jumping genes**. **Unlike plasmids, transposons do not contain genetic information necessary for their own replication**, and their replication, therefore, depends on their physical integration with a bacterial replicon.

DNA probes

DNA probes are radiolabelled or chromogenically labelled pieces of single-stranded DNA which can be used for the detection of homologous DNA by hybridization.

Development of DNA probe

All microorganisms, simple or complex, contain some unique sequences of nucleic acid within their genome that distinguish them from all other organisms. The method of developing a DNA probe is to cut or isolate those sequences from the nucleic acid of the cell using a set of enzymes known as restriction endonucleases, reproduce them in large quantities and attach a reporter molecule to them so that they can be incorporated into a hybridization reaction. **Hybridization** is the process whereby two single strands of nucleic acid come together to form a stable double-stranded molecule. However, they will bind and stay together only if the sequences of bases along each stretch of nucleic acid are complementary (adenine opposite thymine and cytosine opposite guanine).

Hybridizations are accomplished in tubes or by spotting the unknown organisms on a filter paper such as nitrocellulose paper, lysing them to release the DNA, and denaturing in mild alkali to single strands. The probe can then be added and after thorough washing to remove any unbound probe, the tube or probe is examined for evidence of hybridization. Formalin-fixed, paraffin-embedded tissues can also be probed particularly for viral DNA sequences. DNA probes can also be designed that bind to RNA and this procedure has been used particularly to locate ribosomal RNA.

Applications of DNA probes

- In the diagnostic laboratory, DNA probes are being used for culture confirmation as an alternative to conventional, time-consuming or labour-intensive methods.
- Probe technology may also be used for detection of fastidious organisms directly in clinical specimens. Examples are *Neisseria gonorrhoeae* and *Chlamydia trachomatis*.

Polymerase chain reaction (PCR)

Kary Mulis invented this method in 1989. He was awarded Nobel Prize in 1993. Polymerase chain reaction is a primer-mediated, temperature-dependent technique for the enzymatic amplification of a specific sequence (target sequence) to such an extent that it can be detected. The technique can be used to detect very small amounts of specific nucleic acid material in clinical specimens where bacterial, viral or fungal agents are thought to play a causative role. The fundamental basis of this technology is that each pathogenic organism possesses a unique 'signature sequence' in its DNA or RNA composition by which it can be identified. It is based on repeated cycles of high temperature template denaturation, oligonucleotide primer annealing, and polymerase mediated extension (Fig. 6.5).

To multiply a strip of genetic material, four ingredients are placed together in a small vial:

1. Target DNA.
2. Short strands of DNA called primers which tag the section to be copied.
3. Polymerase – an enzyme that promotes gene replication in all living cells.
4. Nucleotides – the building blocks for making DNA.

PCR is carried out in three steps:

1. Heat at 94°C is applied to the target DNA, breaking the bonds that hold the strands together. This is known as **denaturation**.
2. The temperature is then reduced to 55°C, promoting the primers to attach themselves to either end of the target strip. This is known as **annealing of primers**.

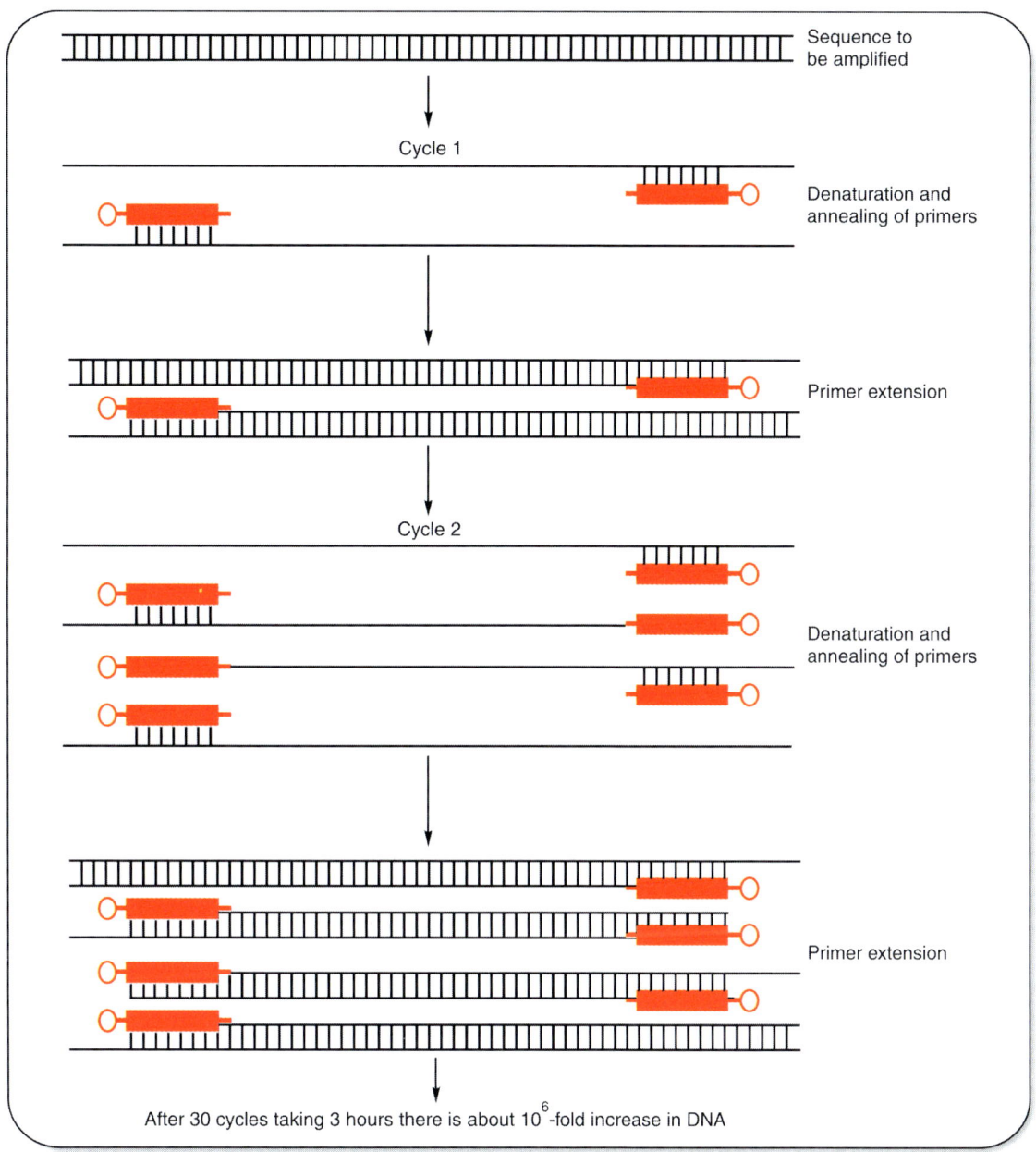

Fig. 6.5. Polymerase chain reaction.

3. Then polymerase enzyme triggers the formation of new DNA strand from the nucleotides. Extension of the primers is done by a thermostable *Taq* polymerase (purified from *Thermus aquaticus*, a thermophilic bacterium that lives in hot springs at temperatures of 70–75°C). This is known as **primer extension**. When the temperature is again raised, the new strands separate and the process begins again.

These three steps are repeated again and again by manipulating the temperature, a process that is automated by the PCR machine (Table 6.1). A cycle takes about 3–5 minutes and after 30 cycles, taking about 3 hours, a single copy of DNA can be increased up to 1,000,000 copies, a sharp contrast

Table 6.1. Programming of cycles in polymerase chain reaction

Step	Temperature	Time	Cycle
Initial denaturation	94°C	5 minutes	First cycle
Denaturation	94°C	30 seconds	
Annealing of primers	55°C	1 minute	30 cycles
Primer extension	72°C	1 minute	
Final primer extension	72°C	7 minutes	Last cycle

to the days required by conventional amplification method (culture).

Amplified sequences of target DNA can be detected by a variety of methods. If enough amplified DNA is present, it can be visualized by:

1. Gel electrophoresis and ethidium bromide staining.
2. Southern blot and dot-blot analysis with either radioactive or nonradioactive probes.
3. Oligomer restriction.
4. Oligomer hybridization.
5. Reverse dot-blot.

Applications of PCR

The development of PCR or gene amplification method is a major methodological breakthrough in molecular biology. Within a short span, this method has found its way into nearly every type of laboratory from forensic to ecology and from diagnosis to pure research. Applications of PCR in clinical laboratory are given in Table 6.2.

• **In diagnosis of inherited disorders:** The PCR technology is being widely used to amplify gene segments that contain known mutations for diagnosis of inherited diseases such

Table 6.2. Applications of PCR in clinical laboratory

Diagnosis of infections due to:

A. *Viruses:* HIV-1, HIV-2, HTLV-1, cytomegalovirus, human papillomavirus, herpes simplex viruses, hepatitis B virus, HCV, HDV, HEV, rubella virus, Epstein-Barr virus, varicella-zoster virus, human herpesvirus 6 and 7, parvovirus B19, enteroviruses, coxsackieviruses, echoviruses, rhinoviruses, measles virus, rotavirus, adenovirus, respiratory syncytial virus

B. *Bacteria:* Mycobacterium tuberculosis, Mycobacterium avium complex, *Legionella pneumophila, Chlamydia trachomatis, Mycoplasma pneumoniae, Helicobacter pylori, Burkholderia pseudomallei, Campylobacter* spp., *Corynebacterium diphtheriae, Leptospira interrogans, Streptococcus pyogenes, Streptococcus pneumoniae, Yersinia enterocolitica*

C. *Fungi: Candida* spp., *Cryptococcus neoformans, Aspergillus* spp., *Pneumocystis jirovecii*

D. *Protozoa: Toxoplasma gondii, Trypanosoma cruzi, Entero-cytozoon bieneusi, Encephalitozoon hellem, Plasmodium* spp.

as sickle cell anaemia, β-thalassaemia, cystic fibrosis, etc. PCR is especially useful for prenatal diagnosis of inherited diseases, where cells obtained from the foetus by amniocentesis are very few.

• **In cancer detection:** Identification of mutations in oncosuppressor genes such as retinoblastoma gene can help to identify individuals at high risk of cancer.

• **In medicolegal cases:** PCR allows DNA in a single cell, hair follicle or sperm to be amplified enormously and analyzed. The pattern obtained is then compared with that of various suspects.

Other types of PCR

Other types of PCR include reverse transcriptase PCR (RT-PCR), nested PCR, multiplex PCR and real time PCR.

RT-PCR

In this technique target is RNA instead of DNA. Complementary DNA (cDNA) is first produced from RNA with the help of enzyme reverse transcriptase and then cDNA is amplified by PCR.

Nested PCR

This increases the sensitivity and specificity of PCR by using two pairs of amplification primers. One pair of primers is used in the first round of PCR to amplify the desired sequence. The amplified product of the first round is then subjected to second round of PCR with the second set of primers which anneal to the sequences of the first round products.

Multiplex PCR

In this technique two or more primer sets are used for amplification of different targets. It helps in amplification of more than one target sequence in a clinical specimen.

Real time PCR

In this technique amplified products are detected as they accumulate after each cycle, in contrast to standard PCR where these are detected at the end of procedure. Therefore, a positive result can be obtained, while the assay is still running. It uses a fluorescent reporter dye. Real time PCR instrument has the ability to measure the increase in reporter fluorescence as PCR products accumulate.

7

Bacteria in Health and Disease

Skin, alimentary tract and other mucous membranes are continually contaminated by microorganisms from the environment. Based on their relationship they can be divided into saprophytes and parasites.

Saprophytes

Saprophytes (*sapros* decayed, and *phyton* plant) are free-living microbes that live on dead or decaying organic matter. They are found in soil and water. They are, generally, incapable of multiplying on living tissues. However, sometimes when host resistance is lowered some saprophytes like *Bacillus subtilis* may cause infection.

Parasites

Parasites are the microorganisms that can enter and multiply in the host. They are of two types – **microparasites** which include viruses, bacteria, fungi and protozoa, and **macroparasites** which include helminths.

Pathogens

Pathogens (*pathos:* suffering, and *gen:* produce, i.e., disease-producing) are the microorganisms which are capable of producing disease in man and animals. They are of two types – opportunistic pathogens and primary pathogens.

Opportunistic pathogens

Opportunistic pathogens rarely cause disease in individuals with intact immunological and anatomical defences. In immunocompromised hosts these bacteria are able to cause disease. Coagulase-negative staphylococci are normally carried on the human skin where they cause no harm. However, introduction of these organisms into anatomical sites in which they are not normally found may lead to infection. Similarly, *Escherichia coli* is normally carried in human intestine. If they enter into urinary tract they lead to urinary tract infection.

Primary pathogens

Primary pathogens are the organisms which are capable of causing disease in previously healthy individuals with intact immunity.

Commensals

Commensals (organisms of normal flora) are the microorganisms which live in complete harmony with the host without causing any damage to it.

INFECTION

The lodgement and multiplication of a parasite in or on the tissue of a host is known as infection.

TYPES OF INFECTION

1. Primary infection

Initial infection with a parasite is known as primary infection.

2. Reinfection

Subsequent infection with the same parasite in the same host is known as reinfection.

3. Secondary infection

When the primary infection lowers the resistance of the host and the latter gets infection with another organism it is known as secondary infection.

4. Cross infection

When a patient already suffering from a disease acquires a new infection it is known as cross infection.

5. Nosocomial infection

When cross infection is acquired by the patient during his stay in the hospital it is known as hospital-acquired, healthcare-associated or nosocomial infection.

6. Iatrogenic infection

When the infection is acquired during therapeutic or investigative procedures, it is known as iatrogenic or physician-induced infection.

7. Subclinical infection

When the clinical symptoms of an infection are not apparent it is known as subclinical infection.

8. Latent infection

When a parasite, after infection, remains in a latent or hidden form for some time and it proliferates and produces clinical disease, when the host resistance is lowered, it is known as latent infection.

SOURCES OF INFECTION

Infections may be endogenous, due to the organisms of the normal flora, and exogenous, due to the organisms derived from a source outside the body.

Endogenous infections

These are also referred to as autoinfections. Organisms of normal flora are usually nonpathogenic but occasionally they may lead to infection. The most important autoinfections are:

1. **Viridans streptococci** are the normal flora of the mouth but when there is abnormality of the heart, like rheumatic heart disease and injury to the oral cavity like tooth extraction or fractured mandible, these organisms enter into the blood stream and settle down on the heart leading to infective endocarditis. In both the above examples, two conditions are fulfilled – the organism initiating infection does so in an area of the body remote from its normal habitat and infection develops only where there is some tissue abnormality lowering local tissue resistance.

2. *E. coli* **and** *Enterococcus faecalis*, which are the normal flora of the intestines, may cause urinary tract infection particularly when there is some abnormality of the urinary tract like congenital malformation, urinary calculi and ureteric and prostatic obstruction. These conditions lower the local tissue resistance.

Exogenous infections

Most of the infections are exogenous in origin. The sources of exogenous infections are as under:

1. Human cases and carriers.
2. Animal cases and carriers.
3. Insects.
4. Environment.

1. Human cases and carriers

The commonest source of human infection is man himself who may be a patient or a carrier. Infections due to some organisms are acquired mainly or exclusively from ill persons, e.g., AIDS, syphilis, gonorrhoea, pulmonary tuberculosis, leprosy, whooping cough, hepatitis B and C, measles, mumps, influenza, poliomyelitis, etc.

A **carrier** is a person who harbours the pathogenic microorganisms without suffering from it. There are several types of carriers:

- *Healthy carrier:* One who harbours the pathogen but has never suffered from the disease caused by it.
- *Convalescent carrier:* One who has recovered from the disease but continues to harbour the pathogen on his body.
- *Temporary carrier:* When carrier state lasts for less than six months.
- *Chronic carrier:* When carrier state lasts for years or may be for the life of the patient.
- *Paradoxical carrier:* Who acquires the organisms from another carrier.
- *Contact carrier:* Who acquires the organisms from a patient.

Carriers are very important source of infection. For example, a person acquires organisms from a patient of meningococcal meningitis and becomes a contact carrier. He is then a source of infection for other persons (patient → carrier → patient).

2. Animal cases and carriers

Certain pathogens are capable of causing infection in both man and animals. Therefore, animals may act as a source of infection of such organisms. The infection may be acquired by contact with the animal, animal bite and ingestion of milk or meat. Infection in animals may be asymptomatic and these animals may serve as reservoir for human infections. These are known as **reservoir hosts**. Infectious diseases transmitted from animals to man are known as **zoonoses**. For example:

- *Bacterial:* Bovine tuberculosis, bubonic plague, *Salmonella* food poisoning, anthrax.
- *Viral:* Rabies, yellow fever.
- *Protozoal:* Leishmaniasis.
- *Helminthic:* Hydatid disease.
- *Fungal: Microsporum canis, Trichophyton verrucosum.*

3. Insects

Blood-sucking insects such as mosquitoes, ticks, mites, flies, and lice act as a source of a number of human and animal infections. Insects transmitting pathogens are known as **vectors**.

4. Environment

This includes soil, water and food. A few infective diseases of man are caused by saprophytic microbes derived from soil and vegetation. Some pathogens can survive in the environment for very long periods. For example, spores of tetanus and gas gangrene bacilli remain viable in the soil for several decades and serve as a source of infection. The normal habitat of these organisms is the human and animal intestines and they enter the soil through their faeces.

Fungi causing mycetoma, sporotrichosis and histoplasmosis survive in soil and cause human infection. Eggs of parasites like roundworms and hookworms survive and develop in the soil and cause human infection. Water contaminated with *Shigella*, *Salmonella*, *Vibrio cholerae*, poliovirus, hepatitis A and E viruses and cyclops containing larvae of guinea worm acts as a source of these infections.

Contaminated food acts as a source of organisms causing food poisoning, gastroenteritis, diarrhoea and dysentery.

MODES OF SPREAD OF INFECTION

Pathogenic organisms can spread from one host to another by a variety of mechanisms. These include:

1. Inhalation

Respiratory infections such as common cold, influenza, measles, mumps, tuberculosis and whooping cough are acquired by inhalation. These organisms are shed into the environment by patients in secretions of nose or throat during sneezing, coughing, talking and other forceful expiratory activities.

2. Ingestion

Intestinal infections like enteric fever, cholera, dysentery, food poisoning, poliomyelitis, hepatitis A and E, and most of the parasitic infections are acquired by ingestion. The source of these infections is the faeces of the patients or carriers. The faeces containing pathogens may contaminate food or drinks.

3. Contact

Infection may be acquired by direct or indirect contact with the patient. Sexually transmitted diseases (STD) such as syphilis, gonorrhoea, lymphogranuloma venereum, lymphogranuloma inguinale, trichomoniasis, herpes simplex type 2, hepatitis B and C, and AIDS are acquired by direct contact. The term **contagious disease** is used for the disease acquired by direct contact, and disease acquired by other modes, through inanimate objects, as **infectious disease**.

4. Contamination of wounds

The infections may be caused by:

- Organisms present in the nose or throat of the patient himself or of nurses or doctors. Pathogenic staphylococci and streptococci derived from respiratory tract are important causes of wound and burn infection.
- Airborne spread of organisms from the infected wounds of other patients.
- Contact with infected hands, clothing or other articles.

- In some instances pathogens may be inoculated directly into the tissues of the host, for example, rabies virus which is present in the saliva of a rabid animal, usually dog, is inoculated directly into the host tissue.
- Spores of *Clostridium tetani* and *C. perfringens* are present in the soil. These get inoculated into the host tissue following severe wounds leading to tetanus and gas gangrene respectively.

5. Blood-sucking arthropods

In some diseases, blood-sucking insects play an important role in the spread of infection from one individual to another. Table 7.1 shows common arthropods and diseases transmitted by them.

Table 7.1. Common arthropods and diseases transmitted by them

Arthropod	Diseases transmitted
1. **Mosquitoes**	
• Anopheles	Malaria, filariasis
• *Culex*	Filariasis, Japanese encephalitis, West Nile fever
• *Aedes*	Yellow fever, dengue, chikungunya haemorrhagic fever, Rift Valley fever, filariasis
• *Mansonia*	Brugian filariasis
2. **Flies**	
• House fly	Typhoid and paratyphoid fever, diarrhoea, dysentery, cholera, gastroenteritis, amoebiasis
• Sand fly	Kala-azar, oriental sore, espundia, oroya fever
• Tsetse fly	African trypanosomiasis
3. Louse	Epidemic typhus, relapsing fever, trench fever
4. Rat flea	Bubonic plague, endemic typhus, *Hymenolepis diminuta* infestation
5. Black fly	Onchocerciasis
6. Reduviid bug	Chagas' disease
7. **Ticks**	
• Hard ticks	Spotted fever group, viral encephalitis, Colorado tick typhus, tularaemia, human babesiosis
• Soft ticks	Q fever, relapsing fever, Kyasanur Forest disease
8. **Mites**	
• Trombiculid mite	Scrub typhus
• Gamasid mite	Rickettsial pox
• Itch mite	Scabies
9. Body and head lice	Epidemic typhus, relapsing fever
10. Cyclops	Dracunculosis, diphyllobothriasis
11. Cockroaches	Same as in case of house fly

Insects normally become infected by biting a human or animal host in whose blood the causative organism is present. After this there is an interval, known as **extrinsic incubation period**, during which the insect is incapable of transmitting the infection. During this period the organisms multiply in the body of the insect. *Ticks which transmit certain rickettsial and arbovirus infections, and mites which transmit scrub typhus are unusual in that the infective agent can be transmitted from one generation of the insect to the next through the ovum.*

6. Iatrogenic and laboratory infections

If meticulous care in asepsis is not taken, infections like AIDS, and hepatitis B, C and D may sometimes be transmitted during therapeutic and investigative procedures such as injections, lumbar puncture, blood transfusion, dialysis, and heart and kidney transplant surgery. These are known as **iatrogenic or physician-induced infections**. Laboratory personnel handling infectious material and doing mouth-pipetting are particularly at risk.

7. Congenital

Some microorganisms like *Toxoplasma*, rubella virus, cytomegalovirus, herpes simplex virus, *Treponema pallidum*, human immunodeficiency virus, malaria parasites, etc. can cross the placental barrier and infect the foetus in utero. This is known as **vertical transmission**. This may result in abortion, miscarriage or stillbirth. Live babies may be born with manifestations of the disease.

FACTORS PREDISPOSING TO MICROBIAL PATHOGENICITY

Pathogenicity denotes the ability of a microbial species to cause disease, while the term **virulence** refers to the same property in a strain of the species.

DETERMINANTS OF VIRULENCE

1. Adhesion

Many bacteria possess on their surface colonization factors or adhesins. These usually occur on fimbriae. Through adhesins bacteria attach specifically on the receptors present on the host cells. They are, therefore, responsible for tissue tropism. Adhesion is necessary to avoid innate host defence mechanisms such as peristalsis in the gut and the flushing action of mucus, saliva and urine which remove nonadherent bacteria. Loss of adhesins may render a strain avirulent.

2. Invasion of tissues

Invasiveness signifies the ability of an organism to penetrate a tissue after it adheres to a cell surface. Some bacteria can invade tissues in the absence of physical injury, e.g., *N. meningitidis* in nasal epithelium and salmonellae in intestinal epithelium. These organisms are endocytosed by epithelial cells, transported across these cells within vacuoles and released into the submucosal space, from which they invade the underlying tissues. *Shigella* and enteroinvasive *E. coli* are also endocytosed by intestinal epithelial cells but do not penetrate the basement membrane.

3. Capsules

Cell wall in many bacteria is enclosed by a protective gelatinous covering layer known as capsule. It contributes to the virulence of the bacteria by inhibiting phagocytosis.

4. Streptococcal M protein

The M protein present on the surface of *S. pyogenes* binds both fibrinogen and fibrin to the bacterial cell wall, thus masking the bacterial receptors from complement.

5. Bacterial toxins

These are substances produced by or present in bacteria, which have a direct toxic action on tissue cells. Two major types of toxin have been described – endotoxins and exotoxins (Table 7.2).

Endotoxins

They are components of the outer membrane of Gram-negative bacteria. They are lipopolysaccharide (LPS) in nature and are released from the bacterial surface by natural lysis of the bacteria or by disintegration of the organisms *in vitro*. The endotoxic activity of LPS resides in its lipid A moiety. The latter is not destroyed by autoclaving, hence infusion of a sterile solution containing endotoxin can cause serious illness. They are poor antigens and the toxicity is not completely neutralized by the homologous antibodies. They cannot be toxoided. Endotoxins exert a wide spectrum of effects on the host, the most dramatic of which are fever and the shock syndrome associated with Gram-negative bacterial sepsis. Man is particularly sensitive to minute amounts of endotoxins and often a mild Gram-negative bacterial infection will cause fever. Larger amounts of endotoxin may cause irreversible shock seen in association with a fulminating Gram-negative bacteraemia.

Exotoxins

They are produced extracellularly by both Gram-positive and Gram-negative bacteria. They are highly potent even in small amounts and constitute some of the most poisonous substances known. **Botulinum toxin is the most poisonous followed by tetanus toxin.** Minimum lethal dose for botulinum toxin for a mouse is 0.03 ng and for humans may be 1 μg. It has been estimated that 3 kg of this toxin can kill all the inhabitants of the world. Exotoxins are heat-labile, protein in nature and have

Table 7.2. Differences between exotoxins and endotoxins

Exotoxins	Endotoxins
1. Proteins with high molecular weight ranging from 10,000 to 900,000.	Lipopolysaccharide in nature. Lipid A portion is probably responsible for the toxicity.
2. Heat-labile. The toxicity is destroyed by heating above 60°C.	Heat-stable; can withstand heat over 60°C without losing toxicity.
3. Highly antigenic; stimulate formation of antitoxin which neutralizes toxin.	Weakly antigenic; do not stimulate the formation of antitoxin. Antibodies against only polysaccharide component are raised.
4. Actively secreted by the cells; diffuse into the surrounding medium.	Form integral part of the cell wall; do not diffuse into surrounding medium. These can be obtained only by cell lysis.
5. Converted into toxoid by formaldehyde.	Cannot be toxoided.
6. Action often enzymic.	No enzymic action.
7. Specific pharmacological effect for each exotoxin.	Non-specific action of all endotoxins.
8. Highly specific for particular tissue, e.g., tetanus toxin for CNS.	Non-specific in action.
9. Very high potency (one mg of botulinum or tetanus toxin can kill more than one million guinea-pigs).	Low potency (one mg of extracted somatic antigen can kill one mouse).
10. Do not produce fever in the host.	Usually produce fever in the host.
11. Produced by both Gram-positive bacteria and Gram-negative bacteria.	Produced by Gram-negative bacteria only.
12. Frequently controlled by extrachromosomal genes (e.g., plasmids).	Synthesis directed by chromosomal genes.

enzymatic activity. Some exotoxins can be partially denatured by treatment with formaldehyde to generate toxoids which lack toxicity but retain antigenicity inducing protective immunity when used as vaccines. Some exotoxins like diphtheria toxin and enterotoxins of cholera vibrio and *E. coli* consist of two fragments A and B. The toxin binds to the specific receptors, on the host cell surface, through fragment B (binding) and then toxic or enzymatic A fragment causes cell damage.

6. Resistance to killing by phagocytic cells

Some pathogens like tubercle bacilli can be readily ingested (phagocytosed) by macrophages and other phagocytes but they resist intracellular killing by preventing fusion of phagosome with lysosome. These organisms rather multiply inside these cells. Other bacteria such as *S. aureus* and *N. gonorrhoeae* are able to resist the action of lysosomal components following fusion.

8

Immunity

Immunity refers to resistance of a host to pathogens and their toxic products. It is of two types:

  I. Innate immunity
 (a) Non-specific
 (b) Specific   ] Species, Racial, Individual
  II. Acquired immunity
 (a) *Active*
  • Natural
  • Artificial
 (b) *Passive*
  • Natural
  • Artificial

I. INNATE IMMUNITY

It is due to genetic and constitutional make-up of an individual. Prior contact with microorganisms or their products is not essential. It may be specific against a particular organism or non-specific. Innate immunity may be further divided into species, racial or individual immunity.

Species immunity

It is total or relative resistance to a pathogen shown by all the members of a species. For example, all human beings are resistant to plant pathogens and many animal pathogens. Rat is strikingly resistant to diphtheria whilst guinea-pig and man are highly susceptible. This is due to physical and biochemical differences between the tissues of different host species which determine if a pathogen can multiply in them.

Racial immunity

Within a species, there may be marked racial differences in resistance to infection, e.g., Algerian sheep is highly resistant to anthrax as compared to European sheep. In the USA, Negroes are more susceptible to tuberculosis than whites. Racial differences in immunity are known to be genetic in

origin. A hereditary (genetic) abnormality of red blood cells (sickling) confers immunity to infection by *Plasmodium falciparum* because such RBCs cannot be parasitized by these parasites. This may provide survival advantage to such individuals in malaria-infested areas.

Individual immunity

Different individuals in a race differ in their resistance to microbial infections. The genetic basis of individual immunity is apparent from the observation that if one homozygous twin develops tuberculosis, there is a 75% chance that the other twin will develop overt tuberculosis. In contrast, for heterozygous twins, there is only 33% chance that the second twin will contract overt disease.

Factors influencing innate immunity

1. Age

In general, very young and very old are more susceptible to infectious diseases than persons in other age groups. This appears to be due to the immaturity of immune system in very young and gradual waning of immune response in very old. Foetus in utero is protected from maternal infection by placental barrier. But some pathogens such as HIV cross this barrier leading to foetal infection, while others like *Toxoplasma gondii*, rubella and cytomegalovirus lead to congenital malformations.

2. Hormonal influences and sex

There is an increased susceptibility to infection in endocrine disorders such as diabetes mellitus, hypothyroidism and adrenal dysfunction.

3. Nutritional factors

Both antibody-mediated and cell-mediated immunity are lowered in malnutrition. Protein calorie malnutrition:

- lowers C3 and factor B of the complement system,
- decreases the interferon response, and
- inhibits neutrophil activity.

Similarly, deficiency of vitamin A, vitamin C, folic acid and zinc predisposes to certain infections.

Mechanism of innate immunity

1. Mechanical barriers and surface secretions

The intact skin and the mucous membranes provide a high degree of protection against pathogens. If skin is damaged, as in case of injury or burns, infections may be a serious problem. Skin is a very effective barrier because of unusual structure of outermost epithelial layer, which is composed mainly of keratin, which is indigestible by most micro-organisms, and thus, protects the living cells of the epidermis from microorganisms and their toxins.

We have a **specialized epithelial lining in our respiratory and gastrointestinal tract to minimize infection**. Mucous membrane is composed of specialized epithelial cells which secrete a sticky substance called mucus. This traps dust. In respiratory tract there are also ciliated cells, which move the dust-laden mucus up and out of respiratory tract (**mucociliary escalator**) enabling it to be swallowed or coughed out. When swallowed they are destroyed in the stomach's highly acidic environment and digestive juices. Should a pathogen survive in stomach, it usually cannot penetrate mucous membrane lining the entire gastrointestinal tract and if it escapes the respiratory mucociliary escalator, it would be met by phago-cytes lining the alveoli.

The mouth is constantly bathed in **saliva** which has an inhibitory effect on many microorganisms. Nevertheless viruses, bacteria, fungi and protozoa have developed strategies to circumvent these defences.

Gastrointestinal tract

Four factors protect gastrointestinal tract from infection:
1. **Physical barrier** produced by mucus-secreting epithelial cells.
2. **Secretory IgA antibodies** produced here.
3. **Highly acidic environment** of stomach may hydrolyze microbial invaders.
4. Already established **normal flora** such as *Escherichia coli* serves to inhibit invasion and repopulation by pathogenic microorganisms. However, normal flora is a double-edged weapon. If body resistance is lowered it may lead to opportunistic infections.

Urogenital tract

Kidneys produce sterile urine which travels down the ureter to the bladder and passes out through the urethral opening. Although, urethra has normal flora, invading microorganisms usually do not gain access to the bladder. It is mainly due to frequent flushing of urethra by sterile urine. However, if organisms have mechanism to attach to epithelial cells lining the tract even frequent flushing might not evacuate them. Because of short urethra, bladder infection is more common in females than in males.

Conjunctiva

Conjunctiva is continually being assaulted by microbe-laden dust. Whenever the dust hits the conjunctiva we blink and tears are produced. Tears mechanically wash away the particles and a hydrolytic enzyme, lysozyme, destroys most viruses and bacteria. However, some microorganisms such as chlamydiae have a special ability to attach to the conjunctival surface. In addition to tears, lysozyme is present in tissue fluids and in nearly all secretions except CSF, sweat and urine.

2. Humoral defence mechanisms

Many microbicidal substances are present in the tissues and body fluids. These are non-specific. There is no specific recognition of the microorganism and the response is not enhanced by re-exposure to the same antigen. They are responsible for innate immunity. Following are the bactericidal substances present in the tissues and body fluids:

Lysozyme

This is a basic protein of low molecular weight (approximately 20,000 daltons) found in high concentrations in polymorpho-nuclear leucocytes as well as in most tissue fluids except CSF, sweat and urine. It has bactericidal action by splitting certain polysaccharide components of the cell walls of susceptible bacteria.

Basic polypeptides

Several basic proteins, derived from tissues and blood cells, possess antibacterial activity. These include spermine and spermidine which can kill tubercle bacilli and some staphylo-cocci. Other antibacterial substances include arginine and lysine-containing proteins, protamine and histone. Basic poly-peptides such as leukins extracted from leucocytes and plakins from platelets have antibacterial effect.

Interferons

These are a family of antiviral agents produced by cells stimulated by live or killed viruses and certain other inducers. A number of molecules have been described. α and β interferons are part of innate immunity, and γ interferon is produced by T cells as part of acquired immunity.

3. Cellular defence mechanisms

Microparasites that penetrate the physical barriers are confronted, in addition to humoral defence mechanism, by non-specific cellular defences. Cellular defence against microparasites is provided by **phagocytes** and a subpopulation of lymphocytes known as **natural killer (NK) cells**. Phagocytes are classified into microphages and macrophages.

Microphages are polymorphonuclear leucocytes and **macrophages** consist of histiocytes which are the wandering amoeboid cells seen in tissues, fixed reticuloendothelial cells and monocytes of blood. In connective tissue they are known as histiocytes, in kidneys as mesangial cells, in bones as osteoclast, in brain as microglial cells, in lungs as alveolar macrophages, in liver as Kupffer cells, and in spleen, lymph nodes and thymus as sinus lining macrophages.

Phagocytic cells reach the site of inflammation in large numbers. They engulf, kill and digest bacteria. On the other hand, viral invasion is countered by NK cells. Residing in the peripheral lymphoid organs, NK cells recognize virus-infected cells, bind to them, and subsequently, lyse them. NK cells have also been implicated in host defence against cancers. They are thought to recognize the changes in the cell membranes of transformed cells in a mechanism similar to that used to combat virus infection. Fungi are confronted by polymorphonuclear leucocytes, macrophages and NK cells.

Phagocytic cell engulfs microparasite by extending pseudopodia around it. These fuse and microorganism is internalized into a vacuole (**phagosome**) which fuses with lysosomes found in the cell to form **phagolysosome** (Fig. 8.1). Microparasites are subjected to the lytic enzymes in the phagolysosome and are destroyed. The macrophages present in the walls of capillaries and vascular tissues in spleen, liver, lungs and bone marrow serve a very important role in clearing the blood stream of foreign particulate material such as bacteria. Some microorganisms such as **mycobacteria and brucellae resist intracellular digestion and may actively multiply inside the phagocyte**. Phagocytosis in such instances may help to disseminate infection to different parts of the body. However, these organisms can be digested by activated macrophages.

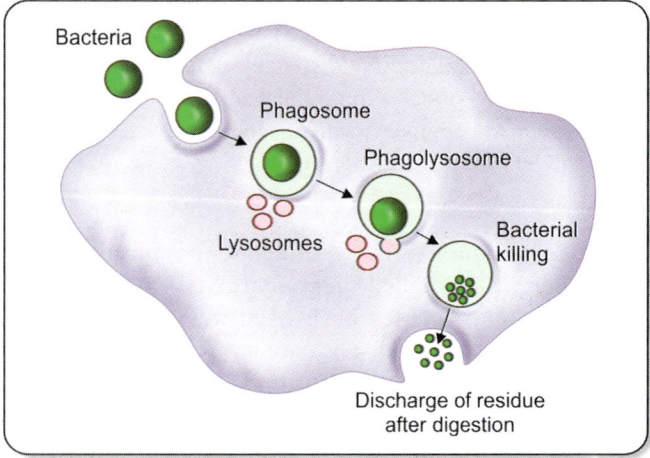

Fig. 8.1. Events of phagocytosis.

Eosinophils are polymorphonuclear leucocytes with cytoplasmic granules and bilobed nucleus. Their number in the blood of normal individuals is 3–5%. But **in patients with parasitic infections and allergies their number increases**.

They are not efficient phagocytic cells. However, their granules possess molecules that are toxic to parasites. Large parasites such as helminths cannot be internalized. Therefore, they must be killed extracellularly. Eosinophils possess Fc receptors (that bind to the Fc fragment of different classes and subclasses of immunoglobulins) and complement receptors that bind the antibody and complement coated parasites. The granule contents of the eosinophils are then released into the space between the cell and the parasite. Eosinophil granules contain enzymes and toxic molecules that are active against helminths.

4. Fever

A rise in temperature following infection is a natural defence mechanism. It inhibits or kills the infecting organisms.

5. Inflammation

It is the cellular and vascular response to injury such as invasion by an infectious agent, exposure to a noxious chemical or physical trauma. The signs of inflammation are redness, swelling, heat, pain and disturbed or altered functions. Inflammation leads to vasodilation, increased vascular permeability and cellular infiltration. **Polymorphonuclear leucocytes** escape into the tissues by diapedesis and accumulate in large numbers attracted by the chemotactic substances released at the site of injury. They then phagocytose microorganisms and their products. Because of increased vascular permeability, there is an **outpouring of plasma** which helps to dilute the toxic products present. In addition, plasma contains a number of non-specific (complement, properdin, beta lysin, leukins and plakins) and specific (antibodies) inhibitors.

II. ACQUIRED IMMUNITY

Most potential pathogens are checked by innate immunity before they establish an overt infection. If these defences are breached the acquired immune system is called into play. The resistance that an individual acquires during his life-time is known as acquired immunity. It is antigen-specific and may be antibody-mediated or cell-mediated. It is of two types – active immunity and passive immunity (Table 8.1 and Fig. 8.2).

Both active and passive immunity may be further divided into natural and artificial.

Active immunity

This involves the active involvement of the person's own immune apparatus leading to the synthesis of antibodies and/or the production of immunocompetent cells (ICCs). It appears only after a **lag (latent) period**, i.e., the time required for generation of antibodies and ICCs. During development of active immunity there is often a negative phase during which the level of measurable immunity may actually be lower than

Table 8.1. Differences between active and passive immunity

Active immunity	Passive immunity
• Produced actively by host's immune system as a result of antigenic stimulation.	• Received passively by the host. No participation of host's immune system.
• Induced by infection or by contact with antigens.	• Conferred by administration of antibodies.
• Long lasting.	• Transient.
• Immunity effective only after a lag period, i.e., time required for generation of antibodies and immunocompetent cells.	• Immunity effective immediately.
• During development of active immunity, there is often a negative phase, during which the level of measurable immunity may actually be lower than before antigenic stimulus. This is due to antigen combining with the pre-existing antibodies and lowering its level.	• No negative phase.
• Immunological memory present, therefore, subsequent challenge (secondary response) is more effective.	• No immunological memory. Subsequent administration of antibodies is less effective due to immune elimination.
• More effective and confers better protection.	• Less effective and provides inferior immunity.
• Not applicable in immunodeficient individuals.	• Applicable in immunodeficient individuals.

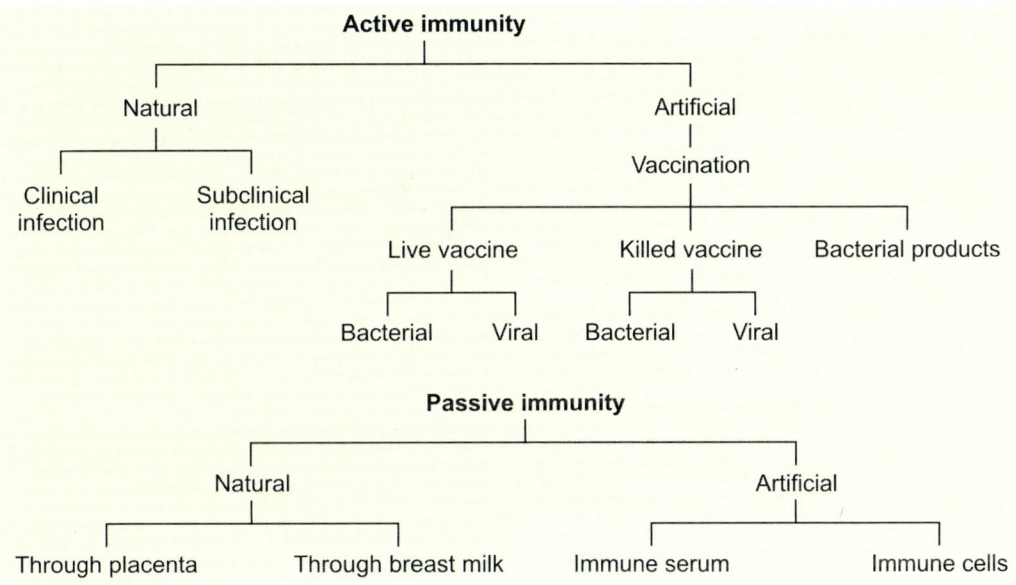

Fig. 8.2. Types of immunity.

before antigenic stimulus. This is due to antigen combining with pre-existing antibodies and lowering its level.

If an individual who has been actively immunized against an antigen, experiences the same antigen subsequently, the immune response occurs more quickly and more abundantly than during the first encounter. This is known as **secondary response**.

Immune system is able to retain the memory of a prior antigenic exposure for long periods and produces a secondary type response when encountered with the same antigen. This is known as **immunological memory**.

Natural active immunity

Natural active immunity results either from a subclinical or clinical infection. A large majority of adults in the developing countries possess natural active immunity to poliomyelitis due to repeated subclinical infections with poliovirus during childhood. Some infections like diphtheria, whooping cough, measles and mumps induce long-lasting immunity. Others such as common cold and influenza confer immunity which lasts for a short time.

Artificial active immunity

This is the resistance induced by vaccines which are preparations of live or killed microorganisms or their products.

I. Bacterial vaccines
(a) *Live:*
  • B.C.G. for tuberculosis
  • Ty 21a for typhoid

(b) *Killed:*
- TAB for enteric fever.
- Cholera
- Pertussis

(c) *Bacterial products*
- Tetanus toxoid
- Diphtheria toxoid
- Capsular polysaccharide of meningococci
- Capsular polysaccharide of *Haemophilus influenzae* type b

II. Viral vaccines

(a) *Live:*
- Sabin vaccine for poliomyelitis or oral polio vaccine (OPV)
- 17D vaccine for yellow fever
- MMR vaccine for measles, mumps, rubella
- Varicella-zoster

(b) *Killed:*
- Salk vaccine for poliomyelitis
- Neural and non-neural vaccines for rabies
- Influenza
- Hepatitis A
- Hepatitis B
- Japanese encephalitis

Live vaccines initiate a sort of mini infection without causing disease. The immunity following vaccination, therefore, parallels that following natural infection. However, it is of lower order than that induced by infection. Since live vaccines undergo limited multiplication in the body, therefore, number of organisms required in a dose is less; single doses may be sufficient and they are relatively cheaper. Live vaccines may be administered orally (e.g., Sabin vaccine for poliomyelitis). They provide more effective and more lasting immunity than killed vaccines. Some of them can be given as combined vaccines, e.g., measles, mumps, rubella (MMR) vaccine.

Killed vaccines have the advantage of stability and safety. These can be given in combination in polyvalent vaccines, e.g., diphtheria, pertussis, tetanus (DPT) vaccine. These are, generally, less immunogenic than live vaccines and protection lasts only for a short period. Therefore, they have to be administered repeatedly. At least two doses are required. First dose is known as **primary** and subsequent doses as **booster doses**. In killed vaccines since the organisms are killed, therefore, larger number of these are required in each dose. Oral route for killed vaccines is, generally, not effective. Antibody response to killed vaccines is improved by addition of adjuvants, for example, aluminium phosphate adjuvant vaccine for cholera.

Passive immunity

The immunity that is transferred to a recipient in a ready-made form is known as passive immunity. Here the recipient's immune system plays no active role. There is no lag or latent period, the immunity is effective immediately after passive immunization. There is no negative phase. It confers only transient immunity lasting usually for days or weeks till the antibodies are metabolized and eliminated. There is no secondary type response. Rather subsequent administration of antibodies is less effective due to **immune elimination**.

Following first injection of antibody, its elimination is only by metabolic breakdown but during subsequent injections its elimination is much quicker because metabolic breakdown is combined with immune elimination as it combines with antibodies to horse serum that would have been produced following first injection. This happens when horse (foreign) serum is used. Immune elimination is not a problem when human serum is used. Because of its immediate action it is employed where instant immunity is required as in case of protection against tetanus, gas gangrene and diphtheria following exposure.

Natural passive immunity

This is the resistance transferred from mother to foetus through placenta. IgG antibodies can cross placental barrier to reach the foetus. After birth, immunoglobulins are passed to the newborn through the breast milk. Human colostrum is rich in IgA antibodies which are resistant to digestion in stomach and small intestine, hence confers immunity in the neonate up to three months of age. Human foetus acquires some ability to synthesize IgM antibodies from twentieth week of gestation, but its immunological capacity is still inadequate at birth. It is only by the age of three months that the infant acquires a satisfactory level of immunological independence. Until then, maternal antibodies give passive protection against infectious diseases of the infant.

Transport of antibodies across placenta is an active process, therefore, the concentration of antibodies in foetal blood may sometimes be higher than that seen in the mother. These antibodies are generally against all common infectious diseases in the locality. Therefore, most paediatric infections are commoner after the age of three months when maternal immunoglobulins disappear. By active immunization of mother during pregnancy the immune status of the neonate can be improved. Therefore, immunization of pregnant women with tetanus toxoid is recommended in countries where neonatal tetanus is common.

Artificial passive immunity

This is the immunity transferred passively to the recipient by administration of antibodies. This is done by administration of hyperimmune sera of man or animals. For example, tetanus antitoxin is prepared in horses by active immunization of horses with tetanus toxoid, bleeding them and separating the serum. Similarly, diphtheria antitoxin and gas gangrene antitoxin are also prepared. However, since these antitoxins are foreign proteins and are liable to cause serious or even fatal hypersensitivity reactions, these should be administered only after testing for hypersensitivity. After first administration, it is removed by metabolism and following subsequent injections by metabolism and immune elimination. Therefore, immunity conferred is short-lived.

Sera collected from patients convalescing from infectious diseases contain high levels of specific antibodies. Convalescent sera have, therefore, been employed for passive immunization against viral infections such as measles and rubella. Sera of healthy adults contain antibodies against infectious agents prevalent in a community. Therefore, sera from a large number of individuals can be collected and used for passive immunization. Placenta provides a convenient source of human immunoglobulins. Human immune serum does not lead to any hypersensitivity reaction, there is no immune elimination and its half-life is more than that of animal sera. However, with human serum there is a grave risk of transmission of human immunodeficiency virus and hepatitis B, C and D viruses.

Indications of passive immunization

- To provide immediate protection to a non-immune individual exposed to an infection, when there is insufficient time for active immunization, e.g., administration of tetanus antitoxin and gas gangrene antitoxin to a non-immune individual with crushing road-side injury, and administration of diphtheria antitoxin to a non-immune child exposed to diphtheria.
- Administration of anti-Rh(D) IgG to Rh-negative mother, bearing Rh-positive baby at the time of delivery to prevent Rh isoimmunization.

Combination of active and passive immunization may also be employed. For example, a person exposed to tetanus may be injected tetanus antitoxin on one arm and tetanus toxoid on the other with separate syringes followed by full course of tetanus toxoid. Diphtheria antitoxin and diphtheria toxoid can also be practised similarly.

ADOPTIVE IMMUNITY

Injection of immunologically competent lymphocytes is known as adoptive immunity. Instead of whole lymphocytes, an extract of immunologically competent lymphocytes known as transfer factor can be used. This has been attempted in the treatment of lepromatous leprosy.

LOCAL IMMUNITY

This means immunity at a particular site, generally, the site of invasion and multiplication of pathogen. For example, in case of poliomyelitis, parenteral vaccine provides systemic immunity. The antibodies neutralize virus only after blood invasion. It does not prevent multiplication of the virus at the site of entry, the gut mucosa, and its faecal excretion. However, when live oral vaccine is given it leads to local immunity. Similarly, live influenza vaccine administered intranasally provides local immunity while killed influenza vaccine evokes humoral antibody response. Local immunity is conferred by secretory IgA antibodies produced locally by plasma cells present on mucosal surfaces or in secretory glands.

HERD IMMUNITY

Overall level of immunity in a community is known as herd immunity. When a large number of individuals in a community (herd) are immune to a pathogen the herd immunity to a pathogen is said to be satisfactory. When herd immunity is low, epidemics are likely to occur on the introduction of the pathogen. This is due to the fact that a larger number of individuals are susceptible.

9

Antigens

Antigens (*anti*body *gen*erators) are substances that can stimulate an immune response and, given the opportunity, react specifically by binding with the effector molecules (antibodies) and effector cells (lymphocytes) produced. Most antigens are proteins, but some are carbohydrates, lipids or nucleic acids. Some antigens are more immunogenic or capable of eliciting an immune response, than others. Some antigens such as proteins may possess a number of small chemical groups that are called antigenic determinants or **epitopes** which can bind specifically to antigen binding site (**paratope**) of the antibody molecule (Fig. 9.1) and T cell receptors. Each determinant can stimulate the formation of a particular kind of antibody or effector cell. Thus, a pure protein antigen may give rise to many distinct antibodies and effector cells. The size of epitope is around 25–35 Å and a molecular weight of 400–1000.

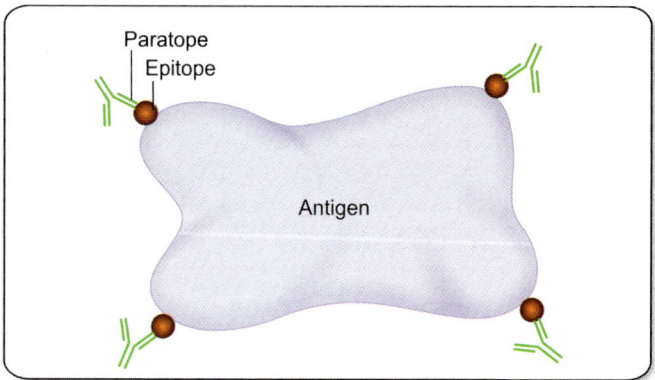

Fig. 9.1. Epitopes of antigen and paratopes of antibody.

Incomplete antigen or hapten

This is a chemical substance of low molecular weight that cannot induce an immune response by itself. Nevertheless, haptens can induce a response if combined with larger molecules (normally proteins) which serve as carriers. This response requires assistance from T helper (Th) lymphocytes. In contrast to complete antigens, haptens contain a single epitope. In response to hapten carried on carrier particle, antibodies are produced not only against the hapten but also against the carrier particle. Haptens are of two types:

1. Complex haptens

These can combine with specific antibodies to form precipitate, e.g., capsular polysaccharide of pneumococci.

2. Simple haptens

These combine with specific antibodies but no precipitate is formed (non-precipitating). This is due to univalent character of simple hapten, whereas complex haptens are polyvalent, since it is assumed that precipitation requires the antigens to have two or more antibody combining sites.

Immunogenicity

This refers to the ability of an antigen to stimulate an immune response.

Determinants of antigenicity

1. Size

Antigenicity depends upon the molecular weight. Generally, molecules with a molecular weight less than 5,000 are nonantigenic or feebly so. Low molecular weight substances may be rendered antigenic by absorbing them on large inert particles such as bentonite or kaolin. Some low molecular weight substances such as picryl chloride and penicillin may be antigenic when applied on the skin, probably by combining with tissue proteins.

2. Foreignness

Only antigens which are foreign to the individual (non-self) induce an immune response because host distinguishes self from non-self and normally does not respond to self. The healthy body is immunologically tolerant to nearly all self antigens, that would be immunogenic in a foreign host. However, under certain circumstances tolerance may be broken leading to **autoimmunity**. *Antigenicity of a substance is related to the degree of its foreignness*. Antigens from other individuals of the same species are less antigenic than those from other species.

3. Chemical nature

Proteins and polysaccharides are most antigenic. Lipids and nucleic acids are less antigenic. Their antigenicity is enhanced by combination with proteins. However, all proteins are not antigenic. A well-known exception is gelatin. The presence of an aromatic radical appears to be essential for antigenicity and the absence of aromatic amino acids such as tyrosine in gelatin is responsible for its nonantigenicity.

4. Susceptibility to tissue enzymes

Only those substances which can be metabolized and are susceptible to the action of tissue enzymes behave as antigens. Antigens introduced into the body are degraded by the host into the fragments of appropriate size containing antigenic determinants. Phagocytosis and intracellular enzymes appear to play an essential role in breaking down antigens into immunogenic fragments. Substances insusceptible to tissue enzymes such as polystyrene latex and synthetic polypeptides which are not metabolized in the body, are not antigenic.

Antigenic specificity

It is determined by chemical grouping and acid radicals. Antigenic specificity varies with the position of antigenic determinant, i.e., whether it is in *ortho*, *meta* or *para* positions. However, antigenic specificity is not absolute. Cross reactions can occur between antigens which bear stereochemical similarities.

Species specificity

Tissues of all individuals in a species contain species-specific antigens. However, some degree of cross-reactivity is seen between antigens from related species. **Species-specific antigens possess forensic applications in the identification of species of blood and seminal stains.**

Isospecificity

Isoantigens are antigens found in some but not all members of a species. On the basis of isoantigens a species may be divided into different groups. The best example of isoantigens is human blood group antigens on the basis of which all humans can be divided into different groups – A, B, AB and O. Each of these groups may be further divided into Rh-positive or Rh-negative. **This carries clinical importance in blood transfusion, isoimmunization during pregnancy and disputed paternity.**

Histocompatibility antigens

These are the antigens present on the cells of each individual of a species. Histocompatibility typing is essential in organ/tissue transplantation from one individual to another within a species. These antigens are associated with plasma membrane of tissue cells and are responsible for evoking immunological response against graft unless it is antigenically identical to that of the recipient. These antigens are encoded by genes known as *histocompatibility* genes which collectively constitute **major histocompatibility complex** (MHC). These are located on short arm of chromosome 6. MHC products present on the surface of leucocytes are known as **human leucocyte-associated (HLA) antigens**. These have been studied extensively in organ transplantation. Major histocompatibility antigens in man and mouse are known as HLA and H2 respectively.

Autospecificity

Autologous or self antigens are ordinarily non-antigenic. However, hidden or sequestered antigens that are not normally found free in circulation or tissue fluids are not recognized as self antigens. For example, **lens protein**, which is normally confined within the capsule of the lens, and antigens that are absent during the embryonic life and develop later, such as **spermatozoa**, are also not recognized as self antigens. But if these antigens are released into the tissues, as for instance following injury to lens or damage to the testis, antibodies are produced against them. This is one of the mechanisms of pathogenesis of autoimmune diseases. Cells or tissues may undergo **antigenic alteration** as a result of infection or irradiation and may thus become immunogenic leading to **autoimmunity**.

Organ specificity

Some organs such as brain, kidney and lens protein of different species share the same antigens. These are known as organ-specific antigens. The **neuroparalytic complications** following antirabic vaccination, with neural vaccines, are a consequence of brain-specific antigens shared by sheep and man.

Heterogenetic (heterophile) specificity

Same or closely related antigens occurring in different biological species, classes and kingdoms are known as heterogenetic or heterophile antigens. The best example of such heterophile antigens is the **Forssman antigen** which is a lipid carbohydrate complex widely distributed in man, animals, birds, plants and bacteria. It is absent in rabbits, therefore, anti-Forssman antibody can be prepared in these animals. Examples of tests based on the principle of heterophile antigens used in diagnostic serology are as under:

(i) Weil-Felix reaction

It is an agglutination test in which patient sera are tested for agglutinins to O antigens of non-motile strains of *Proteus* OX2, OX19 and OXK. Cross reaction between O antigen of these strains of *Proteus* and certain rickettsial antigens is the basis of this test.

(ii) Paul-Bunnell test

In patients with infectious mononucleosis heterophile antibodies appear in the serum of the patient. These antibodies agglutinate sheep erythrocytes. This test is known as Paul-Bunnell test.

(iii) Cold agglutinin test

Agglutination of human O group erythrocytes at 4°C by the sera of patients suffering from primary atypical pneumonia.

(iv) Agglutination of Streptococcus MG

Agglutination of *Streptococcus* MG by the sera of the patients of primary atypical pneumonia.

Tolerogens

Antigens do not always exhibit immunogenicity or evoke antibody formation. In some instances an antigen presented at one concentration might induce specific immunological unresponsiveness or tolerance, while at another concentration it might promote immunity. **An antigen that induces tolerance is referred to as tolerogen.** One important manifestation of tolerance occurs during foetal development. Therefore, an individual's immune system does not normally react against self antigens. Burnet suggested that during foetal life a large number of lymphocytes capable of reacting with different antigens are formed. But cells with immunological reactivity with self antigens are eliminated. This process is known as **clonal deletion**. Their persistence or development in later life leads to **autoimmunity**.

Superantigens

Superantigens is a class of molecules that can interact with antigen-presenting cells (APCs) and T cells in non-specific manner. This activity does not involve the endocytic processing required for typical antigen presentation but instead occurs by concurrent association with MHC class II molecules of the APCs and the Vβ domain of the T cell receptor (Fig. 9.2). This interaction activates a large number of T cells (10%) than conventional antigens (about 1%), explaining the massive cytokine expression and immunomodulation. Various super-antigens include staphylococcal enterotoxins, staphylococcal toxic shock syndrome toxin, staphylococcal exfoliative toxin, streptococcal pyrogenic exotoxin and some viral proteins.

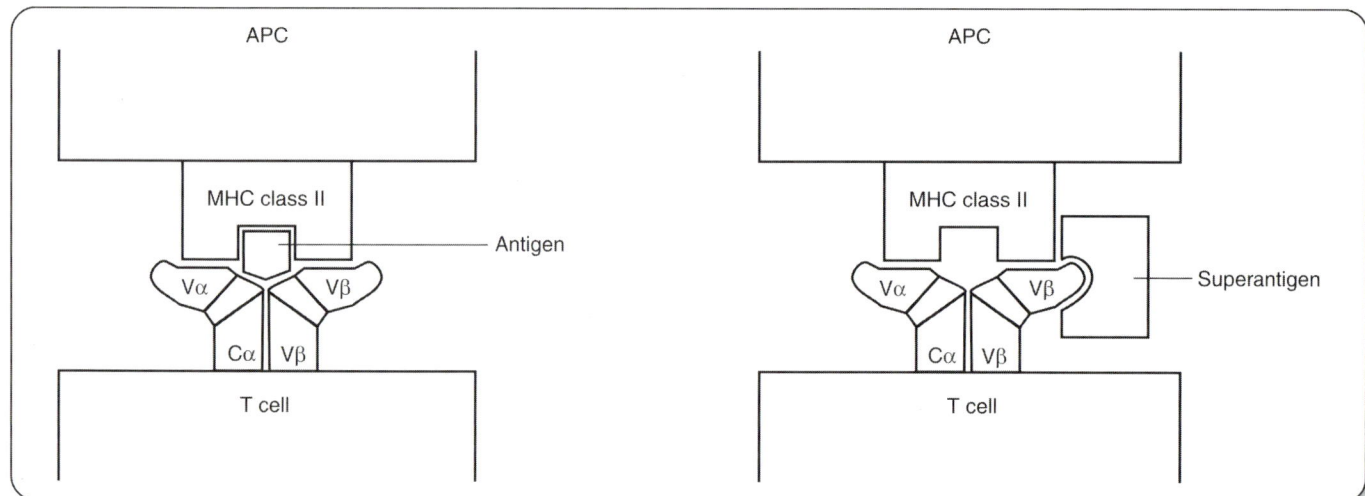

Fig. 9.2. Binding of antigen and superantigen by MHC and T cell receptor.

10

Antibodies

Antibodies or immunoglobulins (Igs) are γ globulins which are produced in response to antigenic stimulation. These react specifically with the antigens which stimulated their production. Igs are produced by plasma cells and to some extent by lymphocytes also. All antibodies are Igs, but all Igs (e.g., myeloma proteins) are not antibodies. On the basis of physicochemical and antigenic structure Igs can be divided into five distinct classes or isotypes namely IgG, IgA, IgM, IgD and IgE.

ANTIBODY STRUCTURE

IgG has been studied extensively and serves as a model of basic structural unit of all Igs. It is a Y-shaped four polypeptide chain molecule. Of the four chains, two each are light (L) and heavy (H). These are held together by disulphide bonds (Fig. 10.1). L chain has a molecular weight of 25,000 daltons and H chain 50,000 daltons. H chains are structurally and antigenically distinct for each class and are designated with Greek letters α (alpha), δ (delta), ε (epsilon), γ (gamma) and μ (mu) in IgA, IgD, IgE, IgG and IgM respectively. L chains are of two types – κ (kappa) and λ (lambda). A molecule of Ig may have either κ or λ chains but never both together. κ and λ chains occur in a ratio of about 2 : 1 in human serum.

IgG when treated with proteolytic enzyme papain in the presence of cysteine cleaves it into three fragments. Two identical fragments (45,000 daltons each) still possess the antigen-binding sites and are thus named **fragment antigen binding (Fab)**. These two fragments represent bivalency of IgG molecule. The third fragment (50,000 daltons) which lacks the ability to bind to antigen can be crystallized. It is, therefore, known as **fragment crystallizable (Fc)**.

Functions of Fc

- Binds complement leading to complement fixation.
- Binds to cell receptors (FcRs).
- Determines passage of IgG across the placental barrier.
- Determines skin fixation and catabolic rate.
- Antigenic determinants that distinguish one class of antibody from another are also located on Fc fragment.

Treatment of the IgG antibody molecule with proteolytic enzyme pepsin cleaves H chains on the carboxyterminal side of the interchain disulphide bonds of the hinge region. Therefore, 2 Fab fragments remain united (100,000 daltons). This fragment is designated as **F(ab')₂** with two antigen-binding sites. It is about 10% larger than the two Fab fragments from a papain digestion of antibody. Pepsin also degrades part of the Fc portion to small peptides and leaves a dimer of the carboxyterminal quarter of the chain, termed **pFc'**.

When IgG is treated with reducing agent such as mercaptoethanol in the presence of urea, the disulphide bonds are reduced releasing four peptide chains – two heavy and two light.

Immunoglobulin domains

Two H chains are always identical in a given molecule and the same is true of L chains. Each H chain of IgG contains 440 amino acids while each L chain contains 220 amino acids. H chain has four domains of 110 amino acids each, while L chain has two domains of 110 amino acids each (Fig. 10.2). The antigen combining sites of the molecule are at its amino-terminal end. These are composed of both H and L chains. Of the 220 amino acids, those that constitute carboxyterminal half of L chain occur in a constant sequence. This part of the chain is called **constant region** (C_L). Only two sequence patterns are seen in constant region of κ and λ chains. On the other hand, amino acid sequence in aminoterminal half of the L chain is highly variable; the variability determines the immunological specificity of the antibody molecule. It is, therefore, called **variable region** (V_L).

A similar pattern is seen in H chains. The variable region of H chain, however, is only 25% as long as constant region. The

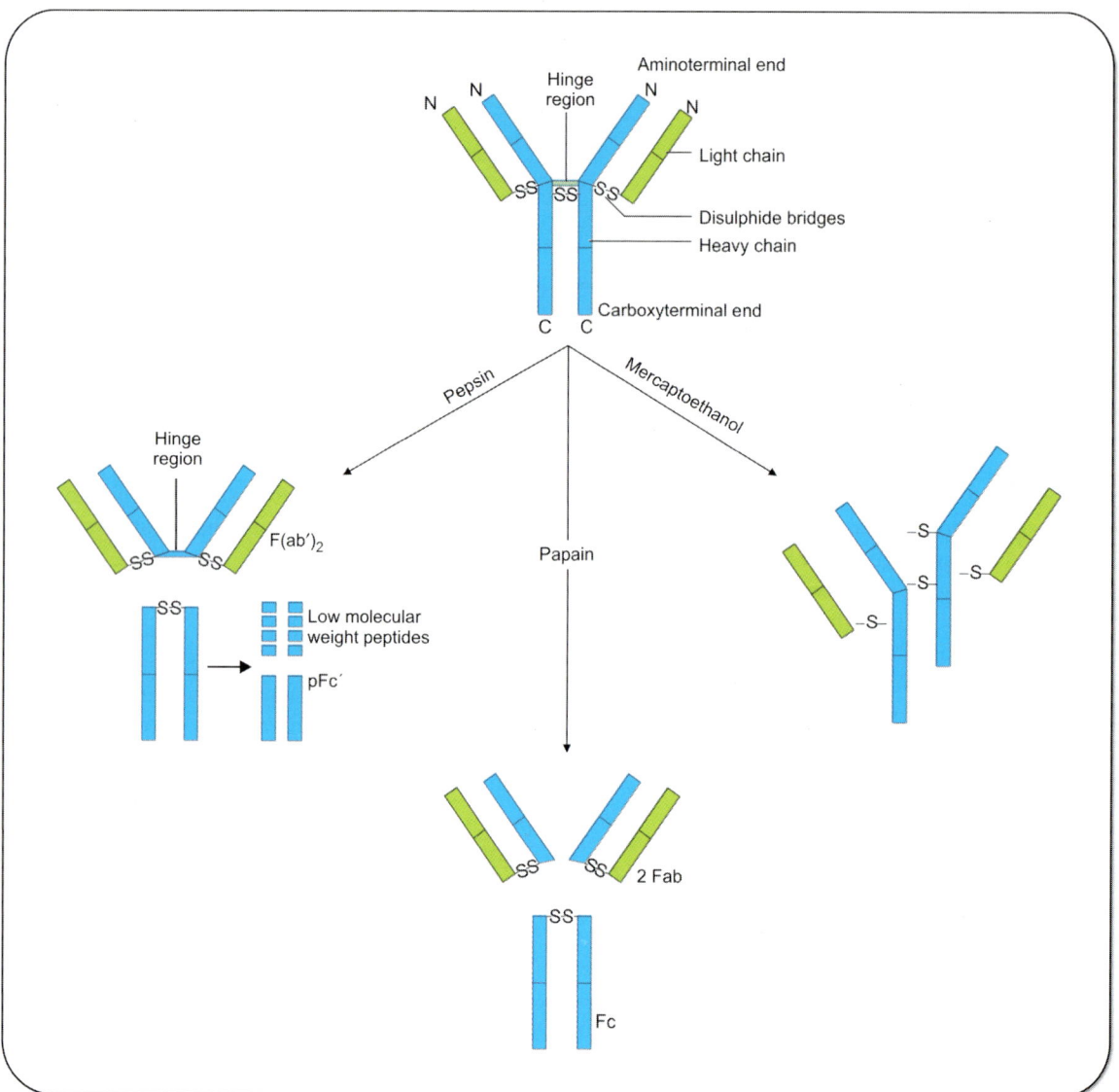

Fig. 10.1. Basic immunoglobulin structure.

variable region of H chain like that of L chain has highly variable sequence of amino acids and is known as V_H. The constant region of H chain is divided into three portions, C_H1, C_H2 and C_H3. The infinite range of specificity of Igs depends upon the variability of amino acid sequences at the variable regions of H and L chains which form antigen combining sites.

Fd piece

It is the portion of H chains present in Fab fragment. H chains carry a carbohydrate moiety which is distinct for each class of immunoglobulins.

Each Ig peptide chain has internal disulphide links in addition to interchain disulphide bonds which bridge H and L chains. These intrachain disulphide bonds form loops in the peptide chain and each of the loops is completely folded to form a globular domain and each domain has its separate

function. Variable region domains V_L and V_H are responsible for the formation of a specific antigen-binding site. C_H2 region in IgG binds C1q in the classical complement sequence and C_H3 domain mediates adherence to monocyte surface. The area of H chain in the C region between C_H1 and C_H2 is the **hinge region**. It is more flexible and is more exposed to enzymes and chemicals.

IMMUNOGLOBULIN CLASSES

Human serum contains five classes of immunoglobulins – IgG, IgA, IgM, IgD and IgE. Table 10.1 shows their differentiating features.

Immunoglobulin G

This is the most abundant class of Ig in the body constituting approximately 75% of the total Igs. This is distributed equally

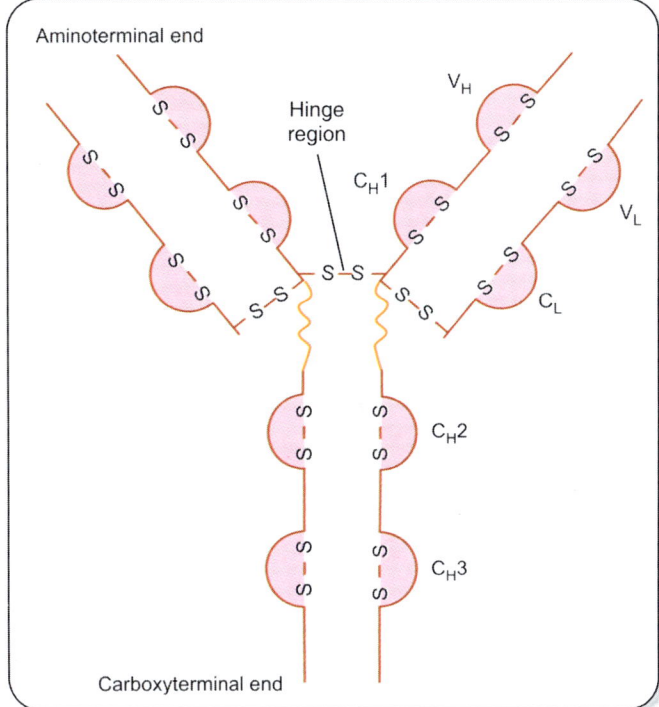

Fig. 10.2. Variable and constant domains of immunoglobulin molecule.

within the intravascular and extravascular pools. Very little IgG is produced during the early stages of the primary response to antigen, but it is the major form of antibody produced during the secondary response. It is not synthesized by the foetus in any significant amount. IgG is also most commonly seen **myeloma protein**. It has a half-life of 21 days. The normal serum concentration of IgG is about 12 mg/ml. It is a glycoprotein with a molecular weight of 150,000 daltons.

There are **four subclasses** of human IgG (IgG1, IgG2, IgG3 and IgG4). Each subclass possesses a distinct type of γ chain which can be identified with specific antiserum. They constitute about 59%, 30%, 8% and 3% respectively of the total human IgG. All normal humans possess all four subclasses of IgG, just as they possess all classes of Igs. IgG binds complement in classical pathway. IgG3 is most effective in binding complement followed by IgG1 and IgG2. It can bind to protein A (from *Staphylococcus aureus*) and protein G (from group G streptococci). *IgG is the only class of Igs that can cross the placenta and is responsible for the protection of the infant during first few months of life. However, subclass IgG2 does not cross the placenta.* IgG is also found, along with IgA, in milk during the first few weeks after birth, providing additional protection if the infant is breast-fed.

Macrophages and monocytes bear Fc receptors (FcRs) which bind to the Fc portion of IgG1 and IgG3 in C_H3 domain. Such binding permits these cells to exhibit antibody-dependent cellular toxicity. IgG usually exhibits high affinity for antigens leading to efficient neutralization of toxins. Among null cells, a distinct subpopulation of cytotoxic cells has been recognized which also possesses FcRs for Fc part of IgG. They are capable of lysing or killing target cells sensitized with IgG. They are known as **killer cells**. They are responsible for **antibody-dependent cell-mediated cytotoxicity (ADCC)**. Platelets also possess FcRs for Fc portion of IgG leading to aggregation, degranulation and release of histamine. IgG is the only Ig which has the property of fixing to guinea-pig skin.

Catabolism of IgG is unique in that it varies with its serum concentration. When its level is raised, as in chronic malaria, kala-azar or myeloma, the IgG synthesized against a particular antigen will be catabolised rapidly and may result in the particular antibody deficiency. Conversely, in hypogammaglobulinaemia, the IgG given for treatment will be catabolised slowly.

Table 10.1. Properties of various immunoglobulin classes

	IgG	IgA	IgM	IgD	IgE
1. Molecular weight in kDa	150	160,385*	900–1,000	180	190
2. Sedimentation coefficient (S)	7	7, 11	19	7	8
3. Carbohydrate content (%)	3	8	12	13	12
4. Heavy chain	$\gamma_1, \gamma_2, \gamma_3, \gamma_4$	α_1, α_2	μ	δ	ε
5. Light chain	κ or λ	κ or λ	κ or λ	κ or λ	κ or λ
6. Serum concentration (mg/ml)	12	2	1.2	0.03	0.00004
7. Half-life (days)	21	6	5	3	2
8. Complement binding	Classical pathway	Alternative pathway	Classical pathway	None	None
9. Binding to tissue	Heterologous	None	None	None	Homologous
10. Secretion from serous membranes	No	Yes*	No	No	Yes
11. Placental passage	Yes	No	No	No	No
12. Heat stability (56°C)	Yes	Yes	Yes	Yes	No

* Secretory IgA.

IgG participates in most immunological reactions such as complement fixation, precipitation and neutralization of toxins and viruses. Passively administered IgG suppresses the homologous antibody synthesis by a feedback process. This property is utilized for prevention of isoimmunization of Rh-negative mother bearing Rh-positive baby by administration of anti-Rh (D) IgG at the time of delivery.

Immunoglobulin M

It is so named because it is a macroglobulin at least five times larger than IgG. It is a glycoprotein with molecular weight of 900,000–1,000,000 daltons (millionaire molecule). It is present on the surface of virtually all uncommitted B cells. About 10% of normal serum Igs consist of this class. The normal serum level of IgM is 1.2 mg/ml. It has a half-life of about 5 days. IgM normally exists as a pentamer, consisting of 5 Ig subunits (Fig. 10.3).

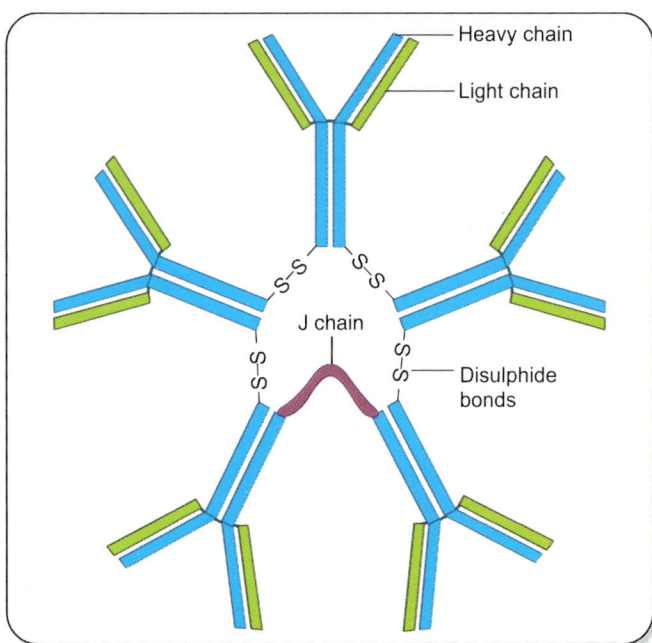

Fig. 10.3. IgM immunoglobulin.

In contrast to IgG, IgM remains almost exclusively in the serum and is not usually found extravascularly in body cavities or secretions. Therefore, IgM is believed to be responsible for protection against blood invasion by microorganisms. Pentameric IgM is apparently too large to cross the placenta. The Hμ chain has four C_H domains rather than three as seen in H chains of IgG. H chains are held together by disulphide bonds. There is an additional peptide chain called the **joining (J) chain**. The J chain may be largely responsible for the polymerization process, which occurs shortly before the molecule is secreted by plasma cell.

IgM contains 10 Fab fragments, and thus 10 antigen-binding sites. Therefore, theoretically it can bind to 10 antigen molecules. However, it appears that many antigens are so large that when bound to one site, they physically prevent the binding of another antigen molecule to an adjacent binding site. Thus, generally, IgM is capable of binding as few as five molecules of antigen.

Phylogenetically IgM is the oldest Ig class. It is usually the first antibody to appear following stimulation by an antigen. However, IgM synthesis is usually not prolonged, and IgG antibodies soon become the most prevalent class. IgM is also the earliest to be synthesized by foetus beginning by about **20 weeks of gestation**. As it cannot cross the placental barrier, the presence of IgM in the foetus or newborn indicates intrauterine infection. Its detection is, therefore, useful for the diagnosis of congenital syphilis, rubella, HIV infection and toxoplasmosis. IgM antibodies are relatively short-lived, hence their demonstration in the serum indicates recent infection. Treatment of serum with 0.12 M 2-mercaptoethanol selectively destroys IgM without affecting IgG antibodies. This provides a simple method for differential estimation of IgG and IgM antibodies.

IgM is much more efficient than IgG in its ability to fix complement, promoting lysis and death of most Gram-negative bacteria. This greater efficacy is due to the fact that complement may bind to several Fc regions of pentameric IgM simultaneously, thus initiating complement cascade and target cell lysis with a single molecule.

Isohaemagglutinins (anti-A and anti-B), and antibodies to *Salmonella* Typhi O antigen and Wassermann reaction antibodies in syphilis are usually IgM. In certain disease states such as lupus erythematosus and rheumatoid arthritis, IgM may occur in monomeric form in high concentration. Monomeric IgM has lower avidity for antigen than does the pentameric form. A single molecule of IgM can bring about haemolysis, whereas 1000 IgG molecules are required for the same effect. IgM is also more effective than IgG in opsonization, bactericidal action and in bacterial agglutination. However, in neutralization of toxins and viruses, it is less active than IgG.

Immunoglobulin A

The basic structure of IgA is similar to that of IgG. It contains two identical light chains (either κ or λ) and two heavy α chains. It is the second most abundant class, constituting about 15% of human serum Igs where it exists as a monomeric Ig. More important form is the dimeric form, known as **secretory IgA (sIgA)**. It is the predominant class of Igs in secretions such as milk, tears, nasal secretions, saliva, perspiration, genitourinary secretions and seromucous secretions.

On mucus surfaces sIgA form an antibody paste and is believed to play an important role in local immunity against respiratory and intestinal pathogens. sIgA is relatively resistant to the digestive enzymes and reducing agents. Many infectious organisms cause disease by attaching to glycoproteins on the surface of epithelial cells of secretory gland. If this adhesion is sufficiently strong, the organism will divide, establish a colony and cause disease by any of a number of mechanisms, e.g., secretion of toxins that cause local and systemic injury. Secretory IgA when present in the secretions prevents attachment of organisms to epithelial cells, thus preventing adhesion, colonization and infection.

Serum IgA is principally a monomeric 7S molecule with a molecular weight of 160,000 daltons. Secretory IgA is synthesized by plasma cells in the subepithelial tissue and secreted as a dimer containing four heavy chains, four light chains and one J chain which is similar to J chain found in pentameric IgM (Fig. 10.4). sIgA also possesses an additional structural unit called secretory component (SC). It is synthesized not in lymphoid cells but in epithelial cells of glands of intestine, and the respiratory tract and is attached to IgA molecules at their Fc portions producing 11S dimer with a molecular weight of 385,000 daltons. sIgA is relatively resistant to digestive enzymes, which may be due to the secretory component. IgA does not fix complement in classical pathway but can activate the alternative complement pathway. It promotes phagocytosis and intracellular killing of micro-organisms.

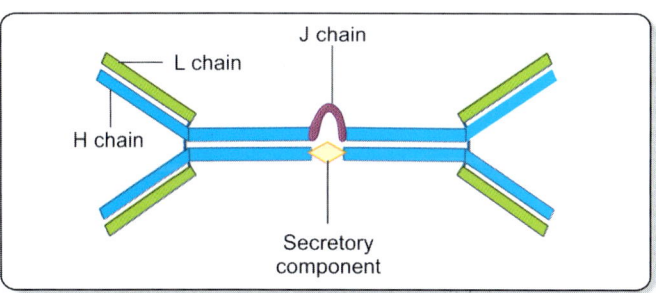

Fig. 10.4. Secretory IgA.

There are two subclasses of IgA in humans – IgA1 and IgA2. In serum, IgA1 constitutes 80–90% of IgA while sIgA consists of about equal amounts of the two subclasses.

Certain streptococci and pathogenic *Neisseria* produce proteases that specifically cleave the heavy chain of IgA1. IgA2 is resistant to such cleavage because it has a shorter hinge region and lacks the proline-rich site cleaved by the proteases.

Immunoglobulin D

Like other monomeric antibodies IgD is composed of two light and two heavy chains. The latter are designated as δ chains. It contains about 13% carbohydrate. Its molecular weight is 180,000 daltons. It does not bind complement. It does not cross placenta and does not bind to cells via Fc region. IgD is present on the surface of B lymphocytes which are

destined to differentiate into antibody-producing plasma cells and its serum concentration is very low (0.03 mg/ml). Reaction of antigen with surface immunoglobulin may lead to cell differentiation and antibody synthesis.

Immunoglobulin E

It resembles IgG structurally. Its molecular weight is 190,000 daltons. Its half-life is about two days. It does not fix complement or cross placental barrier. In contrast to other Igs it is heat-labile and gets inactivated by heating it at 56°C for 30 minutes. It is susceptible to 2-mercaptoethanol. It is chiefly produced in the linings of the respiratory and intestinal tracts. It is present in extremely low concentrations (0.00004 mg/ml) in the serum. But raised serum levels are seen in atopic (type I hypersensitivity) conditions like asthma and hay fever.

Most of a person's IgE is fixed to the surface of mast cells and basophils, and when a specific antigen binds with IgE bound to mast cell or basophil membrane, the reaction results in the release of pharmacologically active substances such as histamine and serotonin, which dilate capillaries, increase vascular permeability and cause bronchial constriction. Fc portion of IgE binds to the Fc receptors present on the surface of mast cells and basophils leaving antigen-binding sites free to react with specific antigen.

So far, no beneficial effect of IgE has been identified. It has been observed that IgE levels may rise following infections with parasites especially helminths. It has been suggested that mast cell-bound IgE reacts with antigens on the parasite followed by release of histamine. This results in increased vascular permeability followed by influx of plasma and cells (particularly eosinophils) and destruction of parasite. IgE mediates Prausnitz-Küstner reaction.

From available information it appears that:

IgG : Protects the body fluids
IgA : Protects the body surfaces
IgM : Protects the blood stream
IgE : Mediates type I hypersensitivity
IgD : Present on the surface of B lymphocytes which are destined to differentiate into antibody-producing cells

ABNORMAL IMMUNOGLOBULINS

Abnormal immunoglobulins are structurally similar proteins. These are found in serum in certain pathological conditions such as **multiple myeloma** and sometimes even in healthy persons. **Bence-Jones (BJ) protein** was the earliest abnormal protein described in 1847. It is typically found in multiple myeloma. These proteins are light chains of immunoglobulins, hence occur as κ or λ forms. But in a patient, it may occur as κ or λ forms but never in both forms. It can be identified in urine by its characteristic property of coagulation when heated to 60°C but redissolving at 70°C.

Multiple myeloma may affect plasma cells synthesizing IgG, IgA, IgD and IgE. Similar involvement of IgM-producing cells is known as *Waldenström's macroglobulinemia*. In this condition, there is excessive production of the respective myeloma proteins (M proteins) and that of their light chains (BJ proteins).

Heavy chain disease is a different disorder. It is a lymphoid neoplasia characterized by the overproduction of the Fc parts of the heavy chains of immunoglobulins.

Cryoglobulinemia is the condition in which the serum from the patient precipitates on cooling and redissolves on warming. It may not always be associated with disease but is often found in patients with myelomas, macroglobulinemias, and auto-immune conditions such as systemic lupus erythematosus. Most cryoglobulins consist of either IgG or IgM or both.

The Complement System

The term **complement** (C) is applied to a system of components present in the serum of man and animals. It consists of nine different proteins denoted C1–C9. The fraction C1 occurs in serum as calcium ion dependent complex, which on chelation with EDTA yields three protein subunits called C1q, C1r and C1s. Thus, C is made up of 11 different proteins. Complement proteins differ in their electrophoretic mobility and molecular weight having sedimentation coefficient ranging from 4S to 11S. These differences permit their separation by physical methods. Though some of its components are stable, C as a whole is heat-labile undergoing spontaneous denaturation slowly at room temperature and in 30 minutes at 56°C. Serum deprived of C activity by heating it at 56°C for 30 minutes is said to be inactivated.

The amount of C present in the serum cannot be increased by immunization. It is, biologically, of considerable importance as an amplifier of immune reactions involving humoral antibodies and is believed to play an important role in the defence of the body against microbial infections. C does not bind to free antigen or antibody but only to antibody which has combined with its antigen. C binding site is located on the C_H2 domain of the Fc portion of IgM and IgG molecules only. These sites are not exposed when antibodies are in the uncombined state. However, after antibody combines with antigen the C binding site is exposed.

A single molecule of IgM can sensitize red cells to C lysis. On the other hand, sensitization by IgG requires that at least two molecules should be bound at adjacent sites on red cell surface. If IgG binding sites are too far apart, as in Rh system, C binding and lysis cannot occur.

C is normally present in the body in an inactive form but can be activated to form an enzyme cascade. The cascade is a series of reactions in which the preceding components act as enzymes on the succeeding components cleaving them into dissimilar fragments. The larger fragments join the cascade and the smaller fragments are released which often possess biological effects which contribute to defence mechanism by:

- Initiating an inflammatory response.
- Causing the destruction of parasites, bacteria, virus-infected cells or red blood cells.
- Clearing dead cells and immune complexes.
- Detoxifying endotoxins.
- Effecting release of histamine from mast cells.

There are two **activation mechanisms** through which complement system executes its role. These are known as classical pathway and alternative or properdin pathway. The former requires the presence of antibody for activation. In contrast, the alternative pathway does not need antibody and can be triggered by the mere presence of bacterial or viral components. For example, the lipopolysaccharide layer of Gram-negative bacterial cell wall is enough to activate alternative pathway. However, both these pathways lead to the same physiological consequences, i.e., opsonization, cellular activation and lysis. But the initiation process is different. Component C3 forms the connection between the two pathways and the binding of the molecule to the surface is the key process in complement activation.

Classical pathway of complement activation

Activation of classical pathway of complement requires the presence of antibody, either IgM or IgG, bound to cell surface antigen or as an antigen-antibody immune complex. All the 11 proteins of the complement comprise the classical complement pathway. All are designated by C followed by the number of the component (complement's protein). Inactive components are described as C1, C2, C3 and so on. Activated forms are designated by placing a bar over the number, for example, $\overline{C2}$ represents activated C2 which is actually C2b.

The classical pathway (Fig. 11.1) is initiated when C1 interacts with the Fc portion of either cell-bound Ig (IgG or

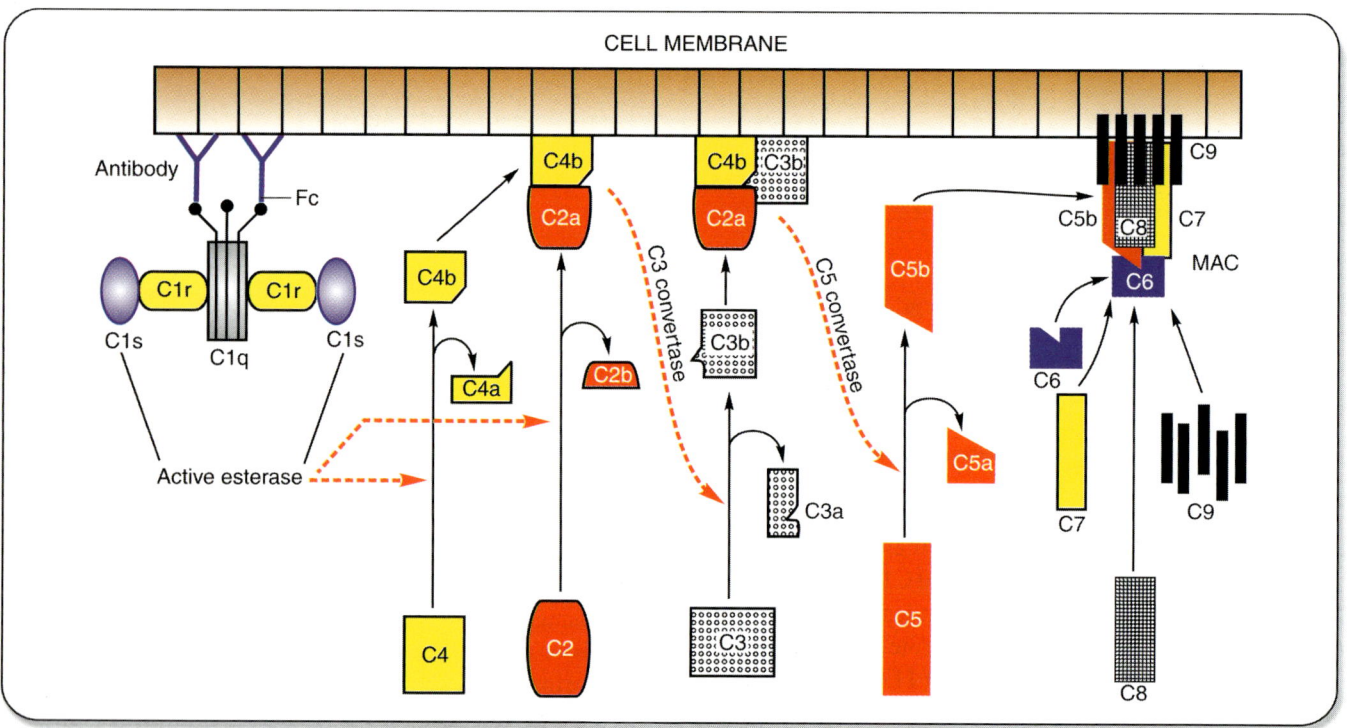

Fig. 11.1. Classical pathway of complement activation.

IgM) or immune complex. This interaction results in the sequential activation of C4, C2 and C3 and leads to the formation of complex cleaving enzymes. Activation of C5, C6, C7, C8 and C9 then completes the cascade and results in the formation of the **C5 to C9 membrane attack complex (MAC)**, which can lyse the cell. C1 is composed of one molecule of C1q, and two molecules each of C1r and C1s. C1q binds to Fc portion of the antibody molecule. Binding of this component of C1 causes a conformational change in the C1 complex that leads to the autoactivation of C1r.

This then converts C1s into an active esterase that acts on C4 to produce C4a and a reactive C4b. C4a is released and less than 1% of the C4b becomes attached to the cell membrane. Unbound molecules of C4b are rapidly inactivated. C1s also cleaves C2 into two components – C2a, larger component, and C2b, smaller component. C2a attaches itself to membrane-bound C4b to form a new active protease, C4b2a , which is called C3 convertase since it can bind and cleave the next inactive complement component in the sequence, C3.

The newly formed C3 convertase, $\overline{C4b2a}$ cleaves C3 into two fragments, C3a and C3b. The larger C3b fragment attaches to both the cell membrane and $\overline{C4b2a}$ complex, while the smaller fragment, C3a, is released to the body fluids. C3a has chemotactic and anaphylatoxic properties. $\overline{C4b2a3b}$ is termed C5 convertase. It cleaves C5 into two products, C5a and C5b. C5a which is a powerful chemotactant of neutrophils and monocytes and has anaphylatoxic activity is released when

formed and C5b attaches to the cell membrane. The binding of $\overline{C5b}$ leads to the uncovering of a binding site for C6 and C7 on the molecule, producing a stable complex $\overline{C5b67}$.

This trimolecular complex attaches to the membrane surface and enables C8 to join. C8 then binds several C9 molecules. About 10–18 protein units of C9 attach to $\overline{C5b678}$ base to form a long hollow tube. This is a stable complex and is referred to as membrane attack complex (MAC). This creates a membrane pore or lesion, that is 100 Å in diameter leading to cell death. Pores in the cell membrane created by MAC may also permit degradative enzymes in the area to enter and destroy cellular organelles contributing to target cell death.

Alternative or properdin pathway of complement activation

This pathway does not require the presence of specific antibodies. C3 is the major component of C. In the classical pathway, activation of C3 is achieved by the C3 convertase ($\overline{C4b2a}$). *The activation of C3, without the prior participation of C142, is known as the alternative or properdin pathway of complement activation.* The overall result of this pathway is the same as that of classical pathway but the C3 and C5 convertases for alternative pathway are different from those of classical pathway. A wide range of chemically unrelated substances are known to activate alternative pathway. These (other than antigen-antibody complexes) include:

- Yeast cell walls.
- Bacterial endotoxins.
- Rabbit (not sheep) RBCs.
- Snake venom proteins.
- A protein termed 'nephritic factor' found in the serum of patients with diseases such as glomerulonephritis.

The fact that these products can activate the alternative pathway directly, without the need of antibody is of considerable importance because it allows for defence against infection prior to initiation of an immune response.

There are at least three normal serum proteins that, when activated together with C3, form a functional C3 convertase and a C5 convertase. These are factor B, factor D and properdin. These are normal serum proteins, and the alternative pathway is routinely being activated in the absence of any stimulus. In the absence of initiators, the initial complexes of the alternative pathway are rapidly destroyed. In the presence of the initiators, such complexes are stabilized and complement is activated to form the MAC as in case of classical pathway.

Intrinsically, C3 undergoes a low level of hydrolysis of an internal thioester bond to generate C3b. Nonimmune activators, such as repeating polysaccharide units or the lipopolysaccharide found on the cell walls of some microbes split up C3 into C3a and C3b. There are a wide variety of pathogens that can be recognized within minutes after they come in contact with plasma. Organisms sensitive to attack by the alternative pathway include bacteria, fungi, certain viruses, virus-infected cells, parasites and certain tumour cells. C3b, in the presence of Mg^{++}, binds to these foreign surfaces and interacts with plasma protein factor B forming C3bB (Fig. 11.2).

The factor B portion of C3bB complex is split by factor D into two fragments, Ba and Bb. Ba is released during reaction and Bb remains bound to C3b forming C3bBb. The newly formed $\overline{C3bBb}$ is a C3 convertase of alternative pathway. $\overline{C3bBb}$ splits more C3 to C3a and C3b. The newly formed C3b binds more factor B. This continues until the membrane surface is saturated with $\overline{C3bBb}$. The result is opsonization of the cell or particle by neutrophils. The soluble C3a, that is released upon cleavage of C3, has chemotactic and anaphylatoxic activity, which can initiate an inflammatory response. C3 convertase ($\overline{C3bBb}$) can bind additional C3b to produce C5 convertase ($\overline{C3bBb3b}$). This activates terminal lytic complement sequence, C5 to C9.

Thus, activation of either classical or alternative pathway leads to the formation of C3 convertases ($\overline{C4b2a}$ or $\overline{C3bBb}$). These cleave C3 into C3a and C3b. The latter combines with C3 convertases forming C5 convertases ($\overline{C4b2a3b}$ or $\overline{C3bBb3b}$). These split C5 into C5a and C5b. C5b then binds C6, C7, C8 and several molecules of C9 to form MAC which initiates lysis of target cells in both pathways.

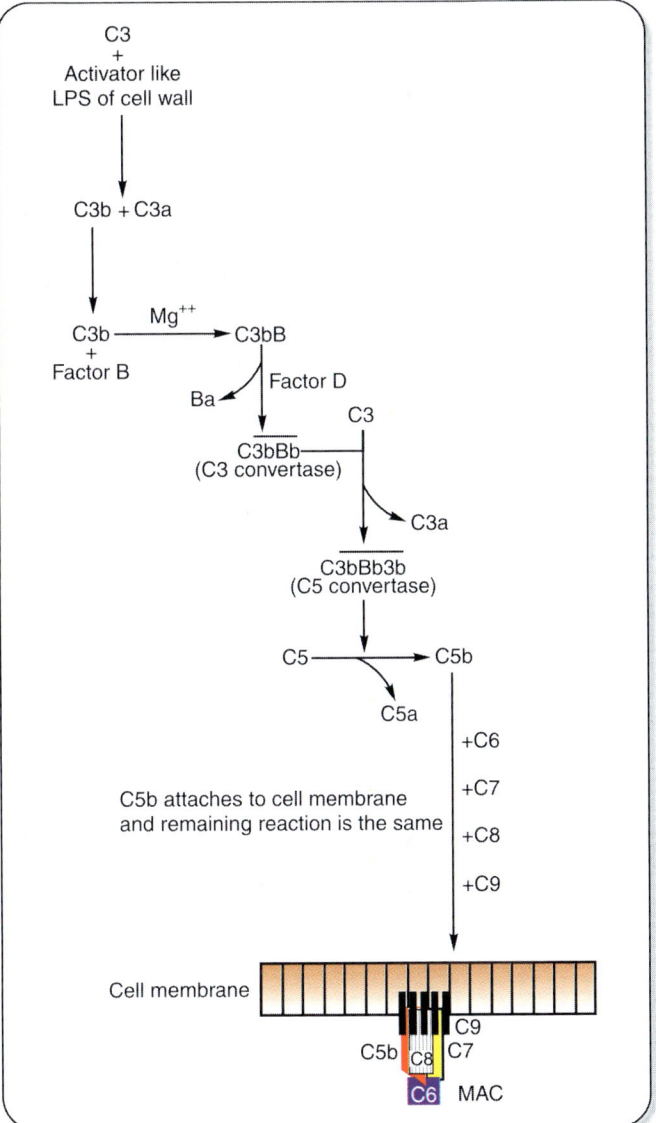

Fig. 11.2. Alternative pathway of complement activation.

Biological effects of complement

1. Complement mediates **immunological membrane damage**. This results in bacteriolysis and cytolysis. Different cells vary in their susceptibility to complement-mediated lysis. Gram-negative bacteria are generally sensitive to lysis, while Gram-positive are killed without lysis. Neutralization of certain viruses requires the participation of C, e.g., neutralization of herpes virus by IgM antibody requires the binding of C1, C4 and possibly C3 too.

2. C fragments released during cascade reaction help in **amplifying the inflammatory response**. Proteolytic cleavage of C3 and C5, in either the classical or alternative pathway, generates two potent mediators of inflammation, C3a and C5a. Mast cells and basophils possess receptors

for C3a and C5a. Binding of C3a or C5a to these receptors causes these cells to release histamine. This may lead to contraction of the uterus, trachea, arteries, atrium of the heart and intestines, and increased vascular permeability leading to oedema. C5a, in addition exerts a series of unique effects on white blood cells. These include:

- Degranulation and lysosomal enzyme release.
- Promotes adherence of granulocytes to the endothelium.
- Induces chemotactic migration of granulocytes.

$\overline{C5b67}$ is also chemotactic. C4a has weak anaphylatoxic activity. It is weakly spasmogenic and increases vascular permeability. Therefore, redness, pain, swelling and heat of inflammation is due to the action of C4a, C3a, C5a and histamine.

3. Phagocytes such as macrophages, monocytes and neutrophils possess surface receptors for C3b. If immune complexes have activated the complement system, the C3b bound to them facilitates their recognition and ingestion by these phagocytes. This facilitated phagocytosis is referred to as **opsonization**.

4. Complement participates in **type II (cytotoxic)** and **type III (immune complex) hypersensitivity** reactions. The destruction of erythrocytes, following incompatible blood transfusion is an example of type II hypersensitivity. Participation of C is required for the production of immune complex diseases such as serum sickness and Arthus reaction (type III hypersensitivity).

5. Several serum C components are lowered in many autoimmune diseases such as systemic lupus erythematosus and rheumatoid arthritis. These may, therefore, be involved in the pathogenesis of autoimmune diseases. C plays a major role in the pathogenesis of autoimmune haemolytic anaemia, paroxysmal nocturnal haemoglobinuria and hereditary angioneurotic oedema.

6. C3 and C6 participate in coagulation process.

7. C bound to antigen-antibody complexes adheres to erythrocytes. This is known as **immune adherence**. It contributes to defence against pathogenic microorganisms as such adherent particles are rapidly phagocytosed. C3 and C4 are necessary for immune adherence.

Antigen-Antibody Reactions

When an antigen is mixed with its specific antibody, in the presence of electrolytes at a suitable temperature and pH, they combine with each other in an observable manner.

Precipitation reactions

Precipitation

When a soluble antigen is mixed with its specific antibody in the presence of electrolytes at a suitable temperature and pH, the antigen-antibody complex forms an insoluble precipitate. This precipitate usually settles down at the bottom of the tube. Precipitation can take place in liquid media and in gels such as agar, agarose and polyacrylamide. The process of precipitation can be hastened by electrically driving the antigen and antibody.

Flocculation

When, instead of sedimenting, the precipitate remains suspended as floccules, the reaction is called flocculation.

Zone phenomenon

If a series (10–12) of tubes is set up (Fig. 12.1), each containing a constant amount of antiserum, and increasing amounts of antigen are added to the tubes in the row, precipitation will be found to occur most rapidly and abundantly in one of the middle tubes, in which antigen and antibody are in optimal or equivalent proportion. In the preceding tubes, in which the antibody is in excess, and in the later tubes, in which the antigen is in excess, the precipitation will be weak or absent. Therefore, the amount of precipitation will be seen to increase along the row, reaching a maximum and then falling off with higher antigen concentration.

If the amounts of precipitate in different tubes are plotted on a graph, the resulting curve will have **three phases** – an ascending part (**prozone** or **zone of antibody excess**), a peak (**zone of equivalence**), and a descending part (**postzone** or **zone of antigen excess**). This is called **zone phenomenon**.

Assay of supernatant solution will show that those tubes containing too little antigen still contain free antibody and in the tubes with antigen excess, little precipitate forms, although soluble immune complexes and free antigens are present in the supernatant fluid. Only in tubes of maximum precipitation is all antibody removed from solution. *The prozone is of importance is clinical serology, as sera rich in antibody may sometimes give a false negative result, unless several dilutions are tested.*

If immune complexes form in serum, monocytes, neutrophils and eosinophils attempt to remove them. Complexes formed at equivalence or antibody excess are easily removed. However, small, soluble complexes formed in antigen excess are more difficult to remove. These might gain entrance to tissues, such as glomeruli of kidneys or become deposited within vessel walls causing varying degree of damage.

Applications of precipitation and flocculation reactions

Some of the precipitation and flocculation tests which have application in diagnostic bacteriology are as under:

Ring test

This test is done by layering antigen solution over a column of antiserum in a capillary tube. After a short while a ring of precipitate forms at the interface. *Typing of streptococci and pneumococci, C-reactive protein test* and *Ascoli's thermo-precipitin test* for the diagnosis of anthrax, are some of the uses of ring test.

Slide test

This is an example of flocculation test. When a drop each of antigen and antiserum are placed on a slide and mixed by shaking, floccules appear. *VDRL, a most widely used test* for the diagnosis of syphilis, is an example of slide flocculation test.

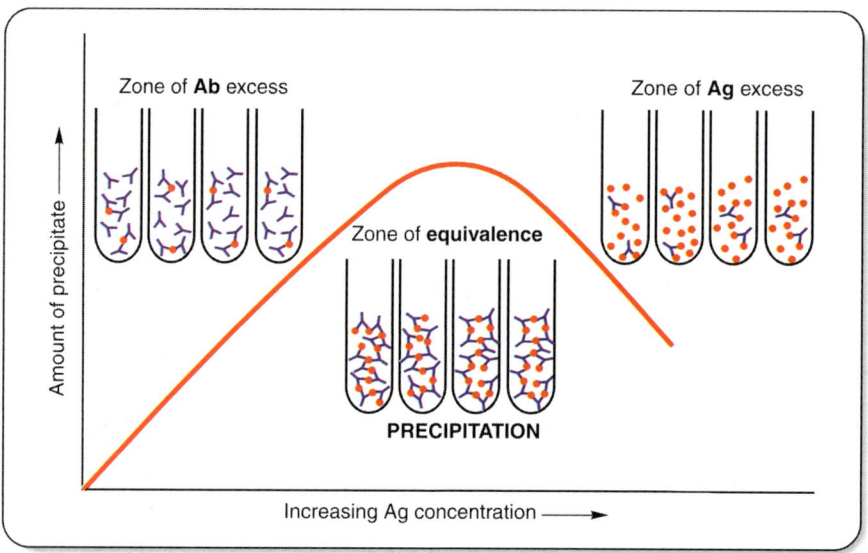

Fig. 12.1. Zone phenomenon.

Tube test

Flocculation test can be carried out in the tubes also. *Kahn test* for the diagnosis of syphilis, and *standardization of toxins and toxoids* are examples of tube flocculation.

Immunodiffusion (precipitation in gel)

When an antibody and its antigen are placed in an agar gel they diffuse towards each other and form an opaque band of precipitation at the junction of their diffusion front. Precipitation in gel has several advantages over precipitation in liquid medium:

- The reaction appears as a distinct band of precipitation which can be stained for better visibility and preservation.
- Since each antigen-antibody reaction gives rise to one line of precipitation, therefore, different number of antigens in a mixture can be detected.
- This technique also indicates *identity*, *cross-reaction* and *nonidentity* between different antigens.

Types of immunodiffusion tests

1. Single diffusion in one dimension (Oudin procedure)

Antibody is incorporated in agar gel in a test tube. Antigen solution is then layered over it. The antigen diffuses down-wards and wherever it reaches in optimum concentration with antibody a line of precipitation is formed (Fig. 12.2A). As more antigen diffuses, the line of precipitation moves down-wards. Number of lines of precipitation indicates the number of antigens and antibodies present.

2. Double diffusion in one dimension (Oakley-Fulthorpe procedure)

Antibody is incorporated in agar gel in a test tube. Above this is placed a column of plain agar which, in turn, is overlaid with antigen, either as liquid or incorporated into agar (Fig. 12.2B). Antigen and antibody diffuse (double diffusion) towards each other (in one dimension) through the intervening column of plain agar and form a band of precipitation where they meet in optimum concentration.

3. Single diffusion in two dimensions (radial immunodiffusion)

This method is used to quantitate the amount of a specific antigen present in a sample and can be used for many antigens. The most widely used diagnostic application of this procedure is to measure the amount of various Ig classes (IgG, IgA, IgM, IgD and IgE) in patient serum.

Here monospecific antiserum (antiserum containing only antibody against the antigen which is to be assayed) is incorporated in agar gel. It is poured on a glass slide or a petri dish and a number of wells are punched into it, and different dilutions of the antigen are placed into various wells. As the antigen diffuses from the well, a ring of precipitate forms at that position where antigen and antibody are in optimal proportions. Larger the concentration of antigen, the farther it diffuses to be in optimal proportions with the antibody incorporated in the gel. Therefore, the diameter of the ring gives the estimate of the concentration of the antigen (Fig. 12.2C).

Using known concentrations of the antigen in question, one can prepare a standard curve by plotting the diameter of the precipitin ring versus antigen concentration. With this standard plot, one needs only to measure the diameter of the precipitin ring formed with the unknown antigen to calculate its concentration. Radial immunodiffusion is used for the laboratory diagnosis of multiple myeloma or agamma-globulinaemia.

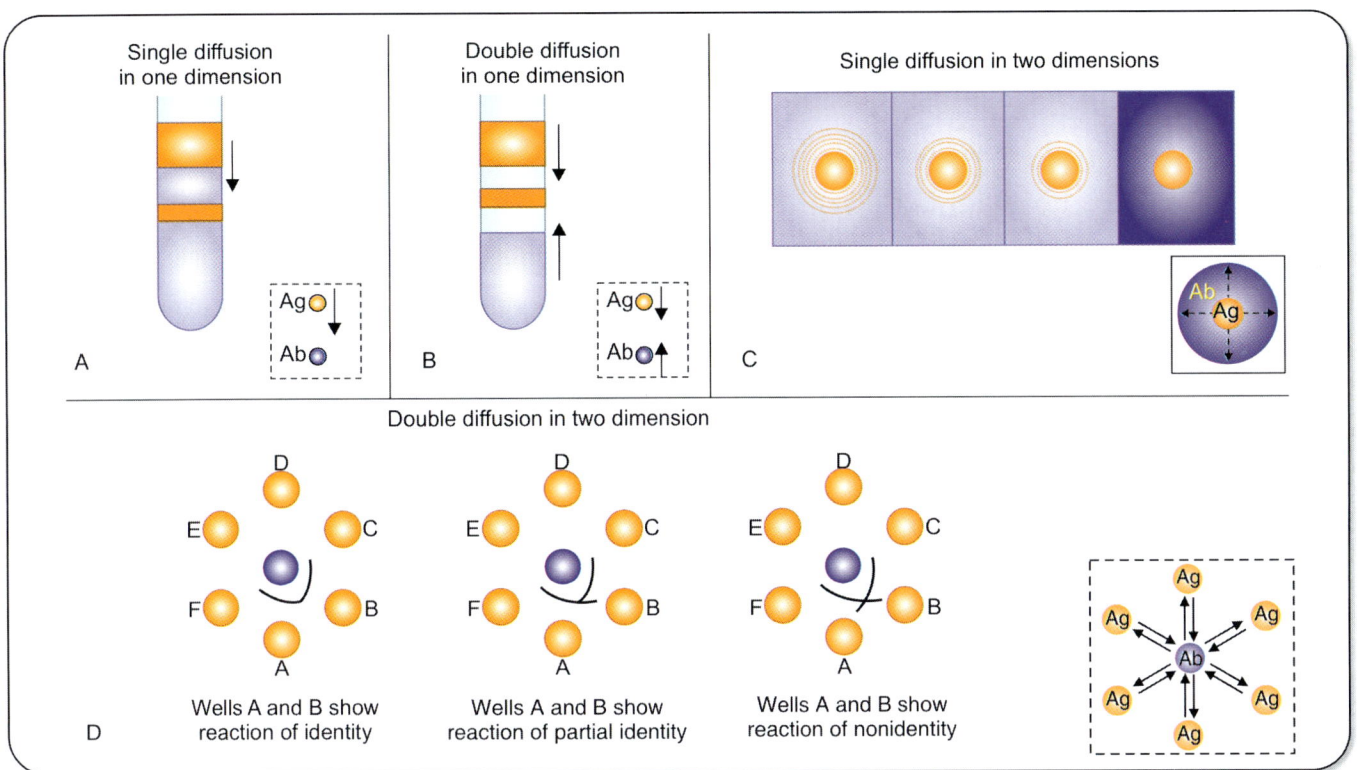

Fig. 12.2. Immunodiffusion tests.

4. Double diffusion in two dimensions (Ouchterlony procedure)

Agar is poured on the slide and wells, usually seven, are punched in it using a template. The known antiserum is placed in the central well and different antigens in surrounding wells. One of these contains known positive antigen. It acts as a positive control. This technique is also useful for comparing different antigens for the presence of identical or cross-reacting components. The samples are placed in adjacent wells, and the corresponding antibody is placed in the central well.

1. **Reaction of identity:** If two precipitin bands fuse completely (Fig. 12.2D), the pattern is termed reaction of identity. It indicates that the antigens in the adjoining wells are identical.
2. **Reaction of nonidentity:** If unrelated antigens are placed in adjacent wells, they diffuse towards central well containing antibodies for both, the two precipitin bands form independently and cross each other. This is known as reaction of nonidentity.
3. **Reaction of partial identity:** If the antigens in the two adjacent wells are cross-reacting (partial identity), the precipitation bands fuse but form a spurlike projection. This is known as reaction of partial identity.

A special variety of double diffusion in two dimensions is the **Elek's test** for toxigenicity of diphtheria bacilli (see chapter 22).

5. Immunoelectrophoresis

Immunoelectrophoresis combines electrophoresis and immunodiffusion (immune precipitation in gel). This method can be used for analyzing complex antigens in biological fluids. A glass slide is covered with molten agar or agarose. A well for antigen and a trough for antiserum is cut on it (Fig. 12.3). Antigen well is filled with antigen mixture (human serum). The slide is then placed in an electric field for about an hour to allow for the electrophoretic migration of various antigens. Different antigens will migrate at different rates or even in different directions, depending upon their size and charge and the conditions of electrophoresis.

After the completion of electrophoresis, antiserum trough is filled with appropriate antiserum (antiserum to whole human serum). Antigens and antibodies diffuse towards each other, resulting in the formation of precipitin bands, for individual antigens and antibodies, whenever they are both in zones of optimal proportions, in 18–24 hours. Because immunoelectrophoresis uses electric charge in addition to diffusion, it is more likely to separate antigen than is simple diffusion alone. By this method, over 30 different antigens can be identified in human serum. This technique is useful for detection of normal and abnormal serum proteins.

6. Electroimmunodiffusion

Immunodiffusion is a slow process. The development of precipitin lines can be speeded up by electrically driving anti-

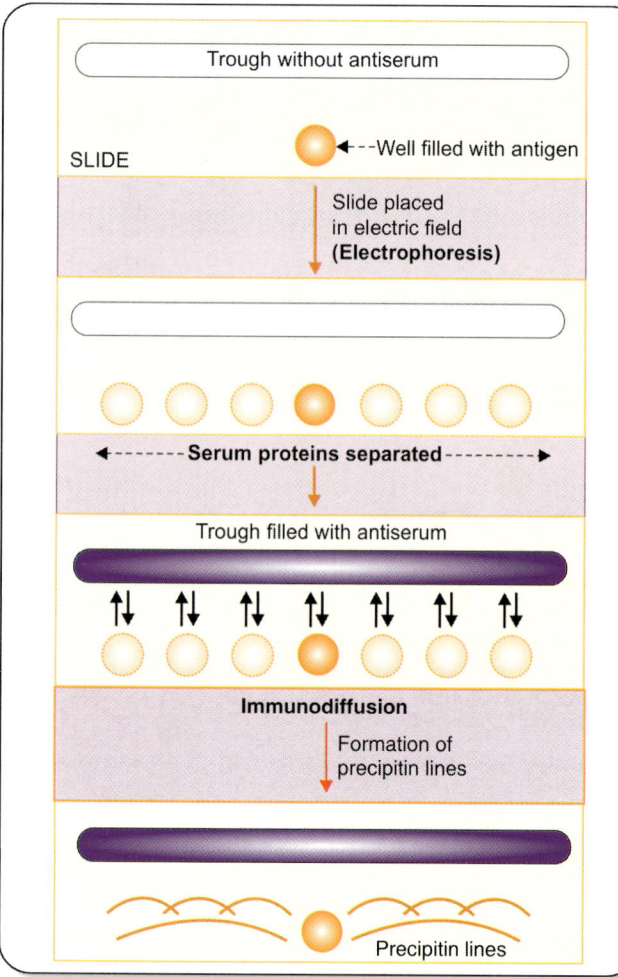

Fig. 12.3. Immunoelectrophoresis.

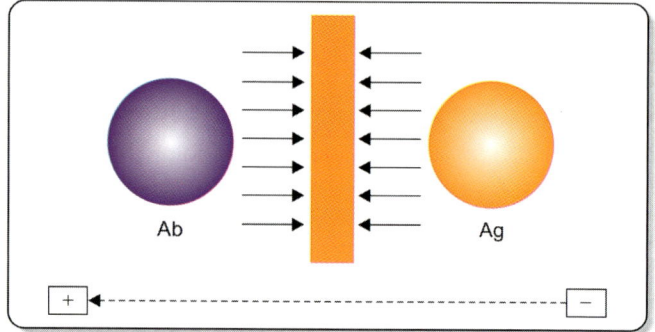

Fig. 12.4. Counterimmunoelectrophoresis.

gens and antibodies in a gel, rather than simply allowing them to come in contact by diffusion. Of these, one dimensional double electroimmunodiffusion and one dimensional single electroimmunodiffusion are used frequently in the clinical laboratory.

I. *One dimensional double electroimmunodiffusion (counterimmunoelectrophoresis or CIE):* This method can be used for those antigens and antibodies that migrate in opposite directions in electric field. The wells are punched about 1 cm apart in an agar slab on a glass plate. Antigen and antibody solutions are placed in wells towards cathode and anode sides respectively. Electric field is then applied electrophoresing both antigens and antibodies from separate wells. The antigen migrates towards antibody and antibody migrates towards antigen. A precipitin band is formed, in between the two wells, where they meet in optimum proportions (Fig. 12.4). This method has several advantages over simple diffusion in agar:

• The electrophoresis focuses the reactants into a small area allowing the detection of small quantities of antigens and antibodies. Therefore, **it is 10 times more sensitive than simple diffusion in agar**.

• It is a rapid assay. Precipitin bands may form in just 30 minutes.

This method is used for detection of various antigens such as:

• hepatitis B surface antigen (HBsAg) and alpha-fetoprotein in serum;

• meningococcal and cryptococcal antigens in CSF; and

• anti-DNA antibody in the serum of patients with several autoimmune disorders.

II. *One dimensional single electroimmunodiffusion (rocket electrophoresis):* As in case of radial immuno-diffusion, wells are cut in an agarose gel slab on a glass plate. Agarose contains the antiserum to the antigen of interest. The antigen, in increasing concentrations, is placed in wells. The antigen is then electrophoresed into the agarose containing antibody that does not migrate. The pattern of immuno-precipitation resembles a rocket (hence the name), since precipitation occurs along the moving boundary of antigen, as it migrates into the agarose (Fig. 12.5). The height (distance from the antigen well to the top of the precipitin band) is proportional to the antigen concentration. The main application of this technique, therefore, is for quantitative estimation of antigen.

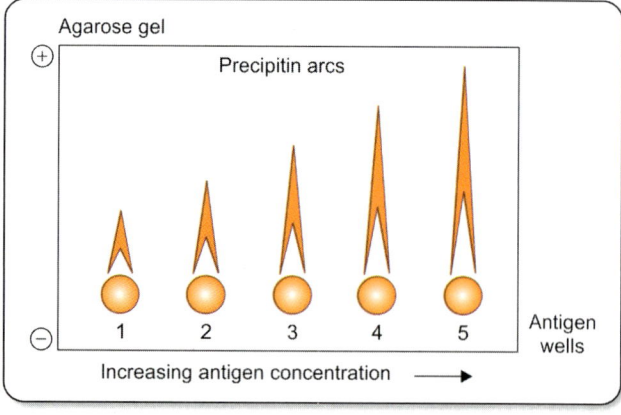

Fig. 12.5. Rocket electrophoresis.

Agglutination reactions

When a particulate antigen or an antigen present on the surface of a cell (red cell or bacterium) or an inorganic particle (e.g., polystyrene latex coated with antigen) is mixed with its antibody in the presence of electrolytes at a suitable temperature and pH, the particles are clumped or agglutinated. Agglutination reaction is more sensitive than precipitation for detection of antibodies.

Prozone phenomenon

False negative agglutination reactions can occur with some antisera in antibody excess (first few dilutions). This is known as prozone phenomenon. Unagglutinated cells in prozone actually have antibody molecules adsorbed on their surface, with both sites of bivalent antibody attached to the same cell resulting into poor or no lattice formation.

Blocking antibodies

Occasionally, antibodies (e.g., anti-Rh and anti-*Brucella*) are formed that react with the antigenic determinants on a cell but do not cause agglutination. Such antibodies are called blocking antibodies, because they inhibit agglutination by complete antibody added subsequently.

Applications of agglutination reactions

Slide agglutination

A drop of saline is placed on a clean glass slide and a small amount of culture from a solid medium is emulsified in it by means of inoculating loop. It is then examined through a hand lens or low-power microscope that the suspension is even and bacteria are not autoagglutinable. Then with a platinum loop a drop of specific antiserum is placed on the slide near the bacterial suspension. The serum and the bacterial suspension are then mixed and examined with naked eye or with hand lens or under low-power microscope for the evidence of agglutination within a minute. Slide agglutination test is rapid and convenient, but in order to obtain rapid agglutination serum is used undiluted or in low dilutions.

Uses:
- Identification of bacterial isolates (e.g., *Salmonella* spp., *Shigella* spp. and *Vibrio cholerae*) from clinical specimens. This method is practicable only when clumping of organisms occurs instantaneously or within a minute because clumping occurring after a minute may be due to drying of the fluid.
- Blood grouping and cross matching.

Tube agglutination

This is done in round-bottomed test tubes or perspex plates with round-bottomed wells. A fixed volume of a particulate antigen suspension is added to an equal volume of serial dilutions of the patient serum in test tubes or perspex plates. Following several hours of incubation at 37°C, agglutination

is seen at the bottom of the tubes. **The titre of the serum is given as the reciprocal of the highest dilution that causes clumping.** Thus, the serum that agglutinates at a dilution of 1 : 256 is reported to have a titre of 256 and if the test has been carried out in 1 ml volumes, the titre of the serum is 256 units/ml of serum.

Uses:

Serological diagnosis of:
- Enteric fever (Widal test)
- Brucellosis
- Typhus fever (Weil-Felix reaction)
- *Streptococcus* MG agglutination
- Cold agglutination
- Paul-Bunnell test

In the **Widal test** used for the diagnosis of enteric fever, two types of antigens are used – the flagellar (H) antigen and somatic (O) antigen. H antigen is a formolised suspension of the organisms which on combination with antibody, forms large, loose and fluffy clumps resembling wisps of cotton-wool. For H agglutination conical (Dreyer's) tubes are used. O antigen is prepared by treating the bacterial suspension with alcohol. On combination with antibody it forms fine granular deposit resembling chalk powder at the base of round-bottomed (Felix) tubes, whereas, negative reaction shows a compact button-like deposit (Fig. 12.6).

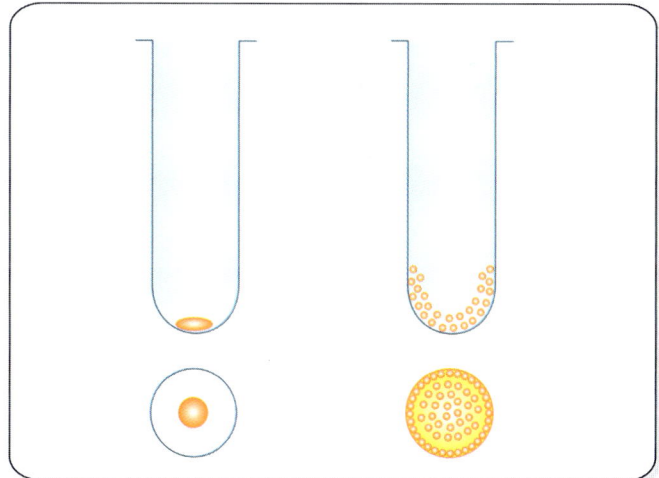

Fig. 12.6. Tube agglutination test.

Heterophile agglutination

Weil-Felix reaction for serodiagnosis of typhus fever and *Streptococcus* **MG agglutination** for the diagnosis of primary atypical pneumonia are the examples of **heterophile agglutination test**. Red blood cells are used as antigens in **cold agglutination** and **Paul-Bunnell test**. IgM antibodies capable of agglutinating human red cells at 0–4°C (cold agglutinins) are sometimes found in certain human diseases including primary atypical pneumonia, malaria, trypano-somiasis and acquired haemolytic anaemia. Sera of the patients suffering from infectious mononucleosis agglutinate sheep RBCs (see Chapter 10).

Antiglobulin (Coombs') test

Anti-Rh antibodies are of IgG type, but they normally do not agglutinate Rh-positive RBCs (incomplete antibodies). The inability of these antibodies to agglutinate is perhaps due to the presence of insufficient antigenic determinants on the RBCs to permit the antibody to overcome the normal electro-static repulsion that exists among RBCs. When sera containing incomplete anti-Rh antibodies are mixed with Rh-positive red cells, the antibody coats the surface of erythrocytes but they are not agglutinated. When such antibody-coated erythrocytes are washed to free all unattached protein and are treated with anti-human gammaglobulin (**antiglobulin or Coombs' serum**), the cells are agglutinated.

Coombs' test is of two types – direct and indirect.

1. **Direct Coombs' test:** The sensitization of erythrocytes with incomplete antibodies takes place *in vivo* as in case of haemolytic disease of newborn due to Rh incompatibility. Therefore, when washed RBCs from such patient are mixed with antiglobulin or Coombs' serum, agglutination takes place.
2. **Indirect Coombs' test:** The sensitization of RBCs with incomplete antibodies is performed *in vitro*. Rh-positive RBCs are mixed with the serum to be tested for Rh-anti-bodies and then after a short incubation and washing, anti-globulin or Coombs' serum is added. If the test serum contained anti-Rh antibodies, agglutination will take place.

Uses of Coombs' test

- Detection of anti-Rh antibodies
- Demonstration of nonagglutinating antibodies in brucellosis

Passive (indirect) agglutination

A precipitation reaction can be converted into agglutination reaction by coating soluble antigen onto the surface of carrier particles such as RBCs, latex, bentonite and gelatin particles. Such test is more convenient and more sensitive for detection of antibodies. Most polysaccharide and lipopolysaccharide antigens may be adsorbed by simple mixing with the cells. For adsorption of protein antigens, tanned red cells are used. Some of the examples of passive agglutination are given below:

- In rheumatoid arthritis, **RA factor** (an antigammaglobulin autoantibody) appears in the serum of the patient. It acts as an antibody to human IgG. Latex polystyrene beads coated with denatured human IgG when mixed with patient serum leads to agglutination of latex polystyrene beads.
- Latex particles coated with antibodies to meningococci, *Haemophilus influenzae* type b and pneumococci can be

used to detect corresponding antigens in cases of **pyogenic meningitis**.

- Latex agglutination tests are also widely used for detection of hepatitis B, antistreptolysin O, C-reactive protein, human chorionic gonadotropin hormone and many other antigens.
- One of the most widely used passive agglutination tests employing erythrocytes is *Treponema pallidum* **haem-agglutination (TPHA)** for serological diagnosis of treponemal infection.
- For the detection of **anti-HIV antibodies**, gelatin particles can be sensitized (coated) with inactivated HIV antigen. When these sensitized particles are mixed with the patient serum or plasma these particles are agglutinated if the anti-HIV antibodies are present in the sample. The test procedure is extremely simple using a microtitre technique and is particularly suitable for mass screening of specimens. The test is time-saving and results are readable by the naked eye after about two hours.

When, instead of antigen, antibody is adsorbed on the carrier particles in tests for estimation of antigens, the technique is known as **reversed passive agglutination**.

Coagglutination

This is based upon the principle that most strains of *Staphylococcus aureus* (especially Cowan strain I) possess protein A on their surface. Protein A binds IgG molecules, non-specifically, through Fc region leaving specific Fab sites free to combine with specific antigen. When suspension of such sensitized staphylococcal cells is treated with homo-logous (test) antigen, the antigen combines with free Fab sites of IgG attached to staphylococcal cells leading to visible clumping of staphylococci within two minutes. This is known as coagglutination (COA).

COA test can be used for detecting the presence of bacterial antigens in serum, urine and CSF. For example, typhoid bacillus antigen is consistently present in the blood in the early phase of disease, and also in the urine of the patients. This antigen can be detected by COA test. Similarly, meningococcal, pneumococcal and *Haemophilus* antigens can be detected by COA test in the CSF. Identification of *Neisseria gonorrhoeae* and serogrouping of b-haemolytic streptococci A, B, C, D and G can also be carried out by COA test.

Complement fixation test (CFT)

The ability of antigen-antibody complexes to fix complement is made use of in complement fixation test (CFT). This is a very versatile and sensitive test. This can detect as little as 0.04 µg of antibody nitrogen and 0.1 µg of antigen. CFTs include **Wassermann reaction** and **Reiter protein comple-ment fixation test (RPCFT)** for the serodiagnosis of syphilis. Similarly, CFTs for the identification of various viral antigens are also available.

In most of the cases fixation of complement with antigen-antibody complex causes in itself no visible effect. Therefore, it is necessary to use an indicator system consisting of sheep red cells coated with anti-sheep red cell antibody. Complement lyses antibody coated red cells. CFT, therefore, is performed in two stages.

Stage 1: Test serum (for the detection of antibody) and the antigen are mixed in the presence of carefully measured amount of complement and then incubated at 37°C for 1 hour. If the test serum contains antibody then antigen-antibody complexes are formed and complement gets fixed on it.

Stage 2: Indicator system, antibody-coated sheep red cells, is added to determine whether the complement has been fixed in stage 1 reaction or not. If the complement has been taken up during stage 1 reaction then it will not be available to lyse the red cells. Therefore, a positive CFT is indicated by absence of lysis of red cells whilst a negative test, with unused complement, is shown by lysis of the red cells (Fig. 12.7).

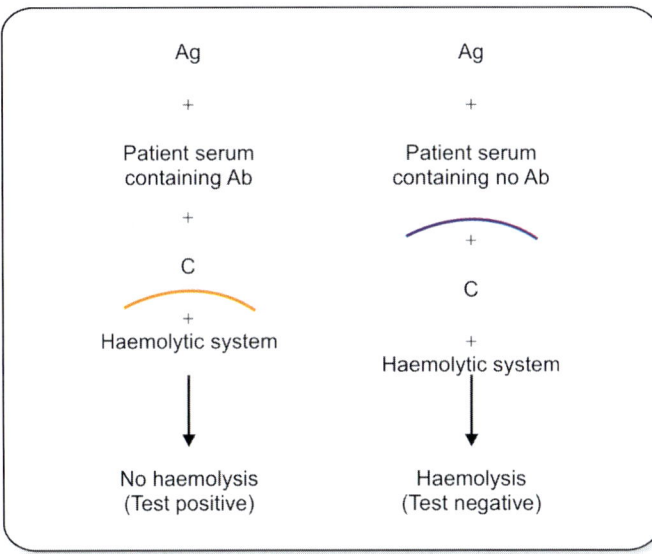

Fig. 12.7. Complement fixation test.

Neutralization tests

These are of two types – virus neutralization tests and toxin neutralization tests.

Virus neutralization tests

Neutralization of viruses by their antibodies in a patient serum may be quantitated by their ability to reduce the infectivity of a stock virus preparation. The test serum is diluted serially, incubated with a known amount of virus and the mixture is then added to indicator systems – animals, embryonated hen's egg and tissue culture. The highest dilution of serum ablating infectivity in 50% of virus-serum mixtures tested is taken as the titre. Neutralization of bacteriophages can be demonstrated by plaque inhibition test. When bacteriophages are seeded in appropriate dilution on lawn cultures, plaques of lysis are produced. Specific antiphage serum inhibits plaque formation.

Toxin neutralization

Bacterial exotoxins are highly antigenic and their activity may be completely neutralized by appropriate concentrations of specific antibody. Antibody to bacterial exotoxin is usually referred to as antitoxin. Bacterial endotoxins are poorly antigenic and their toxicity is not neutralized by antisera.

The neutralizing capacity of an antitoxin can be assayed by neutralization test, in which mixture of toxin and antitoxin is injected into a susceptible animal, and the least amount of antitoxin that prevents death or disease in the animal is estimated. In case of diphtheria toxin, which in small doses causes cutaneous reaction, neutralization test can be carried out on the human skin. The Schick test is based on the ability of circulating antitoxin to neutralize the diphtheria toxin given intradermally. Neutralization (no reaction) indicates immunity, and erythema and induration indicates susceptibility to diphtheria.

If a toxin has a demonstrable *in vitro* effect, this effect can be neutralized by specific antitoxin. For example, **antistreptolysin O**, present in the serum of the patient suffering from *Streptococcus pyogenes* infection, neutralizes the haemolytic activity of the streptococcal O haemolysin. Another example of *in vitro* toxin-antitoxin neutralization is **Nagler's reaction**. *Clostridium perfringens* produces α-toxin which is a phospholipase (lecithinase-C). This produces opalescence in serum or egg yolk media. This reaction is specifically neutralized by the antitoxin.

Opsonization

A substance, such as complement or antibody, that can bind to the surface of a cell or a particle, making it more readily phagocytosed is known as opsonin. Enhanced complement-mediated phagocytosis can occur either in the presence or absence of antibody. Phagocytes such as macrophages, monocytes and neutrophils possess surface receptors (CR1) for C3b and Fc receptors for antibody. If immune complexes have activated the complement system then Fc and CR1 receptors, present on the phagocyte, bind Fc region of antibody and C3b bound on immune complexes respectively, thus facilitating their phagocytosis. This facilitated phagocytosis by antibody and complement is known as **immune opsonization** (Fig. 12.8).

In contrast, **nonimmune opsonization** requires only C3b (opsonin) for opsonization. Bacteria in the blood stream can activate the alternative pathway and generate C3b, which coats the bacteria. C3b binds to CR1 receptors present on the phagocytes, thus facilitating their phagocytosis. Viruses, soluble immune complexes and tumour cells are also opsonized and removed by the same mechanism (Fig. 12.8).

Immunofluorescence

Fluorescent dyes absorb invisible UV light between 290–495 nm and emit visible longer wavelength (525 nm) green light. Therefore, if microorganisms or tissue cells are stained with

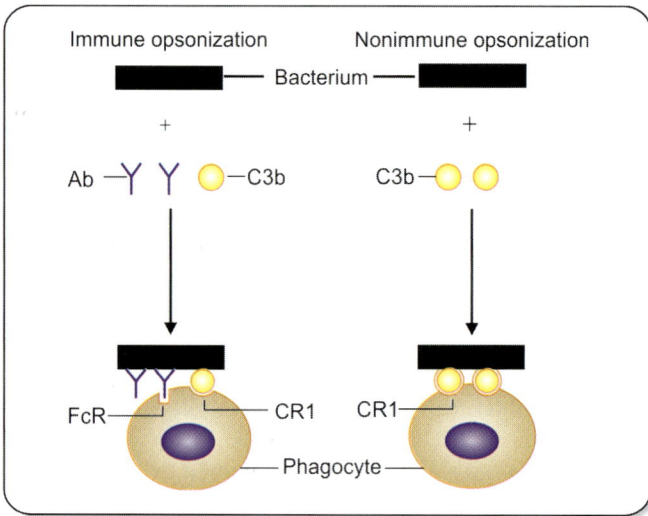

Fig. 12.8. Opsonization.

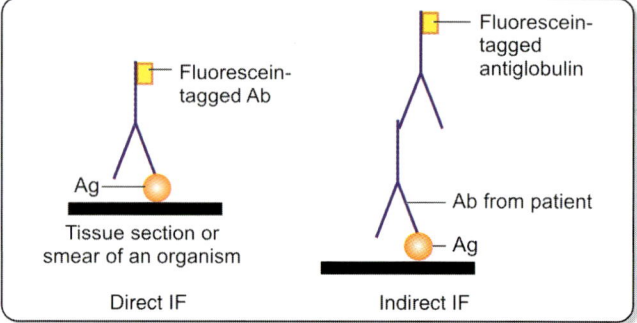

Fig. 12.9. Immunofluorescence.

a fluorescent dye and examined under the microscope with UV light instead of visible light, they are seen as bright objects against a dark background. This principle is used in fluorescence microscopy. Coons and his colleagues (1942) showed that fluorescent dyes, such as fluorescein isothiocyanate (FITC), can be conjugated to antibodies (without affecting their specificity) permitting their ready detection, when attached to an antigen associated with a cell. Immunofluorescence (IF) is now used extensively to detect:

- Tissue antigens.
- Antibodies to tissues including autoantibodies.
- The antigens of infecting organisms in the body.
- Antigen-antibody complexes.

It is more sensitive than precipitation and complement fixation test. Fluorescence can be observed under a fluorescence microscope (FM), which contains a high intensity UV light source (mercury lamp) instead of visible light. Two types of filters are fitted in the FM:

1. *Primary filter:* It is fitted close to the lamp. This ensures the maximum emission of radiation (UV light) of the required wavelengths.
2. *Secondary filter:* It is placed in the eyepiece to cut out UV rays which might damage the observer's eye.

Fluorescence-staining techniques are of two types – direct and indirect (Fig. 12.9).

Direct IF

This consists of bringing fluorescein-tagged antibodies in contact with antigens (bacteria, viruses and other antigens) fixed on a slide (e.g., in the form of a tissue section or a smear of an organism), allowing them to react, washing off excess antibody and examining under FM. The site of union of the labelled antibody with its antigen can be seen by the apple-

green fluorescent areas on the slide. Direct IF is routinely used as a sensitive method of diagnosing rabies, by detection of **rabies virus antigens** in brain smears. **A disadvantage of this method is that separate fluorescent conjugates have to be prepared against each antigen to be tested.**

Indirect IF

This method can be used for detection of specific antibodies in sera or other body fluids and also for identifying antigens. The disadvantage of direct IF, mentioned above, is overcome by this method. An example of this method is the **fluorescent treponemal antibody test for the diagnosis of syphilis.** Here a drop of the patient serum is placed on a smear of *T. pallidum* on a slide and after incubation, the slide is washed well to remove all free serum, leaving behind only antibody, if present, coated on the surface of the treponemes. Whether or not the patient serum contains antibodies to *T. pallidum* is shown by means of a fluorescein-tagged antihuman gammaglobulin (antiglobulin).

If patient serum contains anti-treponemal antibodies fluorescein-tagged antiglobulin will react with it. After washing away all the unbound fluorescent conjugate, when the slide is examined under FM the treponemes will be seen as bright objects against a dark background. If the patient serum is negative for anti-treponemal antibodies, there will be no antibody coating on the treponemes and, therefore, they will not take up the fluorescent conjugate. Therefore, they will not fluoresce. **The advantage of this technique is that a single antihuman gammaglobulin fluorescent conjugate can be employed for detecting human antibody to any antigen.** Indirect IF is also a convenient method for detecting autoantibodies that have bound to membrane antigens, *in vivo*.

The direct method is simple and rapid to perform with fewer nonspecific reactions, however, it is less sensitive. The indirect method is more sensitive and gives brighter fluorescence, however, due to increased cross-reactivity it is less specific.

Radioimmunoassay (RIA)

RIA is a very sensitive and specific method. It involves the use of either antiserum or more usually antigen labelled with

^{125}I. The amount of radioactive label bound to antigen-antibody complex can be measured, and hence the concentration of antigen or antibody in a specimen can be determined. RIA permits measurement of analytes up to picogram (10^{-12} gram) quantities.

Enzyme-linked immunosorbent assay (ELISA) (Fig. 12.10)

1. Indirect ELISA

The principle of this test can be illustrated by outlining its application for detection of anti-HIV-1 and anti-HIV-2 antibodies in the patient serum. The wells of the polystyrene microtitre plate are coated with purified HIV-1 and HIV-2 antigens or synthetic peptides representing immunodominant epitopes of HIV-1 and HIV-2, which constitutes the solid-phase antigen. Diluted test serum or plasma sample is added to such a well and incubated. If antibodies specific for HIV-1 and/or HIV-2 are present in the test sample they will form stable complexes with antigens coated on the well. Well is then washed and a conjugate of goat antihuman immunoglobulin, which has been labelled with the enzyme horseradish peroxidase, is added. If the antigen-antibody complex is present, the peroxidase conjugate will bind to the complex and remains in the well. The conjugate fraction remaining free in the well is removed by washing and the presence of enzyme immobilized on the complexes is shown by incubation in the presence of a colourless enzyme substrate (ortho-phenylene-diamine dihydrochloride solution). Incubation with enzyme substrate produces a yellow-orange colour in the test well. If the sample contains no anti-HIV-1 and/or anti-HIV-2, then the labelled antibody cannot be found and no colour

develops. The absorbance value of each well is read by an ELISA plate reader at wavelength of 492 ± 2 nm.

2. Competitive ELISA

The principle of this test too can be illustrated by outlining its application for detection of anti-HIV antibodies in the patient serum. The wells of the polystyrene microtitre plate are coated with HIV antigens which constitutes the solid-phase antigen. The test sample and human anti-HIV, which has been labelled with the enzyme horseradish peroxidase, are incubated in such a well. When the sample contains no anti-HIV, solid-phase antigen/labelled antibody complex will be formed. The incubation with enzyme substrate produces a yellow-orange colour in the test well. If anti-HIV is present in the test sample, it competes with the labelled antibody for the available solid-phase antigen and no colour or reduced colour develops. Competitive ELISA takes less time than indirect ELISA and no predilution of test serum is required.

3. Sandwich ELISA

The most frequently used ELISA for detecting microbial antigen is the sandwich solid-phase ELISA. It is of two types:

(i) Single antibody or direct sandwich ELISA

Antibody is attached to the solid-phase. The test sample is then exposed to the solid-phase antibody, to which the antigen, if present, will bind. The solid-phase antibody-antigen complex is then rinsed free of unbound test sample and exposed again to antibodies reactive against the test antigen and conjugated with the enzyme. The conjugated antibody will react with the antigen held to the solid-phase by the first antibody, forming an antibody-antigen-antibody sandwich on the solid-phase. The solid-phase sandwich is again separated from unreacted test sample by rinsing. The second antibody (conjugated to an enzyme) can be detected with an appropriate substrate. This is a single antibody or direct sandwich ELISA.

(ii) Double antibody or indirect sandwich ELISA

In the double antibody ELISA the second antibody as above is not conjugated with the enzyme. The second antibody can be detected by treating it with an antiimmunoglobulin-enzyme conjugate. In the double antibody ELISA, the second antibody of the sandwich must be from a different species than the solid-phase antibody, otherwise, the antiimmunoglobulin conjugate reacts with the solid-phase antibody, producing high background activity.

ELISA is a simple and versatile technique. It needs only microlitre quantities of reactants. ELISA kits are commercially available for the detection of anti-HIV, hepatitis B surface antigen and rotavirus.

Chemiluminescence immunoassay (CLIA)

Chemiluminescence refers to a chemical reaction emitting energy in the form of light. As radioactive conjugates are

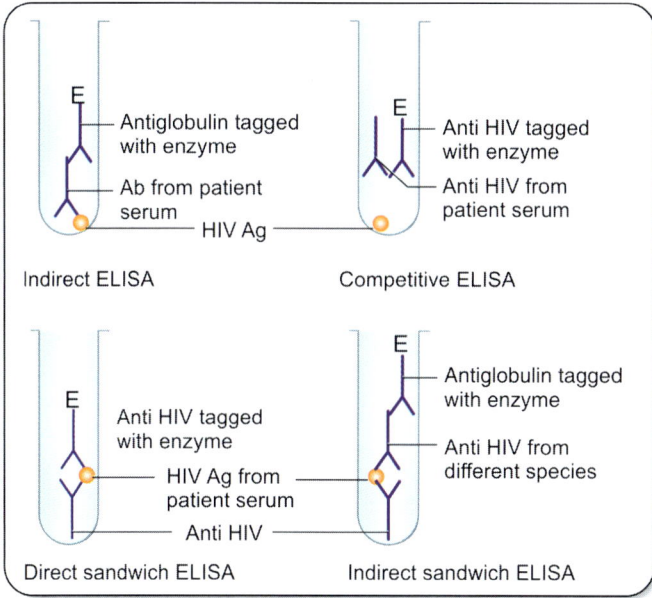

Indirect ELISA
- E — Antiglobulin tagged with enzyme
- Ab from patient serum
- HIV Ag

Competitive ELISA
- E — Anti HIV tagged with enzyme
- Anti HIV from patient serum

Direct sandwich ELISA
- E — Anti HIV tagged with enzyme
- HIV Ag from patient serum
- Anti HIV

Indirect sandwich ELISA
- E — Antiglobulin tagged with enzyme
- Anti HIV from different species
- Anti HIV

Fig. 12.10. ELISA.

employed in RIA, fluorescent conjugates in fluorescence microscopy and enzymes in ELISA, chemiluminescent compounds such as luminol or acridinium esters are used in CLIA as the label to provide the signal during the antigen-antibody reaction. The signal (light) can be amplified, measured and the concentration of analyte calculated. The method has been fully automated.

Western blotting

Western blotting is analogous to Southern blotting, for isolated DNA, and Northern blotting, for isolated RNA. In Western blotting, protein antigens are separated according to their electrophoretic mobility and molecular weight by polyacrylamide gel electrophoresis, then blotted onto nitrocellulose paper by standard blotting procedure. The patient serum is allowed to react with the blot.

Antibodies attached to separated viral antigens on the nitrocellulose paper are detected by enzyme tagged-antihuman gammaglobulin. Enzyme substrate is, subsequently added, which indicates positive test. The substrate changes colour in the presence of enzyme and permanently stains the nitrocellulose paper. The position of the band on the paper indicates the antigen with which the antibody has reacted.

Immunoelectron microscopy

When the virus particles, for example, rotavirus and hepatitis A virus in stool, are scanty in the specimen they can be treated with specific antisera. It leads to clumping of virus particles, which can be seen under electron microscope. This is known as immunoelectron microscopy and it finds application in detection of some viruses causing diarrhoea.

Architecture of the Immune System

Immune responses are mediated by a variety of cells, and by the soluble molecules which they secrete. Lymphocytes (B cells and T cells), phagocytes (mononuclear phagocytes, neutrophils and eosinophils), and auxiliary cells (basophils, mast cells and platelets) are the cellular components of immune system. *Antibodies produced by B cells, cytokines produced by T cells and mononuclear phagocytes, complement produced by mononuclear cells, inflammatory mediators produced by basophils, mast cells and platelets, and interferons produced by infected tissue cells are the soluble mediators of immune system.*

Immune response to an antigen is of two types:

- **Humoral** or **antibody-mediated immunity** (AMI) which is mediated by antibodies produced by plasma cells.
- **Cell-mediated immunity** (CMI) which is mediated directly by sensitized lymphocytes.

Lymphoid organs can be classified into primary (central) lymphoid organs and secondary (peripheral) lymphoid organs. Thymus and bursa of Fabricius are primary lymphoid organs. They are responsible for cellular and humoral immune response respectively. The equivalent of the avian bursa of Fabricius, in mammals, is bone marrow.

The capacity to respond to immunologic stimuli resides mainly in lymphoid cells. During embryonic development, blood cell precursors are found in foetal liver and other tissues; in postnatal life, the stem cells reside in bone marrow. They can differentiate in several ways. In liver and bone marrow, stem cells may differentiate into cells of red cell series or into cells of lymphoid series. Lymphoid stem cells evolve into two main lymphocyte population, B cells and T cells. If a stem cell is to become a T cell, it leaves the bone marrow and emigrates to the thymus, where it differentiates further under the influence of the thymic microenvironment and soluble factors produced by the thymic epithelium. The resulting T cells are responsible for specific cell-mediated immunity.

However, if the lymphoid stem cell is destined to become a B cell it remains in the bone marrow (in case of birds it emigrates to bursa of Fabricius, a gut appendage) where it undergoes several more differentiative steps before it gains the ability to produce and secrete antibody in response to the presence of infectious organisms. After acquiring immuno-competence, both T and B cells leave their primary site of differentiation and emigrate to the peripheral lymphoid organs (Fig. 13.1). These include lymph nodes, spleen, gut-associated lymphoid tissue (GALT), appendix, tonsils and adenoids.

B cells seed into outer cortex in germinal follicles and medullary cords of peripheral lymph nodes and germinal centre and mantle layer of spleen. These areas are known as **bursa-dependent** or **thymus-independent areas**. T cells seed into paracortical areas of lymph nodes and white pulp of spleen around the central arterioles. These areas are known as **thymus-dependent areas**. Here, in the peripheral lymphoid organs, they encounter with infectious organisms that have escaped the innate defence system.

PRIMARY LYMPHOID ORGANS

Thymus

It is a bilobed, greyish, lymphoepithelial organ located just above the heart and extending into the neck on the front and sides of trachea. It develops from the epithelium of third and fourth pharyngeal pouches at about the sixth week of gestation. The embryonic thymus consists of epithelial cells surrounded by a thin capsule. In utero, precursor cells (prothymocytes or progenitor lymphocytes) differentiate from the lymphoid stem cell, emigrate from bone marrow and infiltrate the thymus, wedging between the epithelial cells to form a meshwork of branched epithelial cells and lymphocytes. The peripheral epithelium, called the cortex, becomes heavily populated with the resulting thymocytes, whereas the central area, termed the medulla contains few lymphocytes, some of which are derived from the cortical thymocytes.

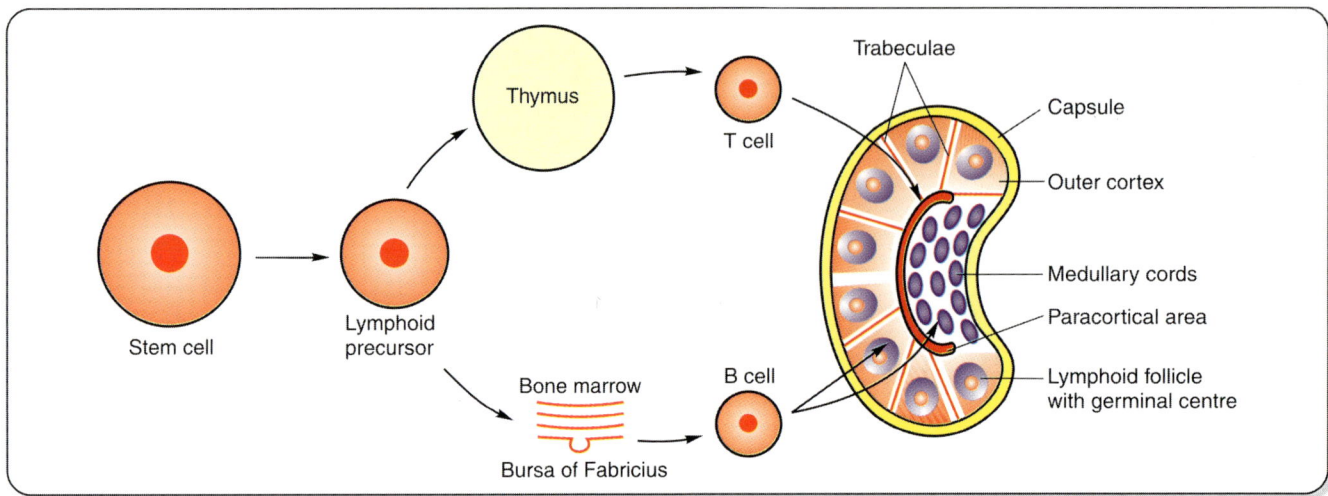

Fig. 13.1. Development of T and B cells.

Histologically, each lobe of thymus is divided into a series of lobules each containing a cortex and a medulla. Prothymocytes, from the bone marrow, migrate through blood stream, enter the cortex and begin dividing rapidly. It is the major site for lymphocyte proliferation in the body. However, most cells die in the process. Of the lymphocytes produced only 5% leave the thymus as viable cells. The reason for this apparent wasteful process is not known. However, some believe that this apparent waste may represent the elimination of lymphocyte clones that react against self. In the thymus, the lymphocytes acquire new surface antigens (*Thy antigens*). Lymphocytes produced in the thymus are called **thymus-derived lymphocytes** or **T lymphocytes** or **T cells**. Unlike lymphocytes proliferation in the peripheral organs, in the thymus, it is not dependent on antigenic stimulation.

The thymus confers immunological competence on the lymphocytes during their stay in the organ. Here they are educated, so that they become capable of mounting cell-mediated immune response against appropriate antigen. This is effected under the influence of the thymic microenvironment and several hormones, such as thymosin and thymopoietin produced by thymic epithelium. Differentiation of thymocytes to T cells, in the thymus, is immediately followed by emigration of these T cells to the peripheral lymphoid organs as mature cells that are precommitted to their function and antigen specificity. These are selectively seeded into paracortical areas of peripheral lymph nodes and into the white pulp of the spleen around the central arterioles. These regions are known as **'thymus-dependent'** and after neonatal thymectomy it is found grossly depleted.

The thymus reaches peak activity in childhood and attains its largest size at puberty. Thereafter, the thymus begins to atrophy without any apparent effect on T cell function and is extremely small in old age. This is probably due to the fact that T cells are very long-lived and can circulate in the resting state for long periods of time.

Bursa of Fabricius

The bursa is a lymphoepithelial organ arising as a pouch from the dorsal part of the cloaca in birds. Like thymus, it is also a site of lymphocytic proliferation and differentiation. Stem cells from yolk sac, foetal liver and bone marrow enter the bursa, proliferate and develop into immunocompetent **bursal lymphocytes** or **B lymphocytes** or **B cells** (B for bursa or bone marrow). These B cells now migrate and seed outer or superficial cortex of the germinal follicles and medullary cords of peripheral lymph nodes and lymphoid follicles of spleen. These are known as **'bursa-dependent'** or **thymus-independent areas**. Following appropriate antigenic stimulation, B lymphocytes transform into plasma cells and secrete antibodies. Surgical removal of bursa (bursectomy) from newly hatched chickens destroys their subsequent ability to produce antibodies but does not affect their ability to mount cell-mediated immune response. Like thymus, the bursa starts to shrink or atrophy at puberty.

Bone marrow

The mammalian equivalent of the bursa of Fabricius appears to be the bone marrow. Therefore, mammalian bone marrow is the site not only of haemopoiesis but also of initial differentiation of stem cells to B cells.

PERIPHERAL LYMPHOID ORGANS

Lymphocytes differentiate and mature in the primary lymphoid organs and proceed via circulation to the secondary lymphoid organs. Here they have an opportunity to bind antigen and undergo further antigen-dependent differentiation. Once in the secondary lymphoid tissues, the lymphocytes do not remain there but move from one lymphoid organ to another through the blood and lymphatics. The advantage of this lymphocyte recirculation is that during the course of a natural infection the continual trafficking of lymphocytes enables many different lymphocytes to have access to antigen. The passage of lymphocytes through an area where antigen has been localized and concentrated on the dendritic processes of macrophages or on the surface of antigen-presenting cells facilitates the induction of an immune response.

Lymph nodes

Lymph nodes are small bean-shaped organs that act as filters. They form part of lymphatic network distributed throughout the body. They are surrounded by connective tissue capsules from which trabeculae penetrate into the nodes. They consist of an outer cortex and an inner medulla. The cortex consists of several rounded aggregates of lymphocytes called lymphoid follicles. The follicle has a pale-staining germinal centre surrounded by small dark-staining lymphocytes. The follicles contain besides proliferating lymphocytes, dendritic macrophages, which capture and process the antigen.

The deeper region of the cortex or paracortex is the zone between the peripheral cortex and inner medulla. The medulla is predominantly composed of cords (medullary cords) of lymphocytes. Lymphoid follicles and medullary cords contain B lymphocytes and constitute **bursa-dependent areas** while paracortex (paracortical area) contains T lymphocytes and constitute **bursa-independent areas**. Each lymph node has a number of lymph channels called afferent lymph channels, that drain into it and a single large lymph vessel, called efferent lymph channel that carries the lymph fluid and lymphocytes to the thoracic duct, which empties into a large vein in the neck.

Spleen

Spleen is a large, encapsulated, lymphoid organ within which antibody synthesis to most blood-borne antigens takes place. There are two types of tissues in the spleen, referred to as the lymphoid or white pulp of the cortex consisting primarily of lymphocytes and macrophages and the erythroid, or red pulp, of the medulla consisting of erythrocyte-rich blood. Arteries entering the spleen are surrounded by a sheath of T cells and macrophages. This is known as periarteriolar sheath. Within this sheath are present lymphoid follicles known as primary follicles of B cells similar to those occurring in lymph nodes. Blood-borne antigens entering the spleen are phagocytosed and processed by macrophages and fixed phagocytic mononuclear cells. Presentation of antigens, on the surface of such cells, to the splenic lymphocytes results in the formation of secondary follicles containing germinal centres of dividing and differentiating B cells.

Mucosa-associated lymphoid tissues

Mucosa lining the alimentary, respiratory, genitourinary and other surfaces are constantly exposed to numerous antigens. These areas possess rich collection of lymphoid tissues. These collections of lymphoid tissues are known as mucosa-associated lymphoid tissue (MALT). Tonsils, adenoids and

Peyer's patches of the small intestine are known as gut-associated lymphoid tissue (GALT). Peyer's patches are small patches of organized lymphoid tissue along the intestine containing B cells (in germinal centre) and T cells. They play a primary role in defence against infectious organisms entering via digestive tract.

CELLS OF THE IMMUNE SYSTEM

Lymphocytes

Of the many cells involved in specific response to antigen, lymphocytes are the most important effector cells. They are small, round, 5–15 μm in diameter and are found in peripheral blood, lymph, lymphoid organs and in many other tissues. In peripheral blood, they constitute 20–40% of the leucocyte population, while in lymph and lymphoid organs they form the predominant cell type. They may be small (5–8 μm), medium (8–12 μm) and large (12–15 μm). The small lymphocytes are most numerous. They may be short-lived (life-span about two weeks) or long-lived (life-span three years or more or even for life). Short-lived cells are effector cells in immune response, while long-lived cells act as memory cells. Long-lived cells are mainly thymus-derived. Lymphopoiesis takes place in the bone marrow, central lymphoid organs and peripheral lymphoid organs.

Lymphocytes possess antigen recognition mechanism on their surface, enabling each cell to recognize only one or a small number of antigens. Two major classes of lymphocytes are recognized which are designated **T cells** and **B cells**. T and B cells are indistinguishable by conventional light microscopy.

Classification of lymphocytes on the basis of surface markers makes use of two important characteristics:

1. Cluster of differentiation or cluster determinant (CD).
2. Antigen recognition receptors.

1. Cluster of differentiation or cluster determinant

CDs represent families of surface glycoprotein antigens that can be recognized by specific antibodies produced against them. Thus, a cell displaying CD1 is identified by the binding of antibodies against CD1. Each class of leucocyte displays a diagnostic pattern of CDs, for example:

- CD3 is expressed only by T cells.
- CD19 is expressed only by B cells.
- CD64 is expressed only by monocytes.
- CD66 is expressed only by granulocytes.
- CD68 is expressed only by macrophages.
- On the other hand, CD18 and CD45 are expressed by a variety of leucocyte types.
- A total of more than 150 CDs are known.

2. Antigen recognition receptors

These include membrane-bound (surface) immunoglobulins (mIgs or sIgs) in B cells, and T cell receptors (TCRs) in T cells. In contrast to CDs, which can serve as diagnostic feature for all leucocytes, antigen recognition receptors are limited to B and T lymphocytes only. These receptors are required for B and T cells to be antigen reactive. Both mIgs and TCRs serve as specific surface receptors, recognizing and interacting with only single antigenic determinant on the antigen. Reaction of antigens with mIgs and TCRs activates B cells and T cells respectively, leading to proliferation and differentiation.

Thus, the antigen specificity of the mIgs in B cells and TCRs in T cells is predetermined, and the sole effect of antigen is to select out a cell with appropriate surface receptor and induce it to clonally expand and differentiate into a cell that will produce the antibody, it has been predetermined to make or produce specific clones of effector T cells respectively.

B lymphocytes

Lymphocytes possessing mIgs are termed B cells. They arise from pleuripotent stem cells in bone marrow, they mature in bone marrow itself and then emigrate to the peripheral lymphoid organs where, upon contact with antigen, they can differentiate into antibody-producing **plasma cells**. Antibodies are formed by clonal selection. Each individual has a large pool of different B lymphocytes (about 10^9) that have life-span of days or weeks and are formed in the bone marrow, lymph nodes, and gut-associated lymphoid tissue (e.g., tonsils or appendix). Each B cell possesses about 10^5 mIg molecules, primarily of IgM and IgD classes. Following activation, immunoglobulins of other classes might also reside on B lymphocyte membranes. Immature B cells do not possess mIg receptors.

A single B cell or a clone of B cells possess mIg receptors specific for only one (monospecific) antigenic determinant. Thus, billions of B cells display a diversity of receptors capable of reacting with any antigenic determinant that might be encountered. Receptor immunoglobulin and secreted immunoglobulin of a single cell or clone of cells are identical in the variable regions of the antibody molecule.

Most B cells and macrophages, and certain activated T cells express class II major histocompatibility gene products or immune associated (Ia) antigens in the mouse, and HLA-DR antigens in humans. Receptors for the Fc portion of IgG (FcR) are found on all B cells, macrophages and certain subsets of T cells. Some cells express receptors for other classes of immunoglobulin as well. These receptors bind antigen-antibody complexes. Receptors for C3 component of complement are found on most B cells. These are known as complement receptors (CRs). These receptors are thought to play a role in the regulation of the B cell response to antigen. Because of the presence of CRs on the surface of B cells they bind to sheep RBCs which have been coated with antibody and complement forming EAC rosettes. They undergo blast transformation on treatment with bacterial endotoxins.

T lymphocytes

Pleuripotent stem cells in the bone marrow give rise to precursor T cells, which migrate to the thymus (Fig. 13.2). Once they enter the cortex of the thymus they are known as **thymocytes**. As T cells mature, their surface antigens including CDs and TCRs change. Monoclonal antibodies are used to identify the antigenic subsets of T cells. Approximately 65% of mature T cells that leave the thymus display CD2+CD3+CD4+CD8–TCR+ phenotype (CD4+ cells), while approximately 35% display CD2+ CD3+CD4–CD8+TCR+ phenotype (CD8+ cells). A very small number express neither CD4 nor CD8 and consequently have a phenotype of CD2+CD3+ CD4–CD8–TCR+ (CD4–CD8– cells).

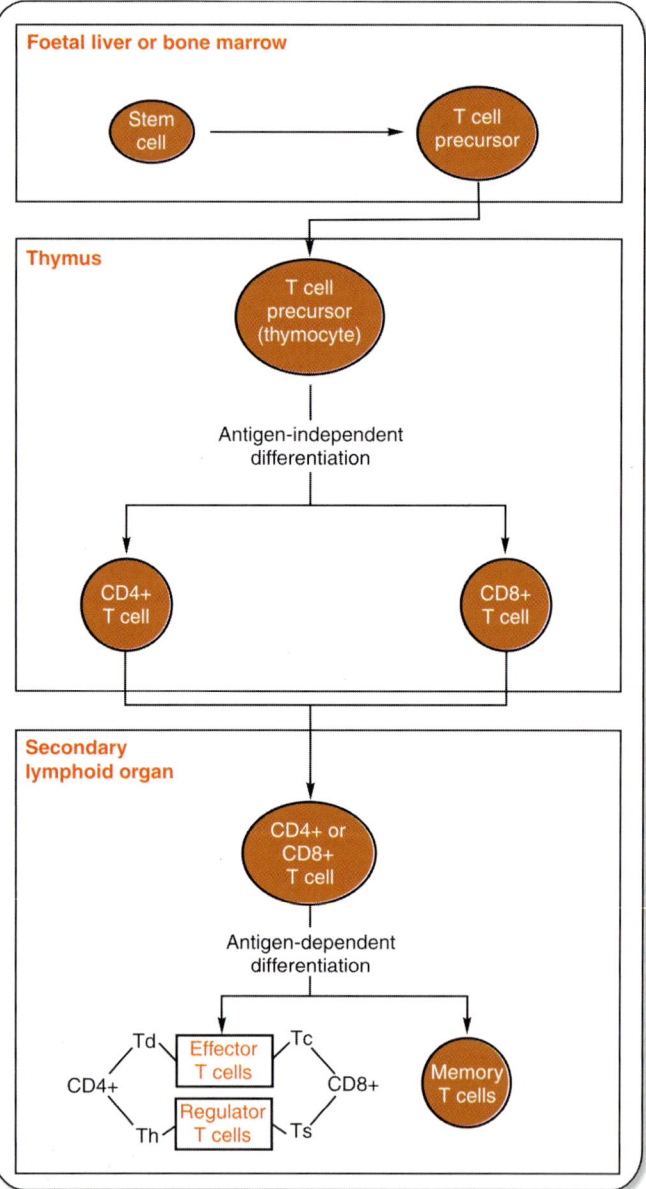

Fig. 13.2. T cell differentiation.

T cell subsets

Four distinct subsets of T cells are known. Two each of these are regulator and effector cells.

Regulator cells

1. *Helper T cells (Th cells):* They possess CD2, CD3 and CD4 surface antigens. They help in the antigen-specific activation of B cells and effector T cells. Th cells have two different profiles of cytokine production (Th1 and Th2) and these patterns select between the two basic types of response mediated by Th cells. Th1 cytokines include interferon-γ (IFN-γ), IFN-β, and interleukin-2 (IL-2) and Th1 cells are involved in cell-mediated inflammatory reactions. Several Th1 cytokines activate cytotoxic inflammatory and delayed hypersensitivity reactions. By contrast, Th2 cells are typified by the production of IL-4 to 6, IL-9, IL-10 and IL-13. Th2 cells encourage production of antibody especially IgE, and Th2 cytokines are associated with regulation of strong antibody and allergic responses. Cytokines from Th1 cells inhibit the actions of Th2 cells and vice versa.
2. *Suppressor T cells (Ts cells):* They possess CD2, CD3 and CD8 surface antigens. They suppress expression of immune response by other lymphocytes.

Effector cells

1. *Delayed-type-hypersensitivity T cells (Td cells):* They possess CD2, CD3 and CD4 surface antigens. They are involved in delayed hypersensitivity and cell-mediated immune responses.
2. *Cytotoxic T cells (Tc cells):* They possess CD2, CD3 and CD8 surface antigens. They are also involved in cell-mediated immune responses and lyse target cells by direct cell-cell contact.

Immune response is regulated by mutually opposing influence of Th and Ts cells. **Overactivity of Th or decreased activity of Ts causes abnormal immune responses as seen in autoimmunity. Diminished Th function or increased activity of Ts leads to immunodeficiency.**

During maturation and differentiation in thymus, T cells also learn to recognize self-major histocompatibility (MHC) antigens. CD4+ cells recognize class II MHC antigens and CD8+ cells recognize class I MHC antigens.

T cells bind to sheep RBCs at 37°C forming SRBC or E rosettes while B cells do not. They undergo blast transformation, evidenced by enhanced DNA synthesis, on treatment with mitogens such as phytohaemagglutinin (PHA) and concanavalin A (Con A).

Table 13.1 summarises differences between T cells and B cells.

Null cells

A small proportion (5%) of lymphocytes that lack distinguishing phenotypic markers characteristic of T or B

Table 13.1. Differences between T and B lymphocytes

Property	T cell	B cell
Antigen recognition receptors	TCRs	mIgs
Surface glycoprotein antigens	CD3	CD19
Receptors for Fc piece of immuno-globulins (FcR)	–*	+
Receptors for C3 component of complement (CRs)	–	+
EAC rosette	–	+
E rosette	+	–
Thymus specific antigens	+	–
Blast transformation on treatment with	PHA and Con A	Bacterial endotoxins

*Certain subsets of T cells possess FcR

lymphocytes are known as null cells or non-T and non-B lymphocytes. They do not possess TCRs or mIgs. A few null cells in the circulation might be immature T or B cells.

Killer cells or K cells

A subpopulation of null cells possess surface receptors for Fc part of IgG. They are capable of lysing or killing target cells sensitized by IgG antibody. They are known as killer or K cells. **They are responsible for antibody-dependent cell-mediated cytotoxicity (ADCC) in contrast to the action of cytotoxic T lymphocytes which are independent of antibody.**

Natural killer or NK cells

Another subpopulation of null cells is natural killer or NK cells. These are large lymphocytes containing azurophilic granules in the cytoplasm. They are, therefore, known as large granular lymphocytes (LGL). **NK cells are capable of non-specific killing of virus-transformed target cells and are involved in allograft and tumour rejection.** They differ from K cells in being independent of antibody.

Plasma cells

Plasma cells are fully differentiated antibody-synthesizing cells. Antigenically stimulated B cells undergo blast transformation, becoming successively plasmablasts, intermediate transitional cells and plasma cells. It is an oval cell, about twice the size of a small lymphocyte. It has an eccentric nucleus, abundant rough endoplasmic reticulum, numerous mitochondria and prominent Golgi apparatus. Plasma cells are end cells and have a short life-span of two or three days. A plasma cell secretes an antibody of a single specificity of a single antibody class and of a single light chain type. However, in primary antibody response plasma cell produces IgM initially and later it may switch onto IgG production. Lymphocytes, lymphoblasts and transitional cells may also synthesize immunoglobulins to some extent.

Antigen-presenting cells (APCs)

A number of different cell types have been described as APCs. In addition to presenting antigen to effector lymphocytes, many of these cells perform non-specific immunological functions such as phagocytosis and cytotoxicity. Induction of humoral or cell-mediated immunity cannot occur efficiently in the absence of APCs, i.e., with lymphocytes alone. APCs include dendritic cells that are found in skin (Langerhans' cells), thymus, lymph node, spleen and other secondary lymphoid organs and macrophages which include monocytes as blood macrophages and histiocytes as tissue macrophages.

The processing and presentation of antigen by macrophages to T cells require that both the cells possess surface determinants coded by the same MHC genes. T cells can accept the processed antigen only, if it is presented by macrophages carrying on its surface, the self-MHC determinant known as immune-associated or Ia antigen. When the macrophage bears a different Ia antigen, it cannot cooperate with T cell. This is known as **MHC restriction**.

Functional activity of macrophages may be enhanced by lymphokines, complement components and interferon. Activated macrophages are not antigen specific. They secrete a number of biologically active substances like interleukin-1. They can bind immune complexes by means of FcRs or CRs, which are present on their surface, and then engulf and digest them. Macrophages can also exhibit ADCC reactions. Role of macrophages in innate immune response is discussed in Chapter 8.

Other cells involved in immunological responses

Neutrophils

Approximately 60% of the circulating leucocytes in humans are neutrophils. Their primary function is phagocytosis of foreign or dead cells and pinocytosis of pathological immune complexes. They can also exhibit ADCC. They are capable of rapid activation and mobilization in response to chemotactic stimuli such as bacterial products or activated components of complement (C5a). A variety of receptors, e.g., FcRs, CR1 and CR2 are increasingly displayed following activation. They constitute predominant cell type in inflammation.

Eosinophils

These are granulocytes containing prominent acidophilic granules. They account for 3–5% of the white blood cells. During allergic conditions and during certain parasitic infections the number of eosinophils may increase dramatically. They can engulf and remove immune complexes by phagocytosis/pinocytosis. They possess FcRs and can mediate ADCC. They can bind to worm larvae such as schistosomulae coated with IgG, degranulate and release toxic proteins which are damaging to the parasites.

Basophils and mast cells

Basophils comprise less than 1% of white blood cells. Basophils and their tissue counterparts, mast cells, possess basophilic granules. These granules contain pharmacological mediators of type I hypersensitivity. IgE antibodies get attached to FcRs present on the surface of mast cells and basophils. When stimulated with allergen, granules release their contents. Basophils also possess FcRs for IgG and CRs for C3a, C3b and C5a.

14

Immune Response

Specific reactivity following an antigenic stimulus is known as the immune response. It is of two types:

1. Humoral or antibody-mediated immunity (AMI).
2. Cell-mediated immunity (CMI).

AMI provides defence against most extracellular bacterial pathogens and helps in defence against viruses that infect through the respiratory and intestinal tract. It also participates in immediate (types I, II, III and V) hypersensitivity reactions and certain autoimmune diseases.

CMI protects against fungi, most of the viruses and intracellular bacterial pathogens like *Mycobacterium leprae*, *M. tuberculosis*, *Brucella* and *Salmonella*, and parasites like *Leishmania* and trypanosomes. It also participates in allograft rejection, graft versus host reaction, delayed hypersensitivity and certain autoimmune diseases. It provides immunological surveillance and immunity against cancer.

HUMORAL OR ANTIBODY-MEDIATED IMMUNE RESPONSE

The antibody response to stimulation by antigen can be described as primary humoral response and secondary humoral response.

Primary humoral response

Phases

Antibody production follows characteristic phases (Fig. 14.1):

1. **Lag phase:** After first injection of the antigen there is a long lag phase of several days before antibody appears. The lag phase depends upon the kind and amount of antigen given, the route of administration, species of animal and its health.
2. **Log phase:** As the lag period ends, the titre of antibody gradually increases over a period of a few days to a few weeks.
3. **Plateau or steady state:** There is equilibrium between antibody production and catabolism.

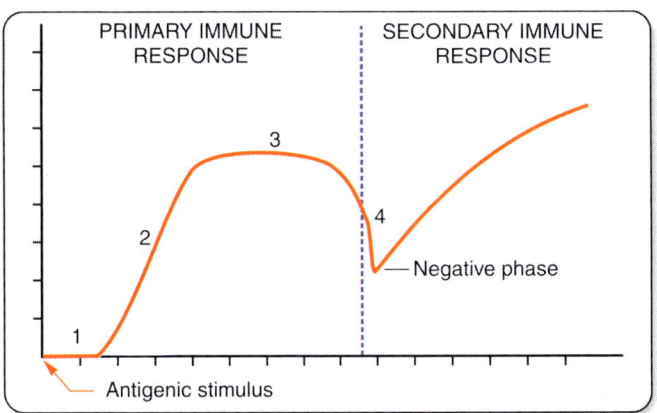

Fig. 14.1. Immune response.

4. **Phase of decline:** Catabolism exceeds the production of antibody and the titre falls.

Secondary humoral response

If the same animal is subsequently exposed to the same antigen there occurs a temporary fall in the level of antibodies due to the combination of the antigen with pre-existing antibody. This is known as **negative phase**. After two to three days a marked increase in antibody level becomes evident. This goes on increasing for several days, thus exceeding the initial level. This is also known as **booster response**. The booster response is attributed to the persistence of antigen sensitive 'memory cells' following the primary response.

The antibody formed in primary response is predominantly IgM and in secondary response IgG. The first dose is known as **priming dose** and subsequent injection as **booster dose**. Both these doses are particularly essential in case of killed vaccines. *With live vaccines a single dose is usually sufficient as multiplication of organisms in the body provides a continuing antigenic stimulus that acts both as priming and booster doses.*

Fate of antigen in tissues

Antigens introduced subcutaneously are mainly localized in the draining lymph nodes, only a small amount being found in the spleen. On the other hand, antigens introduced intravenously are rapidly localized in the spleen, liver, bone marrow, kidneys and lungs. 70–80% of these are broken down by reticuloendothelial (R.E.) cells and excreted in the urine.

Production of antibodies

Antigen processing and presentation

Antigens are presented to **immunocompetent cells (ICCs)** by antigen-presenting cells (APCs) (macrophages and dendritic cells). With many antigens (T cell dependent antigens such as proteins and erythrocytes), processing by macrophages is prerequisite for antibody formation. But for T cell independent antigens, such as polysaccharides, antibody production does not require T cell participation. APC can ingest antigen, degrade it and present it to T cell. T cell is able to recognize only when the processed antigen is presented on the surface of APC, in association with MHC molecules to the T cell carrying the T cell receptor (TCR) for the epitope.

The antigen has to be presented complexed with MHC class II in case of CD4 (helper T/Th) cells and for CD8 (cytotoxic T/Tc) cells with MHC class I molecules.

T and B cell activation

The activation of Th cell requires two signals for activation. The first signal is a combination of the TCR with the MHC class II-complexed antigen. The second signal is interleukin-1 (IL-1) which is produced by the APC. The activated Th cell produces IL-2 and other cytokines required for B cell stimulation. These include IL-4, IL-5 and IL-6 which act as B cell growth factor (BCGF) and B cell differentiation factor (BCDF). They activate B cells which have combined with their respective antigens to clonally proliferate and differentiate into antibody secreting plasma cells. A small proportion of B cells, instead of being transformed into plasma cells, become long-lived memory cells producing a secondary type of response to subsequent contact with the antigen. B cells carry surface receptors which consist of IgM or other immunoglobulin classes. A plasma cell secretes an antibody of a single specificity of a single antibody class (IgM, IgG or any other single class). However, in primary humoral response, plasma cells secrete IgM and later switch over to form IgG.

CD8 (cytotoxic T/Tc) cells are activated when they come into contact with antigens presented along with MHC class I molecules. They also need a second signal IL-2, which is secreted by activated Th cells. On contact with a target cell carrying the antigen on its surface, the activated Tc cells release cytokines that destroy the target, which may be virus infected or tumour cells. Some T cells also become memory cells.

Clonal selection theory of antibody production

This theory was proposed by Burnet (1957). This theory states that during immunological development a large number of lymphocytes capable of reacting with different antigens are formed. Cells with immunological reactivity with self-antigens are eliminated during embryonic life. Such clones are known as **forbidden clones**. *Their persistence or development in the later life leads to autoimmunity*. Each ICC is capable of reacting with one antigen. Contact with specific antigen leads to cellular proliferation to form clones which synthesize antibodies. This theory is more widely accepted than other theories.

Monoclonal antibodies

Principle

If an antigen is injected into an animal, the latter produces different types of antibodies against various epitopes of the antigen. The antibodies, thus generated are polyclonal in nature. This means different clones of antibody secreting cells are simultaneously synthesizing the antibody. Different molecules will have different specificities and affinities. In all microbial infections, body reacts with polyclonal antibody production. When these polyclonal antisera are used in bacterial test systems, **cross reactivity** often occurs.

A single antibody-forming cell or clone produces antibodies directed against specific epitope of the antigen. Such antibodies produced by a single clone and directed against a single antigenic determinant are called **monoclonal antibodies (MCA)**. In nature, MCA are produced in multiple myeloma where only one clone secretes a particular type of antibody. MCA can be generated in the laboratory. The theory of MCA production is based on clonal selection hypothesis of Burnet (1959) and the method for production of MCA was described by Kohler and Milstein in 1975, for which they were awarded Nobel Prize for Medicine in 1984.

The main breakthrough was not that a single line of monoclonal antibody producing cells could be isolated, but rather that the mouse splenic lymphocytes could be fused with mouse myeloma cells to produce **hybrid cells (hybridoma)**. Among the two cell types chosen for fusion, one provides the hybrid cell immortality (**myeloma cell**) while the other (**splenic plasma cell**) provides the antibody producing capacity. Such hybridomas can be maintained indefinitely in culture and continue to form MCA.

Technique

- Lymphocytes from the spleen of a mouse immunized with desired antigen are fused with mouse myeloma cells grown in culture which is deficient in the enzyme hypoxanthine phosphoribosyl transferase (HPRT) (Fig. 14.2).
- The fused cells are placed in a basal culture medium containing hypoxanthine, aminopterin and thymidine (HAT medium).

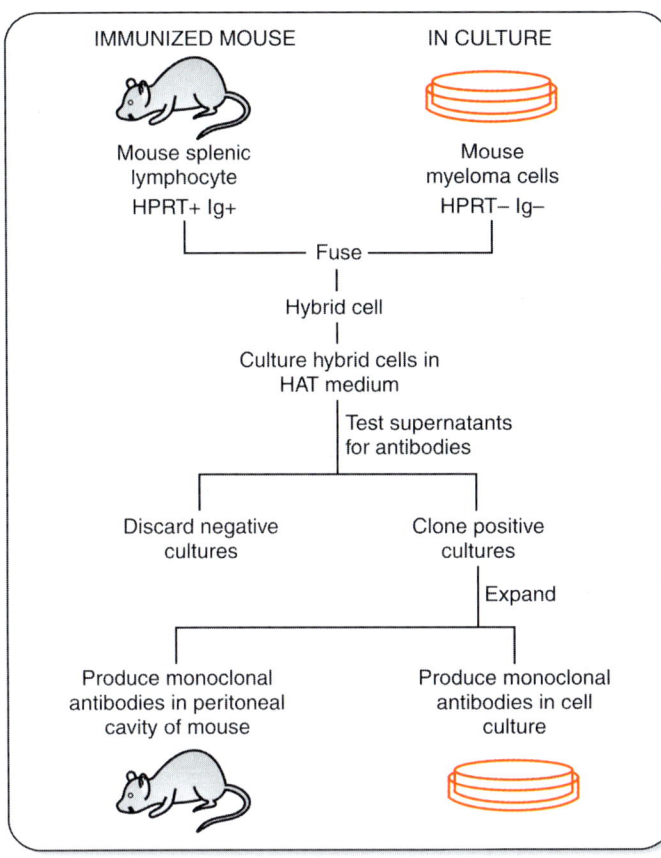

Fig. 14.2. Production of monoclonal antibodies.

- Only hybrid cells possessing properties of both the splenic lymphocytes (HPRT+) and myeloma cells (HPRT−) can grow in culture. Normal lymphocytes cannot replicate indefinitely and unfused myeloma cells are killed by the aminopterin in HAT medium.
- The peritoneal cavity of mice, preferably of the same strain that was used for initial immunization step, can be used to grow the selected hybrid cell clone. First, the peritoneal cavity is injected with an organic irritant such as pristane to produce chemical peritonitis. Next the selected hybrid cell line is injected into the peritoneal cavity. Within days, a tumour known as hybridoma develops. This tumour produces large quantities of MCA that can be harvested by aspirating ascitic fluid from mouse's peritoneal cavity.
- A tumour-bearing mouse will survive for 4–6 weeks, during which time large quantities of antibody can be recovered.
- Hybridomas can also be grown in tissue cultures where highly purified antibodies are produced without contamination from serum, ascites proteins or the cross-reactivity of histocompatibility antibodies derived from mouse tissues.

Applications of monoclonal antibodies

Monoclonal antibodies have been produced for specific epitopes of a wide variety of viruses, bacteria (including myco-

bacteria), parasites and fungi. Many of the commercial systems using direct fluorescence and enzyme-linked assays utilize monoclonal antibody conjugates.

CELL-MEDIATED IMMUNE RESPONSES

Cell-mediated immunity (CMI) normally refers to specific acquired immunity, which is accomplished by effector T cells and macrophages rather than B cells and antibodies. This includes allograft rejection, delayed hypersensitivity (DH) and cytotoxic reactions against intracellular parasites. As in case of antibody-mediated immune response, cell-mediated immune response can also be divided into primary and secondary cell-mediated immune responses.

Primary cell-mediated immune response

This is produced by initial contact with a foreign antigen. Foreign antigen is presented by antigen-presenting cells (APCs) to T cells leading to their activation. T cells possess antigen recognition receptors known as T cell receptors (TCRs) that recognize foreign antigen and a self-MHC molecule on the surface of the APC (Fig. 14.3). Because of the specificity of the TCRs only particular cells become activated. These cells proliferate and produce specific clones of effector T cells (Th, Tc, Td and Ts). Cell-mediated immune response develops after several days of antigenic challenge.

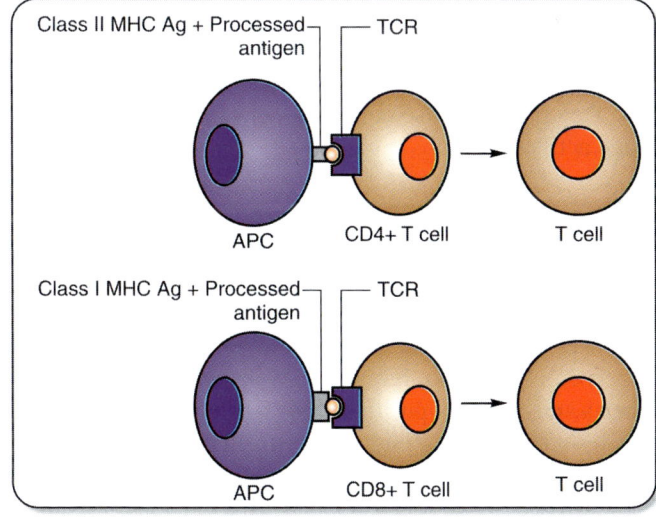

Fig. 14.3. Cell-mediated immune response.

Secondary cell-mediated immune response

If the same host is subsequently exposed to the same antigen, then the secondary cell-mediated immune response is usually more pronounced and occurs more rapidly. Because of the availability of specific memory cells, an increased number of effector cells are produced.

T cell differentiation

APCs, such as macrophages, phagocytose the antigen and degrade it. Subsequently, portions of antigen become associated with MHC antigens and are expressed on APCs surface. Two modes of processing are known (Fig. 14.3):

- One mode is seen in case of processing of phagocytosed material such as bacteria. The antigenic material dissociated from the bacteria is associated with class II MHC molecules probably within the phagosome. MHC-antigen complex then expresses on the surface of the APC.
- Second mode is seen in processing antigens derived within the cell, for example, viral antigens synthesized in infected cell. However, this antigenic determinant associates with class I MHC molecule probably in the endoplasmic reticulum. MHC-antigen complex then expresses on the surface of the APC.

CD8+ cells recognize the combination of foreign antigen and class I MHC antigen and differentiate into Tc and Ts lymphocytes while CD4+ cells recognize the combination of antigen and class II MHC antigen and differentiate into Th and Td cells.

Lysis of target cell

Tc cell recognizes foreign antigen and class I MHC antigen and gets attached to the target cell expressing these on their surface. This stimulates Tc cells to release **cytolysins**. This leads to calcium-dependent lysis of the target cell. Subsequently, the Tc cell can detach from the target cell and repeat this process with another. Recognition of target cells also stimulates Tc cells to synthesize and secrete **interferon-γ**, and thus, they probably also contribute to some extent to macrophage activation.

Delayed hypersensitivity

Delayed hypersensitivity (DH) or **type IV hypersensitivity** is the clinically observable outcome of cell-mediated immune reaction in the tissues of a sensitized individual. The immune response to proteins of the tubercle bacillus, observed by Robert Koch in 1880, has served a general model for DH. When a small dose of purified antigen (tuberculin) is injected intradermally in an individual sensitized to tuberculoprotein by prior infection or immunization, an indurated inflammatory reaction develops at the site of inoculation within 48–72 hours. It is characterized by erythema due to increased blood flow to the damaged area and induration due to infiltration with a large number of mononuclear cells, mainly T lymphocytes and about 10–20% macrophages.

Mechanism

On initial exposure the antigen is engulfed by the macrophage. It then presents the antigen to specific T lymphocytes that can recognize the foreign antigen on its surface. These T cells

clone, and two subsets (Td and Tc) are created. On subsequent exposure to the antigen, Td cells secrete lymphokines. These are glycoproteins which exert a regulatory effect chiefly on macrophages. These include **chemotactic factor** (CF) which attracts macrophages, **migration inhibiting factor** (MIF) which impedes their movement from the site of infection, **macrophage stimulating factor** (MSF) which stimulates macrophage migration to the site of antigen and **macrophage activating factor** (MAF) which keeps them at the site of infection and causes them to actively phagocytose and destroy foreign cells at the site of infection. Activated macrophages release their degradative lysosomal enzyme into the tissues where the antigen is located, thus leading to localized inflammatory response. This can lead to necrosis and fibrosis of the host tissue and destruction of infecting agents.

A second subset of T cells, Tc lymphocytes, is also generated. They also play a role, as described above, under lysis of target cells.

Cytokines

These are biologically active substances produced by cells that influence other cells. They are referred to as **lymphokines** if they are derived from lymphocytes and **monokines**, if they are derived from monocytes and macrophages. Interleukins are a family of cytokines that function primarily as growth and differentiation factors. Cytokines have been named based on the biological effects they produce. Various cytokines are given in Table 14.1.

Detection of CMI

Development of CMI can be detected by following methods:

1. Skin test for DH.
2. Transformation of cultured sensitized T lymphocytes on contact with antigen.
3. Target cell destruction: Killing of cultured cells by T lymphocytes sensitized against them.
4. Migration inhibiting factor (MIF) test (Fig. 14.4).

MIF test is most commonly employed. If a piece of capillary tube containing peritoneal exudate cells (macro-

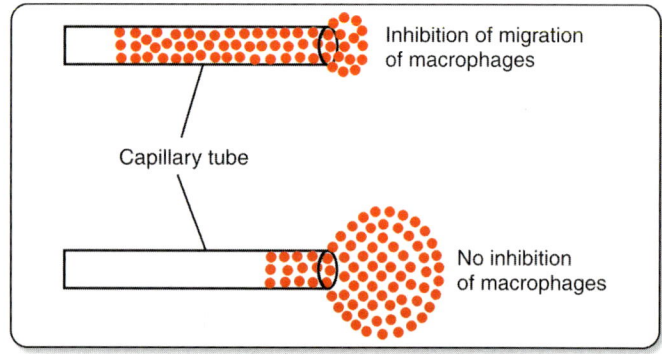

Fig. 14.4. Migration inhibiting factor (MIF) test.

Table 14.1. Source and activity of cytokines

Cytokine	Source	Activity
Macrophage stimulating factor (MSF)	Td cells	Stimulates macrophage migration to the site of action
Macrophage activating factor (MAF)	Td cells	Restricts macrophage movement and increases phagocytic activity
Migration inhibiting factor (MIF)	Td cells	Inhibits migration of macrophages
Chemotactic factor (CF)	Td cells	Stimulates chemotaxis of macrophages
Interferon-gamma (IFN-γ)	Th, Td and NK cells	Increases cytotoxicity of NK cells and macrophages
Interleukin-1 (IL-1)	NK cells, APCs, B cells and T cells	Promotes growth and expression of fibroblasts, NK cells, B cells and T cells
Interleukin-2 (IL-2)	Th cells	Promotes B cell differentiation and T cell growth
Interleukin-3 (IL-3)	Th cells	Acts as a growth factor for bone marrow stem cell
Interleukin-4 (IL-4)	Th cells	Acts as a growth factor for macrophages, mast cells, B cells and T cells
Interleukin-5 (IL-5)	Th cells	Promotes B cell growth, antibody production and maturation of eosinophils
Interleukin-6 (IL-6)	Macrophages	Promotes B cell growth
Interleukin-7 (IL-7)	Bone marrow stroma cell	Stimulates B cell and T cell proliferation
Interleukin-8 (IL-8)	Mononuclear cells, endothelial cells and skin fibroblasts.	Stimulates chemotaxis of neutrophils and T cells
Interleukin-9 (IL-9)	Activated T cells	Stimulates proliferation of IL-3 dependent myeloid cells and mast cells
Interleukin-10 (IL-10)	Th cells	Inhibits production of IFN and mononuclear cell functions
Interleukin-11 (IL-11)	Bone marrow and stromal cells	Induces acute phase proteins
Interleukin-12 (IL-12)	T cells	Activates natural killer (NK) cells
Interleukin-13 (IL-13)	T cells	Inhibits mononuclear cell functions
Interleukin-14 (IL-14)	T cells	Stimulates proliferation of activated B cells, inhibits immunoglobulin production
Interleukin-15 (IL-15)	Monocytes	Proliferation of T cells and activated B cells
Interleukin-16 (IL-16)	Eosinophils, CD8+ T cells	Chemoattraction of CD4+ T cells
Interleukin-17 (IL-17)	CD4+ T cells	Release of IL-6, IL-8
Interleukin-18 (IL-18)	Hepatocytes	Induces production of interferon-γ, enhances NK cell activity

phages and a few lymphocytes) is placed in a tissue culture chamber containing tissue culture fluid and no antigen, the macrophages migrate out of the open end of the tube into culture fluid to form a fan-like pattern. However, if the macrophages are obtained from a guinea-pig sensitized to tuberculoprotein, addition of tuberculin to the culture chamber will inhibit migration.

Transfer factor

Lawrence (1954) reported transfer of CMI in man by injection of extract from the leucocytes from immunized individual. The extract from the leucocytes contains a soluble factor called transfer factor (TF). The transferred immunity is specific in that CMI can be transferred only to those antigens to which the donor is sensitive.

TF is a nucleopeptide with a molecular weight of 2,000–4,000 daltons. It is non-antigenic. It is resistant to trypsin but gets inactivated by heating at 56°C in 30 minutes. The mode of action of TF is not known. It appears to stimulate the release of lymphokines from sensitized T lymphocytes. It does not promote antibody synthesis. TF has been used in patients with:

- T cell deficiency (Wiskott-Aldrich syndrome).
- Disseminated infections associated with deficient CMI (lepromatous leprosy, tuberculosis and mucocutaneous candidiasis).
- Malignant melanoma and other types of cancer.

Immunological tolerance

Immunological tolerance may be defined as a state of unresponsiveness to specific antigens. This unresponsiveness is specific to antigens to which the individual is tolerant. Response to other antigens is unaffected. Two forms of tolerance can be identified – natural tolerance and acquired tolerance.

Natural tolerance

It is nonresponsiveness to self-antigens. This arises during foetal development, when the immune system is being formed and maturing. If this tolerance breaks down and body responds to self molecules then an autoimmune disease will develop. Dizygotic cattle twins, which are genetically dissimilar, share the same placental circulation in utero. As adults, each twin fails to mount immune response to histocompatibility antigens on the cells of the other twin. Thus, they accept transplants from each other. This could be accounted for by induction of specific immunological tolerance during foetal life. Based on this observation of Owen (1945), Burnet and Fenner (1949) suggested that the unresponsiveness of individuals to self-antigens was due to the contact of the immature immuno-logical system with self-antigens during embryonic life.

Any antigen that comes into contact with the immuno-logical system during its embryonic life would be recognised as a self-antigen and would not induce any immune response. They postulated that tolerance could be induced against foreign antigens, if they were administered during embryonic life. Medawar and his colleagues (1953) proved it experi-mentally. When skin graft from one inbred strain of mice (CBA) is applied on a mouse of another strain (A), it is rejected. But if CBA cells are injected into foetal or newborn A strain mice, the latter when grow up will freely accept skin grafts from CBA mice.

Certain strains of mice that are genetically deficient in the C5 complement component make vigorous antibody response when immunized with pure C5 taken from normal animals. Normal animals (which are not deficient in C5) do not respond to similar immunization.

Acquired tolerance

It arises when a potential immunogen induces a state of unresponsiveness to itself. This has consequences for host defences since the presence of a tolerogenic epitope on a pathogen may compromise the ability of the body to resist infection. For acquired tolerance to be maintained the tolerogen must persist or be repeatedly administered. This is probably necessary because of the continuous production of new B and T cells that must be rendered tolerant.

A number of factors influence the induction of tolerance. These include species and immunocompetence of the host, physical nature, dose, and route of administration of antigen. Rabbits and mice can be rendered tolerant more rapidly than guinea-pigs and chickens. Higher the degree of immuno-competence of the host, the more difficult it is to induce tolerance. Therefore, embryos and newborns are particularly susceptible for induction of tolerance.

It is easier to induce tolerance to a soluble macromolecule than to an aggregated antigen. For example, when human gammaglobulin is heat aggregated, it is highly immunogenic in mice, but when de-aggregated it is tolerogenic. This is probably due to the fact that aggregated antigens are readily phagocytosed by macrophages, where they can be presented to antibody-forming cells, thus, inducing antibody synthesis. On the other hand, soluble antigens are not so easily processed and may be more effective in inducing the Ts suppressor circuit.

The induction of tolerance is dose-dependent. Generally, high doses of antigen tolerize B cells, while minute doses given repeatedly tolerize T cells. A moderate dose of the same antigen might be immunogenic. The route of administration is also important. Intravenously administered antigens have faster contact with more cells at the highest concentration of tolerogen. Moreover, an intravenous injection rapidly reaches the spleen to which Ts cells migrate leading to tolerance.

Tolerance can be overcome spontaneously or by injection of cross reacting immunogens. For example, tolerance to bovine serum albumin in rabbits can be abolished by immuni-zation with cross reacting human serum albumin.

Mechanism of tolerance

Tolerance can arise through three possible mechanisms:

1. **Clonal deletion:** In embryonic life clones of B and T cells, possessing receptors that recognize self-antigens, are selectively deleted or eliminated and, therefore, no longer available to respond upon subsequent exposure to that antigen. This is known as clonal deletion.
2. **Clonal anergy:** Clones of B and T cells expressing receptors that recognize self-antigen might remain but they cannot be activated. This is known as clonal anergy.
3. **Suppression:** Clones of B and T cells expressing receptors that recognize self-antigens are preserved. Antigen recognition might be capable of causing activation, however, expression of immune response might be inhibited or blocked through active suppression.

15

Hypersensitivity

Hypersensitivity is an abnormal immune response which produces physiological or histopathological damage in the host. It may be divided into five types:

Type I   Anaphylactic
Type II   Cytotoxic
Type III   Immune complex
Type IV   Cell-mediated or delayed
Type V   Stimulatory or antireceptor

Type I, II, III and V hypersensitivity depend on the interaction of antigen with humoral antibodies and are known as immediate type reactions, although, some are more immediate than others. Immediate hypersensitivity reactions develop in less than 24 hours after reexposure to an antigen. Type IV hypersensitivity or delayed hypersensitivity is mediated by T lymphocytes. Delayed hypersensitivity reactions develop in 24–48 hours.

TYPE I HYPERSENSITIVITY: ANAPHYLACTIC

It is **mediated by IgE antibody** and is due to the powerful effects of histamine and other vasoactive amines. Hypersensitivity may be local or generalized, depending upon the amount of histamine released, the site of its release and route of stimulating antigen. Generally, small amount of antigen administered to mucous membrane or skin will induce local anaphylaxis, whereas larger amounts may induce a generalized reaction and antigen administered systemically may cause generalized anaphylaxis. Local anaphylaxis is exemplified by such conditions as hay fever and asthma. Systemic anaphylaxis is a shocklike condition that can occur in individuals who are intensely allergic to such things as bee venom, penicillin and horse serum.

An antigenic substance that can trigger the allergic state is known as **allergen**. It may be a protein or chemically complex low molecular weight substance. Most allergens are considered weakly immunogenic and most people do not respond to them adversely. However, an allergic person is often sensitive to several different allergens.

Mechanism of type I hypersensitivity

In order to produce type I hypersensitivity an individual must first come in contact with an antigen and produce IgE antibodies. These antibodies bind to mast cells and basophils (Fig. 15.1). Basophils are found in the circulation while mast cells (or fixed basophils) are located in lymphoid regions of respiratory tract, gastrointestinal tract, reproductive tract, skin and lining of blood vessels including capillaries. They have large number of vesicles containing pharmacologically potent compounds like histamine and serotonin.

Thus, **after first exposure** allergen-specific IgE is fixed to the mast cells and basophils, thereby sensitizing them. The part of the IgE molecule that binds to the surface of mast cells and basophils is the Fc portion. These cells possess high affinity receptors specific for Fc portion of IgE antibodies. Thus, Fab portion of IgE remains exposed. IgE antibodies can remain attached on these cells for up to six weeks. Such an individual is said to be **sensitized**.

After a second exposure the allergen travels to the mast cells and basophils, where it binds to antigen-binding site on IgE molecule. Antigen-antibody binding triggers the process of degranulation through which the mast cell explosively discharges its pharmacologically active agents. These include histamine, serotonin, bradykinin, slow-reacting substance of anaphylaxis (SRS-A), platelet-activating factors, eosinophil chemotactic factor of anaphylaxis and prostaglandins.

Histamine

Histamine is the most abundant and fastest acting. It induces smooth muscle contraction, release of mucus, vasodilation and increased capillary permeability. All these reactions can have profound effects. For example, excessive smooth muscle contraction and release of mucus in respiratory tract can close

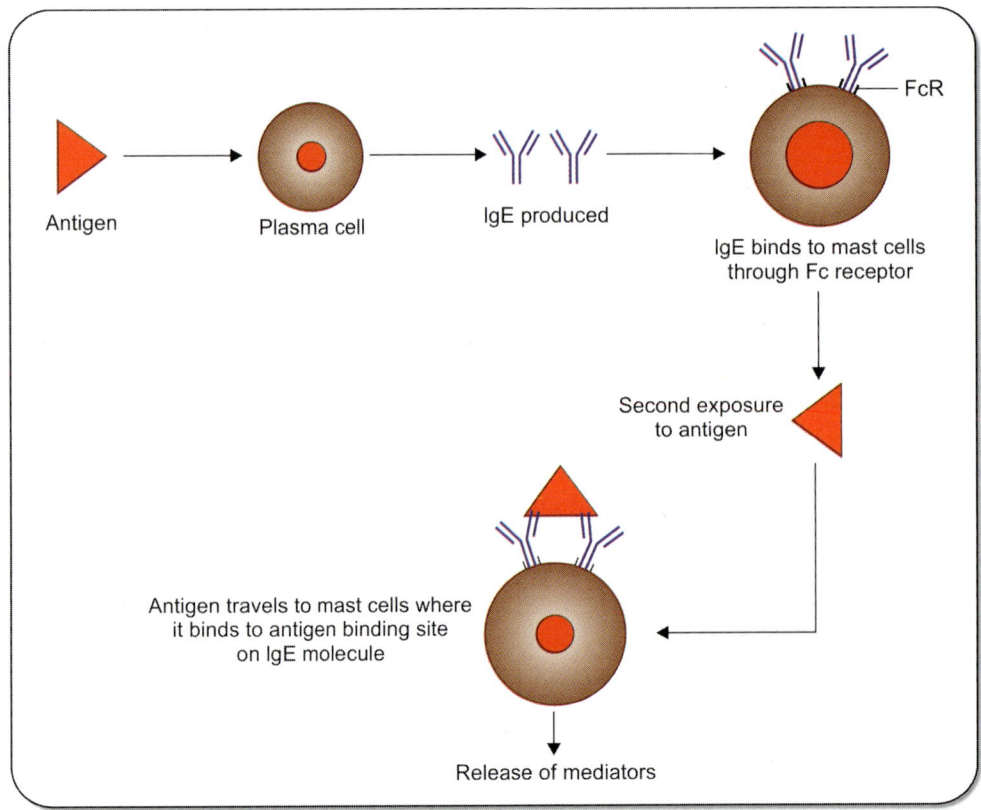

Fig. 15.1. Antigen-induced mediator release from mast cell.

the air passages of trachea and bronchi, causing asphyxiation and death by suffocation.

Another target area is the uterus. Pregnant women who are severely allergic may abort the foetus during an attack of histamine release and subsequent smooth muscle contractions in the uterus. Histamine also induces increased capillary permeability leading to oedema. Thus, there is extensive loss of blood fluids into the tissues. This may lead to circulatory shock and death.

Cutaneous anaphylaxis

If a person is suspected to be allergic to a particular substance, a **skin test** can be done. In this test a small dose of allergen is injected intradermally. In less than 30 minutes results can be read. If the individual is allergic, there will be a **wheal and flare response** at the site of injection. Wheal is a pale central area of puffiness due to oedema (caused by increased capillary permeability) which is surrounded by flare (caused by hyperaemia due to vasodilation). Since the injection site is small, it is possible to test for hypersensitivity to hundreds of substances on a person's back. The wheal and flare response can be used to determine the specific substance to which the atopic person is sensitive.

Prausnitz-Küstner (PK) reaction

Prausnitz and Küstner in 1921 demonstrated transmission of

IgE-mediated type I hypersensitivity by injecting serum containing IgE antibodies from allergic person into the skin of a normal or nonallergic person. Serum from Küstner, who was hypersensitive to certain species of cooked fish, was injected intracutaneously in Prausnitz (normal) followed 24 hours later by an intracutaneous injection of cooked fish, to which Küstner was sensitive, into the same site in Prausnitz. This led to wheal and flare reaction within 20 minutes. As IgE antibody is homocytotropic, the test has to be carried out on human skin, therefore, there is risk of transmission of hepatitis B virus and human immunodeficiency virus.

Passive cutaneous anaphylaxis (PCA)

PCA is similar to PK reaction. This is used to assay IgE antibodies in experimental animals. In this procedure, serum from an anaphylactically sensitized animal is injected intradermally into the skin of a normal animal. Forty eight hours later, this animal is challenged with allergen (to which the first animal was sensitive) and Evans blue dye, injected intravenously. If IgE is present in the serum (from first animal), the allergen will bind to IgE on the mast cell and cause degranulation and the release of vasoactive amines.

The blood capillaries in the area become permeable and allow the Evans blue dye to leak out into the dermis of the skin leading to immediate blueing at the site of intradermal injection. The area of blueing can be related to the quantity of

IgE present in the serum. PCA can be used to detect the human IgG antibody which is heterocytotropic (capable of fixing to cells of other species) but not IgE which is homocytotropic (capable of fixing to cells of homologous species only).

Anaphylaxis *in vitro* (Schultz-Dale phenomenon)

In 1910, Schultz and Dale demonstrated that sensitized strips of smooth muscle contract, *in vitro*, following exposure to antigen. Thus, intestinal and uterine muscle strips from a sensitized animal (guinea-pig) held in Ringer's solution bath contract vigorously on addition of specific antigen. Smooth muscle strips can be passively sensitized by bathing them in serum from a hypersensitive animal. The actual test is done by adding the antigen and observing subsequent contractions.

Atopy

The term atopy refers to chronic human allergic states. These include **hay fever**, **allergic asthma**, **atopic dermatitis (urticaria)** and **food allergies**. The antigens commonly involved in atopy are inhalants (pollen, house dust, animal dander or other types of fine particles suspended in air) or ingestants (milk, milk products, eggs, meat, fish or cereal). Some of them are contact allergens, to which the skin and conjunctiva may be exposed. The mechanism of development of atopy is essentially the same as that of systemic anaphylaxis. Atopy is likely to develop when allergen is localized or absorbed slowly, on the other hand, systemic anaphylaxis is likely to develop if large quantities of allergen are quickly distributed throughout the body.

Hay fever (allergic rhinitis)

It is an IgE-mediated allergic reaction that affects the mucosal surfaces of upper respiratory tract. It leads to nasal congestion, headache, running nose, watery eyes, itching and sneezing. The specific stimuli that cause allergic rhinitis include antigenic components of grass, weed and tree pollens, dust, mites, animal dander, organic dusts, components of tobacco smoke, and noninfectious components of fungal and bacterial allergens. If the allergen cannot be removed, then antihistaminics are the pharmacological agents of choice for the treatment of allergic rhinitis since histamine seems to be the major mediator of this allergy.

Allergic asthma

It is a severe form of respiratory allergy. It leads to contraction of the trachea and bronchi. The specific stimuli that cause allergic asthma include airborne allergens. In addition, asthma-producing foods such as milk, milk products, eggs, meat, fish or cereal may also precipitate allergic asthma. Some patients may even be sensitive to normal microbial flora leading to endogenous asthma. The main mediators of this allergy are serotonin and SRS-A. Therefore, antihistaminics are not able to reverse the smooth muscle contraction. The drug of choice for the treatment of this allergy is adrenaline (epinephrine). It is dispensed as atomizers for quick delivery. In addition, corticosteroids and cromolyn sodium have proved beneficial in treating attacks of allergic asthma.

Atopic dermatitis (urticaria)

Allergic skin eruptions in the form of wheals (whitish swelling), hives (red lesions), or eczema (scaly sores) may develop from varied sources such as foods, drugs, chemicals and clothing materials. Avoidance of these is the treatment. If it is not possible then antihistaminics are indicated.

Food allergies

Food allergy occurs in infants and children, but is uncommon in adults. Certain foods such as eggs, milk, peanuts, seafoods, citrus fruits and chocolate are frequent causes of food allergy. Consumption of the food in a patient with food allergy leads to nausea, vomiting, diarrhoea and cramps with typical urticaria and wheezing or upper airways congestion. Best cure for food allergy is to avoid that food unless it is a common ingredient of prepared foods such as flour.

TYPE II HYPERSENSITIVITY: CYTOTOXIC

This involves the combination of IgG and IgM serum antibodies with foreign antigenic components on a cell surface. Alternatively, a free foreign antigen or hapten such as a drug or microbial product may be adsorbed onto a cell membrane, which subsequently combines with antibody. Two different antibody-dependent mechanisms are involved in this type of hypersensitivity.

1. Complement-mediated cytotoxicity

Some of the cytotoxic reactions are complement dependent. After the antibodies become membrane bound, complement may be activated. Activation of classical complement pathway leads to the lysis of the cell through generation of membrane attack complex (MAC) (Fig. 11.1). Activation of complement cascade also leads to the formation of C3a and C5a fragments. These fragments are chemotactic for phagocytic cells. Fab portions of the antibodies bind to the cell bound antigens and complement gets fixed at the Fc portions of the antibody molecules. The phagocytes, which arrive at the site by the chemotactic activity of C3a and C5a possess complement receptors (CRs) and lead to the phagocytic response (Fig. 15.2).

2. Antibody-dependent cell-mediated cytotoxicity (ADCC)

This is the second possible mechanism involved in type II reactions. Fc portions of IgG or IgM absorbed onto the target cell through Fab interact with Fc receptors (FcRs) of NK cell which, in this context of ADCC, is often referred to as a K

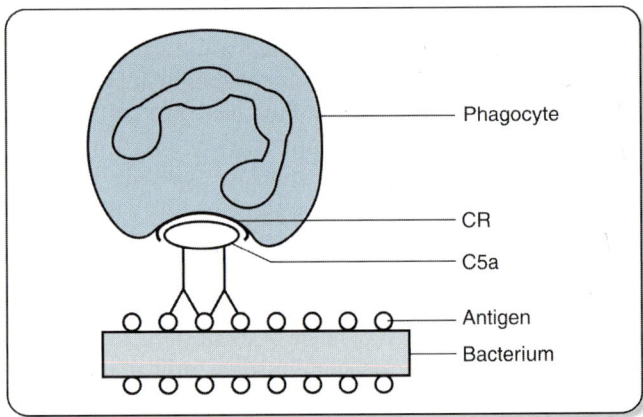

Fig. 15.2. Complement-mediated cytotoxicity.

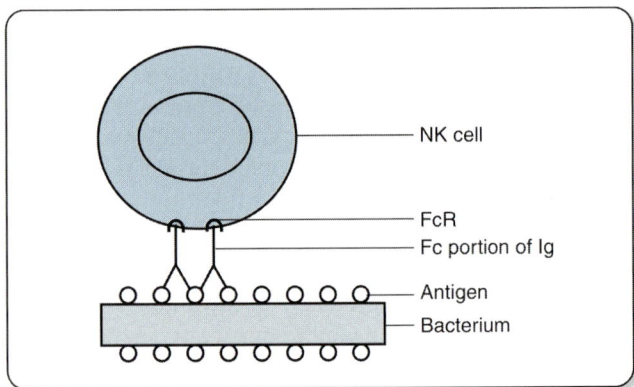

Fig. 15.3. Antibody-dependent cell-mediated cytotoxicity.

cell. Macrophages and eosinophils also indulge in this type of activity. This leads to lysis of target cells (Fig. 15.3). Lysis of target cells requires contact with K cells but does not involve phagocytosis or fixation of complement.

Clinically, antibody-mediated reactions occur in following situations:

1. Drug-induced immune haemolytic anaemia

A type II hypersensitivity reaction involving haemolytic anaemia may be induced by administration of certain drugs. Drugs such as antibiotic penicillin, and alpha-methyldopa for the treatment of hypertension can bind to the surface of red blood cell and form an antigenic complex with the surface of these cells. This can bring about the production of complement-fixing antibody to the drug. Reaction of this antibody with the RBC-bound drug activates the complement system, resulting in RBC lysis and anaemia.

2. Transfusion reactions

When a person receives incompatible blood transfusion, the antibodies normally present in recipient's serum agglutinate and lyse donor RBCs with the liberation of free haemoglobin into the plasma. This leads to jaundice, fever and failure of kidney function. Serum of the donor may also agglutinate and lyse recipient's RBCs. For example, transfusion of group O whole blood or plasma to group A or group B or group AB recipients may lead to haemolysis. But this reaction is mild since the donor's serum gets considerably diluted in the circulation of the recipient.

3. Rh incompatibility

Rh antibodies are major cause of **haemolytic disease of newborn (HDN)**. When an Rh-negative woman carries an Rh-positive foetus, she may be immunized against Rh antigen by passage of foetal red cells into maternal circulation. Minor transplacental leaks may occur any time during pregnancy, but it is during delivery that foetal cells enter the maternal circulation in large numbers. Therefore, the mother is usually immunized only at first delivery, and consequently, the first child escapes damage (except where the woman has been sensitized already by prior Rh incompatible blood transfusion). During subsequent pregnancy, Rh antibodies of IgG class pass from the mother to the foetus and damage its erythrocytes. The clinical features of HDN may vary from a mere accentuation of the physiological jaundice in the newborn to erythroblastosis fetalis or intrauterine death due to **hydrops fetalis**.

4. Autoimmune haemolytic anaemia, agranulocytosis and thrombocytopenia

Some persons develop antibodies against their blood elements, resulting in autoimmune haemolytic anaemia, agranulocytosis or thrombocytopenia.

5. Anaemia due to infectious diseases

A variety of infectious diseases due to *Salmonella* and mycobacteria are associated with haemolytic anaemia. Studies in *Salmonella* infections have revealed that the haemolysis is due to an immune reaction against a lipopolysaccharide bacterial endotoxin that becomes coated onto the erythrocytes of the patient.

TYPE III HYPERSENSITIVITY: IMMUNE COMPLEX

If an antigen is not cell-bound but is rather small and soluble, the body can encounter severe difficulties if it is repeatedly exposed to that antigen. Antigen-antibody complexes formed under these conditions may lead to type III or immune complex-mediated hypersensitivity. Monocytes and macrophages are very efficient at binding and removing large precipitating antigen-antibody complexes. They can also eliminate the smaller complexes made in antibody excess but are relatively inefficient at removing those formed in antigen excess. The formation of antigen-antibody complexes in serum, with subsequent deposition of the complexes in tissues, is the key event in type III hypersensitivity. Antigen-antibody complexes can then activate serum complement, platelets and phagocytes, all of which lead to tissue damage.

As a result of activation of complement, fragments C3a and C5a are created. Both these fragments are anaphylatoxic since they bind to plasma membrane receptor sites on basophils, mast cells and platelets causing histamine release leading to inflammatory response. C5a fragment also attracts polymorphonuclear leucocytes. These cells release their degradative lysosomal enzymes leading to tissue damage.

The degree and site of damage depends on the ratio of antigen to antibody. At equivalence or slight excess of either component, the complexes precipitate at the site of antigen injection and a mild local type III hypersensitivity or Arthus reaction develops. On the other hand, the complexes formed in large antigen excess become soluble and circulate, causing more serious systemic reactions, i.e., serum sickness or eventually deposit in organs, such as skin, joints, kidneys and heart.

Arthus reaction (local immune complex disease)

Arthus (1903) observed that when rabbits were repeatedly injected subcutaneously with normal horse serum, the initial injections were without any local effect, but with later injections, there occurred intense local reaction consisting of oedema, induration and haemorrhagic necrosis. This is known as Arthus reaction. The tissue damage is due to formation of local precipitating immune complexes which are deposited on the endothelial lining of the blood vessels. Antigen-antibody complexes can then trigger and activate complement leading to inflammation and tissue damage as discussed above.

Passive cutaneous form of the Arthus reaction

In this an antiserum is first injected intravenously into a nonsensitive recipient and the corresponding antigen is then injected into the skin.

Reversed passive Arthus reaction

In this the antiserum is injected into the recipient's skin and the antigen is then injected into the same dermal site or intravenously. Both injections are made at about the same time, so that sufficient amount of antibody will remain near the injection site to precipitate with the antigen and cause local inflammation and necrosis.

Serum sickness (systemic immune complex disease)

This is a systemic form of type III hypersensitivity. This develops in persons who receive a single injection of a high concentration of horse antitoxin against tetanus, gas gangrene, diphtheria, etc. for prophylactic and therapeutic purposes. Seven to 12 days after the injection, patient may develop fever, lymphadenopathy, splenomegaly, arthritis, glomerulonephritis, endocarditis, vasculitis, urticarial rash, abdominal pain, nausea and vomiting. It is due to the immune response to horse antigens and it has also been encountered in allergic reactions to certain drugs. After 7–12 days, antibodies to horse antigens appear while horse antigens are still persisting because a large dose was administered. Initially, they form antigen-antibody complexes in antigen excess. These soluble complexes can circulate and get deposited in various sites throughout the body particularly in skin, joints, kidneys and heart.

Antigen-antibody aggregates can fix complement leading to inflammation and tissue damage as discussed above. The plasma level of complement falls due to massive complement activation and fixation by antigen-antibody complexes. Initially, the circulating immune complexes are in antigen excess and produce inflammatory lesions, but as antibody production rises, the immune complexes increase in size as zone of equivalence is reached. These larger immune complexes are more easily phagocytosed and cleared by the cells of reticuloendothelial system of liver and spleen. Once all immune complexes are removed from the circulation, symptoms are usually resolved within a week.

Raised levels of immune complexes have been demonstrated in many infective and other conditions:

(a) **Bacterial infections**
  - Endocarditis
  - Poststreptococcal glomerulonephritis
  - Lepromatous leprosy
  - Secondary syphilis
  - Infected shunts in children

(b) **Viral infections**
  - Dengue haemorrhagic fever
  - Hepatitis B
  - Cytomegalovirus
  - Infectious mononucleosis
  - Subacute sclerosing panencephalitis

(c) **Parasitic infections**
  - Malaria
  - Toxoplasmosis
  - Trypanosomiasis
  - Schistosomiasis
  - Filariasis

(d) **Drugs**
  - Penicillin
  - Sulphonamides

TYPE IV HYPERSENSITIVITY: CELL-MEDIATED OR DELAYED

Type IV hypersensitivity or delayed hypersensitivity (DH) is the clinically observable outcome of cell-mediated immune reaction in the tissues of a sensitized individual. The reaction is not brought about by circulating antibodies and B lympho-cytes but by sensitized T lymphocytes and macrophages. It is named delayed hypersensitivity because it appears in 24–48 hours after the presensitized host encounters the antigen, while immediate hypersensitivity reactions develop in 1/2 to 12

Table 15.1. Comparison of types I–IV hypersensitivity reactions

Characteristic	Type I	Type II	Type III	Type IV
Approximate time to develop clinical signs	1/2–8 hours	5–12 hours	3–8 hours	24–48 hours
Reaction mediators	IgE, histamine, serotonin, SRS-A, etc.	IgG, IgM and complement	IgG, IgM, complement, neutrophils, eosinophils and lysosomal enzymes	T cells, macrophages and lymphokines
Response to intradermal injection of antigen	Wheal and flare	—	Erythema and oedema	Erythema and induration
Passive transfer with	Serum	Serum	Serum	T cells
Examples	Anaphylaxis, asthma, hay fever, and food and insect allergies	Transfusion reaction, HDN and drug-induced allergy	Arthus reaction and serum sickness	Tuberculin test, contact dermatitis, graft rejection and tumour immunity

hours (Table 15.1). The mechanism of delayed hypersensitivity is given in Chapter 14. Two types of DH are recognized – tuberculin (infection) type and contact dermatitis type.

1. Tuberculin (infection) type

The immune response to the tubercle bacillus, observed by Robert Koch in 1880, has served a general model for DH. When a small dose (1 to 3 units) of tuberculin or purified protein derivative (PPD) is injected intradermally in an individual sensitized to tuberculoprotein by prior infection or immunization, an indurated inflammatory reaction, 10 mm or more in diameter, develops at the site of injection within 48–72 hours. It is characterized by erythema due to increased blood flow to the damaged area and induration due to infiltration with a large number of mononuclear cells, mainly T lymphocytes and about 10–20% macrophages. In unsensitized individuals, the tuberculin injection provokes no response. Cell-mediated hypersensitivity reactions are seen in a number of chronic infectious diseases due to mycobacteria, protozoa and fungi.

2. Contact dermatitis type

Contact dermatitis is cell-mediated allergic reaction that occurs when certain substances like metals (nickel and chromium), dyes (picryl chloride and dinitrochlorobenzene), drugs such as penicillin, and toiletries come in contact with skin. Sensitization is particularly liable to occur when contact is with an inflamed area and when chemical is applied in an oily base. Application of antibiotic ointments frequently provokes sensitization. The substances involved are not anti-genic by themselves but may acquire antigenicity on combination with skin proteins. Subsequent contact with allergen in a sensitized individual leads to contact dermatitis. The lesions vary from macules and papules to vesicles which break down leaving behind raw weeping areas typical of acute eczematous dermatitis.

This hypersensitivity can be detected by **patch test**. The allergen is applied to the skin under an adherent dressing. Sensitivity is indicated by itching, appearing in 4–5 hours and local reaction which may vary from erythema to vesicle or blister formation in 24 hours.

TYPE V HYPERSENSITIVITY: STIMULATORY OR ANTIRECEPTOR

This is an antibody-mediated hypersensitivity. Here antibody reacts with a key surface component such as a hormone receptor and switches on or stimulates the cell. An example of this type of hypersensitivity is the thyroid hyperactivity in Graves' disease due to **thyroid stimulating autoantibody**.

Normally, thyroid stimulating hormone (TSH) from pituitary gland binds to thyroid cell receptors. This activates adenyl cyclase in the membrane which converts ATP to AMP. The latter stimulates activity of thyroid cells, thus secreting thyroxine. **The thyroid stimulating antibody present in the sera of thyrotoxic patients is an autoantibody directed against receptors for TSH.** This antibody, therefore, binds to these receptors and brings about the same effect as that of TSH. Type V hypersensitivity differs from type II, because instead of binding to cell surface components, the antibodies, in type V hypersensitivity, recognize and bind to the cell surface receptors and stimulate the cell.

Autoimmunity

Normally, we do not form potentially destructive antibodies and T cells against our own cells because our body has developed tolerance to self-antigens. However, all mechanisms have a risk of breakdown. The self-recognition mechanisms are no exception, and a number of diseases have been identified, in which there is autoimmunity, due to copious production of autoantibodies and autoreactive T cells. **Self-tolerance** refers to lack of responsiveness to an individual's own antigens, and obviously it underlines our ability to live in harmony with our own cells and tissues. **Autoimmunity may, therefore, be defined as immune response to self-antigens, which can generate autoantibodies and autoreactive T cells.**

An individual may have more than one autoimmune disease, for example, thyroid antibodies occur with a high frequency in pernicious anaemia patients who have gastric autoimmunity. There is an undoubted **familial incidence of autoimmunity**. There is much evidence to suggest that auto-antibodies are important in autoimmunity. A number of diseases have been recognized in which autoantibodies to hormone receptors may actually mimic the function of the normal hormone concerned and produce disease.

- Thyrotoxicosis was the first disorder in which such anti-receptor antibodies were clearly recognized. IgG antibodies from thyrotoxic mothers can cross the placenta leading to neonatal thyrotoxicosis, but the problem spontaneously resolves as the antibodies derived from the mother are cata-bolized in the baby over several weeks.
- A similar phenomenon has been observed with mothers suffering from myasthenia gravis where antibodies to acetylcholine receptors cross the placenta into the foetus and cause transient muscle weakness in the newborn baby.
- Somewhat rarely, autoantibodies to insulin receptors and to β-adrenergic receptors can be found. The latter is associated with bronchial asthma.
- In rare cases of male infertility antibodies to spermatozoa lead to clumping of spermatozoa.

- In pernicious anaemia an autoantibody interferes with the normal uptake of vitamin B_{12}. Vitamin B_{12} is not absorbed directly, but must first associate with a protein called intrinsic factor. It is synthesized by the parietal cells in gastric mucosa. The vitamin-protein complex is then trans-ported across the intestinal mucosa. Plasma cells in the gastric mucosa of patients with pernicious anaemia secrete an autoantibody, specific for intrinsic factor. This antibody combines with intrinsic factor, thus inhibiting its role as a carrier for vitamin B_{12}.
- Autoimmune haemolytic anaemia and idiopathic thrombo-cytopenic purpura result from the synthesis of autoanti-bodies to red cells and platelets, respectively.
- In systemic lupus erythematosus, immune complexes containing DNA and antibody are deposited in the kidney, skin, joints and choroid.

MECHANISM OF AUTOIMMUNITY

There are several possible mechanisms involved in the development of autoimmunity:

1. Forbidden clones

According to clonal selection theory, antibody-forming lymphocytes capable of reacting with different antigens are formed. Clones of cells that have immunological reactivity with self-antigens are eliminated during embryonic life. Such clones are called forbidden clones. Their persistence or development in later life by somatic mutations can lead to autoimmunity.

2. Hidden or sequestrated antigen

Certain self-antigens are present in closed systems and are not accessible to immune system. An example is the **lens antigen of the eye**. The lens protein is enclosed in its capsule and does not circulate in the blood. Therefore, immunological tolerance against this antigen does not develop during foetal life. When the lens protein antigen leaks out, following cataract surgery or injury to the eye, it leads to immune response and damage to the other eye.

Another example of hidden antigen is seen in case of **sperm antigens**. Since sperms develop only at puberty, therefore, the sperm antigens cannot induce tolerance during foetal life. Sperms may enter into blood stream following injury of the testes and mumps. Virus probably damages the basement membrane of seminiferous tubules leading to the leakage of sperms and initiation of an immune response resulting in orchitis.

3. Neoantigens or altered antigens

Cells or tissues may undergo antigenic alteration by physical agents such as irradiation. Photosensitivity or cold allergy may be due to altered antigens by light and cold respectively. Several chemical agents including drugs can combine with cells and tissues and alter their antigenic structure. Skin contact with a variety of chemicals may lead to contact dermatitis. Drug-induced anaemia, leucopenia and thrombocytopenia often have autoimmune basis. Viruses and other intracellular pathogens may induce alterations of cell antigens leading to autoimmunity.

4. Cross reacting antigens

Immunological damage may result from immune response induced by cross reacting foreign antigens. For example, **Semple rabies vaccine** consists of infected sheep brain tissue inactivated with phenol. Its injection elicits an immune response against sheep brain antigens. This may lead to damage to patient's nervous tissue due to cross reaction between human and sheep brain leading to encephalitis.

Immunological injury may be due to cross reacting antigens present on microorganisms causing infection. An important example of this is the **non-suppurative sequelae of *Streptococcus pyogenes*** infection which include acute rheumatic fever and acute glomerulonephritis. M protein of *S. pyogenes* and heart of man share antigenic characteristics. The immune response induced by repeated streptococcal infections can, therefore, damage the heart. Nephritogenic strains of *S. pyogenes* share antigens with renal glomeruli. Therefore, immune response following infection with such strains may lead to acute glomerulonephritis.

Escherichia coli **O14** shares antigen with human colon. This organism has, therefore, been blamed to cause ulcerative colitis. Many patients suffering from syphilis develop haemolytic anaemia. It has been suggested that antibodies raised against *Treponema pallidum* **antigens** cross react with certain blood group antigens bringing about the anaemia. There is also an evidence that antigens common to *Trypanosoma cruzi*, causative agent of Chagas' disease, and human cardiac muscle produce the immunopathological lesions seen in this disease.

5. Mutation

Immunocompetent cells may acquire an unnatural responsiveness to self-antigens by mutation.

6. Activity of helper and suppressor T cells

Helper T (Th) cells facilitate B cell response to many antigens. Suppressor T (Ts) cells inhibit antibody production by B cells. Optimal antibody response depends on the balanced activity of Th and Ts cells. *Overactivity of Th cells or decreased activity of Ts cells may lead to autoimmunity.*

CLASSIFICATION OF AUTOIMMUNE DISEASES

1. Autoimmune anaemias
   (a) Pernicious anaemia
   (b) Autoimmune haemolytic anaemias
2. Autoimmune thrombocytopenia
3. Autoimmune thyroid diseases
   (a) Graves' disease (thyrotoxicosis)
   (b) Hashimoto's disease (hypothyroidism)
4. Addison's disease
5. Autoimmune orchitis
6. Diabetes mellitus
7. Goodpasture's syndrome
8. Multiple sclerosis
9. Myasthenia gravis
10. Systemic autoimmune diseases
    (a) Rheumatoid arthritis
    (b) Systemic lupus erythematosus
    (c) Systemic sclerosis (scleroderma)
    (d) Dermatomyositis
    (e) Polyarteritis nodosa
    (f) Sjogren's syndrome

17

Transplantation Immunology

Transplantation of normal tissues and organs from one animal to another has been extensively studied. Most of the experimental work on transplantation has been done on mice, an animal species easy to breed and handle in the laboratory. The aim of tissue and organ transplantation from one person to another is to replace diseased tissues and organs. The tissue or organ transplanted is known as the **transplant** or **graft**. The individual from whom the transplant is obtained is known as **donor** and the individual on whom it is applied, the **recipient**.

TYPES OF GRAFTS

1. **Autografts:** Grafts from one part of the body to another in the same individual are known as autografts. Autografts survive and function for the life time of the individual.
2. **Isografts:** Grafts between genetically identical individuals (identical twins).
3. **Allografts:** Grafts between members of the same species (allogeneic individuals) but of different genetic constitution.
4. **Xenografts:** Grafts between members of different species.

Except in case of uniovular twins, the transplantation of a tissue from one human to another amounts to an allograft. Grafts between ordinary brothers and sisters or between parents and offsprings, or even between dissimilar twins are examples of allografts. Allografts survive longer than xenografts but are ultimately rejected.

ALLOGRAFT REACTION

When a skin graft from an animal is applied on a genetically unrelated animal of the same species (allograft), for the first few days it behaves as an autograft. It is quickly vascularized and looks healthy. By about fourth day, it slowly becomes dark because of diminished circulation due to stasis followed by thrombosis and haemorrhage. The graft is invaded by lymphocytes and macrophages and in about two weeks, the graft sloughs off due to ischaemic necrosis. In addition, anti-bodies are believed to play a significant role in this process. The sequence of events resulting in the rejection of an allograft is known as **first-set reaction**.

If in an animal, which has rejected a graft by first-set reaction, another graft from the same donor is applied, it will lead to a hyperacute or immediate rejection response. This is accomplished by cytolytic leucocytes and complement-mediated antibody lysis of transplanted cells. The initial vascularisation may not occur, if it does, it is poor and is halted abruptly. Thrombosis of vessels is a feature. The graft is rejected much sooner in three to five days. This is known as **second-set reaction**.

The cells of an individual express a unique set of membrane antigens called **histocompatibility antigens**, which immunologically define a person's cell type as specifically as do fingerprints. The information about the synthesis of these antigens is stored on **histocompatibility genes**. Everyone on earth, with the possible exception of identical twins, has a personal set of histocompatibility genes and gene products (histocompatibility antigens). These genetically defined histocompatibility antigens, some of which are found on the surface of all body cells, serve to discriminate self from non-self.

Only those grafts in which there is a complete identity between the genetic constitution of the donor and the recipient (their histocompatibility genes and antigens are identical) survive and function. The rejection of an allograft has an immunological basis. This is evident from the specificity of the second-set reaction. **Accelerated rejection is seen only if the second graft is from the same donor as the first.** Application of a skin graft from another donor will evoke only the first-set reaction.

Mechanism of allograft rejection

Presentation of foreign cell MHC antigens is one of the initial events of first-set reaction. Once blood vessels communicate with the graft, graft antigens can travel to the lymph nodes where they activate lymphatic T cells. The activated lymphocytes give rise to expanded clones of specific Tc, Th and Td cells. Tc cells can enter the circulation directly, while Td cells remain in the lymph nodes and mobilize phagocytic leucocytes via the release of soluble lymphokines. Tc cells eventually reach the transplantation site, enter the blood vessels of the graft, and proceed to destroy the grafted tissue by repeated cell-to-cell toxicity.

In second-set reactions, the memory of foreign antigenic cells is so vivid that the blood vessels of the second graft are destroyed almost as soon as they are established. This rapid response is brought about primarily by Tc cells which are rapidly activated. The additional participation of circulating complement fixing antibodies and NK cells might contribute to graft rejection. The infiltration of neutrophils, macrophages and Tc cells, which are already present in the circulation, follows soon leading to rapid and irreversible rejection of foreign tissue transplanted to the host a second time.

MAJOR HISTOCOMPATIBILITY COMPLEX

Genes mediating graft rejection in mice are called the histocompatibility genes or H genes or H loci. A large number of H loci exist widely spread throughout the mouse genome. The products of the different H genes differ greatly in their ability to induce graft rejection. The strongest locus is known as major histocompatibility complex (MHC) in contrast to weaker loci (minor histocompatibility loci) which are more than 30. The MHC in mouse is referred to as **H-2 complex**.

The MHC in humans is known as the **human leucocyte antigen (HLA) complex**. The genes that code for the HLA antigens are found on the short arm of sixth pair of chromosome (one paternal and one maternal). The MHC genes are contained within four HLA loci known as A, B, C and D (Fig. 17.1). There are many different alleles at each of HLA-A, HLA-B and HLA-C loci, although any individual will possess a maximum of two at each locus (one on each chromosome). The A locus is associated with segregant series of 24 alleles, the B locus with 52 alleles and the C locus with 11 alleles. The various alleles are assigned the letters signifying the locus followed by a number signifying the allele. For example, HLA-A10 implies an HLA allele number 10 belonging to the locus A.

There are three classes of genes in these HLA loci – class I, class II and class III genes which code for the corresponding molecules (antigens).

MHC class I molecules

In humans the genes encoding the major transplantation antigens are HLA-A, HLA-B and HLA-C loci. The products of these loci are known as class I antigens. Class I antigens are membrane-bound glycoprotein in nature. They are composed of two polypeptide chains (Fig. 17.2). The smaller of the two polypeptide chains is known as β_2-microglobulin (β_2-M). It is not encoded by genes within the MHC, but by the gene located on chromosome 2. It has a molecular weight of 12,000 daltons. The larger polypeptide chain of class I antigen is encoded by a gene present on HLA-A, HLA-B and HLA-C regions. It has a molecular weight of 45,000 daltons. It has five structural domains. Three external globular domains (α_1, α_2 and α_3) held in place by disulphide bonds and non-covalent interactions, a transmembrane portion and a short cytoplasmic tail. β_2-M is non-covalently associated with α_3 domain. The globular protein formed by these two peptides is present on the surface of virtually all nucleated cells, with probable exception of ova, sperms and amniotic cells, in man. They are involved in recognition of target cells by cytotoxic T cells. The cytotoxic T cells recognize antigen only if presented simultaneously with class I antigens.

MHC class II molecules

Class II antigens are encoded by the HLA-DP, HLA-DQ and HLA-DR loci (all of which reside within the HLA-D region of HLA complex), for which there are multiple alleles in the population. They are glycoproteins consisting of two polypeptide chains (α and β) held together by non-covalent interactions (Fig. 17.3). Both these chains are inserted into the cell membrane and have molecular weights of 33,000 and 25,000 daltons respectively. Each chain is composed of two extracellular domains (α_1, α_2 and β_1, β_2), a transmembrane portion and a cytoplasmic tail. The tissue distribution of class II MHC antigens is relatively limited. In man, they are

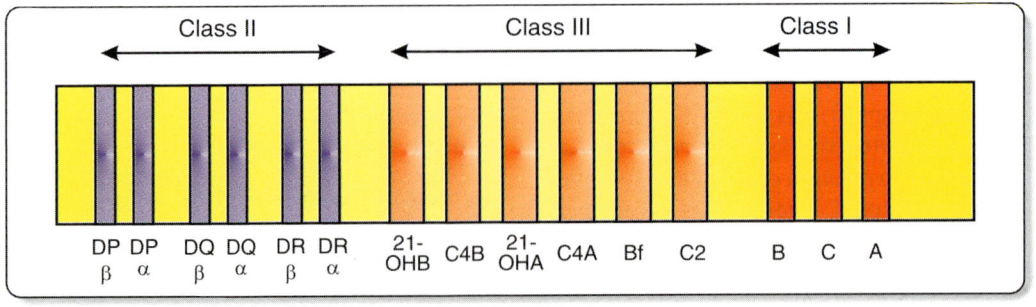

Fig. 17.1. HLA complex.

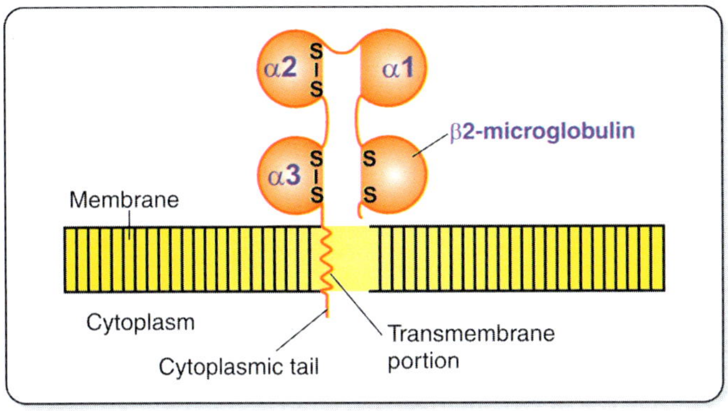

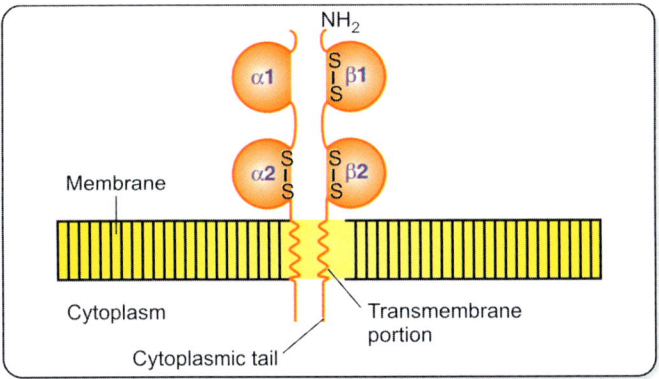

Fig. 17.2. Class I MHC antigens.

Fig. 17.3. Class II MHC antigens.

normally found on immunologically reactive cells such as B lymphocytes, macrophages, monocytes and activated T lymphocytes.

Class I and class II MHC antigens are members of the immunoglobulin superfamily. Both the class I and class II MHC-encoded proteins are structurally related to immunoglobulin and are involved in cell-cell interaction in the generation and regulation of immune responses. As such, they are members of the larger group of proteins called the immunoglobulin superfamily.

MHC class III molecules

The genes coding for the complement components of the classical (C2 and C4) and the alternative (properdin or factor B) pathway also reside in the MHC genes complex located between MHC class I and class II regions (Fig. 17.1).

HISTOCOMPATIBILITY TESTING

For matching of donor and recipient for transplantation following procedures are undertaken:

ABO grouping

When tissue transplantation is anticipated, grouping and cross-matching of blood from donor and recipient are performed as a first step. If there exists any discrepancy in the ABO blood

group, then the use of the prospective donor's tissue is absolutely contraindicated because blood group antigens are strong histocompatibility antigens.

Tissue typing (detection of MHC antigens)

Class I antigens are identified by means of antisera, therefore, the term serologically defined antigens is applied to them. Antisera used to detect class I antigens are obtained from:

- multiparous women,
- individuals who have received multiple blood transfusions,
- individuals who have received and rejected grafts, and
- volunteers who have been immunized with cells from another individual with a different HLA haplotype.

Following methods are used:

(a) Lymphoagglutination test

When lymphocytes are mixed with a panel of specific antisera, agglutination of lymphocytes is seen with specific antiserum.

(b) Lymphocytotoxicity test

Lymphocytes are incubated with a panel of antisera directed against specific class I MHC antigens followed by addition of complement. Lysis of cells is seen with specific antiserum. This can be detected by the addition of eosin or trypan blue which stains only dead cells.

(c) Mixed lymphocyte culture assay

MHC class II antigens are identified by the method known as mixed lymphocyte culture (MLC) assay. This can determine a possible match between donor and recipient class II antigens. In this test, donor and recipient lymphocytes are mixed together in a tube containing a radioactive DNA precursor. Donor or stimulator cells are irradiated to prevent DNA synthesis and proliferation. If the class II antigens are foreign, the responder cells will be stimulated to divide. As the stimulated cells replicate their DNA, they incorporate the radioactive precursor. The amount of radioactivity incorporated into cells can then be easily measured and quantitated.

Uses of HLA typing

HLA typing is used primarily for the following:

- Determination of HLA compatibility prior to transplantation,
- Paternity testing,
- Anthropologic studies, and
- Establishing HLA disease associations.

HLA typing is done to identify HLA compatible donors and recipients for organ transplantation. The collaborative transplant study has demonstrated that the graft survival rate of HLA-identical (two haplotypes) transplants is superior to that of grafts matched for one haplotype. HLA matching has a statistically significant and clinically important impact on the short and long-term graft survival for most of the organ transplants (kidney, liver, bone marrow, etc).

Matching at HLA-D locus has a strong effect on kidney graft survival but in long term (5 years or more) the desirability of reasonable HLA-B, and to a lesser extent HLA-A, matching also becomes apparent. It has now been firmly established that multiple blood transfusions prior to grafting have a significant beneficial effect on survival but its mechanism is still not clear.

In heart transplants, graft survival is significantly influenced by the extent of HLA compatibility. Full HLA matching is of course not practical but single DR mismatch gives 90% survival for three years.

Successful corneal transplants have been performed without recourse to tissue typing or immunosuppression. Cornea is an immunologically privileged site. It lacks lymphatic drainage and the small amount of antigen released into the blood stream from graft is not sufficient to trigger a cellular response. But HLA typing may be very important in corneal transplantation in those cases where the recipient's eye is chronically inflamed.

HLA typing demonstrating that the putative father and child do not share any haplotype is usually accepted by the courts as excluding the possibility that a given male is the father.

GRAFT VERSUS HOST REACTION

Under certain circumstances the immunologically competent cells of the graft react against antigens of the host (recipient), the reverse of the normal transplantation reaction. Such a reaction is known as graft versus host reaction (GVH). Following conditions are necessary for the development of GVH:

1. The host's immunological responsiveness must be either destroyed or so impaired (following whole-body irradiation) that he cannot reject a graft (allograft or xeno-graft).

2. There is HLA incompatibility between the donor and the host (recipient).

3. The graft (bone marrow, lymphoid tissue, splenic tissue, etc.) contains immunocompetent cells. MHC antigens of recipient activate transplanted immunocompetent cells which lead to the production of antibodies, lymphokines, activated phagocytes, Tc cells, etc. They attack the recipient cells leading to the death of the recipient.

MHC RESTRICTION

Limitation imposed upon activation of an immune response, unless antigen presentation occurs in association with either a class I or a class II MHC antigen is known as MHC restriction. Tc and Ts cells recognise the combination of foreign antigen and class I MHC antigens, whereas Td and Th cells recognize foreign antigen in association with class II antigens. Therefore, in addition to transplantation reactions, MHC antigens are involved in immune surveillance, for example in viral infection. Both class I and class II antigens operate in this phenomenon.

Antigen presenting cells (APCs) or virus-infected cells, present viral antigen in association with class I molecules which is recognized by T cell receptors of Tc cell, and in association with class II molecules which is recognized by T cell receptors of Th cells. Binding of class I molecule/viral antigen complex to Tc cell receptors stimulates expansion of cytotoxic cells. Binding of class II molecule/viral complex to Th cell receptors stimulates expansion of Th cells. Release of interleukin-1 (IL-1) from APCs promotes both proliferation and differentiation responses to Tc and Th cells and IL-2, produced by activated Th cells, stimulates clonal expansion of Tc cells. Tc cells then recognize and destroy target cells expressing both self class I molecules and viral antigens.

MINOR HISTOCOMPATIBILITY ANTIGENS IN MAN

Very little is known about minor histocompatibility (mH) in man. However, evidence suggests that mH antigens also play a role in graft rejection because graft rejections have been observed in cases with complete HLA match.

SECTION 2

SYSTEMIC BACTERIOLOGY

Chapter 18   Staphylococcus
Chapter 19   Streptococcus and Enterococcus
Chapter 20   Streptococcus Pneumoniae (Pneumococcus)
Chapter 21   Neisseria, Moraxella and Acinetobacter
Chapter 22   Corynebacterium Diphtheriae
Chapter 23   Bacillus Anthracis
Chapter 24   Clostridium
Chapter 25   Mycobacterium Tuberculosis
Chapter 26   Nontuberculous Mycobacteria
Chapter 27   Mycobacterium Leprae
Chapter 28   Spirochaetes
Chapter 29   Bacteroides, Propionibacterium and Fusobacterium
Chapter 30   Escherichia, Klebsiella, Enterobacter, Serratia, Proteus and Morganella
Chapter 31   Shigella and Salmonella
Chapter 32   Yersinia Pestis
Chapter 33   Vibrio, Pseudomonas and Burkholderia
Chapter 34   Campylobacter and Helicobacter
Chapter 35   Legionella Pneumophila
Chapter 36   Haemophilus and Bordetella
Chapter 37   Brucella
Chapter 38   Mycoplasma and Ureaplasma
Chapter 39   Rickettsia and Orientia
Chapter 40   Chlamydia and Chlamydophila
Chapter 41   Actinomyces and Nocardia
Chapter 42   Gardnerella, Erysiplothrix and Streptobacillus
Chapter 43   Antimicrobial Sensitivity Testing
Chapter 44   Bacteriology of Water, Milk and Air
Chapter 45   Automation in Medical Microbiology

18

Staphylococcus

Genus *Staphylococcus* contains more than 45 defined species, 20 of which are known to be associated with colonization and/or infection of man. Of the 20 species found in man, one (*S. aureus*) is coagulase-positive and 19 coagulase-negative. The name 'staphylococcus' was derived from Greek words *staphyle* (bunch of grapes) and *kokkos* (grain or berry).

STAPHYLOCOCCUS AUREUS

Morphology

They are spherical cocci about 0.8–1.0 μm in diameter. They are arranged characteristically in grape-like clusters. Cluster formation is due to cell division occurring in more than one plane with daughter cells remaining close together. In smear from pus, the cocci appear singly or in pairs, clusters or short chains of three or four cells (Fig. 18.1). They are Gram-positive but old and phagocytosed organisms may be Gram-negative.

Cultural characteristics

They are aerobes and facultative anaerobes. Optimum temperature for growth is 37°C, range being 12–44°C. Optimum pH is 7.5. They can grow well on ordinary media.

1. Nutrient agar

After overnight incubation at 37°C, colonies are 1–2 mm in diameter with a smooth glistening surface. They are opaque and easily emulsifiable. Most strains produce golden-yellow (*aureus*) pigment, though some strains may form white (non-pigmented) colonies.

2. Blood agar

Colonies are similar to those on nutrient agar, but may be surrounded by a narrow zone of haemolysis (Fig. 18.2).

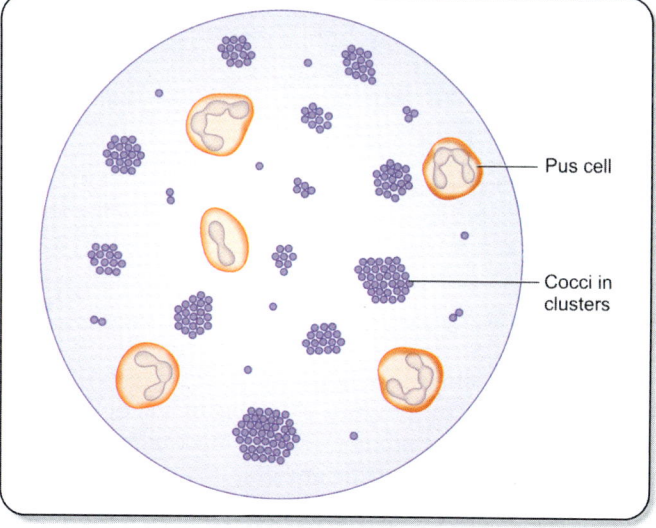

Fig. 18.1. Staphylococci and pus cells.

Pus cell

Cocci in clusters

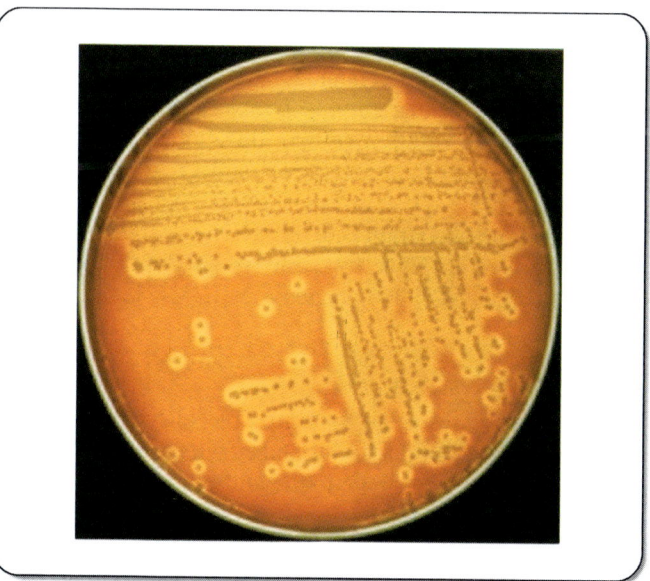

Fig. 18.2. Growth of *Staphylococcus aureus* on blood agar showing haemolysis.

3. Selective salt media

Staphylococci can grow in the presence of 10% or more of sodium chloride, while many other bacteria are inhibited at this concentration. Therefore, 7–10% of sodium chloride may be added to nutrient agar. Salt agar is useful for isolation of staphylococci from food, dust, faeces and pus where mixed bacterial flora are expected. The appearance of colonies on these media is similar to those on nutrient agar.

Bacteriophage typing

Phages of *S. aureus* have a narrow host range and lyse only some other strains of the same species. Therefore, for epidemiological studies and tracing the source of infection, strains of *S. aureus* can be distinguished from one another by their patterns of susceptibility to lysis by an internationally recognized set of 23 standard typing phages (Table 18.1). Lysis of a culture by one phage is often associated with lysis by one or more other phages. Staphylococci can seldom be characterized by lysis by a single phage, but many different patterns of lysis are obtained with a set of phages. Differences between these patterns are used to make fine distinction between staphylococcal strains.

Table 18.1. Typing set of staphylococcal phages

Lytic group	Designation of phages in lytic group
I	29, 52, 52A, 79, 80
II	3A, 3C, 55, 71
III	6, 42E, 47, 53, 54, 75, 77, 83A, 84, 85
IV	—
V	94, 96
Unclassified	81, 95

The strain to be typed is inoculated on a plate of nutrient agar to produce a lawn culture. Drops of various phages at their routine test dilution (RTD) are applied over marked squares. After overnight incubation at 30°C the culture will be observed to be lysed by some phages but not by others. The phage type of a strain is expressed by designation of the phages that lyse it. Thus, if a strain is lysed only by phages 3C, 55 and 71, it is called phage type 3C/55/71.

Determinants of pathogenicity or virulence factors of Staphylococcus aureus

S. aureus possesses a large number of cell wall associated factors, and extracellular toxins and enzymes (Table 18.2 and Fig. 18.3), which contribute to the ability of the organism to overcome the body's defence and to invade, propagate, survive and produce disease in the host.

Cell wall associated factors

1. Capsular polysaccharide

A few strains of *S. aureus* are encapsulated and these tend to be more virulent than the non-capsulated strains. The capsule

Table 18.2. Determinants of pathogenicity or virulence factors of *Staphylococcus aureus*

I. CELL WALL ASSOCIATED FACTORS
1. Capsular polysaccharide
2. Teichoic acid
3. Peptidoglycan
4. Protein A
5. Clumping factor

II. EXTRACELLULAR TOXINS
1. Haemolytic toxins (haemolysins)
   - α lysin
   - β lysin
   - γ lysin
   - δ lysin
2. Leucocidin
3. Epidermolytic toxins
4. Enterotoxins
5. Toxic shock syndrome toxin-1

III. EXTRACELLULAR ENZYMES
1. Coagulase
2. Staphylokinase
3. Hyaluronidase
4. Deoxyribonuclease
5. Lipase
6. Phospholipases
7. Proteases

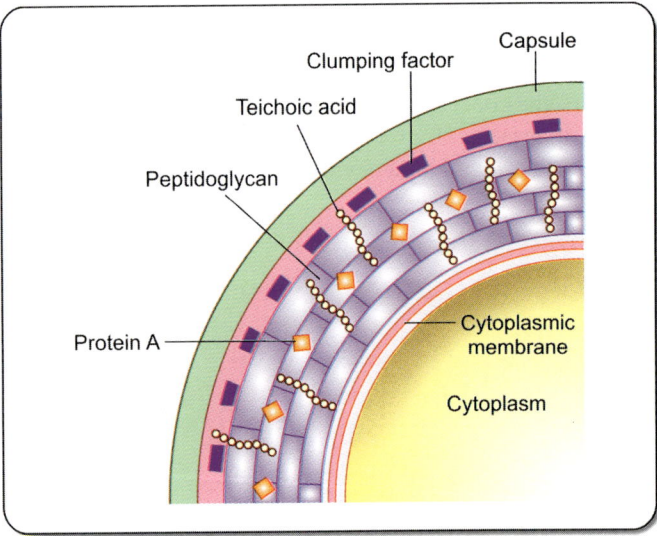

Fig. 18.3. Cell wall associated factors of *Staphylococcus aureus*.

is composed of antigenic polysaccharide. It prevents ingestion of the organism by polymorphonuclear leucocytes. The capsular material may promote the adherence of the organisms to host cells and to prosthetic devices.

2. Teichoic acid

It is a major antigenic determinant of all strains of *S. aureus*. It facilitates adhesion of cocci to host cell surface and protects them from complement-mediated opsonization.

3. Peptidoglycan

It is a polysaccharide polymer which provides rigidity to the cell wall. It stimulates both humoral and cellular immune responses in the host. In addition to their role in providing rigidity and resilience to the staphylococcal cell wall, peptidoglycan and teichoic acid also have several biologic activities that are thought to contribute to virulence.

4. Protein A

Protein A is a group-specific antigen found in the cell wall of about 90% strains of *S. aureus* (especially Cowan I strain). It has a molecular weight of 13,000 daltons. It is chemotactic, anticomplementary, antiphagocytic, mitogenic, potentiates natural killer cells, and elicits platelet injury and hypersensitivity reaction.

Protein A binds IgG molecules, non-specifically, through Fc region leaving specific Fab sites free to combine with specific antigen. When suspension of such sensitized cells is treated with homologous (test) antigen, the antigen combines with free Fab sites of IgG attached to staphylococcal cells leading to visible clumping of staphylococci within two minutes. This is known as **coagglutination** (see Chapter 12).

5. Clumping factor (bound coagulase)

It is a surface component that causes the organisms to clump when mixed with plasma. This factor reacts directly with fibrinogen in plasma, causing rapid cell agglutination. It can be detected by emulsifying a few colonies of the bacteria in a drop of normal saline on a clean glass slide and mixing it with a drop of rabbit plasma. Prompt clumping of the organisms indicates the presence of clumping factor (bound coagulase). Since this factor is detected by performing the test on a slide, therefore, the test is known as **slide coagulase test**.

Extracellular toxins

S. aureus produces a variety of extracellular toxins, including haemolysins, leucocidin, epidermolytic toxins, enterotoxins and toxic shock syndrome toxin-1.

1. Haemolysins

Almost every strain of *S. aureus* produces one or more of four haemolytic, membrane-damaging exotoxins known as α, β, γ and δ lysins. They are antigenically distinct and differ from one another in their activity against the red blood cells of different animal species, lethal activity, dermonecrosis and leucocidal activity.

2. Leucocidin

Leucocidin consists of two protein components. These components act synergistically to damage polymorphonuclear leucocytes and macrophages, and to produce dermonecrosis.

3. Epidermolytic toxins (exfoliative toxins)

Many strains of *S. aureus*, mainly belonging to phage group II, produce two types of epidermolytic toxin (types A and B).

They are proteins with a molecular weight of 30,000 and 29,500 daltons respectively.

4. Enterotoxins

About 40% of all clinical isolates of *S. aureus* produce enterotoxins which are exotoxins that cause food poisoning in man. Enterotoxins are proteins with molecular weights of 26,000–30,000 daltons. These are heat-stable, resisting boiling for 30 minutes. Therefore, once formed enterotoxins might not be destroyed even if food is heated sufficiently to kill all viable staphylococci. These are also not destroyed by gut enzymes. Nine antigenic types (A, B, C_1, C_2, C_3, D, E, H and I) of enterotoxins have been identified. Enterotoxin F is now known as toxic shock syndrome toxin-1. Type A toxin is responsible for the most cases.

5. Toxic shock syndrome toxin-1 (TSST-1)

TSST-1 is produced by certain strains of *S. aureus*. Most of the strains producing TSST-1 belong to phage group I. TSST-1 is a protein with a molecular weight of 22,000 daltons. It is antigenic and most persons over 30 years of age have circulating antibodies.

Extracellular enzymes

1. Coagulase

S. aureus produces an extracellular enzyme called coagulase. It activates a coagulase-reacting factor (CRF) normally present in plasma, causing the plasma to clot by the conversion of fibrinogen to fibrin.

Coagulase (tube coagulase) test

0.1 ml of an overnight broth culture or broth suspension from an agar plate culture made up to the same density is mixed with 0.5 ml of a 1 in 10 dilution of human or rabbit plasma. The mixture is incubated in a water bath at 37°C for three to six hours. If positive, the plasma clots and does not flow when the tube is inverted. If clot does not appear it is left overnight at room temperature and re-examined. On continued incubation, the clot may be lysed by fibrinolysin produced by some strains. Controls with plasma alone, and known coagulase-positive and coagulase-negative cultures must be set up with each batch of tests. Human, rabbit or pig plasma, which are rich in CRF, can be used. Oxalate, EDTA or heparin are suitable anticoagulants. **Citrated plasma should not be used because contaminating Gram-negative bacilli may utilize the citrate and produce false positive reaction.**

For slide coagulase see clumping factor.

2. Staphylokinase (fibrinolysin)

Many strains of *S. aureus* that do not produce β lysin may produce staphylokinase. It is a protein with a molecular weight of 13,000–15,000 daltons. It has fibrinolytic activity.

3. Hyaluronidase

More than 90% strains of *S. aureus* produce hyaluronidase, but the amount varies widely. It hydrolyzes hyaluronic acid present in the intercellular ground substance of connective tissue, thus facilitating the spread of the organisms to adjacent areas.

Pathogenicity

Staphylococcal diseases may be classified as cutaneous and deep infections, exfoliative diseases, food poisoning and the toxic shock syndrome.

Cutaneous infections

These include wound and burn infection, pustules (small cutaneous abscesses), furuncles or boils (large cutaneous abscesses), carbuncles, styes, impetigo and pemphigus neonatorum.

Deep infections

These include osteomyelitis, periostitis, tonsillitis, pharyngitis, sinusitis, bronchopneumonia, empyema, septicaemia, meningitis, endocarditis, breast abscess, renal abscess and abscesses in other organs.

Exfoliative diseases

These lesions are produced by the strains of *S. aureus* which produce epidermolytic toxins. These toxins separate the outer layer of epidermis from the underlying tissues leading to blistering disease. The most dramatic manifestation of these toxins is **scalded skin syndrome** or **Ritter's disease**.

Food poisoning

It is caused by staphylococcal enterotoxin. The enterotoxin is a preformed toxin already present in the contaminated food before consumption.

Patient develops nausea, vomiting and diarrhoea 2–6 hours after consumption of food containing preformed enterotoxin of *S. aureus*. It is a self-limiting condition.

Toxic shock syndrome (TSS)

It is a multisystem illness characterized by high fever, headache, confusion, conjunctival reddening, subcutaneous oedema, vomiting, diarrhoea, scarlatiniform rash and fine desquamation of the hands and feet.

Laboratory diagnosis

Specimens

Specimens to be collected include pus from suppurative lesions, blood from a patient with pyrexia of unknown origin, mid stream urine from a patient with urinary tract infection, sputum from a patient with bronchopneumonia and faeces, food remains and vomit from cases of food poisoning. Nasal and perineal swabs may be collected from suspected carriers.

Microscopy

Examine a Gram-stained smear of pus or wound exudate which may show pus cells and Gram-positive cocci in clusters (Fig. 18.4).

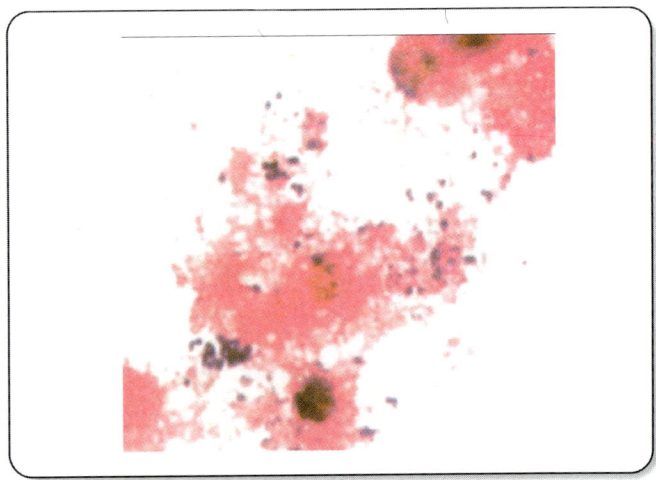

Fig. 18.4. Staphylococci in Gram-stained smear of pus (× 1000).

Culture

The specimens are cultured on a blood agar plate. Specimens, where staphylococci are expected to be outnumbered by other bacteria (e.g., wound swab and faeces), are inoculated on selective media like salt agar. The inoculated media are incubated at 37°C for 24 hours. Next day, the plates are inspected for golden-yellow or white colonies and are confirmed by slide coagulase test. On blood agar plate, look for haemolysis around the colonies (Fig. 18.2).

Methicillin-resistant staphylococci (MRSA)

MRSA is any strain of *S. aureus* that has developed, through the process of natural selection, resistance to beta-lactam antibiotics, which include the penicillins (methicillin, oxacillin, dicloxacillin, nafcillin, etc.) and the cephalosporins. It is also called oxacillin-resistant *Staphylococcus aureus* (ORSA). Strains unable to resist these antibiotics are classified as methicillin-sensitive *Staphylococcus aureus* or MSSA.

MRSA is responsible for several difficult-to-treat infections in humans. It is especially troublesome in hospitals, where patients with open wounds, invasive devices, and weakened immune systems are at a greater risk of infection than general public. The main cause of concern now is the emergence of community acquired MRSA (CA MRSA) which were earlier restricted to the hospital setting hospital associated MRSA (HA MRSA).

Vancomycin-resistant staphylococci

Vancomycin is the drug of choice, and sometimes the only drug available, for serious staphylococcal infections, and thus, the development of vancomycin resistance has been a serious concern. In 2002, isolates of **Vancomycin-resistant *S. aureus* (VRSA)** were reported in the United States, isolated from patients undergoing long-term vancomycin treatment.

COAGULASE-NEGATIVE STAPHYLOCOCCI

Coagulase-negative staphylococci (CoNS) form part of the normal flora of the skin. Some species of CoNS, e.g., *S. epidermidis* and *S. saprophyticus*, can produce human infections. They are morphologically similar to *S. aureus* and the methods for isolation are the same. Their colonies are white (non-pigmented) and they can be distinguished from *S. aureus* by their failure to coagulate plasma and by their lack of clumping factor and DNAse.

19

Streptococcus and Enterococcus

Streptococci are catalase-negative, Gram-positive, non-sporing, spherical or ovoid cells. Based upon their haemolytic properties, streptococci can be classified into three groups:

1. α-Haemolytic streptococci

These cause partial lysis resulting in a greenish discoloration of the area surrounding the colony. The streptococci producing α-haemolysis are also known as **viridans streptococci**. They are widely found as normal flora in upper respiratory tract of humans.

2. β-Haemolytic streptococci

These cause complete lysis of RBCs (2–4 mm wide) resulting in clear area surrounding the colony.

3. Nonhaemolytic streptococci

These organisms do not produce any lysis of RBCs or discoloration on blood agar. Earlier these were termed γ-haemolytic streptococci. However, because no lysis of RBCs occurs, the term γ-haemolytic is confusing.

STREPTOCOCCUS PYOGENES

Morphology

They are Gram-positive, spherical cocci about 0.6–1.0 μm in diameter. They occur in chains of varying lengths. Chain formation is due to the cocci dividing in one plane only and the daughter cells failing to separate completely (Fig. 19.1). In actively spreading lesions within the tissues, diplococcal and individual coccal forms are common, whereas in purulent exudates from walled-off lesions and in artificial culture media, chain formation is a rule. Chains are longer in liquid than in solid media. They are non-motile, non-sporing and some strains produce a capsule of hyaluronic acid, which may be demonstrable during the first 2–4 hours of growth. Because many strains also produce the enzyme hyaluronidase later during the growth cycle, capsules may not be seen in older cultures. Since hyaluronic acid is a normal component of

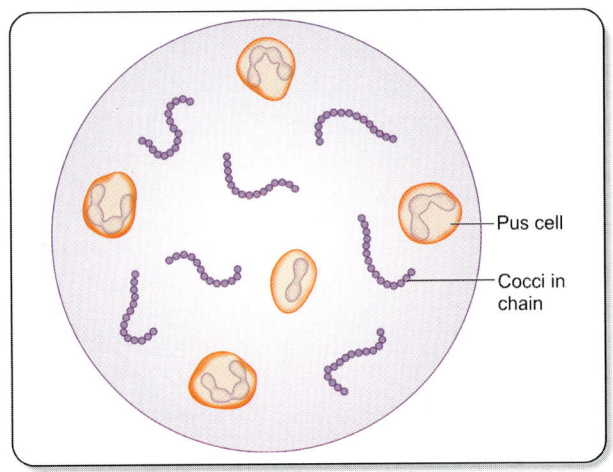

Fig. 19.1. Streptococci in Gram-stained smear of pus.

connective tissue, therefore, anticapsular antibodies are not formed.

Cultural characteristics

They are aerobes and facultative anaerobes. Temperature range is 22–40°C, optimum temperature being 37°C. They can grow on blood and serum agar.

- After 24 hour incubation, colonies of *S. pyogenes* on **blood agar** are small (0.5–1 mm in diameter), semitransparent, grey-white with a matt or glossy surface. The colonies are surrounded by a wide zone of β-haemolysis. Mucoid colonies are formed by strains which produce large capsules. The abundance of hyaluronic acid gives the colony a glistening, watery appearance.
- The addition of 0.0002% crystal violet to blood agar inhibits the growth of some bacteria, notably staphylococci, while permitting the growth of streptococci. **Crystal violet blood agar** is, therefore, a selective medium for isolation of *S. pyogenes*.

Antigenic structure

Several components of bacterial cell of *S. pyogenes* (Fig. 19.2) are antigenic. These include:

1. Capsule

The hyaluronic acid of the capsule is nonantigenic. Capsule has only a weak antiphagocytic effect.

2. Cell wall

Cell wall is composed of an outer layer of protein, a middle layer of group-specific carbohydrate and an inner layer of peptidoglycan.

(a) **Peptidoglycan:** Peptidoglycan is responsible for cell wall rigidity. It also has biologic properties such as pyrogenic and thrombolytic activity.

(b) **Group-specific carbohydrate:** On the basis of group-specific carbohydrate antigen contained in the cell wall, haemolytic streptococci have been divided into 20 groups (A–V except I and J). These are known as Lancefield groups. As this antigen is an integral part of the cell wall, it has to be extracted for grouping by a precipitation test with group antisera. For the test, streptococci are grown in Todd-Hewitt broth and extracted with hydrochloric acid (**Lancefield acid extraction method**) or formamide (**Fuller method**) or by an enzyme produced by *Streptomyces albus* (**Maxted method**) or by autoclaving (**Rantz and Randall method**). The extract and specific antisera are allowed to react in capillary tubes. Precipitation occurs within five minutes at the interface between the extract and the homologous antisera. *S. pyogenes* belongs to Lancefield group A. **All streptococci except the viridans group have a layer of carbohydrate.**

(c) **Proteins:** *S. pyogenes* produces three surface protein antigens (M, T and R) that are useful in serologic typing:

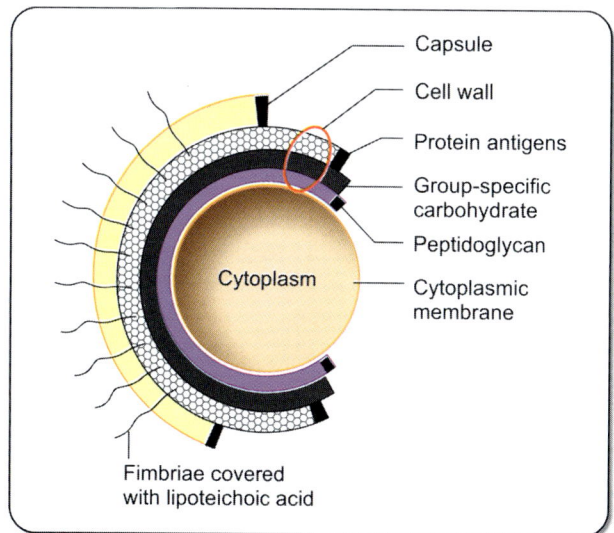

Fig. 19.2. Components of *Streptococcus pyogenes*.

Labels in figure:
- Capsule
- Cell wall
- Protein antigens
- Group-specific carbohydrate
- Peptidoglycan
- Cytoplasm
- Cytoplasmic membrane
- Fimbriae covered with lipoteichoic acid

• **M protein:** It is the most important. It acts as a virulence factor by inhibiting phagocytosis. Specific anti-M antibody develops after infection which enhances phagocytosis. **M protein extends through the capsule as fine fimbriae.** They are covered with lipoteichoic acid. They enable the organism to attach to epithelial cells. M protein is acid- and heat-stable and trypsin-sensitive. It is antigenic and antisera can be raised against it. On the basis of antigenic differences in the M protein, *S. pyogenes* is divided into more than 80 M types. M protein can be extracted by Lancefield acid extraction method and M typing is performed by **capillary tube precipitation tests** using type-specific antisera and acid extract.

• **T protein:** It is resistant to pepsin and trypsin but is heat- and acid-stable. It is present in many serotypes of *S. pyogenes*. T typing is done by slide agglutination test using trypsin-treated whole streptococci.

• **R protein:** It is destroyed by pepsin and not by trypsin. Typing systems employing the R surface antigens are not commonly used.

Toxins and enzymes

S. pyogenes produces several exotoxins and enzymes which contribute to its pathogenicity and identification.

Streptococcal pyrogenic exotoxins (Erythrogenic toxins)

There are three antigenically distinct streptococcal pyrogenic exotoxins A, B and C (streptococcal pyrogenic exotoxins – SPE A, SPE B and SPE C). **These exotoxins are superantigens** and have been associated with streptococcal toxic shock syndrome and scarlet fever.

Dick test: When 0.2 ml of suitably diluted toxin is injected intradermally in the susceptible individual, it causes localized erythematous reaction at least 1 cm in diameter in 12–24 hours. This test is known as Dick test. This test becomes negative during convalescence due to neutralization of toxin by antibody.

Schultz-Charlton test: When the patient serum contains demonstrable antitoxin, an injection of homologous antitoxin intradermally in a patient of scarlet fever causes local blanching of the rash. This is known as Schultz-Charlton test.

Haemolysins (streptolysins)

S. pyogenes produces two types of haemolysins. One of these is oxygen-labile hence designated as streptolysin O (SLO) and the other is oxygen-stable and soluble in serum hence designated as streptolysin S (SLS).

Streptokinase

Streptococci of groups A, C and G produce a substance called streptokinase which is actively fibrinolytic for human fibrin (blood clot) and can be recovered in streptococcal culture filtrates. This acts on plasminogen, a factor present in normal plasma, which is converted into plasmin, an active proteolytic enzyme that lysis fibrin. It is thought to be at least partially responsible for the rapid spread of streptococcal infection by preventing the formation of a fibrin barrier around the infected site. It is an antigenic protein and neutralizing antibodies appear in convalescent sera. Antistreptokinase antibody provides retrospective evidence of streptococcal infection. It is given intravenously for the treatment of early myocardial infarction and other thromboembolic disorders.

Deoxyribonucleases (streptodornases)

S. pyogenes also elaborates enzymes that degrade DNA. Four immunologically and electrophoretically different types (A, B, C and D) of deoxyribonucleases have been found in streptococcal culture filtrates. Of these, B is most antigenic in man and demonstration of **antideoxyribonuclease B** is useful in the retrospective diagnosis particularly of skin infections, where antistreptolysin O (ASO) titre may be low.

Hyaluronidase (spreading factor)

It is an enzyme which splits hyaluronic acid binding tissue cells together and also that of streptococcal capsules, consequently strains, which produce large amounts of hyaluronidase produce little hyaluronic acid capsule. This enzyme is expected to play a part in the virulence of S. pyogenes by facilitating its spread. It is antigenic and antibodies to the enzyme are formed after infection. Hyaluronidase is produced by strains of groups A, B, C and G streptococci.

Serum opacity factor (SOF)

SOF is an enzyme, lipoproteinase. It exists both as cell-bound and released from it. It produces opacity when applied to agar gel containing horse or swine serum. It is produced by group A streptococci of certain M types. It, thus, provides a means of classifying group A streptococci into two categories – SOF-producing and non-SOF-producing strains.

Nicotinamide adenine dinucleotidase (NADase)

This acts on the coenzyme NAD and liberates nicotinamide from the molecule. It is antigenic and is specifically neutralised by the antibody in convalescent sera. Its role in the virulence of the organisms is not known.

Pathogenicity

S. pyogenes causes:
    I. Suppurative diseases.
    II. Non-suppurative sequelae.

I. Suppurative diseases

1. ***Tonsillitis and pharyngitis:*** The main site of streptococcal infection is the throat where purulent tonsillitis is the most typical lesion.
2. ***Scarlet fever:*** Scarlet fever is a complication of streptococcal pharyngitis that occurs when the infecting strain is lysogenized by a bacteriophage that mediates production of a pyrogenic exotoxin. The disease consists of a combination of a streptococcal sore throat and a generalized erythema, although occasionally, the rash can accompany a streptococcal wound infection.
3. ***Impetigo:*** Impetigo is a skin infection that occurs most often in young children, particularly those living in crowded, low socioeconomic conditions. Streptococcal impetigo is characterized by the occurrence on the skin of a superficial discrete crusted spot seldom exceeding an inch in diameter, which lasts for 1–2 weeks and heals spontaneously without leaving a scar.
4. ***Erysipelas:*** This is an acute, spreading, intensely erythematous skin lesion with a sharply demarcated but irregular edge and sometimes with superficial vesicles and bullae.
5. ***Streptococcal toxic shock syndrome:*** Patients with invasive and bacteraemic S. pyogenes infections, and in particular necrotizing fasciitis, may develop toxic shock syndrome.

II. Non-suppurative sequelae

There is a considerable evidence that S. pyogenes is in some way the cause of acute rheumatic fever (ARF) involving the heart and joints, and acute glomerulonephritis (AGN) involving the kidneys. These conditions differ from suppurative infections in that:

(a) These conditions appear only between 2–3 weeks after infection with S. pyogenes. S. pyogenes is no longer detectable when the complications set in.
(b) Many cases are not preceded by overt streptococcal infection but in many of these, high titres of antibodies to streptococcal extracellular antigens, particularly to streptolysin O, are frequently demonstrable.
(c) Streptococci are not directly demonstrable in the lesions in these conditions.

- **Acute rheumatic fever (ARF):** ARF develops in a small percentage (roughly 3%) of individuals, 2–3 weeks after the onset of acute streptococcal pharyngitis caused by any type of group A streptococci. It is characterized by fever, migrating polyarthritis, and carditis, and is frequently associated with subcutaneous nodules. Recovery from ARF occurs without residual injury to the joints, but permanent damage to the heart may occur. The mechanism by which streptococci produce rheumatic fever is still obscure.

   There have been reports that a common cross reacting antigen exists in some group A streptococci and the heart. In this case, antibodies synthesized in response to the streptococcal infection could react with antigens in the heart, causing cellular destruction and permanent damage. This theory is supported by the observation that following a streptococcal epidemic, most patients who develop ARF have higher titre of antistreptococcal antibodies in their sera than do those who escape the disease. Circulating immune complexes have also been found in serum of the patients with ARF.

- **Acute glomerulonephritis (AGN):** AGN is less frequently a consequence of streptococcal infection than is ARF. It is almost always produced by group A streptococci but group C streptococci may also be involved. In contrast to ARF which occurs only after pharyngitis, AGN may be seen after a pharyngeal or cutaneous infection. Most cases of AGN occur 2–3 weeks following skin infection or pharyngitis caused by certain pyodermal (M types 1 and 12) and pharyngeal (M types 49, 53–55 and 59–61) strains of *S. pyogenes*. These strains are known as nephritogenic strains.

Poststreptococcal AGN probably develops because some components of glomerular basement membrane are antigenically similar to the cell membranes of nephritogenic β-haemolytic streptococci. Therefore, antibodies which are produced by the host against the latter cross react with the former. Alternatively, streptococcal antigen-antibody complexes may lodge in the glomeruli. In either case, the activation of the C3 and C5 components of complement leads to tissue destruction. This is supported by the detection of C3 as well as γ-globulin and streptococcal antigens in the glomerular lesion.

Laboratory diagnosis

In acute infections, diagnosis is established by identification of β-haemolytic streptococci that have been isolated from the patient, while in non-suppurative complications, diagnosis is based on the demonstration of rising titre of antibody to one or more streptococcal antigens.

Specimens

Throat and nasal swabs from cases of sore throat or from suspected carriers, high vaginal swabs from cases of puerperal sepsis, pus or pus swabs from suppurative infections and blood from cases of systemic infections are the usual specimens collected.

Gram staining

The observation of typical Gram-positive cocci arranged in chains on microscopic examination of smear of pus or CSF may indicate the likelihood of the presence of streptococci.

Fluorescent antibody technique

The examination of throat swab by the direct fluorescent antibody technique may be used for rapid identification of group A streptococci.

Culture

Inoculate pus or swab on blood agar plate immediately. Incubate it at 37°C for 24 hours and look for β-haemolytic colonies of streptococci. In case of bacteriological examination of skin lesions, crystal violet blood agar is useful selective medium that inhibits many commensal organisms.

Identification

Streptococcal colonies that produce β-haemolysis are subjected to:

- **Lancefield grouping** and in case the isolate belongs to group A, it is further subjected to **M typing**.
- A rapid method for identification of group A streptococci is based on **Maxted's observation** that they are more sensitive to bacitracin than other streptococci. The plate is inoculated with a pure culture of β-haemolytic *Streptococcus*, a 0.04 units bacitracin disc is placed in the area of inoculation and the plate is incubated at 37°C for 24 hours. The inhibition of growth around the disc is seen with *S. pyogenes* but not with other streptococci. However, this test is not totally reliable as 5–15% of bacitracin-susceptible streptococci recovered from clinical sources may belong to groups other than group A. For example, 6% of group B and 7.5% of group C and G β-haemolytic streptococci are bacitracin-sensitive. About 7.5% of α-haemolytic streptococci are also bacitracin-sensitive.

Serological tests

In ARF and AGN, a retrospective diagnosis of streptococcal infection may be established by serological tests, preferably with paired sera, to detect a rise in antibody titre to one or more of the extracellular products of *S. pyogenes*.

- **Antistreptolysin O** (ASO) test is used most frequently. ASO titres higher than 200 Todd units/ml are indicative of prior streptococcal infection.
- **Antideoxyribonuclease B** (anti-DNase B) estimation is also commonly employed. Titres higher than 300 or 350 are taken as significant.
- **Streptozyme test**, which is a passive slide haemagglutination test using erythrocytes sensitized with a crude preparation of extracellular antigens of streptococci, is a convenient, sensitive and specific screening test.

Group B streptococci

Group B streptococci (*S. agalactiae*) are major streptococcal pathogens in neonates and young children. Infection in the neonate is divided into early-onset-type and late-onset-type.

Early-onset-type

Group B streptococci are present in the vaginal flora of about 25% of all women. Early rupture of the membranes, prolonged labour, prematurity, low birth weight and heavy colonization of mother's vagina by group B streptococci lead to early-onset-type infection. Within first five days of life the neonate develops septicaemia and pneumonia, and in spite of the intensive antibiotic therapy, such infections carry a mortality rate of 50–70%. Meningitis may also develop.

The serotype of group B streptococci isolated from the anterior nares, external auditory meatus, umbilicus and rectum of the neonate, with or without infection, in almost all the cases, is similar to that isolated from the cervicovaginal canal, urethra or rectum of the mother. The fact that some babies delivered by caesarean section become infected indicates that direct spread of the organism to the uterus may take place.

Late-onset-type

This type of infection develops between second to fourth weeks of life. Baby acquires infection from the hospital personnel during nursing procedures. Baby to baby spread may also occur. The infecting organism is rarely found in the mother's vagina. This type of infection is not as severe as early-onset-type, but has a high incidence of residual effects often of a neurological nature.

Group B streptococci may also cause adult infections, including septicaemia, endocarditis, meningitis, and local septic lesions in the female genital tract, the urinary tract, surgical wounds and skin. Occasionally, they may lead to pneumonia, empyema, arthritis and osteomyelitis.

S. agalactiae possesses the enzyme hippuricase, which hydrolyzes sodium hippurate. Another test to identify group B streptococci is the CAMP reaction (so called because it was originally described by Christie, Atkins and Munch-Petersen), which can be demonstrated as an accentuated zone of haemolysis (butterfly appearance) when *S. agalactiae* is inoculated perpendicular to a streak of *S. aureus* (NCTC 1803) on a sheep or bovine blood agar plate (Fig. 19.3). Occasional strains are bacitracin-sensitive.

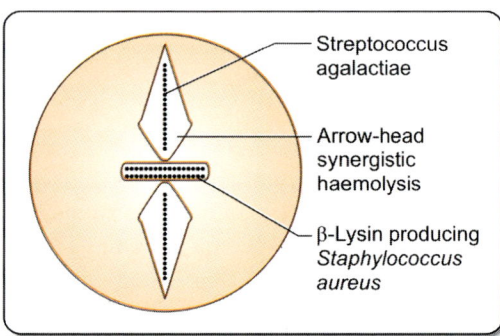

Fig. 19.3. CAMP test.

Group D streptococci

The group D streptococci include *S. bovis* and *S. equinus.* Until the mid-1980s, the group D streptococci were divided into the enterococcal and nonenterococcal groups. Those found in the intestinal tract were part of the enterococcal group and have now been placed in a new genus, *Enterococcus*, but nonenterococcal group remains part of the group D streptococci. Both *Enterococcus* and group D streptococci can grow in the presence of 40% bile and also hydrolyze aesculin to aesculetin and glucose. One or two isolated colonies from blood agar plate are inoculated on a bile aesculin agar slant. If aesculin is hydrolyzed then aesculetin diffuses into the agar

and combines with ferric citrate in the medium to give a black complex. This is known as bile **aesculin hydrolysis test**.

Group D streptococci can be differentiated from enterococci in that they fail to grow in nutrient broth with 6.5% sodium chloride, and are susceptible to penicillin. They are α-haemolytic or nonhaemolytic on sheep blood agar and do not hydrolyze hippurate (Table 19.1). They may cause bacterial endocarditis, urinary tract infections, septicaemia, and other diseases, such as abscesses and wound infections. An association has been reported between bacteraemia resulting from *S. bovis* and the presence of gastrointestinal tumours.

Table 19.1. Differences between group D streptococci and *Enterococcus* spp.

	Group D streptococci	*Enterococcus* spp.
Haemolysis type	α, none	α, β, none
Aesculin hydrolysis	+	+
Growth in presence of 40% bile	+	+
Growth in nutrient broth with 6.5% sodium chloride	–	+
Susceptibility to penicillin	+	–
Hydrolysis of hippurate	–	–*

* Exceptions may occur

ENTEROCOCCUS

Important characteristics of enterococci are:

1. They are normal flora of the lower intestinal tract and vagina.
2. They are non-motile, non-capsulated, Gram-positive cocci occurring in pairs or short chains.
3. These organisms may be α-, β- or nonhaemolytic on sheep blood agar.
4. On MacConkey agar medium they produce tiny, deep pink colonies.
5. They can grow in the presence of 6.5% sodium chloride, at pH 9.6, and at 45°C.
6. *Enterococcus* and group D streptococci can grow in the presence of 40% bile and hydrolyze aesculin to aesculetin and glucose.
7. They do not hydrolyze hippurate.
8. Most strains of enterococci are resistant to penicillin. They are also resistant to sulphonamides. Recently, they have developed resistance to newer penicillins and cephalosporins, streptomycin and gentamicin.
9. They are relatively heat-resistant, surviving 60°C for 30 minutes.

There are currently 38 species in this genus, however, relatively few species are important human pathogens. The species most commonly associated with human disease is *E.*

faecalis, but infections caused by *E. faecium*, *E. durans*, *E. avium* and other enterococci also occur. Identification of various species of *Enterococcus* is made on biochemical grounds. *E. faecalis* ferments mannitol with gas production. It is VP positive and can grow on blood tellurite agar producing black colonies.

Enterococci may cause urinary tract infection, wound infection, infective endocarditis, biliary tract infection, peritonitis, suppurative abdominal lesions and septicaemia.

Viridans streptococci (oral streptococci)

Viridans streptococci are a heterogeneous group of α-haemolytic and non-haemolytic streptococci. Most isolates of viridans streptococci do not possess a group-specific carbo-hydrate; hence they cannot be classified under Lancefield classification of streptococci. They are constantly present as commensals in the mouth and oropharynx.

At least five species of viridans streptococci have been recognized. These include *S. salivarius*, *S. sanguis*, *S. mutans*, *S. mitior* (*mitis*) and *S. milleri*. Viridans streptococci, chiefly *S. mutans* and to a lesser extent *S. sanguis*, are involved in the production of **dental caries**. They break down dietary sucrose, producing acid and a tough adhesive dextran. The acid damages dentine and the dextran binds together food debris, epithelial cells, mucus and bacteria to form **dental plaques** which lead to caries.

In persons with predisposing factors, such as valvular disease of heart, they may cause **infective endocarditis** (**IE**). *S. sanguis* is the most common causative agent of infective endocarditis. Tooth extraction and injury of the oral cavity in such persons is dangerous, because from oral cavity they may enter into the blood stream and cause IE. Tooth extraction in such individuals should be done under antibiotic cover. Other organisms which may also cause IE include *E. faecalis* and other enterococci, *S. aureus*, coagulase-negative staphylo-cocci, *Coxiella burnetii* and some fungi.

Diagnosis of IE is established by repeated blood cultures. Viridans streptococci can be recognized by their α-haemolytic colonies on blood agar, their failure to grow on MacConkey medium and their sensitivity to penicillin. When isolated from mouth, throat and respiratory tract, they are regarded as harmless commensals and when isolated from blood or a closed lesion they are likely to be pathogenic. These strepto-cocci are generally susceptible to penicillin, though some strains may be resistant. Therefore, antibiotic sensitivity of these organisms should also be carried out.

Streptococcus MG

This belongs to group F streptococci. It has been isolated from the sputum of normal individuals and those suffering from primary atypical pneumonia. These patients frequently have in their sera agglutinins to *Streptococcus* MG.

20

Streptococcus Pneumoniae (Pneumococcus)

Morphology

The pneumococcus is a non-motile, non-sporing, Gram-positive coccus. In the material taken from the body, it occurs characteristically in pairs of **flame-shaped cocci** about 1 µm in diameter, the rounded ends of the cocci being adjacent to each other (Fig. 20.1).

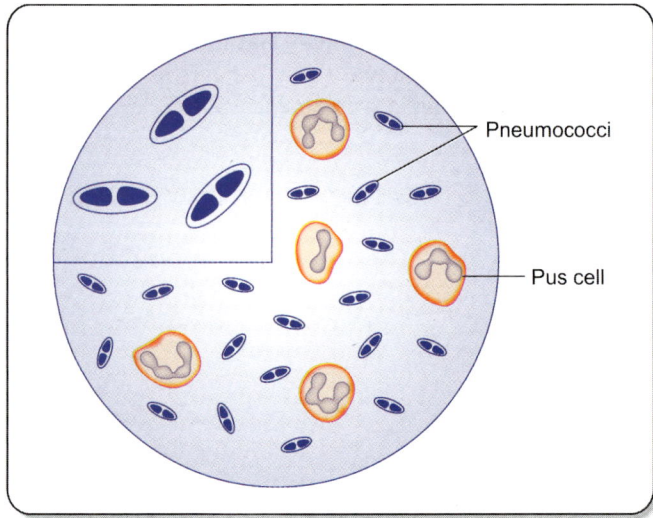

Fig. 20.1. Pneumococci in pus. Inset: enlarged view.

Cultural characteristics

Aerobe and facultative anaerobe, may need 5–10% CO_2 for primary isolation. Optimum temperature 37°C (range 25–40°C), pH 7.8 (range 6.5–8.3) and grows only on enriched media.

On **blood agar**, after 18–24 hour incubation at 37°C, virulent strains with abundant capsular polysaccharide produce small (0.5–1 mm in diameter), round, dome-shaped, transparent colonies. The colonies are surrounded by a 2–3 mm zone of α-haemolysis. On further incubation, the colonies develop a central depression because of autolysis with raised rim (**draughtsman colony**).

Tests to differentiate pneumococcus from viridans streptococci

Following are the tests to differentiate pneumococcus from viridans streptococci, both of which produce α-haemolysis on blood agar.

1. Fermentation of inulin

Fermentation of inulin by pneumococci is a useful test for differentiating them from streptococci which do not ferment it. They are catalase and oxidase negative.

2. Bile solubility test

Pneumococci are **bile soluble** while viridans and other strepto-cocci are not. Bile salts, (sodium deoxycholate and sodium taurocholate) lyse pneumococci when added to actively growing cultures. Pneumococci produce autolytic enzymes leading to autolysis in older cultures. The addition of bile salts is thought to accelerate this process.

For bile solubility test, inoculate the test organism in 5 ml serum digest broth or infusion broth, incubate it at 37°C for 18 hours. While still warm, add 0.5 ml of 10% sodium deoxycholate solution and reincubate at 37°C. Within 15 minutes initially turbid culture becomes clear and transparent due to the lysis of pneumococci. Alternatively, touch a suspected pneumococcal colony on blood agar plate with a loopful of 2% sodium deoxycholate solution at pH 7, incubate the plate at 37°C for 30 minutes. The colony disappears, leaving an area of α-haemolysis.

3. Optochin sensitivity test

Pneumococci are highly sensitive to killing by optochin (ethyl hydrocuprein hydrochloride). For testing, a filter paper disc containing 5 µg of optochin is applied to the surface of a blood agar plate streaked with a lawn of pure culture. Plate is incubated at 37°C in air with 5–10% CO_2. Pneumococcus shows a zone of inhibition of 14 mm or more around the 6 mm optochin disc or 16 mm or more if 10 mm disc is used. Viridans streptococci grow right up to the disc. The differences between *S. pneumoniae* and viridans streptococci are given in Table 20.1.

Antigenic structure

1. Capsular antigen

The most important of pneumococcal antigens is the capsular polysaccharide on the basis of which the pneumococci are divided into more than 90 serologic types named 1, 2, 3, etc. As this polysaccharide diffuses into the culture medium or infective exudates and tissues, it is also known as **specific soluble substance (SSS)**.

The typing of individual isolates can be performed by:

- **Quellung reaction** in which the capsules of pneumococci are made more easily visible when acted upon by specific antisera. It is performed by mixing equal quantities of specimen (sputum, pus or sediment of CSF) or light suspension of the test organisms with type-specific pneumococcal antiserum. After waiting for 15–30 minutes, for the reaction to occur, the mixture is examined microscopically using a 100X objective. If Quellung reaction is positive, the capsule of the pneumococci will appear quite prominent as compared with those in the same specimen mixed with saline solution as a control.
- **Agglutination** of the cocci with the type-specific antiserum.
- **Precipitation** of SSS with the specific antiserum.

2. Somatic antigen

Pneumococcal cell wall contains a species-specific carbohydrate hapten. It is referred to as **pneumococcal C substance**. This appears to be analogous to (though antigenically different from) the group-specific C antigens of β-haemolytic streptococci.

3. M protein

Type-specific protein antigens analogous to the M protein of *Streptococcus pyogenes*, but immunologically distinct, are present in pneumococci. **Antibodies to the pneumococcal M protein do not inhibit phagocytosis and are, therefore, not protective.**

4. C-reactive protein (CRP)

CRP is an abnormal protein (β-globulin). It appears in acute phase sera of cases of pneumonia but disappears during convalescence. It also appears in some other pathological conditions. It is known as C-reactive protein because it precipitates with C antigen of pneumococci. It is tested by:

- Capillary precipitation of patient serum with antiserum prepared in rabbits against purified CRP; and
- Passive agglutination using latex particles coated with anti-CRP antibody.

Pathogenicity

S. pneumoniae causes **pneumonia, either a lobar pneumonia or a bronchopneumonia**. The latter is characteristically a disease of young children and older adults over 50 years, while lobar pneumonia is almost exclusively a disease of the age group 10–50 years. Other pneumococcal lesions are **acute bronchitis, sinusitis, otitis media, mastoiditis, meningitis, endocarditis, suppurative arthritis** and **peritonitis**.

Laboratory diagnosis

The diagnosis is carried out by demonstration of pneumococci in sputum, exudate, blood and cerebrospinal fluid (CSF) by Gram staining, culture and by demonstration of pneumococcal

Table 20.1. Differences between *Streptococcus pneumoniae* and viridans streptococci

	S. pneumoniae	Viridans streptococci
1. Morphology		
• Shape	Flame-shaped cocci	Round or oval cocci
• Arrangement	In pairs	In chains
• Capsule	Present	Absent
2. Cultural characteristics		
• On blood agar medium	After 24 hour incubation, colonies are small (0.5–1 mm), round, dome-shaped, transparent and surrounded by 2–3 mm zone of α-haemolysis. On further incubation, the colonies develop a central depression with raised rim (**draughtsman colonies**)	After 24 hour incubation, colonies are dome-shaped, opaque and surrounded by a narrow zone (1–2 mm in diameter) of α-haemolysis
• In liquid medium	Uniform turbidity	Granular turbidity, powdery deposit
3. Bile solubility	Positive	Negative
4. Inulin fermentation	Positive	Negative
5. Optochin sensitivity	Positive	Negative
6. Animal pathogenicity (Intraperitoneal inoculation in mice)	Fatal, death of mice in 1–3 days	Non-pathogenic

antigen by coagglutination (COA), latex agglutination (LA) and counterimmunoelectrophoresis (CIE).

Microscopy

The sputum is homogenized by agitating the specimen for 30 minutes in a mechanical shaker with an equal quantity of distilled water and a small number of glass beads. Gram-stained smears are prepared from homogenized sputum and examined. In acute otitis media, *S. pneumoniae* may be demonstrated in fluid aspirated from the middle ear. In meningitis, the presumptive diagnosis may be made from Gram-stained films of centrifuged deposit of CSF. Gram-positive diplococci may be seen both inside the polymorphs and extracellularly (Fig. 20.2).

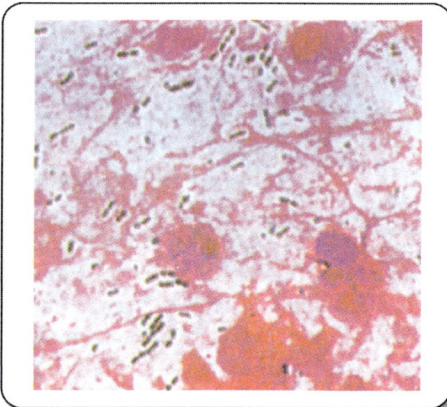

Fig. 20.2. Gram-stained sputum smear showing Gram-positive, encapsulated, extracellular diplococci from a patient of pneumococcal pneumonia (×1000).

Culture

The sputum, after homogenisation, if necessary, is inoculated onto blood agar and heated blood agar media and incubated in air with 5–10% CO_2 for 18–24 hours. If the sputum is unobtainable, as in young children, a serum-coated laryngeal swab is taken and processed. The organisms isolated are identified by their morphological and biochemical characters.

Typing of pneumococcus

The growth of *S. pneumoniae* may be typed with appropriate antisera. Typing can also be done by Quellung reaction in wet films of sputum, pus or sediment of CSF.

- **Blood culture:** Since many healthy individuals carry pneumococci in their throats, therefore, demonstration of organisms in sputum or throat culture is not necessarily indicative of pneumococcal disease. Many pneumococcal infections are associated with a bacteraemia or septicaemia. Therefore, if pneumococci are isolated from patient's blood, the diagnosis of a severe pneumococcal infection can be made with certainty. In all cases of suspected acute bacterial pneumonia sample of blood obtained by venipuncture, prior to administration of antimicrobial drugs, should be cultured immediately in beef infusion broth and thioglycollate broth.
- **Cerebrospinal fluid:** In case of suspected meningitis, a centrifuged deposit of CSF should be examined immediately in a Gram-stained film, cultured on blood agar and heated blood agar and incubated in air with 5–10% CO_2 for 18–24 hours.

Antigen detection

In some cases, particularly if antibiotics have been given before collection of the specimen, viable cocci may not be there in the specimen and culture may be negative. In such cases, pneumococcal antigen is often detectable in CSF by COA, LA or CIE. COA test for antigen gives positive result in larger proportion of specimens than either a Gram-stained film or culture. Moreover, by COA test, result is available within a short time. In addition to CSF, capsular polysaccharide can be demonstrated in blood and urine by CIE.

Mouse inoculation

In specimens where the organisms are scanty, isolation may be obtained by intraperitoneal inoculation in mice, even if culture is negative. Inoculated mice die in 1–3 days, and *S. pneumoniae* may be demonstrated in the peritoneal exudate and heart blood.

21

Neisseria, Moraxella and Acinetobacter

Neisseria meningitidis (meningococcus)

Morphology

They are Gram-negative cocci, 0.6–0.8 μm in diameter. They usually occur in pairs with adjacent sides flattened or concave and long axes parallel. They are typically seen in large numbers inside polymorphonuclear leucocytes (Fig. 21.1).

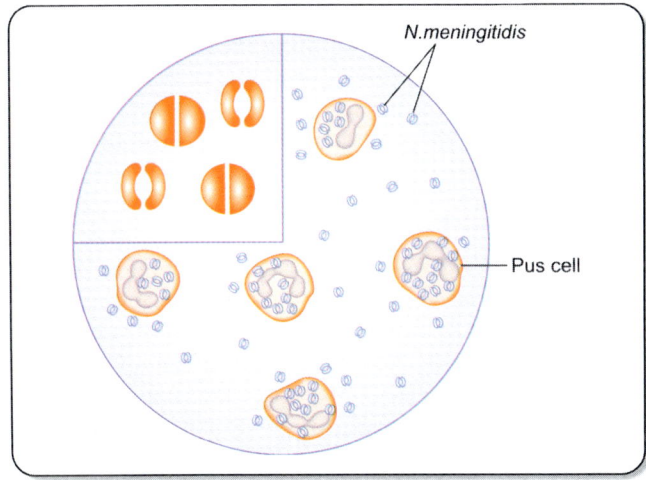

Fig. 21.1. *Neisseria meningitidis* in CSF. Inset: Enlarged view showing adjacent sides flattened or concave and long axes parallel.

Cultural characteristics

Meningococci have exacting growth requirements and do not grow on ordinary media. Growth occurs on media enriched with blood or serum. The growth is facilitated by 5–10% CO_2 and high humidity. The optimum temperature and pH for the growth of meningococci are 35–36°C and 7.0–7.4 respectively.

- On **blood agar**, after 24-hour incubation, the colonies of meningococci are small about 1 mm in diameter, round, convex, grey, nonhaemolytic and translucent. After 48 hours incubation, colonies are larger with an opaque raised centre and thin transparent margins which may be crenated.
- On **heated blood agar (chocolate agar)**, colonies of meningococci are slightly larger than those on ordinary blood agar.

Biochemical characters

Meningococci are catalase- and oxidase-positive.

Oxidase test

When 1% solution of oxidase reagent (tetramethyl-para-phenylenediamine dihydrochloride) is poured on culture plate, *Neisseria* colonies quickly turn deep-purple. This **prompt oxidase reaction** helps in the identification of meningococci and gonococci in mixed cultures. This test may also be done by rubbing a few colonies with a glass rod on a strip of filter paper moistened with oxidase reagent. A deep-purple colour develops immediately.

Meningococci utilize glucose and maltose by oxidative method with the production of acid but no gas. They do not attack lactose or sucrose. Indole and hydrogen sulphide are not produced and nitrates are not reduced.

Antigenic structure

N. meningitidis possesses a polysaccharide capsule and on the basis of immunologic specificity of capsular polysaccharide it has been subdivided into 12 serogroups – A, B, C, X, Y, Z, 29E, W-135, H, I, K and L. Most meningococcal infections are caused by strains of groups A, B and C with a small proportion of infections being due to strains of serogroups Y and W-135. Groups X, Z and 29E are only rarely associated with some form of immune deficiency.

Pathogenicity

The meningococcal disease can be divided into three stages:

1. First stage

The organisms appear in nasopharynx leading to **nasopharyngeal infection**, which is usually asymptomatic but might result in a minor inflammation.

2. Second stage

In a small percentage of cases, the meningococci may enter the blood stream from posterior nasopharynx, probably by way of the cervical lymph nodes. This stage is known as **meningococcaemia**. The patient develops **fever, malaise and petechial skin lesions** due to foci of infection in the capillaries.

3. Third stage

Meningococci infect the meninges causing the major symptoms of severe headache, stiff neck and vomiting accompanied by delirium and confusion.

Laboratory diagnosis

Specimens

CSF, blood, aspirate from skin lesions and nasopharyngeal swabs. Swabs should be transported in Stuart's transport medium. All specimens where meningococcal infection is suspected must be submitted to the laboratory immediately.

- **Cerebrospinal fluid:** In meningococcal meningitis, CSF is under pressure and is turbid due to a large number of polymorphonuclear leucocytes present in a typical case. For bacteriological examination, the CSF is divided into three portions.
  - **First portion** is centrifuged and Gram-stained smears are prepared from the deposit. Meningococci (Gram-negative diplococci) will be seen mainly inside polymorphs, but often extracellularly also.
  - **Second portion** of CSF is inoculated on blood agar or chocolate agar and incubated at 35–36°C under 5–10% CO_2. Colonies appear after 18–24 hours which may be identified by colonial morphology and biochemical reactions. The meningococci isolated may be typed by agglutination with polyvalent or monovalent anti-meningococcal serum.
  - **Third portion** of CSF is incubated for 18–24 hours, either as such or after adding an equal volume of glucose broth and then subcultured on blood agar or chocolate agar. This method may sometimes succeed where direct plating fails.
- **Blood culture:** Blood culture is often positive in meningococcaemia and in early cases of meningitis. Specimen of blood is inoculated into blood culture bottle of trypticase-soy broth. It should be incubated at 35–36°C in 5–10% CO_2 for 4–7 days, with daily subcultures on blood agar or chocolate agar. Look for oxidase-positive colonies of Gram-negative diplococci as above.

Polymerase chain reaction (PCR)

Meningococcal DNA in CSF or blood can be amplified and detected by PCR.

Neisseria gonorrhoeae (gonococcus)

Morphology

Morphology and staining characteristics of *N. gonorrhoeae* are similar to those of *N. meningitidis*.

Cultural characteristics

Gonococci are more difficult to grow than meningococci. They are aerobes, but may grow anaerobically also. Addition of 5–10% CO_2 is essential for primary isolation. Growth occurs best at pH 7.0–7.4 and at a temperature of 35–36°C. They can be isolated on media enriched with blood either partially lysed by heat (chocolate agar) or completely lysed by saponin.

Heated blood agar may be made selective for the isolation of pathogenic neisseriae by the addition of vancomycin 3 mg/litre, colistin 7.5 mg/litre and nystatin 12,500 units/litre. This selective medium (**Thayer-Martin medium**) is valuable in isolating gonococci from heavily contaminated specimens. Trimethoprim lactate (5 mg/litre) may be added to Thayer-Martin medium to inhibit swarming *Proteus* species that are occasionally present in cervicovaginal and rectal specimens. This chocolate agar medium containing vancomycin, colistin, nystatin and trimethoprim is known as **modified Thayer-Martin medium**.

Colony morphology

- On **heated blood agar** after 24-hour incubation, colonies are small about 1 mm in diameter, grey, convex and translucent. After 48 hour incubation, colonies are larger 1.5–2.5 mm in diameter, sometimes with an opaque raised centre and thin transparent margins which may be crenated.
- On **Thayer-Martin medium** growth is slower, although, colonies are similar to those on heated blood agar.

Biochemical reactions

N. gonorrhoeae resembles *N. meningitidis* with the exception that the former can utilize only glucose and the latter glucose and maltose with the production of acid only.

Pathogenesis

N. gonorrhoeae causes **gonorrhoea**. It is a sexually transmitted disease that, with few exceptions, is acquired through sexual contact with an infected individual.

After an incubation period of 2–7 days, patient develops purulent urethral or vaginal discharge, dysuria and frequency of micturition. In male, the acute urethritis may extend to the prostate, testes, seminal vesicles, epididymis and sometimes the periurethral tissue. Chronic urethritis may lead to stricture formation. The infection may spread to the periurethral tissues, causing abscesses and multiple discharging sinuses (**watercan perineum**).

In women, the endocervix is the primary site of infection. The urethra may also become infected. *In adult women, the vagina usually escapes because of the acidic pH of the vaginal secretions, but severe vulvovaginitis can occur in prepubertal girls.* The primary infection may spread from urethra, vagina and cervix to Bartholin's glands, uterus, fallopian tubes, ovaries and pelvic peritoneum causing a pelvic inflammatory disease resulting in sterility. Bacteraemia may occur in fulminating cases, in both men and women, and is occasionally complicated by endocarditis, acute purulent arthritis or both.

- Babies born to infected women may contract serious gono-coccal infection of the eye (**ophthalmia neonatorum**) during passage through infected birth canal.
- **Anorectal infection** occurs in both sexes. In men this follows homosexual rectal intercourse. In women, it can follow rectal intercourse, but may also arise as a result of autoinoculation of rectal mucosa with infected vaginal discharge (direct contagious spread).
- **Gonococcal pharyngitis** may follow orogenital contact in either sex.
- **Conjunctivitis** may occur usually by autoinoculation with fingers.
- **Blood-borne dissemination** of *N. gonorrhoeae* occurs in less than 1% of all infections, resulting in purulent arthritis and rarely septicaemia. Fever and a rash on the extremities may also be present.

Laboratory diagnosis

Specimens

I. Specimens in women

1. **Endocervical:** In women, the endocervix is the optimal site for culture. Specimen should be collected under direct visualization through a vaginal speculum because the adjacent vaginal mucosa harbours bacteria that may overgrow in cultures and may contain organisms such as *Candida* species that can inhibit the growth of gonococci. Remove excessive cervical mucous with cotton or gauze. Insert sterile specimen swab into the endocervical canal, move swab gently from side to side, leave in place for 10–30 seconds for adsorption of organisms to the swab surface.
2. **Anal canal:** Insert sterile specimen swab 4–5 cm in anal canal. Move swab from side to side to sample anal crypts, leave in place for 10–30 seconds for adsorption of organisms to the swab surface. If the swab is heavily soiled with faecal matter, a second specimen should be obtained with a fresh swab.
3. **Urethra:** Strip urethra towards orifice to express exudate and collect specimen on sterile loop or specimen swab.
4. **Vagina (in case of paediatric patients):** If hymen is intact obtain specimen from vaginal orifice and if hymen is not intact then use vaginal speculum and collect specimen from posterior vault.
5. **Bartholin's glands:** Purulent material expressed from the Bartholin's ducts should be collected on sterile sample swab.
6. **Oropharynx:** Using a tongue depressor and direct light, rub a sterile specimen swab firmly over the posterior pharynx and the tonsillar crypts.

II. Specimens in men

1. **Urethra:** Purulent discharge may be expressed at the anterior urethra and collected with a swab.
2. **Anal canal**.
3. **Oropharynx**.

The specimens from anal canal and oropharynx of men are collected by the same method as in women.

III. Specimens in both sexes

1. **Synovial fluid:** In case of gonococcal arthritis.
2. **Blood:** In case of gonococcal septicaemia.
3. **Conjunctival swab:** In case of conjunctivitis.

Culture of blood and synovial fluid is done in trypticase-soy broth enriched with 1% isovitalex, 10% horse serum and 1% glucose.

Microscopy

Prepare smear by rolling the swab gently over the surface of a glass slide in one direction only. Do not rub swab, it may distort microscopic morphology. Do the Gram staining and see under oil-immersion lens.

Culture

All specimens received in the laboratory for recovery of *Neisseria* species should be held at room temperature and plated as soon as possible. Media should be warmed to room temperature before inoculation, because *Neisseria* species are susceptible to cold. Roll specimen swab firmly in a 'Z' pattern onto selective medium (**Thayer-Martin** or **modified Thayer-Martin**) and then cross-streak with a sterile wire loop or needle. In case of specimen from normally sterile sites inoculate nonselective medium (heated blood agar). Incubate the cultures immediately at 35–36°C in 5–10% CO_2.

Observation

Examine plates after 18–24 hours incubation and test suspected colonies by touching with a cotton bud soaked in oxidase reagent. Oxidase-positive bacteria turn the contact area of the bud purple within 5–15 seconds. If oxidase-positive, prepare a smear from an identical colony and stain it with Gram stain. Gonococci will appear Gram-negative diplococci which can be further confirmed by biochemical reactions. Incubation of primary isolation plate is continued for 48 hours and cultures are re-examined by above procedures before any specimen can be reported negative.

Moraxella

The moraxellae are stout Gram-negative cocci or short rods. They appear predominantly in pairs and may simulate gonococci. They are non-capsulate, non-flagellate, non-motile, obligate aerobes, oxidase- and catalase-positive and grow best at 32–37°C. After 24 hour-incubation, on blood agar, the colonies tend to be small (less than 0.5 mm in diameter) with poor or no growth on MacConkey agar. They do not form acid from carbohydrates. Most *Moraxella* species are extremely sensitive to low concentrations of penicillin. However, β-lactamase-producing strains have been encountered.

The *Moraxella* spp. of medical importance are *M. lacunata*, *M. nonliquefaciens*, *M. osloensis*, *M. phenyl-pyruvica*, *M. atlantae* and *M. catarrhalis*. *M. lacunata* and *M. nonliquefaciens* may cause chronic angular blepharo-conjunctivitis and endophthalmitis respectively. *M. phenyl-pyruvica* and *M. osloensis* have been isolated from cases of sinusitis, conjunctivitis, bronchitis, endocarditis, meningitis and septicaemia. *M. atlantae* may occasionally cause systemic infections.

Moraxella (syn *Branhamella*) *catarrhalis* are Gram-negative cocci about 0.8 μm in diameter. They occur singly, but more often in pairs with adjacent sides flattened. Occasionally, they are found in groups of four as a result of characteristic division in two successive planes at right angle to one another. Sometimes they may be found inside polymorphonuclear leucocytes. They are aerobes. Optimum temperature for growth is about 36°C but growth of many strains occurs at 22°C. Although, CO_2 may enhance growth there is no absolute requirement. Most strains grow on nutrient agar. After incubation for 24 hours, colonies on blood agar or chocolate agar are 1–2 mm in diameter, nonhaemolytic, often friable, white or greyish, convex with an entire margin later becoming irregular. After 48 hours colonies are larger, more elevated with a raised opaque centre. It may be differentiated from *Neisseria* spp. by positive DNase and tributrin hydrolysis.

M. catarrhalis is a normal commensal of the respiratory tract of man. It is an opportunistic pathogen causing lower respiratory tract infection, particularly when lung function is previously impaired, but also occasionally in the previously healthy respiratory tract. Predisposing factors in the patho-genesis include advanced age, immunodeficiency, neutro-penia, and chronic debilitating diseases such as chronic obstructive pulmonary disease. **M. catarrhalis has been reported as the third most common cause of acute otitis media and sinusitis in children.**

Acinetobacter

This genus contains obligate aerobic, short, stout, non-motile, often capsulated and Gram-negative bacilli. They are 1–1.5 × 1.5–2.5 μm in size, often appearing in pairs, mimicking neisseriae in appearance. They are oxidase-negative, catalase-positive and indole-negative. Some strains produce urease. They do not reduce nitrate and some strains liquefy gelatin slowly.

Two species are the most common clinical isolates – *A. baumannii* and *A. lwoffii*. *A. baumannii* is saccharolytic and produces acid oxidatively from glucose, arabinose, lactose, and xylose. In contrast, *A. lwoffii* is asacchar-olytic.

They can grow well on ordinary media. On blood agar, after 24 hour-incubation, the colonies are 0.5–2.0 mm in diameter, translucent to opaque, convex and entire. A few strains are haemolytic on blood agar. The colonies of *A. lwoffii* tend to be smaller (average 0.5 mm in diameter in 24 hours) than those of *A. baumannii*. They can grow on MacConkey medium, on which saccharolytic strains form pink colonies.

Both species are widely dispersed in soil and water. They can be found colonizing the moist regions of human skin (axilla and groin) in about 25% of normal persons. They may also be commensals in oropharynx and vagina. They are opportunistic pathogens and may lead to bronchopneumonia, endocarditis, meningitis, peritonitis, urinary tract infection, osteomyelitis, synovitis, conjunctivitis and skin and wound infections in compromised patients.

Predisposing factors include the presence of a prosthesis, endotracheal intubation, intravenous catheter and peritoneal dialysis. *A. lwoffii* is less virulent, and its isolation most often indicates contamination or colonization rather than infection. Isolates of *Acinetobacter* spp., particularly *A. baumannii*, are often inherently resistant to many antimicrobial agents, including β-lactam agents (other than carbapenems), aminoglycosides and quinolones.

22

Corynebacterium Diphtheriae

Morphology

They are thin, slender, non-sporing, non-capsulated, non-motile, non-acid-fast, Gram-positive bacilli of varying lengths with an average size of 3 × 0.3 µm. They frequently possess club-shaped swellings at one or both ends, a characteristic feature which is responsible for the name of the genus (*coryne* means club). When dividing, the bacilli snap and bend abruptly and appear as angled pairs resembling letters V or L or parallel rows of 3–4 bacilli (palisades) which resemble Chinese letters (*Chinese letter arrangement* or *cuneiform arrangement*) (Figs. 22.1 and 22.2).

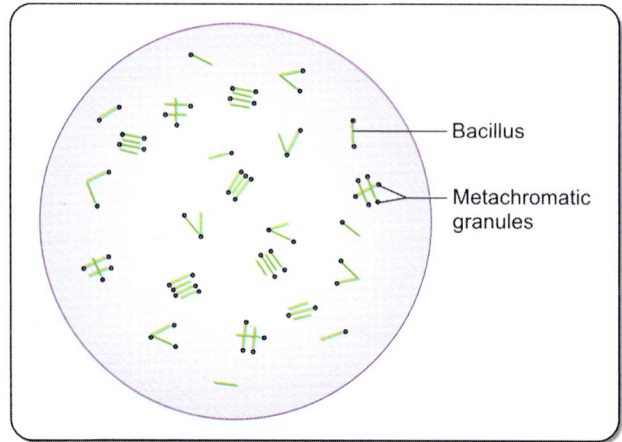

Fig. 22.1. *Corynebacterium diphtheriae* showing metachromatic granules and Chinese letter arrangement.

Although, Gram-positive, *C. diphtheriae* is readily decolourized. Another characteristic of this organism is its granular and uneven staining. When stained with methylene blue or toluidine blue, the granules in the cell stain metachromatically (i.e., granules that stain a colour different from the primary dye colour) bluish black. Most cells contain 2 or 3 of these, and they tend to be on the poles. The granules

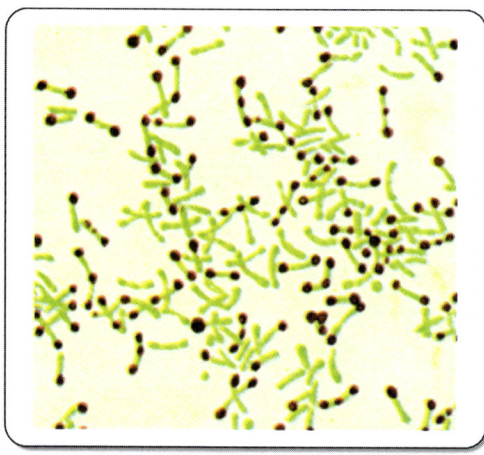

Fig. 22.2. *Corynebacterium diphtheriae* showing metachromatic granules (Albert stain, ×1000).

consist of long-chain inorganic polyphosphates. These granules are known as *metachromatic granules* or *volutin granules* or *Babes-Ernst bodies*. In unstained wet preparations, they appear as round refractile bodies within the bacterial cytoplasm.

With Albert stain, the granules stain bluish-black and the cytoplasm green. The granules are not seen during active growth, but start to appear towards the end of the logarithmic growth period. The granule formation is best seen on Loeffler's serum slope. It appears that they represent storage depots for materials needed to form high-energy phosphate bonds. Their presence in thin slender bacilli helps to distinguish *C. diphtheriae* from short, thick, plumpy, non-pathogenic diphtheroids which lack them.

Cultural characteristics

Diphtheria bacillus is an aerobe and facultative anaerobe, has an optimum temperature for growth of 37°C (range 15–40°C). Two media are useful for this purpose:

1. **Loeffler's serum slope:** Diphtheria bacilli grow rapidly on Loeffler's serum slope, and colonies can be seen in 6–8 hours, long before other bacteria grow. The colonies are at first small, white, opaque discs, but on continued incubation increase in size and may acquire a yellow tint.

2. **Blood tellurite agar (BTA):** The addition of 0.03–0.04% potassium tellurite (K_2TeO_3) to blood agar makes the medium selective for corynebacteria by inhibiting most other pathogenic and commensal bacteria. It may retard the growth even of corynebacteria, so that colonies may be very small after 24 hours, therefore, incubation should be continued for 48 hours. On this medium, colonies of *C. diphtheriae* become grey to black because tellurite or tellurous ions are able to diffuse through the cell wall and membrane and are reduced to tellurium metal, which is precipitated inside the cell. On the basis of colonial morphology on BTA, diphtheria bacilli can be divided into three biotypes – mitis, intermedius and gravis (Table 22.1).

Biochemical reactions

C. diphtheriae ferments glucose, maltose and on rare occasions sucrose with the production of acid without gas. It does not ferment lactose, mannitol and trehalose. For biochemical differentiation of three biotypes of *C. diphtheriae*, starch and glycogen are used. Gravis strains ferment both but intermedius and mitis strains ferment neither.

The fermentation tests are usually done by culture for 24 hours at 37°C in *Hiss's serum water*. Calf or rabbit serum should be used in the medium, because some batches of ox and sheep sera contain a saccharolytic enzyme that gives rise to false positive results.

Most strains of the biotype mitis show β-haemolysis on sheep, rabbit or horse blood, gravis strains are often weakly haemolytic, but intermedius strains are non-haemolytic (Table 22.1).

Toxin production

Toxigenic strains of *C. diphtheriae* produce a potent bacteriophage-encoded protein exotoxin which is an iron-free, crystalline, heat-labile protein. Its molecular weight is 61,150 daltons and is made up of two parts – A and B with molecular weights of 21,150 and 40,000 daltons respectively. Fragment B is required for transport of fragment A into the cell where it inhibits polypeptide chain elongation at the ribosome. Inhibition of protein synthesis is probably responsible for both the necrotic and neurotoxic effects of the toxin. When the toxin is treated with formalin it is converted into toxoid.

Pathogenicity

***C. diphtheriae* causes natural infection only in man.** Infection spreads directly from person to person via nasopharyngeal secretions. Spread is facilitated by intimate contact. Most clinical infections are probably contracted from carriers rather than symptomatic patients. Nasal carriers are particularly dangerous because they shed large number of bacilli which may survive for many weeks in dust and on dry fomites. Children are susceptible after the age of 3–6 months when passive immunity derived from maternal antibodies has disappeared. Incidence is highest among young children, but outbreaks also occur among teenagers and young adults.

Table 22.1. Differentiation of three biotypes of *Corynebacterium diphtheriae*

Character	Gravis	Intermedius	Mitis
1. Morphology	Uniformly stained short rods. Some degree of pleomorphism with irregularly barred tear-drop forms. Few or no granules.	Long, irregularly barred cigar-shaped rods, highly pleomorphic. Poor granulation.	Long, curved, pleomorphic, wispy rods with terminal swellings. Prominent granulation.
2. Colony characters on blood tellurite agar after 18–24 hours incubation	Dull greyish black, opaque colonies, 1.5–2.5 mm in diameter. In 2–3 days, 3–5 mm in diameter flat colony with raised dark centre, radially striated periphery and crenated edge – **'daisy-head'** colony.	Small (0.5–0.75 mm in diameter), grey colony with a darker centre and a shining surface – **'frog's egg'** colony. There is little change in size after 48 hours incubation.	Grey, opaque colonies, 1.5–2.0 mm in diameter with regular margins and glossy smooth surface. On further incubation the colony becomes flat with central elevation and regular margins – **'poached egg'** colony.
3. Haemolysis of sheep, rabbit and horse blood	Weakly haemolytic.	Nonhaemolytic.	β-haemolytic.
4. Growth in broth	Surface pellicle, granular deposit and little or no turbidity.	Uniform turbidity with fine granular deposit.	Uniform turbidity with pellicle later.
5. Fermentation of starch and glycogen	+	–	–
6. Serotypes	13	4	40
7. Toxigenic strains	Almost 100%	95–99%	80–85%
8. Predominant strains in	Epidemic areas	Epidemic areas	Endemic areas

Incubation period is 3–4 days, however, it may be as short as 1 day. When toxigenic diphtheria bacilli become lodged in the throat of a susceptible individual, they first multiply rapidly on epithelial cells and produce an exotoxin (diphtheria toxin) that causes local tissue necrosis. The organisms then multiply in cell debris, produce more toxin leading to enlargement of the lesion. The combination of cell necrosis and an exudative inflammatory response of tissue leads to an accumulation of necrotic cellular material, erythrocytes, fibrin and bacteria, which forms a characteristic **diphtheritic pseudomembrane** (in Latin *diphtheria* means pseudomembrane) varying in colour from white to grey to yellow. Since epithelial cells of the mucosa are incorporated in the pseudomembrane, therefore, attempts to remove it produce bleeding.

Diphtheritic pseudomembrane usually appears first on **tonsils** or **posterior pharyngeal wall**. The infection may then spread either upwards into nasal passages or downwards into the larynx and trachea. In **laryngeal diphtheria**, mechanical obstruction may cause suffocation unless the airway is restored by intubation or tracheostomy.

Diphtheria bacilli do not, as a rule, penetrate deeply in the underlying tissues, or the blood, but they produce a powerful exotoxin. Toxin is absorbed into the blood stream from the site of infection and causes toxaemia and various systemic complications. The toxin has a **special affinity for certain tissues, notably heart muscles**, **nerve endings** and **adrenal glands**. Death often results from cardiac failure, but necrotic and often haemorrhagic lesions are usually seen in many organs at necropsy, and in laryngeal diphtheria, death is due to suffocation caused by mechanical obstruction.

Although, diphtheria is usually a disease of the upper respiratory tract, primary or secondary lesions may occur in other parts of body. The most common nonrespiratory site is the skin (**cutaneous diphtheria**).

Laboratory diagnosis

Diagnosis of diphtheria is based on isolating *C. diphtheriae* from the infected area and demonstrating its toxin-producing ability.

Specimens

Two swabs are taken from the local lesion, which is usually in the throat but may also be in the nose, larynx, ear, conjunctiva, vagina and skin or from the nose and throat of contacts or suspected carriers. No antiseptics, in the form of gargles, etc., must have been applied within 12 hours. The swabs should be rubbed over the affected area and pseudomembrane, if formed, should be scraped with swab stick or where there is no definitely localized lesion the swabs should be rubbed over the mucous membrane of posterior pharyngeal wall and tonsils.

Microscopy and culture

One swab should be inoculated on Loeffler's serum slope, blood tellurite agar and a plate of ordinary blood agar, the last for differentiating streptococcal or staphylococcal pharyngitis, which may simulate diphtheria. All these media are incubated at 37°C. Loeffler's serum slope is examined after 12–18 hours. If an early result is urgently required then culture may be examined after 6–12 hours, but if it is negative the examination must be repeated after 18–24 hours.

The resultant growth is mixed by emulsifying it with a wire loop in the condensation fluid and from this smears are made and stained by Gram and Albert methods. Blood tellurite agar is examined after 24 hours, and after 48 hours if no growth is obtained after 24 hours. The growth is identified by colonial morphology, Gram staining, Albert staining and biochemical reactions (Table 22.1).

With the **second swab**, **two smears** are prepared and stained by Gram and Albert methods, but only in a small proportion of cases can positive results be obtained in this way and cultures should always be made as a routine procedure, irrespective of direct examination. Smear from Loeffler's serum slope may be the first indication of the presence of diphtheria bacillus.

Toxigenicity or virulence tests of C. diphtheriae

The identification of an isolate as *C. diphtheriae* does not mean that the patient has diphtheria. Diagnosis of diphtheria depends on showing that the isolate produces diphtheria toxin. This can be done by either *in vivo* or *in vitro* testing. *In vivo* testing is rarely done because the *in vitro* method is reliable, less expensive, and free from the need to use animal.

I. *In vivo*
- Subcutaneous test
- Intradermal test

II. *In vitro*
- Elek's gel precipitation test

Subcutaneous test: Emulsify the growth from an overnight culture on Loeffler's serum slope in 2–4 ml broth and inject 0.8 ml of the emulsion subcutaneously into two guinea-pigs, one of which has been protected with intramuscular injection of 500 units of diphtheria antitoxin 18–24 hours previously. If strain is virulent, the unprotected animal will die within four days.

Perform autopsy on any of the animals dying within this period. If the isolate is toxigenic then the unprotected animal shows:

- Gelatinous haemorrhagic oedema at the site of inoculation.
- Blood-stained pleural and peritoneal exudate.
- Haemorrhagic inflammation of adrenal glands.

If neither animal dies, the culture is non-toxigenic. If both animals die, the culture is virulent or toxigenic, but not *C.*

diphtheriae. This method is usually not employed because the animal is sacrificed.

Intradermal test: Inoculate one colony of suspected *C. diphtheriae* isolate from BTA on a moist Loeffler's serum slope. Incubate at 37°C for 24 hours. Prepare a dense suspension of culture on this medium in 3 ml broth and inject 0.1 ml of this intradermally into the shaved side of a guinea-pig or rabbit. After four hours, the animal is injected intraperitoneally with 500 units of antitoxin. Thirty minutes later a second sample of the test suspension is injected intradermally on the opposite side.

Non-specific inflammatory reaction may occur at both sites within 24–48 hours, but if toxigenic bacilli are present, only the site injected before the antitoxin was administered will progress to form a characteristic necrotic lesion in 48–72 hours. With this test first injection acts as test and second as control and about five strains (10 injections) can be tested on each animal. Moreover, the animal does not die. Therefore, intradermal test is better than subcutaneous test.

Elek's gel precipitation test: This is a gel precipitation test. Pipette 10 ml of nutrient agar, that has been cooled to 55°C in a water bath and 2 ml sterile calf serum in a petri dish and rotate 20 times to mix. Before the medium solidifies, place a 1 cm × 8 cm filter paper strip that has been soaked in the diphtheria antitoxin 500–1,000 units/ml across the middle of the plate on the surface of the agar. Allow the medium to solidify and then place the plate in the incubator with the lid ajar to allow the surface moisture to evaporate.

Inoculate the plate within 2 hours after drying by streaking a heavy inoculum of the culture to be tested across the plate at right angles to the antitoxin strip. Parallel to this streak, at a distance of about 15 mm from it, streak a known toxigenic strain of *C. diphtheriae* on one side of the test strain and streak a non-toxigenic strain on the other side. Incubate the plate at 37°C and examine after 24 and 48 hours. Look for **white lines of precipitation** a few mm from the paper strip, that extend out from the line of bacterial growth, forming an angle of about 45°.

These white precipitin lines form where the toxin from pathogenic strains of *C. diphtheriae* combines with the anti-toxin in optimum concentration from the paper strip, thus identifying the strains of *C. diphtheriae* that produce the toxin. At 24 hours, the line is best seen with the help of a hand lens, at 48 hours it is more obvious. Look for continuity between the line from unknown culture and that from the known toxigenic culture (Fig. 22.3). This test is very convenient and economical.

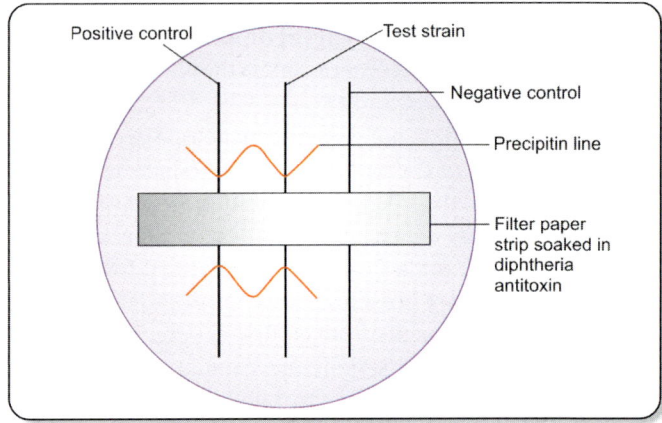

Fig. 22.3. Elek's test.

23

Bacillus Anthracis

Morphology

They are large, Gram-positive, catalase-positive, non-acid-fast, non-flagellate, non-motile, spore-forming bacilli, 4–8 × 1–1.5 μm in size. In smears from infected tissues these are found singly, in pairs and in short chains, the entire chain being surrounded by a **capsule** (Fig. 23.1A). It is polypeptide in nature. It is not formed under ordinary conditions of culture but only if the media contain bicarbonate or are incubated in the presence of 10–25% CO_2.

Spores are formed in culture or in the soil, but never in the animal body during life. Sporulation occurs under unfavourable conditions for growth and is encouraged by distilled water and 2% sodium chloride. It is inhibited by anaerobic conditions and by calcium chloride. **The spores are oval, refractile, central in position and of the same diameter as the bacilli, so that they do not cause bulging of the vegetative cell.** In cultures, the bacilli are arranged end-to-end in long chains. The ends of the bacilli are truncated and somewhat swollen, so that a chain of bacilli presents a **"bamboo-stick" appearance** (Fig. 23.1B).

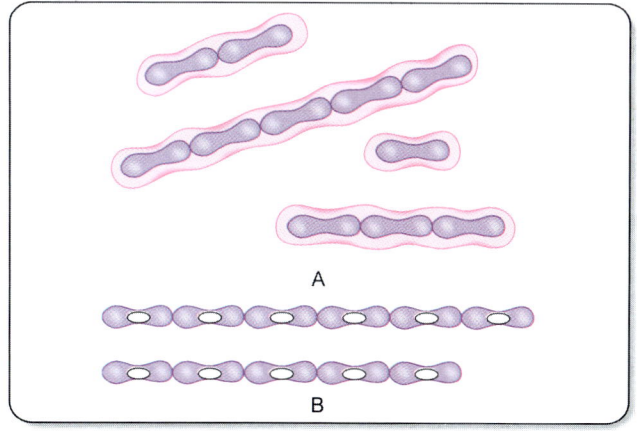

Fig. 23.1. *Bacillus anthracis.*

Cultural characteristics

Anthrax bacilli are aerobes and facultative anaerobes. The optimum temperature for growth is 37°C but growth occurs over a wide temperature range of 12–45°C. Optimum pH for growth is 7–7.4. They can grow on ordinary media.

- On **nutrient agar**, the organisms produce large, raised, opaque, greyish-white colonies, 2–3 mm in diameter with an irregular, fringe-like edge. Under low power of the microscope, the edge of the colony is found to be composed of long, interlacing chains of bacilli, resembling curled hair-lock. This gives them the **'medusa head' appearance**. Virulent capsulated strains form rough colonies, while avirulent strains form smooth colonies. Colonies on blood agar produce very slight haemolysis.

- A selective medium (**PLET medium**) consisting of heart infusion agar with polymyxin, lysozyme, ethylenediamine-tetraacetic acid (EDTA) and thallous acetate has been devised to isolate *B. anthracis* from mixtures containing other spore-bearing bacilli.

- In a **gelatin stab** culture, there is growth down the stab line with lateral spikes that are longest near the surface, giving **'inverted fir tree' appearance** with slow liquefaction commencing from the top.

- When *B. anthracis* is grown on the surface of a **solid medium** containing 0.05–0.5 units of penicillin/ml, in 3–6 hours the cells become large, spherical, and occur in chains on the surface of agar, resembling a string of pearls. This **string of pearls reaction** clearly differentiates *B. anthracis* from *B. cereus* and other aerobic spore bearers. *B. anthracis* is susceptible to gamma phage. This is another useful test which differentiates it from *B. cereus*.

Pathogenicity

B. anthracis causes **anthrax**. It is a **zoonosis** – a disease of animals transmissible to man. It is primarily a disease of cattle and sheep and less often of horses and swines, but experimentally most mammals are susceptible. Bacilli are shed in large numbers from all orifices of the infected animal during the terminal stages of the disease. The organisms sporulate in the soil and remain a source of infection for a number of decades. Animals are infected by ingestion of spores present in the soil. Direct spread from animal to animal is rare.

Man acquires infection through small cuts or abrasions in the skin, by inhalation of spores and rarely by ingestion of infected meat. *Since the release of weaponized B. anthracis spores in the U.S. postal system in 2001, the potential danger associated with this organism has been re-emphasized.* Depending on the mode of infection, anthrax presents in one of the three forms – cutaneous, pulmonary and intestinal.

Cutaneous anthrax

About 95% of human cases of anthrax are cutaneous infections. It is common in farmers and veterinary surgeons handling infected animals, dock workers, factory workers, persons who handle carcasses, hides and animal hair, and those who use shaving brushes prepared from infected animal hair. The lesion starts as a small, pruritic, painless **papule** 1–5 days after contact with infected material. The papule then develops into **vesicle** containing haemorrhagic fluid. Eventually, the vesicle breaks down and is replaced by a **black eschar**, from which it derives its name. *Anthrax in Greek means coal.* Black eschar is later surrounded by a ring of vesicles containing serous fluid and an area of oedema and induration which may become extensive. This has been called a **malignant pustule**. If the lesion is not treated, the organisms may invade the regional lymph nodes and blood stream causing death.

Pulmonary anthrax

It is also known as **wool-sorter's disease** because it used to be common in workers in wool factories, due to inhalation of spores from infected wool. It may also involve workers who handle animal hides which contain spores. This is a haemorrhagic pneumonia with a high fatality rate.

Intestinal anthrax

It is extremely rare and occurs in primitive communities who eat improperly cooked carcasses of animals dying of anthrax. Patient develops haemorrhagic diarrhoea, after a day or so, and dies rapidly from septicaemia.

Laboratory diagnosis

Specimens

B. anthracis can be demonstrated in the material from a malignant pustule, sometimes in sputum from pulmonary anthrax, in gastric aspirates, faeces or food in intestinal anthrax and in the blood in the septicaemic stage of all forms of the disease. Specimens should be taken before antibiotic therapy has been instituted. **All procedures connected with the handling of B. anthracis should be carried out in microbiology laboratory that utilizes Biological Safety Level 2 (BSL2) practices. Laboratory personnel should wear protective gowns, masks and surgical gloves when processing the samples. Safety glasses or eye shields are recommended. After the work is over, all laboratory work benches and surfaces in the safety cabinet must be sterilized with 5% hypochlorite or 5% phenol, and all the instruments used for processing the specimen must be autoclaved.**

In case of malignant pustule, necessary specimens include fluid aspirated from the vesicles surrounding black eschar or material beneath the edge of the black eschar. In early cases, fluid may be obtained by scraping the lesion with a needle.

Microscopy

Prepare smears of each specimen and stain with Gram's method. Examine the stained smears under oil-immersion lens for characteristic Gram-positive anthrax bacilli.

When blood films containing anthrax bacilli are stained with **polychrome methylene blue** for a few seconds and examined under microscope, **an amorphous purplish material** is noticed around the bacilli. This represents the capsular material and is characteristic of anthrax bacillus. This is known as **McFadyean's reaction** and is employed for the presumptive diagnosis of anthrax (Fig. 23.1A). When stained with Giemsa's stain, the bacillus stains purple and capsule red.

Culture

Culture the exudate on nutrient agar, blood agar, PLET medium and nutrient broth. Incubate at 37°C for 24 hours. Examine plates for the medusa-head colonies characteristic of *B. anthracis*. Prepare a smear, stain it by Gram's method and look for tangled chains of large Gram-positive bacilli some of which have central, oval, non-bulging spores. In nutrient broth, look for a pellicle and a deposit.

Animal inoculation

Anthrax bacilli can often be isolated from contaminated tissue by applying them over shaven skin of a guinea-pig. The animal dies in 48–72 hours. Autopsy reveals gelatinous, haemorrhagic oedema at the site of inoculation, petechial haemorrhages in the peritoneum and an enlarged dark red spleen. Make smears from heart blood and spleen, stain by Gram's and McFadyean's methods, and look for typical anthrax bacilli.

Serology

If the sample received is putrid, so that viable bacilli are unlikely, diagnosis may be established by **Ascoli's thermo-precipitin test**. The tissue is ground up in saline, boiled for 5 minutes, filtered and layered over antianthrax serum in a narrow tube. If tissue contains anthrax antigen, a ring of precipitation will appear at the junction of the two liquids within 5 minutes at room temperature.

For further confirmation PCR with specific primers may be carried out.

BACILLUS CEREUS

It is an aerobic, spore-forming, large Gram-positive bacillus resembling *B. anthracis* except that it is motile, non-capsulated, not susceptible to gamma phage and does not react with fluorescent antibody conjugate.

B. cereus produces two different toxins:

1. **Emetic toxin:** This is a heat-stable toxin. Patient develops nausea and vomiting 1–6 hours after ingestion of food that contains this toxin and recovers 6–24 hours after the onset of symptoms. Most of the outbreaks of emetic syndrome have been associated with boiled or fried rice served in oriental restaurants.
2. **Enterotoxin:** It is heat-labile toxin formed in the intestine. Like cholera enterotoxin and labile-toxin (LT) of *Escherichia coli*, it acts on the epithelial cells of small intestine resulting in stimulation of cell-bound adenyl cyclase. This leads to increased levels of cyclic adenosine monophosphate (cAMP) in the gut epithelial cells resulting in active secretion of large volumes of fluid into the intestinal lumen.

This toxin results in symptoms of abdominal pain and profuse diarrhoea (diarrhoeal syndrome) after an incubation period of 10–12 hours. Recovery usually occurs within 12 hours after onset. Implicated foods associated with diarrhoeal syndrome include poultry, meat, mashed potatoes and various soups. In both situations, enormous numbers of organisms (up to 10^{10} per gram) are found in contaminated food.

Laboratory diagnosis

Suspected food, faeces and vomitus are cultured on ordinary media or a special mannitol-egg yolk-phenol red-polymyxin agar (MYPA) medium. *B. cereus* is a motile bacillus, non-capsulated, not susceptible to gamma phage and does not react with fluorescent antibody conjugate. It produces lecithinase and ferments glucose but not mannitol. The inability to recover organisms from fried rice does not necessarily rule out *B. cereus* as cause of the emetic form of illness because flash frying of the fried rice can eliminate the organisms but not the heat-stable toxin.

Anthracoid bacilli

There are several aerobic spore-bearers which are saprophytic and do not ordinarily cause disease in human beings. Morphologically, these resemble anthrax bacilli, and are known as anthracoid bacilli. The important species included in this group are *B. subtilis*, *B. licheniformis* and *B. mycoides*. Unlike anthrax bacilli, anthracoid bacilli are generally motile, non-capsulated, grow in short chains, do not produce medusa-head colonies, produce β-haemolysis and are not pathogenic to laboratory animals. Rarely, some of these may produce human disease. For example, *B. subtilis* which is ubiquitous in nature and a common laboratory contaminant may occasionally cause eye infection and septicaemia, and *B. licheniformis* may cause food poisoning.

24

Clostridium

Clostridium perfringens (Clostridium welchii)

Morphology

They are large, Gram-positive, spore-bearing bacilli, measuring 4–6 × 1 μm with parallel sides and truncated or slightly rounded ends. They occur singly, in pairs or in small bundles. They are non-motile and form capsules in animal body. Spores are oval, subterminal or central and non-bulging (Fig. 24.1A). They are formed under natural conditions, e.g., in the bowel. They are only rarely seen in direct smears from wounds or cultures but can be demonstrated on growth in special media such as Ellner's medium.

Cultural characteristics

It is an anaerobe, but can grow under microaerophilic conditions. Optimum temperature for growth is 37°C. It grows best on media containing carbohydrate such as **glucose blood agar** and forms two main types of colonies. One is round, 2–4 mm in diameter, smooth, regular, convex, amorphous, greyish-yellow and slightly opaque. Other is umbonate with an opaque brownish centre and a lighter, translucent, radially striated periphery with a crenated edge.

Biochemical reactions

It is actively saccharolytic and ferments glucose, maltose, sucrose, lactose and starch with the production of acid and gas.

In **litmus milk medium**, it ferments lactose and produces acid and gas. The acid clots the milk and the gas breaks up the clot resulting in **stormy clot reaction**. Production of acid is also indicated by change in the colour of the litmus from **blue to red**. The culture has sour butyric acid odour. It is indole negative, MR positive, VP negative and H_2S positive.

Gelatin is liquefied but coagulated serum is usually not liquefied. In **cooked meat broth (CMB)**, meat turns pink and is not digested. **It produces phospholipase-C** which gives opalescence around the colonies on egg yolk containing medium.

Toxins

C. perfringens produces **four major lethal, eight minor lethal or non-lethal toxins, and enterotoxin**. Major lethal toxins include α (alpha), β (beta), ε (epsilon) and ι (iota) and minor lethal toxins include γ (gamma), δ (delta), κ (kappa), λ (lambda), μ (mu), η (nu), θ (theta) and ν (eta).

On the basis of four major toxins, *C. perfringens* can be divided into **five types, A–E** (Table 24.1). Typing is done by neutralization tests with specific antitoxins by intracutaneous injection in guinea-pigs or intravenous injection in mice. Strains of *C. perfringens* type A that produce enterotoxin are associated with a mild form of food poisoning.

Alpha toxin is produced by all types of *C. perfringens* but most abundantly by type A strains. It is the most important

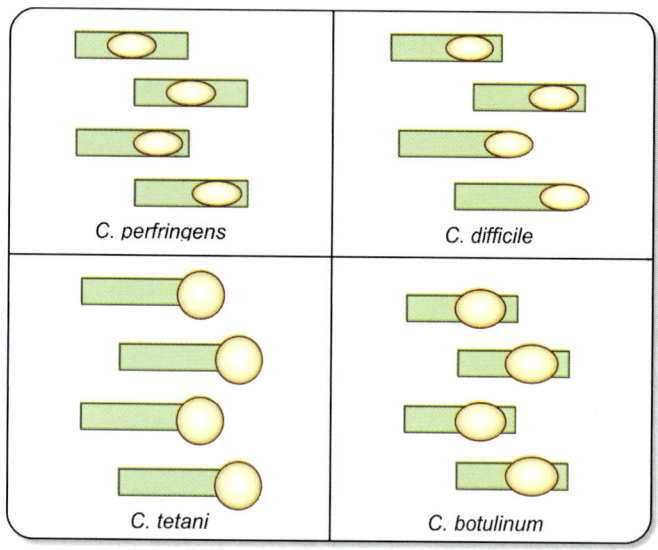

Fig. 24.1. Types of spores in different *Clostridium* species.

Table 24.1. Typing of *Clostridium perfringens*

Type	Toxin produced			
	α	β	ε	τ
A	+	−	−	−
B	+	+	+	−
C	+	+	−	−
D	+	−	+	−
E	+	−	−	+

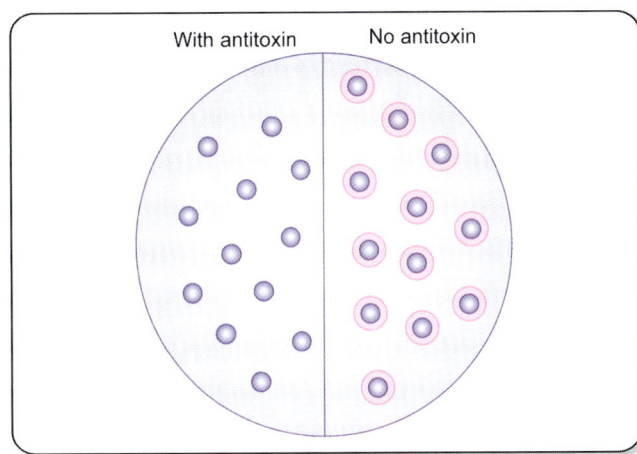

Fig. 24.2. Nagler's reaction.

toxin and is responsible for the profound toxaemia of gas gangrene. In the presence of free Ca^{++} or Mg^{++}, it produces opalescence in serum or egg yolk containing media by splitting phospholipid complexes. This reaction can be inhibited by specific antitoxin. This is the basis of Nagler's reaction.

Pathogenesis

C. perfringens may lead to following infections:

1. Wound infection

C. perfringens occurs normally in the soil, particularly that of manured and cultivated land, and animal and human excreta. The infection usually results from contamination of a wound with these. Wound may get contaminated with patient's own faeces during surgery or after accident. Clostridia may also be present on the normal skin, especially on the perineum and thigh. These may also cause infection.

The presence of devitalized or dead tissue due to crushing of tissues and the severing of arteries in accidental and war injuries, blood clots, extravasated fluid, foreign bodies (bullets, shell fragments and bits of clothing) and coincident

infection with aerobic organisms reduce the oxygen tension with reduction in local Eh. This leads to germination of clostridial spores followed by multiplication of vegetative forms with the production of exotoxins and enzymes into the surrounding environment causing more tissue destruction and resulting in a rapid and fulminating spread of the organism in the necrotic environment. In addition, carbohydrates may be fermented, resulting in production of large quantities of gas in the tissues.

Three types of clostridial wound infections are recognized:

1. ***Wound contamination:*** Here one or more clostridia are present in the traumatized tissue without evidence of infection. Up to 80–90% isolates of *C. perfringens* from hospitalized patients represent simple saprophytic wound contamination.

2. ***Clostridial cellulitis:*** In this condition, infection is confined to local fascial planes in the absence of significant toxaemia. The infecting clostridia are of low invasive power and poor toxigenicity. There is a seropurulent discharge from the wound with an offensive odour and prognosis is good.

3. ***Clostridial myonecrosis or gas gangrene:*** In this condition, there is invasion of healthy muscle tissue and striking systemic intoxication.

The **incubation period of gas gangrene** is 2–3 days. The disease develops with increasing pain, tenderness and oedema of the affected part along with systemic signs of toxaemia. There is a thin watery discharge from the wound, which later becomes profuse and serosanguinous. Accumulation of gas (predominantly hydrogen which is less soluble than carbon dioxide) makes the tissue crepitant.

2. Food poisoning

Enterotoxin producing strains of *C. perfringens* are associated with a mild form of food poisoning. **It is third most common etiologic agent of food poisoning after *Salmonella* spp. and *S. aureus.***

Nagler's reaction

A culture plate containing 6% agar, 5% peptic digest of sheep blood and 20% human serum or 5% egg yolk is prepared. The plate is dried. On one half of the plate, 2–3 drops of *C. perfringens* antitoxin are spread and allowed to dry. The plate is then inoculated with the test organisms or the exudate under study and incubated anaerobically at 37°C for 18 hours. On the section containing no antitoxin, *C. perfringens* colonies show surrounding zone of **opalescence**, i.e., Nagler's reaction, whereas colonies of the remainder half of the plate show no change (Fig. 24.2). It is because of specific neutralization of the alpha toxin. Neomycin sulphate may be added to this medium to inhibit aerobic spore-forming organisms and coliforms. **Willis and Hobbs medium** also incorporates lactose and neutral red to indicate lactose-fermenting organisms, and milk to indicate proteolysis.

Laboratory diagnosis

The diagnosis of gas gangrene must primarily be made upon clinical grounds and initiation of treatment should not await full laboratory report. The function of laboratory is only to provide confirmation of clinical diagnosis.

Specimens

1. Edges of affected muscles,
2. Necrotic tissue, and
3. Exudate from the depth of the lesion, where infection seems to be most pronounced, to be collected with a capillary pipette.

Microscopic examination

Gram smears are prepared. If gas gangrene exists, smear shows typical Gram-positive bacilli often with other bacteria. Thick, stubby, Gram-positive rods suggest *C. perfringens*.

Culture

Aerobic and anaerobic cultures are made on fresh blood agar and heated blood agar. To prevent swarming by some anaerobes, 5–6% agar in plates is used. A plate of human serum or egg yolk agar with *C. perfringens* antitoxin spread on one half of the plate is used for Nagler's reaction. The bacterial isolate is identified by morphology, biochemical reactions and reverse CAMP test (Fig. 24.3).

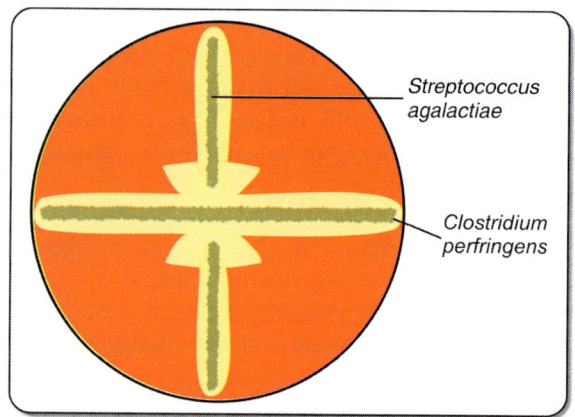

Fig. 24.3. Reverse CAMP test.

Reverse CAMP test

The test is similar to the CAMP test for identifying group B streptococci except that *C. perfringens* is inoculated over the centre of blood agar plate in place of *Staphylococcus aureus*. *Streptococcus agalactiae* is streaked at right angle to it. Positive CAMP test shows butterfly-shaped enhanced haemolysis pointing towards *C. perfringens*.

Clostridium difficile

It is a Gram-positive bacillus, 4–8×0.5–1 µm in size with oval, subterminal or terminal, non-bulging spores (Fig. 24.1B). It is motile by peritrichate flagella. It is an obligate anaerobe and

grows well on blood agar at 37°C. On this medium, after 24 hours incubation, colonies are non-haemolytic, glossy, greyish, low convex, and circular with irregular edges. Cefoxitin cycloserine fructose agar (CCFA) with egg yolk and neutral red, a selective medium, significantly aids in its isolation from faeces.

Pathogenesis

C. difficile is ubiquitous in nature, and has been isolated from soil, water, intestinal contents of various animals, vagina and urethra of humans, and faeces of 40–50% of neonates and only 3% of healthy adults. It has, however, been implicated as a causative agent of **antibiotic-associated diarrhoea** (AAD), **antibiotic-associated colitis** (AAC) and life-threatening **pseudomembranous colitis** (PMC). These conditions have been associated with a number of anti-microbial agents particularly clindamycin and ampicillin. Use of these antibiotics leads to killing of antibiotic-sensitive organisms and overgrowth of *C. difficile* in the intestine leading to these conditions. Most of the cases of PMC are caused by *C. difficile* but infrequently it may also be caused by *S. aureus* and *C. perfringens*.

C. difficile produces disease by the elaboration of two distinct exotoxins:

1. *Toxin A:* It is an enterotoxin that is primarily responsible for diarrhoea. It is capable of producing fluid accumulation in ligated rabbit ileal loop assay.
2. *Toxin B:* It is a potent cytotoxin capable of producing cytopathogenic effects in several tissue culture cell lines.

Laboratory diagnosis

It can be accomplished by demonstrating the toxin in the faeces of the patient by its characteristic effect on HEp2 and human diploid cell cultures or by ELISA. *C. difficile* can also be grown from the faeces of the patient.

Treatment

Discontinue the antibiotic that is presumed to have precipitated the disease, and suppress growth and toxin production of *C. difficile* by giving vancomycin or metronidazole.

Clostridium tetani

Morphology

C. tetani is a slender, Gram-positive bacillus, 2–5 × 0.4–0.5 µm with rounded ends. It tends to be pleomorphic and filamentous. It is non-capsulated and motile by peritrichate flagella. However, type VI strains which do not possess flagella, are non-motile. Young cultures of the organisms usually stain Gram-positive but in older cultures and in smears made from the wounds, they are Gram-variable and even frank Gram-negative. The spores are spherical, terminal and twice the diameter of vegetative cells giving them typical 'drumstick' appearance (Fig. 24.1C). The spores do not take up the Gram stain and appear as colourless round structures.

Cultural characteristics

C. tetani is an obligate anaerobe. The optimum temperature and pH for its growth are 37°C and 7.4 respectively. It can grow well on ordinary media, but its growth is improved by the addition of blood or serum.

- **Colonies on solid media** are irregularly round, 2–5 mm in diameter with fine branching projections. Some strains form colonies with thicker, translucent, yellow brown centre and thin, translucent, colourless periphery. Isolated colonies of *C. tetani* may not be obtained because of the tendency of the organism to swarm over the surface of the medium. However, non-motile variants may produce isolated colonies.
- **On egg yolk agar**, it does not produce opalescence or pearly layer.
- It grows well **in CMB**. The meat is not digested but shows slight blackening on prolonged incubation.

Tetanus toxins

C. tetani produces an oxygen-labile haemolysin (tetanolysin) but all the symptoms in tetanus are attributable to a potent neurotoxin (tetanospasmin).

1. Tetanospasmin

It is a heat-labile protein that may be inactivated by heating at 60°C for 20 minutes. Tetanospasmin is synthesized in the bacterium as a single polypeptide chain with a molecular weight of 150,000 daltons. **It is an extremely powerful toxin second in potency only to the exotoxin of *C. botulinum*.** It has a minimum lethal dose, for a mouse, of 50–75 ng. It gets toxoided spontaneously or in the presence of low concentrations of formaldehyde. It is a good antigen and is specifically neutralized by the antitoxin. The structural gene for toxin production is located on a 75-kilobase plasmid.

2. Tetanolysin

In addition to its neurotoxin, *C. tetani* produces an oxygen-labile haemolysin, antigenically related to streptolysin O and θ toxin of *C. perfringens* and *C. novyi*. There is no evidence that it plays a significant role in pathogenesis.

Pathogenesis

The spores of *C. tetani* are ubiquitous. They occur in the gastrointestinal tracts of man and animals. They are also present in the soil especially in manured soil. Tetanus develops following the contamination of wound with *C. tetani* spores. The source of infection may be soil, dirty clothing or faeces. Germination of spores is dependent upon the reduced oxygen tension occurring in devitalized tissue.

C. tetani remains localized at the site of initial infection and produces tetanus toxin. It is absorbed from the site of its production and ascends to the central nervous system via motor nerves. However, some toxin may be delivered from the site of infection via the blood to all nerves in the body and the subsequent transmission to the central nervous system depends upon uptake through neuromuscular nerve endings and intra-axonal transport. Therefore, the first symptoms in human tetanus appear in head and neck because of the shorter length of the cranial nerves. The **incubation period** of tetanus varies from 2 days to several weeks but commonly it is 6–12 days.

Laboratory diagnosis

The diagnosis is usually based on clinical findings alone because the isolation of the organism can occur in the absence of the disease, and it is also possible to have tetanus and never isolate the organism.

Microscopy

Collect pus or necrotic material from the wound, prepare a smear and stain it by Gram's method. Examine under microscope for typical 'drumstick' bacilli.

Culture

Diagnosis by culture is more dependable. Pus or wound scrapings or excised bits of tissue from the necrotic depths of wound should be plated on one half of a blood agar plate and 3 bottles of CMB. Blood agar plate is incubated anaerobically at 37°C. *C. tetani* produces swarming growth which may be detected on opposite half of the plate after 1–2 days. Of the 3 inoculated CMB bottles, one should be incubated unheated, second is heated in a water bath at 80°C for 5 minutes and third for 20 minutes. The purpose of heating for different periods is to kill non-sporing bacilli, while leaving tetanus spores undamaged, which vary widely in heat-resistance. The heated bottles are also incubated anaerobically at 37°C.

Subcultures from all these bottles are made on half of a blood agar plate daily for 4 days. The plates are incubated anaerobically at 37°C and examined for the swarming edge of *C. tetani*. Incorporation of polymyxin B, to which clostridia are resistant, makes the medium selective.

In vitro toxigenicity test

A blood agar plate containing 4% agar, to minimize swarming, is divided into 2 halves. One half is smeared with tetanus antitoxin. Both halves are then inoculated with growth assumed to be *C. tetani* and incubated anaerobically for 2 days. Colonies haemolytic on the untreated half, but not on the antitoxin half, are of *C. tetani*.

In vivo toxigenicity test

The toxigenicity of the organisms is confirmed by demonstrating the production of tetanospasmin. Two mice, one unprotected and other protected, by giving 1,000 units of tetanus antitoxin intraperitoneally 1 hour before the test, are challenged with an intramuscular injection in the hind leg of

0.1 ml of a 48 hour CMB culture supernate of the isolate. The protected mouse remains well. Signs of ascending tetanus develop in the unprotected animal after several hours, they begin in the inoculated leg and extend to the tail, then the other hind limb is affected and then generalized signs appear. The animal dies within 2 days.

Clostridium botulinum

Morphology

C. botulinum is a straight or slightly curved Gram-positive bacillus with rounded ends. It measures about 5 × 1 μm (range 3.4–8.6 × 0.5–1.3 μm) in size. It is non-capsulated and motile by peritrichate flagella. It produces heat-resistant spores that are oval, subterminal and bulging (Fig. 24.1D).

Cultural characteristics

It is an obligate anaerobe. Optimum temperature for growth is 35°C, but some strains can grow and produce toxin at 1–5°C. It can grow well on routine culture media. Surface colonies are large, irregular, smooth, semitransparent with fimbriate border.

Pathogenicity

C. botulinum is widely distributed in soil and decaying vegetation, thus, many foods, both vegetables and meat, may become contaminated with these organisms. It is non-invasive and its pathogenicity is entirely due to the toxin produced by it. The disease caused by this organism is known as botulism. It is of 3 types:

1. Food-borne botulism

It is due to the ingestion of preformed toxin. The causative organism, *C. botulinum*, multiplies in the food before it is consumed, and produces a powerful soluble toxin. The source of botulism is usually preserved food such as meat and meat products, fish, and vegetables. Food responsible for botulism is usually abnormal in appearance and odour. Bulging of tins and the presence of gas bubbles on opening suggest contamination with *C. botulinum*. However, at times food may look normal.

Symptoms usually begin 18–36 hours after ingestion of food and may include nausea, vomiting, thirst, constipation, double vision, difficulty in swallowing, speaking and breathing. This may be followed by muscular weakness, blurred vision, and death as a result of respiratory failure. Case fatality varies from 25–70%.

2. Wound botulism

C. botulinum has occasionally been isolated from wound in man. Toxin is produced at the site of infection and is absorbed. The symptoms are those of food-borne botulism except those of gastrointestinal system. Symptoms appear 4–14 days after injury, in persons with *C. botulinum* infection.

3. Infant botulism

This entity was recognized in 1976. Affected infants have ranged from 3 weeks to 9 months in age and both sexes have been affected equally. Older children and adults are not susceptible. The infants ingest spores, but not preformed toxin, from soil, household dust, honey, etc. About 10% of honey samples have been shown to contain type A and B spores of *C. botulinum*. **Within the intestine, *C. botulinum* multiplies and elaborates toxin.** After a period of normal development, the infant develops constipation, listlessness, difficulty in sucking and swallowing, weak or altered cry, muscle weakness, ptosis, and loss of head control. Eventually, the baby appears 'floppy' (**floppy child syndrome**) and develops respiratory insufficiency or respiratory arrest. Patient excretes toxin and spores in the faeces.

Laboratory diagnosis

Diagnosis may be made by demonstration of the bacillus or the toxin in suspected residual food or in faeces.

Demonstration of toxin

Botulinum toxin may be demonstrated in the food or faeces. The food is macerated in sterile saline, and the filtrate inoculated into mice or guinea-pigs intraperitoneally. The test animal develops dyspnoea, flaccid paralysis and dies within 24 hours. Control animals protected by polyvalent antitoxin remain healthy. Toxin may also be demonstrated in patient serum.

Demonstration of the organism

Gram-positive sporing bacilli may be demonstrable in smears made from the residual food. For the isolation of *C. botulinum*, the specimen is inoculated on egg yolk agar (EYA), blood agar and three bottles of CMB. Hold one of these three bottles in a water bath at 80°C for 10 minutes and another for 20 minutes and third is unheated. This procedure selects heat-resistant spores and also allows heat-sensitive spores to grow in unheated CMB. The culture media are incubated anaerobically at 30°C for 3–5 days. Cultures in CMB are screened at intervals for toxin production in mice and presence of the organisms may be detected by fluorescent antibody test. Absence of toxin production up to 5 days usually rules out botulism. Subculture toxin-positive CMB culture onto EYA and blood agar. Incubate anaerobically at 30°C for 48 hours. The growth on EYA and blood agar (direct as well as subculture) is identified by Gram staining, fluorescent antibody procedure, colonial morphology and biochemical characters.

25

Mycobacterium Tuberculosis

Morphology

Tubercle bacilli are slender, straight or slightly curved rods with rounded ends. They measure $1–4 \times 0.2–0.8$ μm (average 3×0.3 μm) in size. In sputum and other clinical specimens they may occur singly or in small clumps.

The Ziehl-Neelsen acid-fast stain is useful in staining organisms from cultures or from clinical material. With this stain, the tubercle bacilli stain bright red, while the tissue cells and other organisms are stained blue (Fig. 25.1). Organisms in tissue and sputum smears often stain irregularly and have a beaded or barred appearance, presumably because of their vacuoles and polyphosphate content. However, *M. bovis* appear straight, stout, short uniformly stained rods.

Tubercle bacilli may also be stained with auramine-rhodamine fluorescent stain and smears examined by fluorescence microscopy under low magnification. Tubercle bacilli are seen as yellow luminous organisms in a dark field. When they have been detected under low power, the morphology of the bacilli

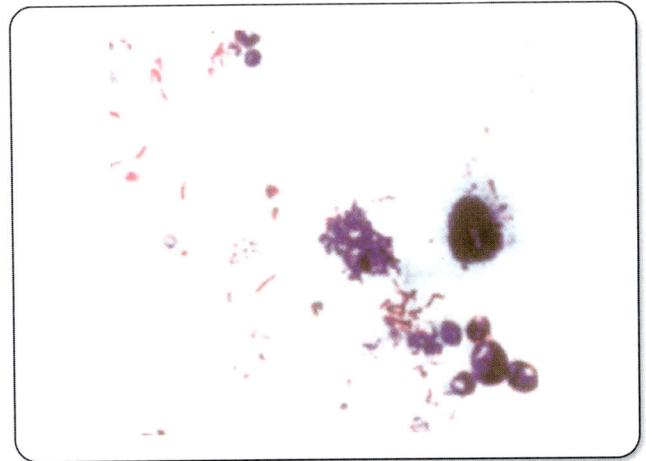

Fig. 25.1. Sputum smear showing acid-fast bacilli (Ziehl-Neelsen staining, ×1000).

is confirmed by observation with an oil-immersion objective. Tubercle bacilli are Gram-positive but it is difficult to stain them with the Gram stain. This is because of the failure of the dye to penetrate the cell wall.

Cultural characteristics

M. tuberculosis is an obligate aerobe while *M. bovis* is microaerophilic on primary isolation, becoming aerobic on subculture. Optimum temperature for growth is 37°C (range 30–40°C) and optimum pH is 7.0 (range 6.0–7.6). Tubercle bacilli can grow on a wide range of enriched culture media but **Lowenstein-Jensen (LJ) medium** is most widely used. This medium consists of whole egg, asparagine, some mineral salts, malachite green and glycerol or sodium pyruvate, and solidified by heating (inspissation). **Malachite green inhibits the growth of organisms other than mycobacteria and provides a colour contrast against which colonies of mycobacteria can be easily seen.** The addition of glycerol improves the growth of *M. tuberculosis*, while it is without any effect or even inhibitory to *M. bovis*. Sodium pyruvate improves the growth of both *M. tuberculosis* and *M. bovis*.

The average generation time of tubercle bacilli is about 14–15 hours, prolonged incubation is, therefore, necessary. *M. tuberculosis* grows well on LJ medium (**eugonic growth**). It produces visible growth on LJ medium, incubated at 37°C, in 2–8 weeks, although on primary isolation from clinical material from patients treated with antituberculous agents, colonies may take up to 12 weeks to appear. It grows as **'rough, tough and buff'** colonies – rough due to dry, irregular growth; tough due to difficulty in lifting the colony from the surface; and buff due to the pale yellow colour. On the other hand, *M. bovis* grows poorly on LJ medium (**dysgonic growth**) forming moist, smooth, flat and white colonies which easily break up when touched.

In **glycerol broth**, the hydrophobic properties of the organisms cell surface result in a whitish wrinkled pellicle and granular deposit. Dispersed, uniform growth can, however, be obtained by subculturing them 2 or 3 times in **Dubos and Davis liquid medium** containing nonionic detergent Tween 80 (polyoxyethylene sorbitan monooleate). It wets the surface, deters aggregation of cells and permits them to grow diffusely. Virulent strains tend to grow as serpentine cords in the liquid media, while avirulent strains grow in a more dispersed fashion.

Pathogenesis

Humans become infected with *M. tuberculosis* most frequently by inhaling infective droplets coughed or sneezed into air by a patient with tuberculosis. Bovine tuberculosis is spread from animal to animal, and sometimes to human attendants, in moist cough spray. About 1% of infected cows develop lesions in the udder and bacilli are excreted in the milk which can then infect people who drink it raw. Thus, primary human tuberculosis due to *M. bovis* usually involves cervical or mesenteric lymph nodes.

Primary tuberculosis

This begins with inhalation of the mycobacteria. Inhaled tubercle bacilli are engulfed by alveolar macrophages in which they replicate to form the initial lesion or **Ghon focus**. It consists of a parenchymal subpleural lesion, often just above or just below the interlobar fissure between the upper and the lower lobes.

Some bacilli are transported by macrophages to the hilar lymph nodes. The Ghon focus together with the enlarged hilar lymph nodes forms the **primary complex**. In addition, the bacilli may be seeded by further lymphatic and haematogenous dissemination in many organs and tissues, including other parts of the lung.

Post-primary (secondary) tuberculosis

It is caused by reactivation of the primary lesion (endogenous), or by exogenous reinfection. Reactivation tuberculosis is particularly likely to occur in immunocompromised individuals including the elderly, transplant recipients and those who are infected with human immunodeficiency virus (HIV). Granulomas of secondary tuberculosis most often occur in the apex of the lungs but may be widely disseminated in the lungs, kidneys, meninges, bones and other organs.

Koch's phenomenon

When a healthy guinea-pig is inoculated subcutaneously with a pure culture of tubercle bacilli, the puncture site heals quickly and there is no immediate visible reaction. But after 10–14 days a hard nodule appears which soon breaks down to form an ulcer that persists till the animal dies of progressive tuberculosis. The regional lymph nodes are enlarged and caseous.

If, on the other hand, virulent tubercle bacilli are injected into a guinea pig which had received an injection of the tubercle bacillus 4–6 weeks previously, an indurated lesion appears at the site of second inoculation in a day or two, which undergoes necrosis in another day to form a shallow ulcer that heals rapidly without involvement of the regional lymph nodes or other tissues. **Koch's phenomenon is a combination of hypersensitivity and immunity**.

Tuberculin test

Principle

Delayed, type IV or cell-mediated hypersensitivity.

Reagents

1. *Old tuberculin (OT):* It was originally described by Robert Koch. It is prepared by autoclaving or boiling a culture of tubercle bacilli, concentrating it 10-fold on a steam bath, filtering off the debris, and adding glycerol as preservative.
2. *Purified protein derivative (PPD):* A slightly more refined tuberculin called purified protein derivative was prepared by Seibert (1941) by growing *M. tuberculosis* in a semisynthetic medium, autoclaving, removing debris by filtration, concentrating the filtrate by ultrafiltration and precipitating several times with 50% saturated ammonium sulphate. The product is mostly a mixture of small proteins (average molecular weight 10,000).

Method

1. *Mantoux test:* 0.1 ml of PPD containing 5 tuberculin units (TU) is injected intradermally into the skin of the volar aspect of the forearm. The site of inoculation is palpated 72 hours later. The development of an area of palpable, firm induration 10 mm or more in diameter is recorded as positive, and those between 5 and 9 mm in diameter as doubtful. The extent of the accompanying erythema is irrelevant and should be ignored.
2. *Heaf test:* This test is done with a multiple puncture apparatus with 6 needles that prick 1–2 mm deep into the skin. A drop of undiluted PPD is spread on the area of skin selected for inoculation. The multiple puncture apparatus is pressed against this area of skin and needles are released. The test is read after 72 hours. Erythema and induration around at least 4 of the punctures is regarded as positive. The equipment must be adequately sterilized between each use to prevent transmission of hepatitis and AIDS.

Uses of tuberculin test

1. To diagnose active infection in infants and young children.
2. To measure prevalence of infection in a community.
3. To select susceptibles for BCG vaccination.
4. Indication of successful BCG vaccination.

False positive

False positive reactions may be seen in patients with infection by related mycobacteria (nontuberculous mycobacteria). These are usually low grade reactions and can be differentiated by testing with tuberculin prepared from these mycobacteria.

False negative (tuberculin anergy)

1. Early tuberculosis.
2. Advanced tuberculosis.
3. Miliary tuberculosis.
4. In patients with measles and other exanthematous reactions.
5. Occasionally after chemotherapy and removal of lung lesion.
6. Advanced age.
7. Immunosuppressive therapy and defective CMI.
8. Lymphoreticular malignancy.
9. Sarcoidosis.
10. Severe malnutrition.

Laboratory diagnosis

Diagnosis of tuberculosis can be established by demonstration of tubercle bacilli in clinical specimens by microscopy and cultural techniques. Only up to 50% of pulmonary and 25% of extrapulmonary tuberculosis can be diagnosed by smear examination.

Collection of specimen

- The specimen most commonly collected is **sputum** which consists of pus and mucus secretions coughed up from the lung. Patient is instructed to cough up the sputum into a clean wide-mouthed container. Disposable waxed cardboard containers are ideal. A morning specimen may be collected. If sputum is scanty, a 24 hour specimen may be collected.
- If no sputum is produced, **laryngeal swab or bronchial washings** are examined.
- In children, stomach washings may be examined as they tend to swallow sputum.
- Depending upon the site of involvement, **cerebrospinal fluid, pleural fluid, urine and aspirated fluid from bone and joint** are centrifuged and the deposits are examined.
- **Tissue biopsies** are homogenized and examined by microscopy and culture.
- In pulmonary and renal tuberculosis, three consecutive specimens of **sputum and urine** should be examined respectively.

Direct microscopy

Pour the sputum in a petri dish and examine. For preparation of smear, select **blood-tinged part** of the sputum, if it is not there then **purulent part** should be selected. The smear is stained by Ziehl-Neelsen technique and examined under oil-immersion lens. Acid-fast bacilli stain bright red against a blue background (Fig. 25.1). To be detected microscopically, there must be 50,000–100,000 bacilli per ml of sputum. A negative report should not be given till at least 300 fields have been examined, taking about 10 minutes. Smears are

graded based on Revised National Tuberculosis Control Programme (RNTCP) recommendations in India. Table 25.1 gives Ziehl-Neelsen smear grading as per RNTCP recommendations.

Table 25.1. Ziehl-Neelsen smear grading as per RNTCP recommendations

If the slide has	Result	Grading	No. of fields to be examined
More than 10 AFB per oil-immersion field	Positive	3+	20
1–10 AFB per oil-immersion field	Positive	2+	50
10–99 AFB per 100 oil-immersion fields	Positive	1+	100
1–9 AFB per 100 oil-immersion fields	Positive	Scanty	100
No AFB in 100 oil-immersion fields	Negative	—	100

Unless care is taken, Ziehl-Neelsen staining may show false positive results due to following reasons:

1. Stained bacilli may be transferred to a negative smear by blotting paper used previously to dry a positive smear. Therefore, a blotting paper should be used only once.
2. If a positive slide is cleaned, all stained bacilli may not be washed away. If such a slide is reused for preparation of a smear from a negative specimen, false result is obtained. Therefore, a new slide should be used for each specimen.
3. Stained bacilli may be transferred from a positive smear to a negative smear by immersion oil on the microscope lens. In such a case, microscopic examination will reveal bacilli floating in the oil over the smear. Fresh smear should be prepared, stained and examined after cleaning the oil-immersion lens.
4. Saprophytic mycobacteria may be present in tap water. These may get into the smear during washing. Most saprophytic species stain uniformly without any barred or beaded appearance and are usually only acid-fast, without being alcohol-fast.

Concentration of specimens

Mycobacteria in a specimen can be decontaminated and concentrated into a small volume without inactivation. Such concentrate can be used for microscopy, culture and animal inoculation. Several methods are in use:

- *Petroff's method:* It is a simple and widely used technique. Equal volumes of sputum and 4% sodium hydroxide are mixed and incubated at 37°C with frequent shaking till it gets liquefied and becomes clear. On the average, it takes 20–30 minutes. It is then centrifuged at 3,000 rpm for 30 minutes. The supernatant fluid is pipetted off and the deposit is neutralized by adding 8% hydrochloric acid in the presence of a drop of phenol red indicator.

Culture

It is very sensitive for detection of tubercle bacilli. It may be positive with as few as 10–100 bacilli per ml of sputum and it is necessary for antimicrobial drug sensitivity testing. **Concentrate of sputum** is inoculated on two slopes of LJ medium. In case of **laryngeal swab**, add enough 5% oxalic acid to the tube to cover the swab and leave it at room temperature for 30 minutes to kill non-acid-fast contaminants. Squeeze the swab against the side of the tube to remove excess fluid and rub it over the surface of two slopes of LJ medium.

In case of **gastric washings**, 15 ml of the specimen is collected in a 25 ml bottle containing 5 ml of 15% trisodium phosphate, which will neutralize the acid. Then cap and shake the bottle. In the laboratory, homogenize and decontaminate the specimen by Petroff's method. Centrifuge and examine the deposit by Ziehl-Neelsen staining and culture on LJ medium.

In case of **renal tuberculosis**, three early morning specimens of urine should be collected. Each specimen should consist of 50–100 ml. It is centrifuged at 1500 g for 30 minutes and treat the deposit by Petroff's method. Prepare a smear and stain by Ziehl-Neelsen staining and inoculate on two slopes of LJ medium.

Tubercle bacilli are usually scanty in **pleural and peritoneal fluids**. Therefore, at least 50–100 ml of either of these should be collected. Centrifuge these fluids and treat the deposits by Petroff's method as above. In case of **CSF**, 3–4 ml is collected and centrifuged. The deposit is used for the smear and culture. **Pus** is directly used for smear and culture.

The inoculated media are incubated at 37°C. The cultures are examined weekly for up to 12 weeks. Growth of most strains of *M. tuberculosis* may appear in 2–8 weeks. But cultures should not be discarded as negative until they have been observed for 12 weeks. Longer incubation is necessary for strains originating from patients treated with antituberculous agents.

The use of liquid medium with **radiometric growth detection**, such as BACTEC 460TB has simplified culture method. It is an automated radiometric method using Middlebrook 7H12 (BACTEC 12B) containing a ^{14}C-labelled substrate (palmitic acid) that is metabolized by mycobacteria, liberating radioactive CO_2 ($^{14}CO_2$) into the head space of a glass vial. The amount of $^{14}CO_2$ liberated is detected by the BACTEC 460TB instrument and interpreted as a "growth index". It is assumed that the release of CO_2 denotes growth of the organisms. The recommended inoculum for the BACTEC 12B 4-ml vial is 0.5 ml of decontaminated concentrated specimen. By this method the growth of *M. tuberculosis* and nontuberculous mycobacteria is detected in 9–14 days and less than 7 days respectively. The time in which the radiometric system detects growth reflects the quantity of viable mycobacteria in the submitted sample, which is indirectly reflected by smear positivity. In smear-positive samples, *M. tuberculosis* may be detected as early as 7–8 days and *M. avium* as early as 5–8 days. In smear-negative samples, *M. tuberculosis* and nontuberculous mycobacteria are usually detected in 14–28 days and 8–12 days respectively.

A disadvantage of BACTEC system is that no colony morphology or pigmentation is available to suggest that the growth is of a mycobacterial species and not that of a contaminant or commensal organism. Other disadvantages of the BACTEC 460TB include radioisotope disposal.

Another method of detection of mycobacterial growth is **mycobacterial growth indicator tube** (MGIT). It is non-radiometric automated method. It consists of tubes containing liquid culture media, and a fluorescent compound is embedded on the bottom of the tube. The fluorescent compound is sensitive to dissolved oxygen in the liquid medium. Therefore, the dissolved oxygen in the uninoculated medium quenches any fluorescence from the compound. However, when the mycobacteria grow, they deplete the dissolved oxygen in the liquid medium and the compound fluoresces brightly which can be detected by observing the tube under ultraviolet light (wood's lamp). The sensitivity and time to positive culture is similar to BACTEC 460TB.

The MB/Bac TAlert 3D system uses a colorimetric carbon dioxide sensor in each tube to detect bacterial growth. The specimen is inoculated in liquid medium vials. If mycobacteria are present in the specimen, carbon dioxide is released by actively proliferating mycobacteria. The elevated levels of carbon dioxide lowers the pH of the medium which produces a colour change in the sensor present in the liquid medium vial. The colour change is detected by the instrument.

Sensitivity testing

With the emergence of multidrug resistance in mycobacteria, it is essential to perform sensitivity testing on tubercle bacilli as an aid and guide to treatment. Drug-resistant mutants continuously arise at a low rate in any mycobacterial population. The purpose of sensitivity testing is to determine whether the great majority of the bacilli in the culture are sensitive to the antitubercular drugs currently in use. Following techniques for sensitivity testing can be used:

- **Resistance ratio method:** This method is most important. Slopes of LJ medium incorporating doubling concentrations of drugs are inoculated with a standardized suspension of the test strain and a known sensitive strain (H37Rv strain of *M. tuberculosis*) or preferably a number of known sensitive strains. After incubation for 3 weeks at 37°C, the slopes are examined for growth and the lowest concentration of antibiotic showing no more than 0–20 colonies is taken as the end point or minimum inhibitory concentration (MIC). The result is expressed as resistance ratio, i.e., the ratio of the MIC of the test strain to the MIC of known sensitive strain or to the average concentration inhibiting a number of known sensitive strains. A ratio of 8 is reported as unequivocally resistant. A strain with a ratio of 4 is regarded as doubtfully resistant and the test should be repeated. Strains having resistance ratio of 1 or 2 are reported as sensitive.

- **Absolute concentration method:** In this method, the MIC of the drug against the test strain only is determined. Therefore, this method is inferior to resistance ratio method.
- **Proportion method:** In this method, the number of colonies growing from a standard inoculum on a drug-containing medium is compared with the colony count from same sized inoculum on a drug-free medium. The strain is regarded as resistant when more than 1% of the bacteria grow in the presence of the drug.
- **BACTEC radiometric method:** In this method, a standardised inoculum is inoculated in liquid media, one containing and other without drug. The medium contains ^{14}C-labelled substrate. The rate and amount of $^{14}CO_2$ produced in the absence or presence of drug is measured by the special instrument and is then compared.
- **Non-radiometric method:** Mycobacterial growth indicator tube (MGIT) can also be used for sensitivity testing of *M. tuberculosis*.

Molecular methods

Polymerase chain reaction (PCR) and ligase chain reaction (LCR) are used as diagnostic techniques. PCR is based on DNA amplification and has been used to detect *M. tuberculosis* in clinical specimens. The restriction fragment length polymorphism (RFLP) is used to type different strains for epidemiological purposes. The principle of this technique is that restriction endonuclease treatment yields nucleic acid fragments of different lengths, the patterns of which are strain-specific.

GeneXpert system – XpertMTB/Rif test

The XpertMTB/Rif test is a cartridge-based fully automated nucleic acid amplification test (NAAT). It purifies, concentrates, amplifies (by rapid, real-time PCR) and identifies targeted nucleic acid sequences in the TB genome, and provides results from unprocessed sputum samples in less than 2 hours, with minimal hands-on technical time.

The most widely used method to detect TB in most disease-endemic countries is the 125 year-old sputum smear microscopy test, which has a number of drawbacks including low sensitivity and inability to determine drug-susceptibility.

Conventional diagnosis of drug-resistant TB, as discussed above, relies on mycobacterial culture and drug-susceptibility testing. It is a slow and cumbersome process requiring sequential procedures for isolation of mycobacteria from clinical specimens, identification of *Mycobacterium tuberculosis* complex and *in vitro* testing of strain susceptibility to anti-TB drugs. During this time patients may be inappropriately treated, drug-resistant strains may continue to spread, and amplification of resistance may occur. In contrast, the XpertMTB/Rif test is a rapid test which identifies both the presence of *M. tuberculosis* and resistance to rifampicin in a single test. This can enable early and appropriate treatment initiation, as well as accelerating the implementation of MDR-TB control measures, and ultimately reducing TB case incidence.

Prophylaxis

Protection from tuberculosis may be afforded by public health measures, BCG vaccination and by chemoprophylaxis. General measures, such as adequate nutrition, good housing and health education are important.

BCG vaccine

It is a live attenuated vaccine. It is available in liquid form and freeze-dried (lyophilized) form. The latter is commonly used. The lyophilized vaccine supplied by BCG vaccine laboratory, Chennai, is reconstituted by sterile physiological saline to make a final concentration of 0.1 mg (moist weight) in 0.1 ml of the vaccine. Once reconstituted, vaccine should be utilized within 3–6 hours. Following injection of 0.1 ml of vaccine intradermally, the organisms grow to a limited extent in the tissues. Immunizing capability of the vaccine depends on this. Dead vaccine or tuberculin is not effective. BCG vaccine should be administered soon after birth failing which it may be given at any time during the first year of life.

A **small nodule** develops at the site of inoculation 2–3 weeks after injection. It increases slowly in size and by about 5 weeks it attains a diameter of 4–8 mm. It then subsides or breaks into a **shallow ulcer** which heals by scarring. Such individuals become **tuberculin-positive** after 4–6 weeks. A few cases have been recorded where BCG has given rise to progressive tuberculosis.

26

Nontuberculous Mycobacteria

Mycobacteria other than tubercle and leprosy bacilli, that normally exist as saprophytes of soil and water (environment) and occasionally cause opportunistic disease in man resembling tuberculosis are known as nontuberculous mycobacteria (NTM), earlier also called anonymous atypical, or MOTT (mycobacteria other than typical tubercle) bacilli. Infection caused by these organisms is known as **mycobacteriosis**. NTM are:

- Acid-fast and alcohol-fast and may resemble or differ in morphology from tubercle bacilli.
- They may be longer and even filamentous.
- They can grow at 25°C and 37°C. Some of them (*M. xenopi*, *M. phlei* and *M. smegmatis*) can grow at 44°C.
- Some of them are rapid growers. They produce visible growth on LJ medium within one week.
- Some of them produce a bright yellow or orange pigment.
- They are resistant to antituberculous drugs such as streptomycin, isoniazid and *p*-aminosalicylic acid. All of them are resistant to at least one of these drugs. However, many strains are sensitive to rifampicin.
- They are niacin and neutral red reactions negative.
- They produce enzyme arylsulphatase.
- They are non-pathogenic for guinea-pig but pathogenic for mouse.
- They occasionally cause opportunistic disease, resembling tuberculosis in man.

Classification

On the basis of production of bright yellow or orange pigment and rate of growth, Runyon (1959) classified nontuberculous mycobacteria into four groups (Table 26.1). These mycobacteria can grow on Lowenstein-Jensen (LJ) medium. All strains of groups I, II and III grow slowly and form colonies in 2–8 weeks. However, group IV (rapid growers) produce colonies within one week.

Table 26.1. Nontuberculous mycobacteria

Runyon group	Name	Species
I	Photochromogens	*Mycobacterium kansasii*, *M. marinum, M. simiae*
II	Scotochromogens	*M. scrofulaceum, M. gordonae, M. szulgai*
III	Non-chromogens	*M. avium, M. intracellulare, M. xenopi, M. ulcerans, M. malmoense, M. terrae, M. triviale, M. nonchromogenicum*
IV	Rapid growers	*M. smegmatis, M. phlei, M. chelonae, M. fortuitum*

I. Photochromogens

They form colourless colonies when incubated in the dark, but when the young culture is exposed to light for one hour in the presence of air (cap of the culture bottle loosened) and re-incubated for 24–48 hours, they develop a bright yellow or orange pigment (beta-carotene). For testing photochromogenesis, test strain is inoculated on two LJ slopes. One of them is wrapped in aluminium foil to exclude light from it and the other is left unwrapped. Both these slopes are incubated in an incubator at 37°C with a lighted 15 watt electric bulb for 14 days. If only the unwrapped, but not wrapped culture shows a bright yellow or orange pigment, the strain is a photochromogen.

This group contains three species – *M. kansasii, M. marinum* and *M. simiae*.

- *M. kansasii* causes chronic pulmonary disease resembling tuberculosis, particularly in old persons with pre-existing lung disease. It has been isolated on several occasions from piped water supplies. It grows well at 37°C on LJ medium yielding a good growth within two weeks and reduces nitrate to nitrite. The bacterial cells are usually elongated and have a distinct beaded appearance. It is usually sensitive to rifampicin and several other antitubercular drugs.

- **M. simiae** was originally isolated from monkeys. Like *M. kansasii*, it grows well at 37°C and causes pulmonary disease. It synthesizes niacin in significant amounts and may, thus be falsely identified as *M. tuberculosis*.

- **M. marinum** was originally isolated from fish. It grows poorly or not at all at 37°C. It grows well at 33°C. It causes superficial granulomatous skin disease of man known as **swimming pool granuloma** or **fish tank granuloma**. It resembles *M. kansasii* in colonial and microscopic appearance. *M. marinum* may, however, be distinguished from *M. kansasii* by its:
  – poor or no growth at 37°C;
  – failure to reduce nitrate to nitrite;
  – failure to produce catalase; and
  – ability to hydrolyze pyrazinamide.

II. Scotochromogens

These organisms form bright yellow or orange pigment in cultures incubated in the dark, though the intensity of the colour may increase on exposure to light.

- **M. scrofulaceum** is an important member of this group which may cause **scrofula** (cervical lymphadenitis) in children. The bacilli may be short or long and filamentous. It is resistant to isoniazid and sensitive to cycloserine and ethionamide.

- **M. gordonae** is often found in water. It is a frequent contaminant of clinical specimens and a rare cause of pulmonary disease.

- **M. szulgai** is a scotochromogen when incubated at 37°C and photochromogen at 25°C. It may occasionally cause pulmonary disease and bursitis.

III. Non-chromogens

They do not form pigment even on exposure to light. Medically important species include *M. intracellulare*, *M. avium*, *M. xenopi*, *M. ulcerans* and *M. malmoense*.

- **M. intracellulare** was formerly known as Battey bacillus as it was first detected in Battey State Hospital for tuberculosis in Georgia, USA. The infection with this organism is common in the Southeast USA, where the organism occurs in soil and water. It causes chronic pulmonary disease indistinguishable from tuberculosis.

- **M. avium** causes tuberculosis in fowls and sometimes in pigs. It can grow at 45°C. *M. avium* and *M. intracellulare* are the **commonest nontuberculous mycobacteria** causing opportunistic infections in man. Colonies of both these species are smooth, non-pigmented and easily emulsifiable.

  Because there is no clear-cut division between *M. avium* and *M. intracellulare*, therefore, they are usually grouped together as *M. avium-intracellulare* (MAI) or *M. avium* complex (MAC). This complex possesses 28 agglutination serotypes. Types 1, 2 and 3 are regarded as *M. avium* and the others as *M. intracellulare*. In man, MAC causes pulmonary disease indistinguishable from tuberculosis, lymphadenitis and disseminated disease, particularly in patients with AIDS.

- **M. xenopi** was first isolated from a skin lesion in a South African toad (*Xenopus laevis*). It is a thermophile and grows well at 45°C. It may cause pulmonary lesions in man. It has a limited geographical distribution. Most of the cases of pulmonary lesions, due to *M. xenopi* have been reported from South London.

- **M. ulcerans**, causative agent of **Buruli ulcer**, was originally isolated from ulcerative skin lesions in Australia in 1948. The name Buruli ulcer is derived from the Buruli district of Uganda where a large outbreak of the disease was extensively investigated. *M. ulcerans* grows slowly at 31–34°C but not at all at 37°C in primary culture. It produces an exotoxin which has been characterized as a high molecular weight phospholipoprotein-lipopolysaccharide complex, which when inoculated intradermally in the guinea-pig, causes inflammation, tissue necrosis and histopathological changes similar to those seen in human lesions. Therefore, this exotoxin may be involved in the pathogenesis of the disease.

- **M. malmoense** causes pulmonary disease and lymphadenitis. It was first isolated from patients from Malmo in Sweden. It is a very slow-growing species. On primary isolation, colonies may not be visible until after 10 weeks incubation. It causes pulmonary disease and lymphadenitis. It is resistant to isoniazid and rifampicin and sometimes also to streptomycin and ethambutol.

- **M. terrae**, **M. triviale** and **M. nonchromogenicum** are rare pathogens which belong to Runyon group III (non-chromogens). They are sometimes grouped as the *Mycobacterium-terrae-trivialenonchromogenicum* group.

IV. Rapid growers

Rapid growers which may be photo-, scoto- or non-chromogens, produce visible growth on LJ medium within one week, usually in 2–3 days. All the chromogenic rapid growers, e.g., *M. smegmatis* and *M. phlei* are saprophytes.

- **M. smegmatis** forms rough colonies, white to buff in colour. The bacilli are slender rods, which may be curved and beaded. Since it is normally present in smegma, a whitish secretion around the orifice of urethra, it is a frequent contaminant of urine specimens. Some strains of *M. smegmatis* are acid-fast but not alcohol-fast, therefore, they are not seen in a Ziehl-Neelsen stained smear if acid-alcohol is used as decolourizer. Other strains are both acid- and alcohol-fast. In such cases, rapid growth on LJ medium and guinea-pig inoculation distinguishes it from *M.*

tuberculosis. M. smegmatis has been implicated in rare cases of pulmonary, skin, soft tissue, and bone infections.

- **M. phlei** is rarely encountered and is non-pathogenic. It grows as rough colonies that at first are buff coloured and later become yellow to orange. It can be differentiated from *M. smegmatis* by its ability to grow at 52°C and survive heating at 60°C for 4 hours.
- Only two of the rapid growers, **M. chelonae** and **M. fortuitum** are human pathogens. Both these are coccoid to filamentous and form white to cream-coloured colonies. The former grows better at 25°C than at 37°C. *M. fortuitum* can further be differentiated from *M. chelonae* in reducing nitrate and assimilation of iron from ferric ammonium citrate. *M. chelonae* was originally identified as turtle and *M. fortuitum* as frog tubercle bacilli. They are found in soil and infection usually follows some injury and can lead to chronic abscess formation. They occasionally cause pulmonary or disseminated disease.

Pathogenicity

As compared to tubercle bacilli, nontuberculous mycobacteria are of low virulence. They may occasionally cause pulmonary disease resembling tuberculosis, lymphadenopathy, skin lesions (Bruli ulcer, nontuberculous swimming pool granuloma) and disseminated disease (Table 26.2).

Laboratory diagnosis

Specimens

Sputum, pus, exudates.

Microscopy

Ziehl-Neelsen staining of smear shows acid-fast bacilli. Repeated smear examination is necessary.

Culture

Several LJ media should be inoculated with the specimen. These are incubated in the dark and in light at different temperatures for distinguishing various species.

Biochemical reactions

Biochemical reactions are performed for distinguishing various species (Table 26.3).

Table 26.2. Disease caused by atypical mycobacteria

Disease	Causative agents
1. Pulmonary disease	*M. kansasii*
	M. simiae
	M. gordonae
	M. szulgai
	M. intracellulare
	M. avium-intracellulare
	M. xenopi
	M. malmoense
2. Lymphadenopathy	*M. scrofulaceum*
	M. avium-intracellulare
	M. malmoense
3. Skin lesions	
• Bruli ulcer	*M. ulcerans*
• Swimming pool granuloma	*M. marinum*
4. Disseminated disease	*M. avium-intracellulare*

Table 26.3. Differential characters of various species of non-tuberculous mycobacteria

Test	Species							
	M. kansasii	*M. marinum*	*M. scrofulaceum*	*M. avium-intracellulare*	*M. fortuitum*	*M. chelonae*	*M. phlei*	*M. smegmatis*
Growth within 7 days	–	–	–	–	+	+	+	+
Growth at								
25°C	+	+	+	±	+	+	+	+
37°C	+	–	+	+	+	+	+	+
45°C	–	–	–	±	–	–	+	+
Pigment production in dark	–	–	+	–	–	–	+	–
Pigment production in light	+	+	+	–	–	–	+	–
Urease production	+	+	+	–	+	+	+	+
Niacin production	–	–	–	–	–	–	–	–
Nitrate reduction	+	–	–	–	+	–	+	+

27

Mycobacterium Leprae

Morphology

Lepra bacilli are straight or slightly curved slender bacilli about the same size as tubercle bacilli (average size: 3 × 0.3 μm). They have pointed, rounded or club-shaped ends. They are non-motile and non-sporing. They are Gram-positive and stain more readily than *M. tuberculosis*. With Ziehl-Neelsen stain, they are less acid-fast than tubercle bacilli, so 5% sulphuric acid, instead of 20%, is employed for decolorization after staining with carbol fuchsin.

The bacilli are seen singly and in groups, intracellularly and lying free outside the cell. Inside the cells they are usually present in parallel bundles of 50 or more organisms bound together by a lipid-like substance, the **glia**. These masses of bacteria are known as **globi** which are seen inside the histiocytes which have a foamy appearance. These are known as **lepra cells** (Fig. 27.1).

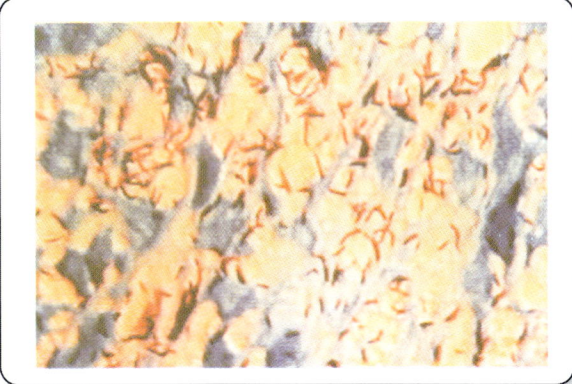

Fig. 27.1. Lepromatous leprosy showing acid-fast bacilli in macrophages (lepra cells) (Ziehl-Neelsen staining, ×1000).

Live bacilli in the smear appear solid and uniformly stained, while dead or dying forms appear fragmented, beaded and granular. The percentage of uniformly stained bacilli in the tissues is known as **morphological index** (MI). This provides a method for assessing the progress of patients on chemotherapy and is more meaningful than the old criterion, the **bacteriological index** (BI). Poorly stained bacilli are probably dead. A continuing fall in the MI is encouraging and a fall succeeded by a rise indicates development of **drug resistance** in the bacteria. Bacteriological index of a smear is the total number of acid-fast bacilli in an oil-immersion field. It can be expressed from 1+ to 6+ by Ridley's scale (Table 27.1).

Table 27.1. Bacteriological index (Ridley's scale)

Bacteriological index	Number of acid-fast bacilli
6+	More than 1000 per oil-immersion field
5+	100–1000 per oil-immersion field
4+	10–100 per oil-immersion field
3+	1–10 per oil-immersion field
2+	1–10 per 10 oil-immersion fields
1+	1–10 per 100 oil-immersion fields

Cultivation

A large number of attempts at cultivation of *M. leprae*, in artificial culture media and in tissue culture, have been made and success has been claimed from time to time, but none has been confirmed so far. One of the best known of such reports came from Indian Cancer Research Centre (ICRC), Bombay (now Mumbai) (1962), where an acid-fast bacillus was isolated from a leprosy patient, employing human foetal spinal ganglion cell culture. This is known as **ICRC bacillus**. It has been adapted for growth on Lowenstein-Jensen medium and taxonomical studies suggest that this organism is not *M. leprae* and belongs to *M. avium-intracellulare* group.

There have been many attempts to transmit leprosy to various experimental animals (Table 27.2).

Table 27.2. Experimental animals which have been used for experimental transmission of leprosy

1. Mice
2. Nine-banded armadillos
3. Slender loris
4. Indian pangolin
5. Chipmunks
6. European hedgehog
7. Monkeys
   • Mangabey
   • Rhesus
   • African green
   • Filipino cynomolgus
8. Chimpanzees
9. Gibbon apes
10. Golden hamsters
11. Rats-Lewis

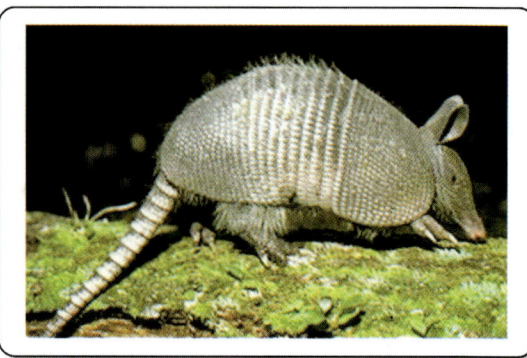

Fig. 27.2. Nine-banded armadillo.

• *M. leprae* can be transmitted from one animal to another without any change in microbe, therefore, an abundant source of *M. leprae*, for research and the preparation of lepromin or of a vaccine, has now become available.
• The yield of *M. leprae* from armadillo skin leproma is 100–1,000 times more than that from human leproma.

Other animals suitable for propagation of *M. leprae* are:

• Chipmunk,
• Indian pangolin,
• Slender loris, and
• European hedgehog.

But the first breakthrough was achieved by Shepard (1960) when he reported a limited localized multiplication of *M. leprae* in the **footpad of mouse** in 1–6 months. Footpad of mouse model can be used for:

• Identification of *M. leprae*.
• To study the susceptibility of organisms to chemotherapeutic agents.
• To study the development of drug resistance in *M. leprae* in patients under treatment.
• To study the properties of bacilli isolated from different forms of the disease.
• To study the efficacy of various vaccines to suppress multiplication of *M. leprae*.
• To determine viability of *M. leprae*.

The disadvantages of the footpad of mouse model are:

• Following intradermal inoculation, there occurs only a limited multiplication of *M. leprae* (1×10^6 bacilli per footpad), therefore, the yield of the bacilli is not sufficient for comprehensive research on *M. leprae*.
• Mice have a short life-span and leprosy has a long incubation period and chronic course. So, it is not possible to study the pathogenesis of the disease.
• The lesion produced is not of lepromatous leprosy type.

Nine-banded armadillo (*Dasypus novemcinctus*) (Fig. 27.2) is highly susceptible to leprosy. This is presumably due to low body temperature. When inoculated with *M. leprae*, about 40% armadillos develop generalized infection with extensive multiplication of *M. leprae*. Involvement of skin, nerves, lymph nodes, larynx and eye is similar to that of man. The advantages of armadillo are:

• Relatively long life-span (12–15 years).
• Relatively low body temperature (32–35°C).
• Unique mode of reproduction by means of monozygous genetically identical quadruplets.

Pathogenesis

Leprosy is an exclusively human disease and the only source of infection is the patient. It is not considered a highly contagious disease. The exact mode of infection is not clear. Very large number of bacilli are shed in nasal secretions (over 10^8 organisms per ml) and in discharges from superficial lesions of the cases of lepromatous leprosy. Organisms may be acquired by a susceptible person by way of skin to skin contact or through respiratory tract. It has also been suggested that insect vectors may have a role in transmission of leprosy.

M. leprae causes **chronic granulomatous lesions** closely resembling those of tuberculosis with epithelioid cells and giant cells but **without caseation**. The organisms in the lesion are predominantly intracellular and like tubercle bacilli can proliferate in macrophages. The organism has predilection for skin, nerves and nasal mucosa though it is capable of affecting any tissue or organ.

• In **cutaneous form** of the disease, large, firm nodules are distributed widely and on the face they create a characteristic **leonine appearance**.
• In the **neural form**, segments of peripheral nerves are involved leading to **localized patches of anaesthesia**. The loss of sensations in fingers and toes increases the frequency of minor trauma, leading to secondary infection and mutilating injuries.

Both forms may be present in the same patient.

Spectrum of leprosy

On the basis of clinical, histopathologic and immunologic findings, Ridley and Joplings (1966) introduced a scale for classifying the spectrum of leprosy into 5 types with hyper-reactive tuberculoid leprosy (TT) at one pole and anergic lepromatous leprosy (LL) at the other.

- **Tuberculoid type:** It is seen in patients with high degree of resistance where cell-mediated immunity is intact. The skin lesions are few and consist of nonelevated hypo- or hyperpigmented macular anaesthetic patches involving the face, trunk and limbs. There are very few acid-fast bacilli (AFB), so that they are generally not seen microscopically (**paucibacillary disease**) and numerous epithelioid cells, giant cells and lymphocytes as in tuberculosis. The local nerves are involved in the early stage, and gradually the infection extends into the bigger nerve trunks which are thickened, hard and tender. In tuberculoid leprosy, lepromin test is positive due to intact CMI. Antimycobacterial and autoantibodies are rarely produced.
- **Lepromatous type:** It is the generalized form of the disease and is found in individuals where the host resistance is low. Patient develops numerous nodular skin lesions (lepromata) on face, ear lobes, hands, feet and less commonly on trunk. Skin lesions contain many macrophages, often seen as large foamy cells packed with AFB (Fig. 27.1). In advanced cases, there may be 10^9 *M. leprae*/g of skin (**multibacillary disease**). Cooler parts of the body, such as ear lobes, are particularly infiltrated by bacilli. Blood stream may be invaded, with resulting foci in the liver, spleen, adrenals, testicles and bone marrow and excretion of the organisms in milk. In addition, there is heavy infection of upper respiratory tract, particularly the nasal mucosa, from which the organisms are shed.

  There is slow and symmetric thickening of nerves and anaesthesia. Nodular skin lesions ulcerate due to repeated trauma as a result of loss of sensation. The ulcerated nodules become secondarily infected that leads to distortion and mutilation of extremities. **Lepromatous leprosy is more infectious than other types and has a poor prognosis.** Because of deficient CMI, lepromin test is negative. Humoral antibodies against mycobacterial antigens are produced in high concentrations which play no protective role. **Autoantibodies are also produced.**
- **Borderline or dimorphous type:** Many patients occupy an intermediate position on the spectrum and are classified as **borderline tuberculoid (BT), mid-borderline (BB) and borderline lepromatous (BL)**. The characteristics of these five forms are shown in Table 27.3.

In all types of leprosy, *M. leprae* organisms invade both sensory and motor nerves and destroy nerve fibres. **No other bacterial species has the capacity to enter nerves.** *M. leprae* invades dermal nerves and nerve trunks, but the most vulnerable sites are parts of the body that either tend to remain

Table 27.3. Characteristics of 5 types of leprosy

	TT	BT	BB	BL	LL
1. AFB in the skin	–	+/–	+	++	+++
2. AFB in nasal secretions	–	–	–	+	+++
3. Granuloma formation	+++	++	+	–	–
4. Lepromin reaction	+++	+	+/–	–	–
5. Antibodies to *M. leprae*	+/–	+/–	+	++	+++

cool or are subject to trauma. The organisms are present in Schwann and perineural cells. The nasal bones are also involved in leprosy and their destruction may lead to **collapse of the nose**. The eye is frequently damaged by direct bacillary invasion or corneal infection secondary to paralysis of the eyelids leading to blindness.

Lepromin test

This reaction was first described by Mitsuda in Japan in 1919.

Lepromins

The lepromins used as antigen in lepromin test may be of human origin (lepromin-H) or of armadillo origin (lepromin-A) and are of two types:

1. **Integral lepromin (Mitsuda lepromin):** This was developed by Mitsuda in 1919 by boiling human lepromatous tissue rich in *M. leprae*. Standard Mitsuda lepromin contains 4.0×10^7 *M. leprae*/ml and has a shelf life of 2 years at 4°C. Mitsuda lepromin is increasingly being prepared from armadillo-derived *M. leprae* (lepromin-A).
2. **Bacillary lepromin:** This contains more of bacillary components and less of tissue. An important example of bacillary lepromin is Dharmendra antigen, which is prepared by floating out the bacilli from finely ground lepromatous tissue with chloroform, evaporating it dry and removing the lipids by washing with ether. The antigen is made up in phenol saline for use.

Procedure

The test is carried out by the intradermal injection of 0.1 ml of lepromin. The response to this is biphasic:

1. **Early or Fernandez reaction:** It is characterized by an acute localized area of inflammation with congestion and oedema, more than 10 mm in diameter, appearing usually in 24–48 hours and tending to disappear in 3–4 days. Histologically, it consists of serous exudate with lympho-cytic infiltration.
2. **Late or Mitsuda reaction:** It appears 1–2 weeks after the injection, reaching peak in 4 weeks. The reaction appears in the form of a nodule that may undergo central necrosis and ulceration. It takes several weeks to heal. Histo-logically, there is infiltration with lymphocytes, epithelioid cells and giant cells.

Fernandez reaction is like tuberculin reaction, a delayed type hypersensitivity (DTH). This reaction indicates that the patient has been infected at some time in the past. On the other hand, Mitsuda reaction is not a measure of pre-existing DTH, but is the **manifestation of cell-mediated immunity**, which the lepromin itself has induced. It, thus, discriminates between persons who are capable of responding to *M. leprae* and those who cannot.

Uses of lepromin reaction

1. To classify the lesions of leprosy patients. The reaction is positive in tuberculoid and negative in lepromatous leprosy patients.
2. To assess the prognosis and response to treatment. A positive reaction indicates a good prognosis and a negative one a bad prognosis. Conversion to lepromin positivity during treatment is the evidence of improvement.
3. To assess the resistance of an individual to leprosy.
4. For recruitment of persons to work in leprosy homes. Only lepromin-positive persons are recommended to be appointed.
5. To verify the identity of candidate *M. leprae*. Cultivable AFB, claimed to be *M. leprae*, should give matching results when tested in parallel with standard lepromin.

Laboratory diagnosis

As a routine, smears are made from affected parts of the skin and nasal mucous membrane. Material for smear is, however, sometimes taken from lymph nodes and affected nerves.

- **In lepromatous cases**, bacilli are always found in large numbers and about equally frequently in skin and nose. However, in the lepromatous cases, under chemotherapy, nasal smears become negative earlier than the smears from skin lesions, consequently, in cases under treatment, skin smears are more frequently positive than the nasal smears.
- **In tuberculoid cases**, as a rule, the bacilli are very few and found with great difficulty, or not at all. The characteristic histologic response in biopsy material is helpful in such cases and is essential for accurate classification of the disease within the disease spectrum.

Skin smears

The selection of site for taking smear is of great importance. Places where leprous lesions are most prominent, such as nodules, thick patches and areas of infiltration, should be selected. In case of patches, smears should be made from the thickened margins. In a patient with only diffuse infiltration, about 5–6 different areas of the skin should be sampled, including the skin over the ear lobes, buttocks, forehead, chin and cheeks. The specimen is obtained by **slit and scrape method**.

Thoroughly clean the selected portion of skin with spirit. This is necessary in order to remove any saprophytic acid-fast bacilli that may be present on the skin surface. Hold the skin pinched up and raised between the thumb and index finger of the left hand. This will squeeze out blood from the part and will minimize bleeding when the cut is made. With a small bladed-scalpel an incision, about 5 mm long and 3 mm deep, is made on the pinched skin. If any blood or lymph appears, wipe it away without releasing pressure on the held skin.

The blade of the scalpel is then turned at right angle to the cut (slit) and the bottom and sides of the slit are scraped with the point of the blade, several times in the same direction, so that tissue fluid and pulp (not blood) collects on one side of the blade. This is gently smeared on glass slide.

Nasal scrapings

Smears from the nose are made by scraping a little material from the nasal septum, particularly from inferior turbinate bones, with a small-bladed knife. While examining smears from the nose, great care is needed because of the presence of weakly acid-fast diphtheroids in that site, which may be mistaken for acid-fast bacilli, especially when the smear is not properly decolourized. **Nasal smears are of great importance in deciding whether a leprosy patient is infectious or not.** They are positive in patients of leprosy of LL and BL type but are negative in all cases of BB, BT and TT. Furthermore, they disappear more rapidly from the nose as a result of chemotherapy, than they do from skin lesions.

When smears dry, these are fixed by passing the slide twice or thrice over a flame with the surface carrying the smears uppermost. The smears are then stained by the Ziehl-Neelsen technique using 5%, instead of 20%, sulphuric acid for decolourization. Bacteriological and morphological indices (as already discussed) are also determined.

Skin and nerve biopsy

Skin biopsy is collected from active edge of the patches, and nerve biopsy from thickened nerve for histological confirmation of tuberculoid leprosy when acid-fast bacilli cannot be demonstrated in direct smear. Skin biopsy is useful in the diagnosis and accurate classification of leprosy lesion but nerve biopsy is not required if a skin lesion is present.

Animal inoculation

- Injection of ground tissue from lepromatous nodules and nasal scraping from leprosy patient into the **footpad of mouse** produces typical granuloma at the site of inoculation in 1–6 months.
- **Nine-banded armadillo** is highly susceptible to leprosy. Such an animal, when inoculated with ground tissue from lepromatous nodules and nasal scrapings from leprosy patient, develops generalized infection with extensive multiplication of bacilli and the lesions produced resemble lepromatous leprosy.

The lesions which develop in the mouse and armadillo can be identified by histological examination and Ziehl-Neelsen staining.

Lepromin test or Mitsuda reaction

It is not a diagnostic test but is a guide to the resistance of the patient to *M. leprae* infection.

Serological test

Serodiagnosis of leprosy may be carried out by detection of antiphenolic glycolipid 1 antibodies by latex agglutination, *M. leprae* particle agglutination and ELISA test.

Polymerase chain reaction (PCR)

PCR can be used for the diagnosis at an early stage, before appearance of clinical symptoms. It is effective even in the diagnosis of paucibacillary leprosy, as **the detection limit of PCR is as low as one bacillus**. The PCR assay can be performed on biopsy specimens, skin scrapings and nasal secretions.

28

Spirochaetes

Spirochaetes are thin, helical, motile and flexible bacteria, twisted spirally along the long axis. They possess a varying number of fine fibrils which are attached subterminally at each pole of the cell and extend towards the opposite pole between outer membrane and peptidoglycan layer of the cell wall. Because of their similarity to other bacterial flagella they are known as **endoflagella**. The number of endoflagella per cell end is a morphologic characteristic of each species, in *Treponema*, that are pathogenic for humans, the number is 3 but occasionally 4, in most *Borrelia* it is 15–20 and in *Leptospira* it is one.

The spiral shape and serpentine motility of the spirochaetes depend upon the integrity of these endoflagella. Motility is of three types:

1. Flexion and extension.
2. Corkscrew-like rotatory movement.
3. Translatory motion.

Some are very actively motile while others are sluggish.

Spirochaetes vary in size from 5–500 µm in length.

The spirochaetes of medical importance belong to three genera – *Treponema*, *Borrelia* and *Leptospira*. The differentiating features of these genera are given in Table 28.1.

Table 28.1. Differentiating characters of *Treponema*, *Borrelia* and *Leptospira*

Character	Treponema	Borrelia	Leptospira
1. Size	6–14 × 0.2 µm	8–30 × 0.2–0.5 µm	6–20 × 0.1 µm
2. Spirals	6–12 regular, close spirals at 1 µm intervals, amplitude of the spirals is 1–1.5 µm. The ends of the spirals are pointed	3–10 loose, open spirals at interval of about 3 µm and amplitude of 1–2 µm	Tightly coiled regular spirals with hooked ends. The interval and amplitude of spirals is 0.5 µm each
3. Number of endoflagella	3–4 at each pole	15–20 at each pole	1 at each pole
4. Motility	Actively motile exhibiting flexion and extension, translatory and corkscrew-like rotatory motility and tendency to bend at right angles near its midpoint	Flexion and extension, cork screw-like rotatory and translatory	Rotation around long axis, forward and backward, and bending and flexion.
5. Staining	Do not take up ordinary stains, can be stained with Giemsa and silver impregnation stains	Readily stain by ordinary methods and are Gram-negative	As in *Treponema*
6. Mode of infection	Sexual contact, intimate cutaneous contact, blood transfusion and transplacental	By insects – ticks and lice	Water contaminated with rodent urine
7. Incubation period	10–90 days	2–14 days	7–14 days
8. Pathogenicity	Syphilis, bejel, yaws and pinta	Relapsing fevers, Lyme disease	Weil's disease

TREPONEMA PALLIDUM

Morphology

It is a thin, delicate, long, motile, flexible organism which is twisted spirally round its long axis. It is 6–14 μm long. Its width is 0.13 μm in dried state, but is about 0.2 μm in the wet living state, which is just great enough for resolution with the light microscope. It has 6–12 coils which are remarkably evenly disposed at 1 μm intervals and the amplitude of spirals is 1–1.5 μm. They have tapering ends. It is actively motile exhibiting flexion and extension, translatory and corkscrew-like motility. As the spirochaete moves across the dark-field of the microscope, it often displays a **characteristic tendency to bend at right angles near its midpoint**. These secondary curves appear and disappear but its primary spirals remain unchanged.

Because of its weak refractility and slender thickness, about the limit of resolution by the light microscope, it is best seen in wet living preparation with the **dark-ground microscope**. In dried preparations, it needs to be thickened by **silver impregnation methods (Fontana's method is useful for staining films and Levaditi's for tissue sections)**. It possesses Gram-negative envelope. It cannot be stained by simple aniline dyes or by Gram's method. By prolonged **Giemsa staining** it stains pale pink. By **immunofluorescence method**, treponemes can be detected in tissues and body fluids.

Ultrastructurally, *T. pallidum* possesses usually three but occasionally four endoflagella attached subterminally at each end of the cell and extend towards the opposite pole between outer membrane and peptidoglycan layer of the cell wall. The endoflagella from the two ends are more than half the length of the organism and interdigitate over the central portion of the organism, so that in transverse section there often appear to be three or four of them in section taken from terminal regions and 4–6 in sections from the central portion.

Cultivation

Pathogenic treponemes cannot be cultivated in artificial media and are maintained by subculture in susceptible animals. **Nichol's strain** of *T. pallidum* has been maintained, in rabbit testis, for several decades by serial testicular passage since it was isolated in 1913 from CSF of a patient with neurosyphilis.

Cultivable treponemes such as *T. phagedenis* (**Reiter treponeme**) and *T. refringens* are non-pathogenic. They can be grown under strictly anaerobic conditions in Smith-Noguchi medium or in digest broth enriched with serum.

Pathogenesis

T. pallidum is a **strict parasite** and its life outside the animal body is short. Most cases of syphilis are **contracted during sexual intercourse**. The treponemes are present in the superficial genital lesions and pass from one partner to the other through **intact mucous membranes or through minor skin abrasions**. The disease may also be transmitted **congenitally**, by close contact with mucous membrane lesions as in **kissing** and through **blood transfusions**. Medical personnel are occasionally infected by an **accidental finger prick** with an infected needle.

In venereal syphilis, the treponemes penetrate mucosal surfaces or abraded skin and multiply at the site of entry and after an incubation period of about a month (range 10–90 days), the clinical disease sets in. The clinical manifestations fall into four stages – primary, secondary, latent and tertiary.

1. Primary syphilis

The primary lesion of syphilis is the **chancre** which is painless, relatively avascular, circumscribed, indurated, 1–2 cm in diameter. It ulcerates in the centre. It is known as **hard chancre** to distinguish it from the non-indurated lesion (**soft sore**) caused by *Haemophilus ducreyi*. The primary lesion of syphilis is also known as **Hunterian chancre**, after John Hunter who produced the lesions on himself experimentally. Histologically, it is oedematous and infiltrated predominantly with mononuclear cells.

Most frequently chancre appears on the external genitalia – prepuce, corona of the penis (Fig. 28.1), labia and vaginal wall. It may also occur on the cervix, perianal area, anal canal or on the tongue (Fig. 28.2), and other oral mucous membranes. In some cases it may be on lips, cheeks and nipples (when it is acquired through kissing). *Chancres usually occur singly but in immunocompromised individuals, such as those infected with human immunodeficiency virus, multiple chancres may develop.*

A large number of treponemes are present in the primary lesion and in the serum that exudes from it. In the early days of infection, the spirochaetes invade the regional lymph nodes (inguinal in males and pelvic in females) and lead to **lymphadenitis**. The lymph nodes are swollen, discrete, rubbery and non-tender. From lymph nodes treponemes enter into the blood stream in large numbers. *Chancre heals spontaneously in about 3–6 weeks even without treatment leaving a thin scar.*

2. Secondary syphilis

This sets in 2–6 months after the primary lesion heals during which period the patient is asymptomatic. The secondary lesions are due to widespread multiplication of the treponemes and their dissemination through the blood. Patient develops marked constitutional symptoms, **diffuse erythematous cutaneous lesions**, particularly on the trunk and extremities, mucous patches in the oropharynx and **condylomata** at mucocutaneous junctions. *Lesions of secondary syphilis undergo spontaneous healing in 4–5 years.*

3. Latent syphilis

After the secondary lesions disappear, the disease becomes latent and can be detected only by serological tests. In many

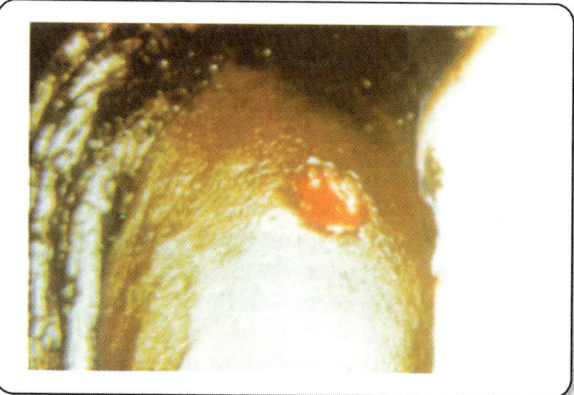

Fig. 28.1. A chancre caused by *Treponema pallidum* on the penis.

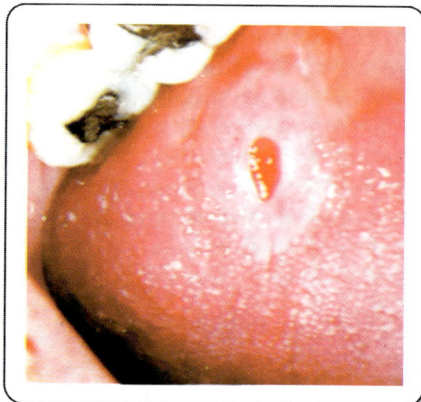

Fig. 28.2. A chancre caused by *Treponema pallidum* on the tongue.

cases, this is followed by natural cure but in others, after several years, manifestations of tertiary syphilis appear.

4. Tertiary syphilis

Decades after the primary infection, patient may develop late or tertiary syphilis. It is a slowly progressive, destructive inflammatory disease that may affect any organ. It may lead to relatively benign ulcerating lesions of the skin, mucous membranes or bones, or **gummata** of the internal organs. More serious are lesions of heart and aorta that may lead to the formation of **aneurysms**, or of the central nervous system, of which **tabes dorsalis** and **general paralysis of the insane** are the most common.

Congenital syphilis

The treponemes can cross the placental barrier. Infection in the foetus usually occurs from primary and secondary infection of the mother.

Laboratory diagnosis (Table 28.2)

The clinical diagnosis of syphilis is confirmed in the laboratory by:

Table 28.2. Methods of laboratory diagnosis of syphilis

A. Demonstration of treponemes in the exudate
1. Dark-ground microscopy
2. Direct fluorescent-antibody staining for *Treponema pallidum* (DFA-Tp)

B. Demonstration of treponemes in tissues
- Immunofluorescence
- Silver impregnation method

C. Demonstration of treponemal antigen in the lesion
- EIA

D. Nucleic acid-based test
- PCR

E. Serological diagnosis of syphilis
1. Nontreponemal tests
   - Wassermann reaction
   - Kahn test
   - VDRL test
   - RPR test
2. Treponemal tests
   - (a) Those using cultivable treponemes
     - RPCF test
   - (b) Those in which pathogenic *T. pallidum* is the antigen employed
     - I. Test using live *T. pallidum*
       - TPI test
     - II. Tests using killed *T. pallidum*
       - TPA test
       - TPIA test
       - FTA, FTA-ABS, IgM FTA-ABS tests
     - III. Tests using *T. pallidum* extract
       - TPHA
       - EIA

A. Demonstration of treponemes in the exudate

1. **Dark-ground microscopy:** To avoid the risk of acquiring infection, it is important to wear gloves and exercise great care in handling the lesions. The surface of the lesion is cleansed carefully with a gauze swab soaked in warm normal saline and the margins are gently scrapped, so that superficial epithelium is abraded. Gentle pressure is applied to the base of the lesion until serum exudes from its surface. If it is blood stained, it should be wiped away and process repeated until a clear fluid is obtained. Wet film is now made on a thin glass slide, covered with a thin coverslip and examined under dark-ground microscope. *T. pallidum* is recognized by its slender structure, regularity of its spirals and slightly pointed ends (Fig. 28.3). It is motile with a to and fro drilling motion and occasional flexion of the body.

2. **Direct fluorescent-antibody staining for T. pallidum (DFA-Tp):** A more definite approach to diagnosis is provided by DFA-Tp. It has the advantage that a smear of the material to be tested is made on a glass slide, fixed in acetone and sent to the laboratory. The smear is then stained with fluorescein-labelled pathogen-specific monoclonal antibody and examined under fluorescence microscope.

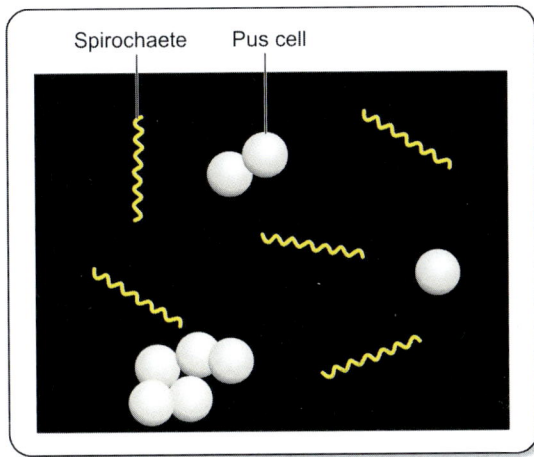

Fig. 28.3. Dark-ground illumination preparation of serous exudate from primary syphilitic chancre.

The treponemes appear distinct, sharply outlined and have an apple-green fluorescence.

B. Demonstration of treponemes in tissues

Treponemes in the tissues can be demonstrated by immuno-fluorescence or silver staining.

C. Demonstration of treponemal antigen in the lesion

T. pallidum antigen in the lesion can be detected by enzyme immunoassay.

D. Nucleic acid-based test

Nucleic acid amplification test (polymerase chain reaction) has been developed for detecting *T. pallidum* in genital lesions, infant blood, and cerebrospinal fluid.

E. Serological diagnosis of syphilis

Depending upon the antigens used, serological tests for syphilis may be divided into the following:

1. **Nontreponemal tests or Standard tests for syphilis (STS)** in which cardiolipin or lipoidal antigen is used.
2. **Treponemal tests** in which treponemes are used as the antigen. These are of two types:
   (a) Those using cultivable treponemes, such as Reiter treponemes (*T. phagedenis*) as the antigen.
   (b) Those in which pathogenic *T. pallidum* is the antigen employed. These tests may further be classified according to whether the treponeme employed is live, killed or extracts of the treponemes.

Nontreponemal tests

Nontreponemal tests that can be employed are Wasser-mann, Kahn, Venereal Diseases Research Laboratory (VDRL) and the rapid plasma reagin (RPR) tests. The antigen used in these tests is an alcoholic extract of beef heart tissue (cardiolipin) to which lecithin and cholesterol are added. Wassermann reaction and Kahn test are complement fixation and tube flocculation tests respectively. Since Wassermann reaction offers no advantage over simple and rapid flocculation tests such as VDRL and RPR, therefore, World Health Organization (1982) recommended that its use should be discontinued. Similarly, Kahn test is rarely done these days.

VDRL test

The test is named after Venereal Disease Research Laboratory, New York, where the test was developed. It is the most widely used simple and rapid test which requires only a small quantity of serum.

VDRL test is performed as a slide test in which inactivated patient serum is mixed with a freshly prepared suspension of cardiolipin-lecithin-cholesterol antigen on a glass slide. The mixture is rotated, usually mechanically, for 4 minutes after which the flocculation (aggregation of antigen-antibody complexes in suspension) can be detected under a low power objective of a microscope.

Method

Preparation of antigen:

1. Pipette 0.4 ml of buffered saline into a 30 ml round bottomed screw cap bottle.
2. Add 0.5 ml of VDRL antigen, with the help of a tuberculin syringe, drop by drop rapidly in 6 seconds while gently rotating the bottle in a circle of 5 cm diameter.
3. Continue rotation of bottle for 10 more seconds.
4. Add 4.1 ml of buffered saline more.
5. Replace the top of the bottle and shake it for 10 seconds.
6. Allow it to stand for 15–30 minutes. The working antigen suspension may be used during the whole working day.

Serum sample: Heat clear serum samples in a water bath at 56°C for 30 minutes. Sera that are excessively haemolyzed, grossly contaminated with bacteria or very turbid are unsatisfactory for testing. Serum samples to be tested more than 4 hours after inactivation should be reheated for 10 minutes.

Qualitative test: It can be carried out on glass slides (7.5 × 5 cm), each with 12 paraffin rings of approximately 15 mm diameter or in a slide with twelve depressions.

1. Pipette 50 μl of inactivated patient serum into the paraffin ring or depression in the glass slide.
2. Pipette 50 μl each of positive and negative control sera into other paraffin rings.
3. Add one drop of working antigen suspension to each of these paraffin rings from a syringe delivering 60 drops in 1 ml.
4. Mix with wooden sticks and rotate slide for 4 minutes with hand on a flat surface in a circular manner in a diameter of about 5 cm or on a mechanical VDRL rotator set at about 180 rpm.

5. Read the test results immediately under a low power objective of a microscope. The antigen particles are seen as small fusiform needles which remain more or less evenly dispersed in case of non-reactive serum. In case of a weak positive test, small clumps of antigen with little or no background clearing and in case of a positive test large clumps of antigen with marked background clearing are obtained. The results of controls should be satisfactory for validity of the results of the tests.

Any specimen giving a weak positive or positive reaction should then be tested quantitatively. It is performed with serial dilutions of patient serum. The highest dilution that can be classified as reactive is reported as the titre.

RPR test

In rapid plasma reagin test, VDRL antigen is adsorbed on finely divided carbon particles and suspended in choline chloride which blocks inhibitory factors in the serum, thus eliminating the need to heat the serum before testing. The antigen is also stabilized with EDTA, allowing it to be used for up to 6 months when stored at 4–10°C. This test is performed by mixing one drop of patient serum or plasma (50 µl) with a drop of this modified antigen (20 µl), on a disposable plastic card (12.5 × 7 cm in size with 10 clearly defined test areas) using a disposable stick. The card is then rocked gently to and fro for 8 minutes and observed under strong source of light. In a positive test, the flocculation of carbon particles (black aggregates) is visible with naked eye. Black aggregates may be deposited at the periphery of the liquid. In a negative test, there is a complete absence of black aggregates with a uniform greyish background. Any specimen giving a positive reaction should then be tested quantitatively using doubling dilutions of serum (1 : 2, 1 : 4, 1 : 8, 1 : 16, 1 : 32, etc.).

Biological false positive (BFP) reactions: Antibodies against cardiolipin may be detected in the absence of *T. pallidum* infection and give what is known as biological false positive (BFP) reaction. In such cases, specific treponemal tests are negative and there is no history of present or past treponemal infection. BFP reactions may occur in 0.3–0.9% of all sera examined and are caused mainly by IgM antibody. These reactions are of two types:

- **Acute or transient BFP reactions** which may develop shortly after an acute febrile infectious disease and will disappear within a few weeks or months after the illness has subsided.
- **Chronic BFP reactions** persist longer than 6 months. These may occur in a wide variety of infectious and noninfectious conditions associated with tissue damage. These include:
  - autoimmune diseases particularly systemic lupus erythematosus,
  - leprosy particularly lepromatous leprosy,
  - malaria,
  - relapsing fever,
  - infectious mononucleosis,
  - hepatitis, and
  - tropical eosinophilia.

Treponemal tests

(a) Those using cultivable treponemes

The antigen used to detect group-specific antibody is derived from *T. phagedenis* (Reiter treponeme). It is protein in nature and the test is known as **Reiter protein complement fixation (RPCF) test**. The principle of this test is the same as that of Wassermann test, but the antigen in RPCF test is extracted from *T. phagedenis*. This is less sensitive than cardiolipin tests in early syphilis but is more sensitive in late or latent syphilis. It is much more specific than cardiolipin tests, but false reactions still occur in a few cases. With the advent of newer treponemal tests such as *Treponema pallidum* haemagglutination assay, RPCF test is rarely done now a days. New ELISA tests based on purified endoflagella of *T. phagedenis* have been developed.

(b) Those in which pathogenic T. pallidum is the antigen employed

A number of specific tests are now available for the definite diagnosis of syphilis. All require live or killed or extracts of *T. pallidum* (Nichol's strain) grown in rabbit testes.

I. Test using live T. pallidum

Treponema pallidum immobilization (TPI) test

This test determines the ability of patient serum to immobilize motile virulent *T. pallidum*. The test serum is incubated anaerobically with a suspension of the treponemes and complement. If antibodies are present, the treponemes will be found to be immobilized, when examined under dark-ground microscope. The test is considered reactive if more than 50% of the treponemes are immobilized, and non-reactive if less than 20% are immobilized. The test is doubtful if 20–50% treponemes are immobilized.

II. Tests using killed T. pallidum

Treponema pallidum agglutination (TPA) test

In this test, a suspension of *T. pallidum*, inactivated by formalin, is mixed with test serum and incubated. The mixture is then examined under dark-ground microscope. In the presence of antibody, treponemes are found to be agglutinated. This test is not very specific and false positive reactions are common.

Treponema pallidum immune adherence (TPIA) test

Suspension of inactivated treponemes is mixed with test serum, complement and fresh heparinised whole blood from a normal individual, and incubated. In the presence of antibodies, the treponemes will be found to adhere to the erythrocytes. In the absence of antibody, immune adherence does not take place. Both TPA and TPIA are not used in diagnostic laboratories, they serve primarily as research tools.

Fluorescent treponemal antibody (FTA) test

It is an indirect immunofluorescence test. Smears of *T. pallidum* are prepared on slides and fixed with acetone. These slides can be stored in the deep freezer for several months. The patient serum is added on the smear and incubated for the antibody to react with the treponemes. The excess serum is then washed off and the antibodies that bind to the fixed organisms are detected by treating the smear with fluorescein-labelled antihuman immunoglobulin. After incubation and washing off the unfixed conjugate, slide is examined under fluorescence microscope. In a positive test, treponemes fluoresce.

Originally, patient serum was used in a dilution of 1 in 5. At this dilution, the test has high sensitivity and poor specificity. Therefore, the dilution of the serum was raised to 1 in 200. In this test, called **FTA-200**, the specificity was improved but sensitivity was decreased. Therefore, this test was further modified to **fluorescent treponemal antibody absorption (FTA-ABS) test**. Here the patient serum is first absorbed with an extract of non-pathogenic *T. phagedenis* (Reiter treponemes) to remove group-reactive antibody. FTA-ABS test has high specificity and sensitivity. It is almost as specific as the more complicated TPI test. Therefore, it is the most widely used serologic test for detection of specific treponemal antibodies. **VDRL and FTA-ABS tests can also be performed on cerebrospinal fluid.** Antibodies do not reach from the blood stream but are probably formed in the CNS in response to treponemal infection.

FTA-ABS test becomes reactive around 3rd week of infection and is positive in 80%, 100% and 95% of primary, secondary and late syphilis respectively. Unlike VDRL test, its reactivity persists after successful therapy. However, occasionally the test may become non-reactive if treatment is given early in the disease. The specificity of this test ranges from 92–99%. **False positive reactions have been observed in patients with rheumatoid arthritis, lupus erythematosus, cirrhosis and hypergammaglobulinaemia and in 1% of normal persons.**

Another modification of this test, the **IgM FTA-ABS test, can detect IgM antibodies in congenital syphilis**, thus distinguishing it from seropositivity due to passively transferred maternal antibodies which are IgG in nature. In addition, in the former repeated tests will show an increase in titre, whereas in the latter titre will fall.

III. Tests using *T. pallidum* extract

Treponema pallidum haemagglutination test (TPHA)

In this test, *T. pallidum* antigen is adsorbed onto the surface of red blood cells. When these red blood cells are mixed with patient serum, specific antibody, if present, causes haemagglutination. As in FTA-ABS test patient serum is pre-absorbed with an extract of Reiter treponemes to remove group-reactive antibody. TPHA reactivity may be detectable around the 4th week of infection. It is less sensitive than FTA-ABS in primary syphilis being positive in 65% of cases, but both give similar results for secondary and late syphilis. After treatment, TPHA invariably remains positive for life. **This test can also be used to detect localised production of anti-treponemal antibodies in cerebrospinal fluid, a marker of neurosyphilis.**

TPHA is very simple to perform, therefore, it was the first of the specific tests suitable for routine screening. Because of greater convenience and lower cost, TPHA may be performed in microtitre plates. This is referred to as **microtitre haemagglutination-T. pallidum (MHA-TP) test**. Both these terms are used synonymously. Combination of a cardiolipin antigen test and TPHA is the most widely used screening procedure.

Enzyme immunoassay (EIA)

Ultrasonicate of *T. pallidum* antigen is coated on tubes or ferrous metal beads as a solid-phase carrier for antigen. Antibody in the patient serum is detected by enzyme immunoassay. Sensitivity and specificity of this test has been reported to be 90% and 98% respectively.

BORRELIA

Borreliae are large, motile, refractile spirochaetes with 3–10 irregular, wide and open coils. Borreliae of medical importance are:

- *B. recurrentis* causing relapsing fever,
- *B. vincentii* causing Vincent's angina, and
- *B. burgdorferi* causing Lyme disease.

RELAPSING FEVER

Relapsing fever is characterized by the occurrence of one or more relapses after the subsidence of primary febrile paroxysm. It occurs worldwide as epidemic or louse-borne relapsing fever, and endemic or tick-borne relapsing fever. The former is caused by *B. recurrentis* and the latter by several *Borrelia* species, including, *B. duttoni*, *B. hermsii*, *B. parkeri* and *B. turicatae*.

Morphology

Various *Borrelia* species causing relapsing fever are morphologically indistinguishable, but exhibit some antigenic differences. They are 8–20 µm long and 0.2–0.5 µm wide. They possess 15–20 endoflagella per cell end and 3–10 loose, uneven spiral coils. Spirals are coarser and more irregular than those of the treponemes or leptospires and can usually be seen with light microscopy in preparations stained with aniline dyes such as Wright or Giemsa stains. The spirochaetes may be demonstrated in the peripheral blood by direct stain. In fresh blood the organisms are actively motile, they move in forward and backward waves and in a corkscrew-like motion.

Cultural characteristics

Borrelia are microaerophilic. Optimum temperature for growth is 28–30°C. These may be grown in fluid media containing blood, serum or tissue, and on chorioallantoic membrane of chick embryo.

Pathogenesis

Relapsing fever is transmitted by infected vectors – body louse (*Pediculus corporis*) in case of *B. recurrentis*, and tick (*Ornithodoros*) in case of *B. duttoni* and others. After an infected blood meal, spirochaetes may be demonstrated in the stomach of the louse for 24 hours. Thereafter, they grow in the haemolymph of the louse but do not invade tissues. They are not found in the salivary glands, the gut or the genital organs. As a result, the excrement of the louse is non-infectious and the **bacterium is not transferred transovarially to the progeny**. However, once the louse is infected, it remains so for the rest of its life (usually about 3 weeks).

The disease is transmitted to man not by the bite of the louse, but by contamination of the wounds made by the bite itself or by scratching, with body fluids of the louse which is crushed by scratching releasing spirochaetes. The latter then enter into the tissues through damaged or intact skin or mucous membranes.

Spirochaetes causing tick-borne relapsing fever invade all the tissues of the tick, including the salivary glands, genitalia and excretory system. Infection is transmitted to man through the bite of the ticks or through their excrements. **Transovarial transmission** to the tick progeny maintains the spirochaete in the tick population.

In both forms of relapsing fever, after an incubation period of 2–14 days, the disease sets in abruptly with high fever (up to 40°C), rigors, headache, myalgia, arthralgia, photophobia and sometimes nausea and vomiting. The spleen and liver are enlarged and tender. Some patients develop jaundice, bronchitis and skin rash. During acute phase, there may be up to 10^5 spirochaetes per ml of blood. The primary illness subsides in 3–9 days. After an afebrile period of 11–15 days during which borreliae are not demonstrable in blood, a **relapse** follows which is less severe and shorter than the primary attack. The borreliae reappear in blood during the relapse of fever. The disease ultimately subsides after 3–4 relapses. In general, tick-borne relapsing fever has shorter febrile and afebrile periods than louse-borne infection.

Each episode of spirochaetaemia is terminated as a result of development of specific antibodies. The borreliae readily undergo **antigenic variation**, particularly in outer membrane protein composition, *in vivo*, and this is believed to be the reason for the occurrence of relapses in the disease. As relapses continue, the borreliae tend to revert back to the antigenic types that caused the original spirochaetaemia, thus clearing the infection.

Laboratory diagnosis

Wet preparation

Blood is collected during pyrexial period and a drop of it is examined as a wet film under the dark-ground or phase-contrast microscope. Borreliae can be detected by their active movements.

Staining

Thick or thin blood smears may be stained with Giemsa or Leishman stain and examined for *Borrelia*.

Animal inoculation

If direct microscopy is negative, 1–2 ml of fresh whole blood or of clot ground up in saline, is injected intraperitoneally into a newborn mouse or rat. The borreliae multiply in the animal and appear in large numbers in peripheral blood within two days. Smears are prepared from blood collected from the tail vein and examined daily for two weeks. The degree of spirochaetaemia in adult animals is much less and may not be detected for several days.

Serology

Because of the occurrence of frequent antigenic variation, serological diagnosis of relapsing fever is unreliable. Serological tests for syphilis are positive in 5–10% of cases of relapsing fever.

BORRELIA VINCENTII

Borrelia vincentii is 7–18 μm long and 0.2–0.6 μm wide, with 3–8 loose, open coils of variable size. It is actively motile. It is easily stained with dilute carbol fuchsin, methyl violet, Giemsa and Leishman stains and is Gram-negative. It is an obligate anaerobe and can be cultured in sealed tubes containing digest broth enriched with ascitic fluid. *B. vincentii* is a normal commensal of mouth but may, under predisposing conditions such as malnutrition or viral infections, give rise to **ulcerative gingivostomatitis** or **oropharyngitis (Vincent's angina)**.

In Vincent's angina, *B. vincentii* is often associated with 'fusiform bacillus' known as *Leptotrichia buccalis* (*Fusobacterium fusiforme*). This symbiotic infection is known as **fusospirochaetosis**. Vincent's angina is characterized by ulcerative lesions of mouth or tonsillar area.

For the diagnosis, smears are made from the ulcerative lesions and are stained with dilute carbol fuchsin. A clinical diagnosis of Vincent's angina is confirmed when a large number of spirochaetes and fusiform bacilli are seen together with many pus cells.

BORRELIA BURGDORFERI

Morphology

It measures 4–30 μm in length and 0.2 μm in diameter. It is flexible, helical and Gram-negative.

Culture

It is a microaerophilic spirochaete. It can be grown on BSK medium which contains *N*-acetyl glucosamine, yeast extract, amino acids, vitamins, nucleotides and serum. Optimum temperature for growth is 34–37°C.

Pathogenesis

B. burgdorferi causes **Lyme disease**. Wild and domestic animals, including mice and other rodents, deer, sheep, cattle, horses and dogs are the natural hosts of *B. burgdorferi*. It is transmitted to man by ixodid ticks that become infected whilst feeding on infected animals. The organisms grow in the midgut of the tick and transmission to man occurs by regurgitation of the gut contents during the blood meal.

Patient develops a small red macule or papule at the site of bite. Three to 22 days later, redness spreads centrifugally surrounded by an induration about 2 cm wide. It is known as **erythema chronicum migrans (ECM)**. The centre of the lesion may become vesicular or necrotic. Commonly affected sites are the thigh, groin and axilla. The organism also spreads to a variety of other organs. In about one-half of the patients, multiple skin lesions develop several days after the appearance of the initial lesion. ECM is frequently accompanied with headache, fever, stiff neck, malaise and lymphadenopathy. Weeks to months later, some patients develop meningo-encephalitis, myocarditis or migratory musculoskeletal pain and intermittent arthritis.

Laboratory diagnosis

The diagnosis of Lyme disease is made mainly on clinical grounds. The presence of an ECM lesion at the site of vector bite, which was followed by an expanding bright red rash would be suggestive of a positive diagnosis. However, a definitive diagnosis can be made by the isolation and identification of *B. burgdorferi* from skin lesions or blood of the infected patient. However, the culture is too slow and gives too low a yield of positive results for routine use. Microscopic detection of borreliae by dark-ground microscopy, phase-contrast microscopy, silver staining and immunofluorescence methods also lacks sensitivity. DNA probes have been developed for a gene encoding a specific outer membrane protein, however, their efficiency in detecting this in tissue samples is yet to be established.

For the **serological diagnosis**, ELISA, indirect immuno-fluorescence and haemagglutination tests are commonly used.

LEPTOSPIRA INTERROGANS

Morphology

L. interrogans are spiral bacteria, 6–20 µm long and 0.1 µm in diameter. They are actively motile and possess tightly coiled spirals and hooked ends. Because of their narrow diameter, leptospires are best observed by dark-ground, phase-contrast and electron microscopy. Leptospires rotate rapidly along their long axes and also glide across the field with either end foremost. They occasionally form secondary coils and then straighten again. They stain poorly with aniline dyes but can be demonstrated by fluorescent antibody technique, and silver impregnation techniques of Levaditi and Fontana. They possess Gram-negative cell envelope.

Cultural characteristics

L. interrogans are obligate aerobes. Optimum pH and temperature for their growth are 7.2 and 28–32°C respectively. They do not grow at 13°C and for primary isolation from infected tissues, incubation at 37°C may be advantageous. *L. interrogans* can be grown in artificial media supplemented with sterile rabbit serum or bovine serum albumin with Tween 80. A semi-solid medium prepared by adding 0.2–0.5% agar to liquid medium may be used for isolation of *L. interrogans* from animal tissues. Leptospires may be grown on the chorioallantoic membrane of chick embryo. They may be demonstrated in the blood of allantoic vessels 4–5 days after inoculation.

Pathogenesis

L. interrogans causes leptospirosis. It is primarily a parasite of vertebrates other than humans, such as rodents, dogs, pigs and cattle. Leptospires localize in the kidneys, colonizing the convoluted tubules and are continuously shed in the urine of some infected animals, thereby contaminating the environment.

Man acquires infection mainly through contact with water, soil or vegetation contaminated with animal urine. The pathogenic leptospires enter the body through cuts or abrasions of the skin. They may also enter through the mucous membranes of the nose, mouth or eyes. The organisms enter the blood and invade various tissues and organs, particularly the kidney, liver, meninges and conjunctiva.

After an incubation period of 1–2 weeks, the patient develops muscular pain, headache, vomiting, photophobia, fever and chills. Jaundice occurs in about 10–20% of cases by second or third day. Purpuric haemorrhages sometimes occur on the skin and mucosa. Albuminuria is a constant feature. Leptospires can be seen in the blood during acute phase of the disease, but can seldom be demonstrated after 8–10 days. However, they persist in internal organs, particularly in the kidneys, so that they may be demonstrated in the urine in the later stages of the disease.

L. interrogans serovar *icterohaemorrhagiae* produces a more severe illness. It is known as **Weil's disease** (infectious jaundice). It has a fatality rate of 25% due to renal failure and hepatic injury. Other serovars, e.g., *australis*, *bataviae* and *pyrogenes* may also cause spirochaetal jaundice.

Laboratory diagnosis

I. Demonstration of leptospires

Leptospires may be demonstrated in (1) the blood, and (2) the urine.

1. **Demonstration of leptospires in the blood:**
   - Leptospires can be demonstrated in the blood, by dark-ground microscopy, especially after differential centrifugation of blood. As leptospires disappear from blood after 8 days, therefore, blood examination is useful only in the early stages of the disease.
   - Inoculate a number of bijou bottles containing 3 ml of modified Korthof's medium with varying amounts of blood ranging from 1–4 drops. Incubate at 28–32°C and examine by dark-ground microscopy every 3 days up to 6 weeks before discarding it as negative. The blood from the patient is also inoculated intraperitoneally into young guinea-pigs, followed some days later by culture of the animal blood obtained by cardiac puncture.

2. **Demonstration of leptospires in the urine:** Leptospires may be present in the urine in the second week of the disease and intermittently thereafter for 4–6 weeks.
   - Centrifuged deposit of fresh urine may be examined by dark-ground microscopy and by culture on Fletcher's semi-solid medium containing neomycin sulphate. Because leptospires are very sensitive to acid urine, therefore, the urine should be examined immediately after voiding.
   - For culture of urine by animal inoculation, 2 ml of fresh urine is inoculated intraperitoneally into young guinea-pigs, followed some days later by culture of the animal blood. The identification of serovar of the isolate is carried out by agglutination and agglutination absorption technique.

II. Serological diagnosis

Antibodies appear in the serum towards the end of the first week of the disease, they continue to rise for several weeks and then begin to decline. Serological tests fall into two categories:

1. Genus-specific tests.
2. Serogroup and serovar-specific tests.

1. **Genus-specific tests:** These tests detect leptospiral infection without indicating the exact infecting serovar. The antigens for these tests are prepared from nonpathogenic *L. biflexa* Patoc 1 strain. These tests include complement fixation test, sensitized erythrocyte lysis and haemagglutination test, and enzyme-linked immunosorbent assay (ELISA) which is capable of detecting IgM and IgG leptospiral antibodies.

2. **Serogroup and serovar-specific tests:** These tests identify the infecting serovar by demonstrating specific antibodies. Macroscopic and microscopic agglutination tests have been widely used.
   - **Macroscopic agglutination test:** In this test, commercially available, formalin-killed suspensions of a number of reference strains are tested for macroscopic agglutination with serial dilutions of the test serum.
   - **Microscopic agglutination test:** In this test, formalinized or live suspensions of well grown cultures are used and the results are read by low-power dark-ground microscopy.

Bacteroides, Propionibacterium and Fusobacterium

Bacteroides

Bacteroides occur as commensals in the mouth, gastro-intestinal and female genital tracts. This genus comprises the most common anaerobes isolated from clinical specimens. They are non-sporing, non-motile, Gram-negative bacilli. They are very pleomorphic, appearing as slender rods, branching forms or coccobacilli. They occur singly, in pairs or in short chains. They grow readily in media such as brain heart infusion agar in an anaerobic atmosphere containing 10% CO_2. They possess capsular polysaccharide which appears to be virulence factor. The capsule confers resistance to phagocytosis and intracellular killing.

They cause peritonitis following bowel injury, pelvic inflammatory disease, abdominal and brain abscesses, and empyema. Pus is often foul smelling. *B. fragilis* is the most frequent of the non-sporing anaerobes isolated from clinical specimens. *B. melaninogenica* forms black-pigmented or brown colonies on blood-containing media. The pigment is an intracellular or cell-associated derivative of haemoglobulin (haemin). It has been isolated from lung or liver abscesses, mastoiditis, and lesions of intestine, mouth and gums.

Propionibacterium

Propionibacteria are pleomorphic, Gram-positive, coryneform rods, non-acid-fast, non-motile and are often arranged in short chains or clumps. They are commonly found on the skin, conjunctiva, external ear, and in the oropharynx and female genital tract. They are aerotolerant, and growth may occasionally be obtained aerobically. Two most commonly isolated species are *Propionibacterium acnes* and *P. propionicum*. *P. acnes* is responsible for two types of infections – (1) **acne vulgaris** in teenagers and young adults, and (2) **opportunistic infections** in patients with prosthetic devices (e.g., artificial heart valves or joints) or intravascular lines (e.g., catheters, cerebrospinal fluid shunts).

Fusobacterium

Fusobacteria are Gram-negative, **strict anaerobic rods** of varied size and morphology. Some species of *Fusobacterium* produce long slender Gram-negative rods that are wide at the centre and taper towards the ends (fusiform), but others produce coccobacilli to very long and filamentous cells. They are usually non-motile and growth is often improved by 5–10% CO_2. They can be isolated on blood agar plates containing neomycin and vancomycin. After 48 hours incubation at 37°C, the colonies are striate or granular with irregular or crenated edge and a raised centre.

F. nucleatum is the most studied species. It may cause infections of head and neck region including dental and periodontal infections and cerebral abscess. *F. necrophorum* is an important animal pathogen. It may, however, sometimes cause infections in man similar to those caused by *F. nucleatum*.

Escherichia, Klebsiella, Enterobacter, Serratia, Proteus and Morganella

ESCHERICHIA COLI

Morphology

It is a Gram-negative, non-sporing bacillus measuring 1–3 µm × 0.4–0.7 µm in size. Most (about 80%) strains are motile by peritrichous flagella.

Cultural characteristics

It is an aerobe and a facultative anaerobe. Optimum temperature for its growth is 37°C (range 10–40°C). It can grow on ordinary media like **nutrient agar** forming large (2–3 mm in diameter), circular, low convex, colourless, opaque or partially translucent colonies after 18 hours incubation at 37°C. Since most strains ferment lactose rapidly the colonies on **MacConkey agar** medium are red or pink in colour (Fig. 30.1).

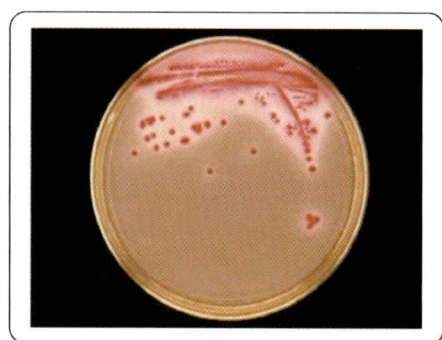

Fig. 30.1. Growth of *Escherichia coli* on MacConkey agar showing lactose fermenting colonies.

On **blood agar**, colonies of some strains of *E. coli* (especially those isolated from pathologic conditions) are surrounded by a complete zone of haemolysis.

Biochemical reactions

Four biochemical tests widely used in the classification of enterobacteria are indole, MR, VP and citrate utilisation tests, generally, referred to by the mnemonic IMViC. *E. coli* is indole and MR positive, & VP and citrate utilisation negative (IMViC++––).

Antigenic structure

E. coli possesses 4 types of antigens:
1. H (flageller) antigens
2. O (somatic) antigens
3. K (capsular) antigens
4. F (fimbrial) antigens.

1. **H antigens:** So far **75 H antigens** have been recognized. These are thermolabile.
2. **O antigens:** These are heat-stable, lipopolysaccharide antigens of cell wall. **One hundred and seventy three different O antigens** have been described which are designated 1, 2, 3, 4, etc.
3. **K antigens:** This term was first used collectively for the surface or capsular antigens that cause O inagglutinability. In the past, these antigens were divided into 3 classes (L, A and B) on the basis of (1) effect of heat on the agglutinability, (2) antigenicity, and (3) antibody-binding power of bacterial strains carrying them.
4. **F antigens:** These are thermolabile proteins and heating the organisms at 100°C detaches their fimbriae.

Toxins

Some strains of *E. coli* produce enterotoxins, Verocytotoxin and haemolysin.

1. Enterotoxins

Enterotoxigenic strains of *E. coli* (ETEC) produce one or both of two different toxins, a heat-labile toxin (LT) and a heat-stable toxin (ST).

2. Verocytotoxin

E. coli O157:H7 produces two cytotoxins – Verocytotoxin 1 (VT1) and Verocytotoxin 2 (VT2). These can be detected by their cytotoxic effect on Vero and HeLa cells.

3. Haemolysin

Many strains of *E. coli* produce a haemolysin which can bring about lysis of RBCs of some species. A larger proportion of strains of *E. coli* recovered from extra-intestinal lesions of man are haemolytic than are those isolated from human faeces.

Pathogenesis

E. coli forms a part of normal intestinal flora of man and animals. It can cause four main types of clinical syndromes:

1. Urinary tract infection.
2. Diarrhoea and dysentery.
3. Pyogenic infections.
4. Septicaemia.

1. Urinary tract infection

E. coli is the commonest organism causing urinary tract infection (UTI). Most frequently encountered O serotypes of *E. coli* in UTI include O1, O2, O4, O6, O7, O18 and O75. These are also known as nephritogenic strains.

2. Diarrhoea and dysentery

E. coli causing diarrhoeal diseases are divisible into six groups. They produce diarrhoea with different pathogenic mechanisms.

- ***Enteropathogenic E. coli (EPEC):*** *It is second most common cause of infantile diarrhoea after rotavirus.* It causes prolonged watery diarrhoea in babies < 1 year in developing countries. Common serogroups of EPEC are O26, O55, O86, O111, O114, O119, O125, O126, O127, O128 and O142.
- ***Enterotoxigenic E. coli (ETEC):*** These strains are associated with diarrhoea in infants and adults in tropical and subtropical climates, especially in developing countries, where it is one of the major causes of infantile bacterial diarrhoea. Common serogroups of ETEC are O6, O8, O15, O25, O27, O63, O78, O115, O148, O153, O159 and O167.
- ***Enteroinvasive E. coli (EIEC):*** These strains invade large bowel, similar to shigellosis. It causes watery diarrhoea with excess of leucocytes, fever and abdominal pain. About 10% patients progress to dysentery. Common serogroups of EIEC are O28, O112, O124, O136, O143, O144, O152 and O164.
- ***Verocytotoxigenic E. coli (VTEC):*** These strains cause **haemorrhagic colitis (HC)** and **haemolytic uraemic syndrome (HUS)**.
- ***Enteroaggregative E. coli (EAEC):*** Enteroaggregative *E. coli* cause acute and chronic diarrhoea in developing countries by adhering to the mucosal surface of the intestine. These strains are found to adhere to HEp-2 cells, packed in an aggregative pattern on the cells and in between the cells.
- ***Diffusely adherent E. coli (DAEC):*** These strains adhere to epithelial cells in a diffuse pattern. Majority of the patients with DAEC develop watery diarrhoea without blood or faecal leucocytes.

Laboratory diagnosis

Urinary tract infection

Collection of specimen

Normal urine is sterile, but during voiding, may become contaminated with genital commensals. Therefore, **clean-voided midstream sample** of urine is employed for culture. The normal flora of anterior urethra must be adequately flushed out by passing some urine before the specimen is obtained.

Microscopy

Microscopic examination of urine is done to detect the presence of increased number of polymorphs (pyuria) which is an indication of UTI. The deposit of the centrifuged urine can be examined under microscope to find out the presence of pus cells, red blood cells and bacteria in it. Presence of more than 3 pus cells per high power field is suggestive of infection. Red blood cells indicate damage to urinary tract hence increased susceptibility to infection.

Culture

Measured quantity of urine (0.001 ml or 1/1000 ml) with the help of standardized loop of nichrome or platinum wire is inoculated on blood agar and MacConkey media and incubated overnight at 37°C. The number of colonies is counted and multiplied by 1000 to get the bacterial count per ml. For example, growth of 100 colonies indicates the presence of 10^5 bacteria/ml of urine (100 × 1000). On the basis of this result, it can be reported whether the patient has significant bacteriuria or not. The identification of the isolate is carried out by cultural characteristics and biochemical reactions.

Diarrhoea and dysentery

Faeces or rectal swab is inoculated on MacConkey agar. For detection of EPEC, *E. coli* colonies are emulsified in saline on a slide and tested by agglutination with polyvalent and monovalent O antisera against enteropathogenic serogroups.

EIEC can be detected by **Sereny test**, in which the organism is instilled into the conjunctival sac of guinea-pig. The animal is examined after 72 hours for the production of **keratoconjunctivitis**.

Pyogenic infections

For the diagnosis of pyogenic infections caused by *E. coli* pus, wound swab, CSF, etc. are inoculated on MacConkey agar and blood agar followed by incubation at 37°C for 24 hours. The isolate is identified by its morphological and biochemical characters.

Septicaemia

Diagnosis of septicaemia caused by *E. coli* depends on the isolation of the organism by blood culture. Five to 10 ml of blood is inoculated into 50–100 ml glucose broth. It is incubated at 37°C for up to 7 days. After overnight incubation, subculture is made on MacConkey agar and blood agar, and processed as above. If no growth is obtained from first subculture, then subcultures should be repeated every other day up to 7 days.

KLEBSIELLA

Morphology

Members of the genus *Klebsiella* are Gram-negative, non-sporing, non-motile bacilli, 1–2 μm long and 0.5–0.8 μm wide with parallel or bulging sides and slightly pointed or rounded ends. They occur either in end to end pairs (diplobacilli, like pneumococci) or are arranged singly.

Freshly isolated strains possess a well-defined polysaccharide capsule. It is produced in greater amounts in media rich in carbohydrates. It can be demonstrated by India ink preparation, Quellung reaction and even by Gram staining. In the Gram-stained smear, capsule appears as an empty halo around the bacterium. Some extracellular polysaccharide is also secreted from the bacteria as loose soluble slime, accumulation of which gives mucoid appearance to the colonies. Non-capsulated and non-slime-forming mutants appear from time to time. They form small and non-mucoid colonies.

The genus *Klebsiella* consists of several species, including *K. pneumoniae* subspecies *pneumoniae*, *K. pneumoniae* subspecies *ozaenae*, *K. pneumoniae* subspecies *rhinoscleromatis*, and *K. oxytoca*. Another species, *K. granulomatis*, has been included in the genus *Klebsiella*. It was previously known as *Calymmatobacterium granulomatis*. It causes donovanosis.

Cultural characteristics

Klebsiellae grow well on ordinary media in a temperature range of 12–43°C with optimum growth at 37°C. On MacConkey agar, the colonies typically appear large, mucoid and red. However, some strains are not mucoid.

Biochemical reactions

Biochemical reactions of different subspecies of *K. pneumoniae* and *K. oxytoca* are given in Table 30.1.

Antigenic structure

Somatic (O) antigen

Klebsiellae possess five O antigens (O1–O5). O1, O3, O4 and O5 are identical with or related to *E. coli* O antigens 19b, 9, 20 and 8 respectively. In capsulated strains, O antigens are masked by K antigens and because the latter are heat-stable at 100°C for 2.5 hours, therefore, O antigens are identifiable only in non-capsulated mutants.

Capsular (K) antigen

On the basis of capsular (K) antigens, the klebsiellae have been differentiated into 80 (1–80) serotypes, which is usually done by the microscopic demonstration of capsule swelling in wet films with capsular antiserum. Capsular type 2 is immunologically similar to type 2 pneumococcus. Human respiratory tract infection is mostly caused by capsular types 1–6.

Methods of typing

As mentioned above, klebsiellae can be typed by serotyping. Other typing methods such as phage typing, biotyping, bacteriocin (klebocin or pneumocin) typing and resistotyping have also been tried. Bacteriocin (klebocin) production in *Klebsiella* has been found to be determined by conjugative (transmissible) plasmids (Arora and Chugh, 1982).

Pathogenicity

Klebsiellae are widely distributed in nature and in the gastro-intestinal tracts of humans and animals. They are found in

Table 30.1. Differentiation of species and subspecies of *Klebsiella*

Property	K. pneumoniae subspecies				K. oxytoca
	aerogenes	*ozaenae*	*pneumoniae*	*rhinoscleromatis*	
Indole	–	–	–	–	+
MR	–	+	+	+	v
VP	+	–	–	–	v
Citrate	+	v	+	–	+
Urease	+	–	+	–	+
Gelatin liquefaction	–	–	–	–	v
Lactose (acid)	+	+	+	–	+
ONPG	+	+	+	–	+
Lysine decarboxylase	+	v	+	–	+
Ornithine decarboxylase	–	–	–	–	–
Growth in KCN medium	+	+	–	+	+

v, variable.

the oropharynx of 1–6% of normal healthy individuals, however, a prevalence as high as 20% may be seen in hospitalized patients. This colonization may prove to be the source of lung infections such as severe bronchopneumonia, sometimes with chronic destructive lesions, pleuritis and multiple abscess formation in the lungs (**Friedlander's pneumonia**). Many of these patients may develop septicaemia with high mortality.

But klebsiellae, in general, are more frequently involved in healthcare-associated (nosocomial) urinary tract infections, wound and burn infections and as secondary invaders in other respiratory infections. In fact, they are the most frequently encountered Gram-negative pathogens causing nosocomial infections of the lower respiratory tract and are second only to *E. coli* as a cause of primary bacteraemia by Gram-negative organisms. They may also cause meningitis and diarrhoea.

K. pneumoniae subsp. *ozaenae* has been associated with atrophic rhinitis, a condition known as **ozaena**, and purulent infection of nasal mucous membrane. *K. pneumoniae* subsp. *rhinoscleromatis* causes a granulomatous disease called **rhinoscleroma**. It is a chronic upper respiratory tract disease. The lesions occur in the nose, larynx, throat and to a lesser extent, in the trachea and consist of granulomatous infiltrations of the submucosa.

ENTEROBACTER

Enterobacter belongs to the tribe Klebsielleae. It can be differentiated from *Klebsiella* because it is motile and ornithine positive. *Enterobacter* is less often and less heavily capsulated than *Klebsiella*. Therefore, the colonies of *Enterobacter* are less mucoid. Genus *Enterobacter* has 12 species of which *E. aerogenes* and *E. cloacae* are most commonly encountered in clinical specimens. Some strains of *E. cloacae* are non-motile.

Pathogenicity

E. aerogenes and *E. cloacae* are widely distributed in water, sewage, soil and on vegetables. They are occasionally found in faeces and the respiratory tract of man. They are also associated with a variety of opportunistic infections involving the urinary tract, respiratory tract and cutaneous wounds. They may occasionally cause meningitis and septicaemia. In recent years, infection of hospital patients with *E. aerogenes* and *E. cloacae* has been reported more frequently, but *Enterobacter* species are a much less important cause of hospital infection than *Klebsiella* species. Aminoglycosides are often effective in the treatment of *E. aerogenes* and *E. cloacae* infections.

SERRATIA

These are small (0.7–1.5 × 0.7 μm), motile, Gram-negative coccobacilli. Several species of *Serratia* have been described. *S. marcescens* is the most important member of this genus.

After 24–48 hours incubation, colonies of *S. marcescens*, on nutrient agar, are usually homogeneous and then may develop a convex, pigmented (red) and relatively opaque centre and colourless, transparent periphery with crenated edge. The red pigment, **prodigiosin**, is insoluble in water and does not diffuse away from the colonies. Therefore, the colonies are red or pink. The pigment is soluble in absolute alcohol, and organic solvents. Many strains grow best at 30–37°C but pigmentation may be poor at such temperatures, whereas, at lower temperatures, e.g., 15–20°C, growth is poorer and pigment formation is abundant. The pigment is formed only in cultures grown aerobically and non-pigmented variant strains may originate by mutation in laboratory cultures. *Serratia* species fail to ferment lactose, therefore, unless pigment is produced, they form pale colonies on MacConkey agar.

Pathogenicity

Serratia is a saprophyte found in water, soil and food. However, it can lead to serious nosocomial infections particularly in the newborn, the debilitated or the patient receiving immunosuppressive drugs. These include infections of wound, urinary and respiratory tracts, meningitis, endocarditis, septicaemia and endotoxic shock.

Serratia is commonly resistant to cephalosporins. Resistance to ampicillin and gentamicin varies from strain to strain. In hospital strains, multiple drug resistance is common.

PROTEUS

Genus *Proteus* has four species – *P. mirabilis*, *P. vulgaris*, *P. myxofaciens* and *P. penneri*.

Morphology

They are Gram-negative coccobacilli, 1–3 μm long and 0.6 μm wide. In young cultures, most of them are long (up to 80 μm) curved and filamentous. They may be arranged singly, in pairs or in short chains. They are actively motile by peritrichous flagella.

Cultural characteristics

They can grow on ordinary media like nutrient agar and culture emits characteristic putrefactive (fishy or seminal) odour. *P. mirabilis* and *P. vulgaris* possess the **ability to swarm** (spread) on solid media. A group of cells at the edge of a developing microcolony migrate to an uninoculated area of the medium. Swarming growth on a plate may eventually appear either as a uniform film of growth extending over the whole plate (**continuous swarming**) or as a series of concentric circles of growth around the point of inoculation (**discontinuous swarming**). Swarming of *Proteus* appears to be due to vigorous motility of the organism, although, the exact cause is not yet established. Swarming can be inhibited by increasing the concentration of agar in the medium from 1–2% to 6%.

On **MacConkey agar** they form smooth, pale or colourless (NLF) colonies and do not swarm on this medium. In liquid medium (peptone water), *Proteus* produces uniform turbidity with a slight powdery deposit and an ammonical odour.

Biochemical reactions

All species of *Proteus* produce acid from glucose. Lactose is not fermented. Other biochemical characters of four species of *Proteus* are given in Table 30.2.

Pathogenicity

P. mirabilis is the most important species (70–90%) recovered from humans, particularly as a causative agent of urinary tract and wound infections. **After *Escherichia coli*, *P. mirabilis* is the most frequently associated bacterium with urinary tract infection (UTI).**

Occasionally, *Proteus* may cause wound infection, bed sores, osteomyelitis and in neonates it may cause infection of the umbilical stump which often leads to bacteraemia and meningitis. *P. penneri* and *P. myxofaciens* are rarely encountered in clinical laboratory.

Laboratory diagnosis

Specimens

- Clean voided midstream urine sample in case of UTI.
- Pus in case of pyogenic infections.

Collection

Specimens should be collected in sterile containers under aseptic conditions and transported immediately.

Culture

Specimens are inoculated on MacConkey agar or blood agar with 6% agar to inhibit swarming. These are incubated at 37°C for 18–24 hours. On MacConkey agar NLF colonies are seen.

Gram staining

Shows Gram-negative coccobacilli.

Hanging drop preparation

Shows actively motile bacilli.

Biochemical reactions

Proteus spp. are PPA and urease positive, and ferment glucose with the production of acid and gas. Other biochemical reactions can be used to differentiate various species of *Proteus* (Table 30.2).

MORGANELLA

This genus has only one species – *M. morganii*. It was first isolated by Morgan and was included in the genus *Proteus* but on the basis of enzyme studies and genetic evidence, it has been assigned a separate genus with a single species. It is motile, but does not swarm on solid nutrient media. Biochemical reactions of this organism are shown in Table 30.2.

M. morganii is frequently found in human faeces and sometimes in the faeces of other animals and reptiles. It has also been isolated from diarrhoeic stools in the absence of other known bacterial enteropathogens. However, its role in the causation of enteritis has not as yet been established. It may also cause nosocomial urinary tract infection, pneumonia and wound infection. Occasionally, it is isolated from blood.

Table 30.2. Differentiation of four species of *Proteus* and *Morganella morganii*

Property	Proteus				M. morganii
	mirabilis	*vulgaris*	*penneri*	*myxofaciens*	
Motility	+	+	+	+	+
Swarming on solid nutrient media	+	+	–	–	–
Indole	–	+	–	–	+
Methyl red	+	+	+	+	+
Voges-Proskauer	v	–	–	+	–
Citrate	v	v	–	v	–
Phenylalanine deaminase test	+	+	+	+	+
Urease	+	+	+	+	+
H$_2$S	+	+	–	+	–
Gelatin liquefaction	+	+	v	+	–
Lipase production	+	+	v	+	–
Ornithine decarboxylation	+	–	–	–	+
Gas from glucose	+	+	v	+	+
Acid from:					
• Mannose	–	–	–	–	+
• Maltose	–	+	+	+	–
• Xylose	+	+	+	–	–
• Trehalose	+	v	v	+	–

v, variable.

Shigella and Salmonella

SHIGELLA

Morphology

Shigellae are non-motile, non-flagellate, non-sporing, non-capsulate, Gram-negative bacilli measuring 1–3 × 0.5 μm.

Cultural characteristics

They are aerobes and facultative anaerobes, growing within a temperature range of 10–40°C, with an optimum temperature of 37°C and pH of 7.4. They can grow on ordinary media.

1. On **nutrient agar** or **blood agar**, colonies are 2–3 mm in diameter, circular, convex, smooth, greyish or colourless and translucent. Colonies of *S. sonnei* are slightly larger and more opaque than those of other shigellae.
2. On **MacConkey agar**, colonies are colourless due to the absence of lactose fermentation. However, colonies of *S. sonnei*, a late lactose-fermenter, become pink when incubation is prolonged beyond 24 hours.
3. Colonies of *Shigella* on **deoxycholate citrate agar** (DCA), a selective medium for isolation of shigellae from faeces, are smaller (1–1.5 mm in diameter) and do not form a black centre. On prolonged incubation, colonies of *S. sonnei* form pink papillae due to late lactose fermentation.
4. **Xylose lysine deoxycholate** (XLD) agar is a better selective medium than DCA because it is less inhibitory to *S. dysenteriae* and *S. flexneri* than DCA. On this medium, colonies of *Shigella* are red and unlike those of most salmonellae, without black centres.

Enrichment media

(a) **Selenite F broth:** Sodium selenite in this enrichment medium inhibits coliform bacilli while permitting salmonellae and many shigellae to grow. Therefore, it is recommended for the isolation of these organisms from faeces.

(b) **Gram-negative (GN) broth:** Because of the relatively low concentration of sodium deoxycholate, GN broth is less inhibitory to *E. coli* and other coliforms.

Classification

On the basis of biochemical reactions and serological specificity, shigellae are classified into four groups (A, B, C and D) or species – *S. dysenteriae*, *S. flexneri*, *S. boydii* and *S. sonnei* (Table 31.1).

Antigenic structure

All *Shigella* species possess somatic (O) antigens, and certain strains may possess K antigens. *Shigella* K antigens, when present, interfere with the detection of the O antigen during

Table 31.1. Differentiation of *Shigella* species

Species	Acid produced in fermentation of					Indole	Lysine decarboxylase	Ornithine decarboxylase	Number of serotypes
	Lactose	Sucrose	Mannitol	Dulcitol	Xylose				
S. dysenteriae	–	–	–	–	–	v	–	–	15
S. flexneri	–	–	+	–	–	v	–	–	6 + 2 variants
S. boydii	–	–	+	v	v	v	–	–	19
S. sonnei	–*	–*	+	–	v	–	–	+	2 phases; 26 colicin types

*, negative at 24 hours, late positive at 2–8 days; v, variable.

serologic grouping. The K antigen is heat-labile and may be removed by boiling the organism in a cell suspension. On the basis of O antigens, shigellae can be subdivided into serotypes. This is carried out by agglutination tests with absorbed specific antisera.

Group A (*S. dysenteriae*): It is subdivided into 15 serotypes.

Group B (*S. flexneri*): Based on type-specific (I–VI) and group-specific (1–8) antigens, they have been classified into 6 serotypes (1–6) and several subtypes (1a, 1b, 2a, 2b, 3a, 3b, 3c, 4a, 4b, 5a, 5b). In addition, 2 antigenic variants called X and Y are recognized, which lack the type-specific antigen (Table 31.2). Serotype 6 is always indole negative and can be subdivided into three biotypes – Boyd 88, Manchester and Newcastle (Table 31.3).

Group C (*S. boydii*): Dysentery bacilli of this group resemble those of *S. flexneri* biochemically but not antigenically.

Group D (*S. sonnei*): It is antigenically homogeneous. It may, however, undergo an antigenic variation that affects the somatic antigens and has been referred to as phase or form variation. These 2 phases or forms of the culture are known as phase S or form I and phase R or form II. The former gives rise to smooth colonies while the colonies of the latter are larger, flatter and irregular. Cultures often contain a mixture of both forms, but the colonies of one form can be selected by addition of antiserum of the other form to the culture medium because form II variant is antigenically different from form I variant. By using 33 indicator strains, Horak (1980) could divide *S. sonnei* into **26 colicin types**.

Toxin formation

1. **Endotoxin:** All shigellae release an endotoxin after autolysis. It is thermostable lipopolysaccharide of the cell wall. It has irritating action on the intestinal wall which causes diarrhoea and subsequent ulcers.

2. **Exotoxin:** *S. dysenteriae* serotype 1, in addition to endotoxin, produces a powerful exotoxin. It is a heat-labile protein and acts as **enterotoxin** and **neurotoxin**. As enterotoxin, it acts on the intestinal mucosa causing transudation of fluid in the lumen and as neurotoxin, it damages endothelial cells of small blood vessels of the central nervous system, which results in neurological complications like polyneuritis, coma and meningism.

3. **Verocytotoxin:** *S. dysenteriae* serotype 1 produces a potent toxin (shiga toxin) very similar to VT1 expressed by strains of Verocytotoxigenic *E. coli* (VTEC).

Pathogenicity

Members of the genus *Shigella* produce a serious illness known as **bacillary dysentery**. It is an acute diarrhoeal disease characterized in the more severe infections by the presence of blood and mucus in the stools. Humans appear to be the only natural hosts for shigellae and they become infected by ingestion of contaminated food or water. **The only source of infection is man – cases or carriers. The infective dose is small – 10–100 organisms.** *Shigella*, unlike *Vibrio cholerae* and most *Salmonella* serotypes, is acid-resistant and survives passage through the stomach to reach the intestine.

After reaching the large intestine, the shigellae multiply in the gut lumen. Many bacteria adhere to the epithelial cells of the gut mucosa and induce these cells to ingest them. They then multiply within the epithelial cells and spread laterally into adjacent cells and deep into the lamina propria. Inflammatory reaction develops with capillary thrombosis, leading to necrosis of patches of epithelium, which slough off, leaving behind **superficial ulcers**. The cellular response is mainly by polymorphonuclear leucocytes which can be seen on microscopic examination of stool, together with red cells and sloughed epithelium.

Table 31.2. Antigens of various serotypes of *Shigella flexneri*

Serotype	Subserotype	Type antigen	Group antigens
1	1a	I	1, 2, 4
	1b	I	1, 2, 4, 6
2	2a	II	1, 3, 4
	2b	II	1, 7, 8
3	3a	III	1, 6, 7, 8
	3b	III	1, 3, 4, 6, 7, 8
	3c	III	1, 6
4	4a	IV	1, 3, 4
	4b	IV	1, 3, 4, 6
5	5a	V	1, 3, 4
	5b	V	1, 7, 8
6		VI	1, 2, 4
X variant		–	1, 7, 8
Y variant		–	1, 3, 4

Table 31.3. Biotypes of *Shigella flexneri* serotype 6

Biotype	Indole	Fermentation of Glucose	Fermentation of Mannitol
Boyd 88	–	⊥	⊥
Manchester	–	+	+
Newcastle	–	⊥ or +	–

⊥, acid only; +, acid and gas.

Laboratory diagnosis

Specimen

The laboratory diagnosis of bacillary dysentery can be made by the isolation of *Shigella* from faeces. It should be inoculated without delay. If this is impossible, the mucus or faeces should be transported in a buffered 30% glycerol saline solution, which prevents the dysentery bacilli from being destroyed by the acid produced during the growth of other organisms. A direct swab may be taken from the ulcer by sigmoidoscopic examination. Rectal swabs which do not allow adequate macroscopic and microscopic examination of faeces should be avoided.

Direct microscopy

Microscopic examination of the faeces or mucus shows numerous erythrocytes and polymorphonuclear leucocytes and a few macrophages. The latter must be carefully differentiated from vegetative forms of *Entamoeba histolytica* which have relatively smaller nuclei with a central karyosome.

Culture

The mucus or faeces are inoculated on MacConkey agar and DCA. XLD medium can also be used. After overnight incubation at 37°C, the plates are inspected for pale (non-lactose-fermenting) colonies on MacConkey agar and DCA, and red and colourless colonies with no blackening on XLD, and SS agar respectively. These are tested for motility and biochemical reactions.

Enrichment media inoculation

Along with the inoculation of plating media, selenite F broth and GN broth (enrichment media) may also be inoculated. Subcultures are made on plating media after 8–12 hours and 4–6 hours respectively and processed as above.

Slide agglutination test

The colonies that give the characteristic biochemical reactions should be identified further by slide agglutination with species-specific sera and then with type-specific sera unless the strain is *S. sonnei*.

SALMONELLA

Morphology

Salmonellae are Gram-negative, non-sporing, non-acid-fast, non-capsulated bacilli measuring $1–3 \times 0.5\ \mu m$. Most strains are motile by means of peritrichous flagella except *S. Gallinarum* and *S. Pullorum* which are non-motile.

Cultural characteristics

Salmonellae are aerobes and facultative anaerobes, growing within a temperature range of 15–41°C (optimum temperature 37°C). They can grow on ordinary media.

1. On **nutrient agar** or **blood agar**, colonies are 2–3 mm in diameter, greyish-white, circular, moist, convex and translucent.
2. On **MacConkey agar**, after overnight incubation at 37°C, the colonies are 1–3 mm in diameter and pale yellow or colourless due to the absence of lactose fermentation.

3. The colonies of *Salmonella* on **deoxycholate citrate agar (DCA)**, a selective medium for isolation of shigellae and salmonellae from faeces, are similar to or slightly smaller in size than those on MacConkey agar. After 48 hours incubation, the colonies may develop a black centre.
4. For the appearance of colonies of *Salmonella* on **xylose lysine deoxycholate (XLD) agar** see cultural characteristics of *Shigella*.

Enrichment media

(a) **Tetrathionate broth:** It enriches salmonellae and sometimes shigellae, but permits the growth of *Proteus*. The latter may reduce the tetrathionate, thus impairing the selectivity of this medium for salmonellae.

(b) **Selenite F broth:** Sodium selenite in this medium inhibits coliform bacilli while permitting salmonellae and many shigellae to grow. It is an excellent enrichment medium for the isolation of *S.* Typhi and *S.* Dublin, but some salmonellae, e.g., *S.* Paratyphi A and *S.* Choleraesuis and some shigellae may fail to grow in this medium.

Biochemical reactions

Salmonellae are indole negative, methyl red reaction positive, Voges-Proskauer negative and citrate positive (except *S.* Typhi and *S.* Paratyphi A which are citrate negative). Most salmonellae give a positive reaction for H_2S in triple sugar iron agar, but exceptions include strains of *S.* Paratyphi A and *S.* Choleraesuis.

Antigenic structure

Salmonellae possess three main types of antigens (Fig. 31.1) on the basis of which they are serologically typed. These are:

- Flagellar (H) antigens.
- Somatic (O) antigens.
- Vi antigen.

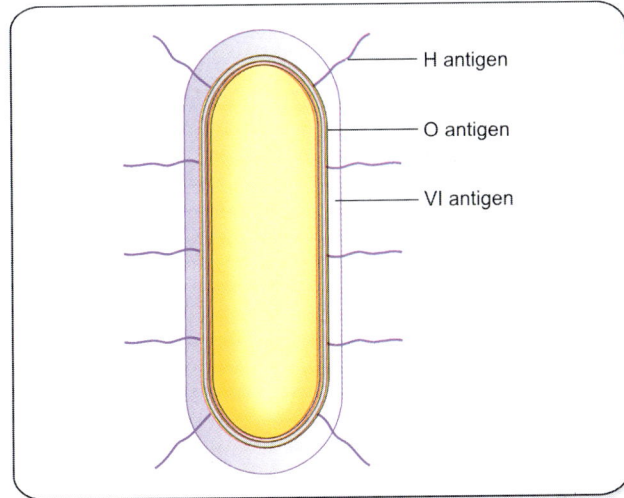

Fig. 31.1. Antigenic structure of salmonellae.

H antigens

These antigens, present on flagella, are heat-labile and alcohol-labile, but are well preserved in 0.04–0.2% formaldehyde. Heating at 100°C for 30 minutes detaches all the flagella.

O antigens

The somatic O antigen is phospholipid-protein-polysaccharide complex, which forms an integral part of the cell wall. It is identical to endotoxin. They can withstand boiling for 2.5 hours. They are also alcohol-stable, withstanding treatment with 96% ethanol at 37°C for 4 hours.

Vi antigen

Almost all recently isolated strains of *S.* Typhi possess surface antigen, known as Vi antigen, enveloping the O antigen. It was originally designated Vi because its presence appeared to determine virulence for mice. It is a heat-labile acidic polysaccharide. It is destroyed by boiling or heating the bacteria at 60°C for one hour. It is also destroyed by treatment with phenol, N hydrochloric acid and 0.5 N sodium hydroxide. It is unaffected by alcohol or 0.2% formaldehyde. It tends to be lost on serial subcultures.

Kauffmann-White scheme

This scheme, first developed in 1934, classifies salmonellae into different O serogroups based on distinctive O antigen factors. Strains possessing factor 2 belong to serogroup A, factor 4 to serogroup B, factor 9 to serogroup D and so on. Each serogroup contains a number of serotypes. Formerly, O serogroups were designated by capital letters A–Z and those discovered later by the number 51–67. Serogroups A–Z and 51–67 represented O antigens 2–50 and 51–67 respectively.

It appears more logical to name each O serogroup by its common O antigen. These numbers are not continuous. Within each O serogroup, the different serotypes are distinguished by identification of phase 1 and 2 flagellar antigens (Table 31.4).

Bacteriophage typing

For epidemiological study, strains within a particular serotype may be differentiated into a number of phage types. Craigie and Yen (1937) observed that a bacteriophage acting on Vi antigen of *S.* Typhi (Vi phage II) is highly adaptable. The parent phage is known as phage A. It could be made specific for a particular strain of *S.* Typhi by serial propagation in that strain. The phage typing is done by determining the sensitivity of the culture to a series of variants of Vi phage II. Type A strains are sensitive to all adaptations of the Vi phage but most other types are sensitive to only one or a few related adaptations. As phage typing of *S.* Typhi depends on the presence of Vi antigens, a proportion of strains (Vi negative) will be untypable. At present, 97 Vi II phage types of *S.* Typhi are recognized. **Phage types E_1, O and A are the most common in India.**

Pathogenesis

Man acquires infection by ingestion of contaminated water or food. Water becomes polluted by the introduction of faeces from any human or animal excreting salmonellae. Infection by food usually results either from ingestion of contaminated meat or by way of the hands of the carrier.

Salmonellae cause the following clinical syndromes in man:

- Enteric fever.
- Septicaemia with or without local suppurative lesions.
- Gastroenteritis or food poisoning.

Enteric fever

Enteric fever is most usually caused by *S.* Typhi (**typhoid fever**) or *S.* Paratyphi A, B and C (**paratyphoid fever**). On

Table 31.4. Kauffmann-White classification of *Salmonella* showing antigenic formulae of some important serogroups and serotypes

O serogroup New	O serogroup Old	Serotype	O antigens (and Vi)	H antigens Phase 1	H antigens Phase 2
2	A	*S.* Paratyphi A	1, **2**, 12	a	–
4	B	*S.* Paratyphi B	1, **4**, 5, 12	b	1, 2
		S. Typhimurium	1, **4**, 5, 12	i	1, 2
7	C1	*S.* Paratyphi C	6, **7** (Vi)	c	1, 5
		S. Choleraesuis	6, **7**	c	1, 5
8	C2	*S.* Muenchen	6, **8**	d	1, 2
		S. Newport	6, **8**, 20	e, h	1, 2
9	D	*S.* Typhi	**9**, 12 (Vi)	d	–
		S. Enteritidis	4, **9**, 12	g, m	–
		S. Gallinarum	1, **9**, 12	–	–
		S. Pullorum	1, **9**, 12	–	–
3, 10	E1	*S.* Anatum	3, **10**	e, h	1, 6

reaching the gut, the bacilli attach themselves to the microvilli of the ileal mucosa by means of adhesins on the bacterial surface, which adhere specifically to mannose-containing receptors on the epithelium. They then penetrate to the lamina propria and submucosa, where they are phagocytosed by neutrophils and macrophages. They resist intracellular killing and multiply within these cells. These cells enter the mesenteric lymph nodes, where after a period of multiplication, the bacilli invade the blood stream via thoracic duct and a transient bacteraemia (**primary bacteraemia**) follows.

During this period, the bacilli are seeded in the liver, gall bladder, spleen, bone marrow, lymph nodes, lungs and kidneys, where further multiplication takes place. After multiplication in these organs, bacilli pass into the blood, causing a **second and heavier bacteraemia**, heralding the onset of clinical illness.

The organisms multiply abundantly in the gall bladder and are discharged continuously into the intestine where Peyer's patches and other gut lymphoid tissues of ileum become involved. These become inflamed, undergo necrosis and slough off, leaving behind characteristic **typhoid ulcers**. Perforation and haemorrhage are occasional associated accidents.

Incubation period is usually 8–15 days, but can be as short as 5 days or as long as 50 days. The clinical course may vary from a mild undifferentiated pyrexia to a rapidly fatal fulminating disease. The onset is usually gradual with headache, malaise, anorexia, a coated tongue and abdominal discomfort with either constipation or diarrhoea. In the untreated case the temperature shows a step-ladder rise over the first week of illness, remains high for 7–10 days and then falls by lysis during third or fourth week.

Physical signs include a relative bradycardia for the height of the fever, hepatomegaly, splenomegaly and often a rash of **rose spots**. These are 2–4 mm in diameter, slightly raised discrete irregular macules. They are most often found on the front of the chest during the second or third week and fade on pressure. They are seldom noticeable in dark-skinned patients.

Laboratory diagnosis

Laboratory diagnosis of enteric fever can be made by:

- Isolation and identification of the causative agent from the patient blood, faeces, urine, bone marrow, rose spots, etc.
- Demonstration of circulating antigen.
- Demonstration of antibodies in the patient serum.

Blood culture

With all aseptic precautions, 5–10 ml of blood is collected by venipuncture and transferred into a culture bottle containing 50–100 ml of 0.5% bile broth. Before transferring blood into blood culture bottle, the cap of the bottle is thoroughly cleaned with spirit. The blood should be transferred through a hole in the cap by inserting the needle of the syringe rather than opening the bottle, thus it avoids contamination from the external environment. As far as possible, sample of blood should be collected before starting treatment.

Blood culture bottle is incubated at 37°C for up to 7 days. After overnight incubation, subculture is made onto MacConkey agar, and blood agar (for organisms other than *Salmonella*) media. These plates are incubated at 37°C for 24 hours and the isolate is identified by its morphological and biochemical characters, and slide agglutination test. If salmonellae are not obtained from first subculture from bile broth, then subcultures should be repeated every other day up to 7 days. If no growth is obtained after 7 days, then the culture is declared as negative.

For slide agglutination test, a loopful of growth from nutrient agar plate or slope is emulsified in two separate drops of saline on a clean slide. One emulsion acts as a control to show that the strain is not autoagglutinable. If the isolate is anaerogenic (i.e., *S.* Typhi is suspected) then a loopful of factor 9 antiserum is added to one drop of bacterial emulsion on the slide. The slide is rocked gently. Prompt agglutination indicates that the isolate belongs to *Salmonella* O serogroup D. Its identity as *S.* Typhi is established by agglutination with the flagellar antiserum (anti-d serum). Sometimes, fresh isolates of *S.* Typhi are in the V form and do not agglutinate with O antiserum. Such strains may be tested for agglutination with anti-Vi serum or the growth is scraped off in a small amount of saline, boiled for one hour and tested for agglutination with O antiserum. If the isolate is nontyphoid *Salmonella*, it is tested for agglutination with O and H antisera for serogroups A, B, C1, C2, etc.

Clot culture

With strict aseptic precautions, 5 ml blood is withdrawn from the patient into a sterile test tube and allowed to clot. The separated serum is removed and used for the Widal test. The clot is broken up with a sterile glass rod and added to a bottle of bile broth containing streptokinase (100 units/ml). Streptokinase causes rapid clot lysis with release of bacteria trapped in the clot. Clot culture with streptokinase yields a higher rate of isolation than whole blood culture as the bactericidal action of the serum is obviated. Another advantage is that a sample of serum also becomes available for Widal test.

Faeces culture

A spoonful of faeces should be collected in a sterile container. Rectal swab is not satisfactory. If there is likely to be a delay of some hours before specimen of faeces for culture reaches the laboratory, the faeces can be placed in a container with 5 ml of **buffered glycerol saline** transport medium. Faecal samples are plated directly on MacConkey agar, DCA and Wilson and Blair's brilliant-green bismuth sulphite agar media. The last is highly selective and should be plated heavily.

On MacConkey and DCA media salmonellae appear as pale yellow or colourless colonies after 18–24 hours incubation at 37°C.

For enrichment, one tube each of selenite F and tetra-thionate broth are also inoculated. These are also incubated at 37°C for 8–12 hours with subsequent subculture on MacConkey and DCA media.

Other materials for culture

Salmonellae may be isolated from several other sources. These include urine, bone marrow, bile obtained by duodenal aspiration, rose spots, pus from suppurative lesions, CSF and sputum. Bone marrow and bile culture are positive in most cases. The latter may be employed for detection of carriers.

Demonstration of circulating antigen

In the early phase of the disease, typhoid bacillus antigens are consistently present in the blood and urine of the patient. *Staphylococcus aureus* containing protein A (Cowan 1 strain) is stabilized with formaldehyde and then coated with *S.* Typhi antibody. When a 1% suspension of such sensitized staphylo-coccal cells is mixed with patient serum on a slide, typhoid antigen present in the serum combines specifically with the antibody attached to staphylococcal cells producing visible agglutination within 2 minutes. This is known as **coagglutination**. The test is rapid, sensitive and specific, but is not positive after the first week of illness.

Demonstration of antibodies in the patient serum

Widal test

It is an **agglutination test** which detects the presence of agglutinins in patient serum against H and O suspensions of the enteric bacteria likely to be encountered, e.g., *S.* Typhi and *S.* Paratyphi A in India. Two types of tubes are used for the test:

1. Dreyer's tube (narrow tube with conical bottom) for H agglutination.
2. Felix tube (short round bottomed tube) for O agglutination.

Equal volumes (0.4 ml) of serial dilutions of the patient serum (1 : 20 to 1 : 640) and H antigens of *S.* Typhi (TH) and *S.* Paratyphi A (AH); and O antigen of *S.* Typhi (TO), are mixed in Dreyer's and Felix tubes respectively and incubated in a water bath at 37°C for 4 hours and read after overnight refrigeration at 4°C. O antigen of *S.* Paratyphi A (AO) may not be employed as it cross reacts with TO. Control tubes containing the antigen and normal saline are set to check for autoagglutination. H agglutination leads to the formation of loose and cotton-woolly clumps, while O agglutination appears as a disc-like granular deposit at the bottom of the tube (Fig. 12.6). **The highest dilution of the serum showing agglutination indicates the titre of the antibody.**

Interpretation of Widal test

1. Agglutinins usually appear by seventh to tenth day of the illness in enteric fever, so that a negative result at an early stage is inconclusive. The titre then increases steadily till the third or fourth week, after which it declines gradually.

2. Demonstration of rising titre, e.g., four-fold or greater rise, between tests made in the first and third weeks is highly significant. However, if the first sample is taken late in the disease, a rise may not be demonstrable. Instead a fall in titre may be seen in some cases.

3. Though, it is generally stated that titres of 1 : 100 or more for O agglutinins and 1 : 200 or more for H agglutinins are significant, the results in a single test by no means prove the presence of enteric fever nor negative results its absence.

Salmonella septicaemia

Certain salmonellae, *S.* Choleraesuis, may cause septi-caemia. It is characterized by suppurative lesions, such as osteomyelitis, deep abscesses, endocarditis, pneumonia and meningitis. Infection occurs by oral route and the incubation period is short. Salmonellae can be isolated from blood or exudate from focal lesions but rarely from faeces.

Salmonella gastroenteritis

Salmonella gastroenteritis or food poisoning is generally a **zoonotic disease**.

Source of infection

It is caused by ingestion of food like meat, egg, milk and sweets contaminated by certain species of *Salmonella* which are primarily animal pathogens. In most parts of the world, *S.* Typhimurium is the commonest (30–40%) species. Other common species include *S.* Enteritidis, *S.* Newport, *S.* Dublin, *S.* Heidelberg and *S.* Indiana. Food contamination may result from droppings of rats, lizards or other small animals. Salmonellae can enter through the shell of the egg if the eggs are left on contaminated chicken feed or faeces, and grow inside.

Pathogenesis

The incubation period is 12–24 hours and the illness is characterised by fever, vomiting, abdominal pain and diarrhoea. It may vary in severity from the passage of one or two loose stools to an acute cholera-like disease. It usually subsides in 2–7 days. There are multiple reports that *Salmonella* serotypes secrete a cholera-like enterotoxin that induces increased levels of cAMP and that some strains produce a heat-stable enterotoxin. A cytotoxin that inhibits protein synthesis in intestinal cells has been described.

Laboratory diagnosis

It is made by isolating the causative agent from faeces and food.

Prophylaxis

- Prevention of food contamination.
- Proper cooking of food.

32

Yersinia Pestis

Morphology

They are Gram-negative coccobacilli or rods with rounded ends and straight or convex sides, about 1.5 × 0.7 µm in size, occurring singly or in pairs or, when in fluid culture, in chains. They are non-sporing, non-acid-fast and non-motile. In exudates from lesions and in cultures grown at 37°C, rather than at the optimum temperature of 27°C, *Y. pestis* exhibits typical capsule. In smears from the tissues stained with Giemsa or methylene blue, the bacilli show characteristic bipolar staining (safety pin appearance), in which the ends of the bacilli stain darker than the central part (Fig. 32.1). In culture, the bipolar staining is less obvious.

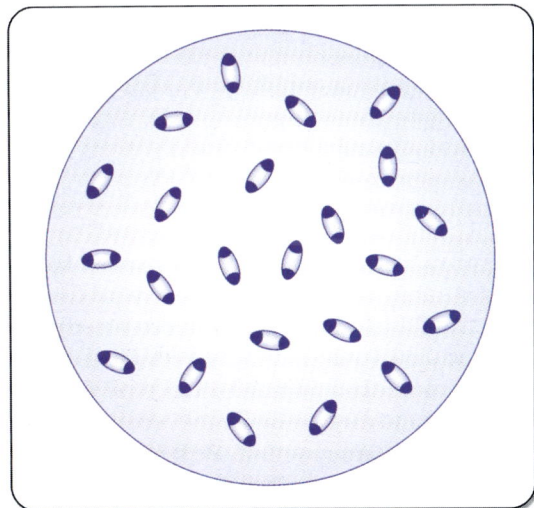

Fig. 32.1. Bipolar staining of *Yersinia pestis*.

Cultural characteristics

Plague bacilli are aerobes and facultative anaerobes. Optimum (and range) pH and temperature for the growth of these organisms are 7.2 (5.0–9.6) and 27°C (14–37°C) respectively.

It can grow on ordinary media.

- On **nutrient agar** medium, after overnight incubation, *Y. pestis* forms transparent, minute, pin-point colonies. On further incubation, they continue to increase in diameter reaching 4 mm in 5 days and become opaque.
- On **blood agar**, colonies are dark brown due to absorption of the haemin pigment.
- Colourless colonies are formed on **MacConkey agar**.
- In **broth**, it produces little turbidity but results in a granular deposit at the bottom and the sides of the tube. On prolonged incubation, a surface pellicle may appear. If a drop of sterile oil is allowed to float on the surface of an inoculated broth and provided the flask is not shaken, a characteristic growth appears which hangs down into the broth from the oil drop resembling stalactites (**stalactite growth**).

Biochemical reactions

Y. pestis is catalase-positive, indole negative, methyl red reaction positive, Voges-Proskauer and citrate negative. It is nitrate reduction positive and urease and gelatin liquefaction negative. It ferments glucose, mannitol and maltose with the production of acid but no gas. Lactose and sucrose are not fermented.

Pathogenesis

Y. pestis is a natural pathogen of rodents. It causes **zoonotic disease** called **plague**. Infection is transmitted from one animal to another by the bite of rat flea. The infection normally does not pass from one animal to another unless a flea carries the organism from one to another.

When a rat flea, commonly *Xenopsylla cheopis*, bites a diseased rat, it sucks about 0.5 ml of blood per feed, which contains about 5,000–50,000 bacilli. These are sufficient to infect flea. In the flea, the bacilli multiply in the stomach and block the lumen of proventriculus. In *X. cheopis* it takes about 3 weeks (**extrinsic incubation period**). When such a flea bites another rodent blood cannot pass through. The hungry flea bites ferociously and bacteria are regurgitated into the site of bite, transmitting the infection.

When the diseased rat dies, the flea leaves the carcass and in the absence of another rat may bite man causing bubonic plague. Infection in man may also be transmitted by contamination of the wound of bite with the faeces of infected fleas. In man plague occurs in three forms – **bubonic**, **septicaemic** and **pneumonic**.

Bubonic plague

After an incubation period of 2–5 days, the lymph nodes draining the site of entry of bacillus become infected. As the plague bacillus usually enters through the bite of infected flea on the legs, the inguinal lymph nodes are involved, hence the name bubonic plague (bubo means enlarged gland in groin). The glands become enlarged and suppurate. Patient develops fever, chills, nausea and malaise. Pain may precede and accompany the bubo. The spread of disease is not stopped by the lymph nodes and hence bacteraemia occurs.

Septicaemic plague

The presence of bacteria in the blood denotes septicaemic plague. Massive involvement of blood vessels occurs resulting in haemorrhages in the skin and mucosa. This manifestation is responsible for the disease being given the name **'black death'**.

Pneumonic plague

Bacterial emboli may become trapped in the lungs causing pneumonic plague. It gives an added dimension to the disease since **it can be transmitted from man to man by droplet infection (airborne route)**. Pneumonic plague may also occur in epidemic form. Patient develops fever, 104°F or more, and cough with expectoration. The sputum at first is mucoid and blood-tinged later. It is loaded with *Y. pestis*. Patient complains of severe chest pain, difficult and rapid breathing. Towards the end, patient develops cyanosis and circulatory failure. Those who develop pneumonic plague die within 2–3 days if not treated vigorously. Death rate from bubonic plague is 50–75%, from pneumonic plague almost 100%, and with treatment it is 5–30%.

Laboratory diagnosis

The diagnosis of plague can be confirmed by demonstrating *Y. pestis* in stained films from bubos in bubonic plague or in sputum in pneumonic plague. In septicaemic plague, the bacilli may be demonstrated in blood cultures or from spleen on postmortem.

Bubonic plague

1. Puncture the bubo with a hypodermic syringe and draw the exudate for examination.
2. Prepare the films of the exudate and stain by Gram staining and methylene blue. Characteristic Gram-negative cocco-bacilli, and bacilli showing bipolar staining with methylene blue are suggestive of plague bacilli.
3. Culture the exudate on blood agar plate, incubate at 27°C. Pick up a single colony and subculture to obtain a pure growth. Carry out biochemical tests to confirm the diagnosis.
4. Inoculate guinea-pigs or white rats subcutaneously with exudate from bubo or with 24 hours broth culture. Infected animals die in 2–5 days. Postmortem reveals marked local inflammatory condition at the site of inoculation, with necrosis and oedema. Regional lymph nodes are enlarged and congested and may show greyish-white patches in the tissue. Prepare films from local lesions, lymph nodes, spleen and heart blood. Stain films with Gram and methylene blue stains and examine under microscope for characteristic *Y. pestis*.

Pneumonic plague

1. Prepare films from sputum and stain by Gram and methylene blue stains. Examine stained films micro-scopically for characteristic Gram-negative and bipolar stained coccobacilli respectively.
2. Inoculate on blood agar plate and proceed further as in case of bubonic plague.
3. Inoculate sputum into guinea-pigs or rats by applying the sputum to the nasal mucosa or to a shaved area of skin. The plague bacilli can enter through microabrasions caused by shaving while other organisms in sputum cannot. Carry out postmortem as in case of bubonic plague.

In the convalescent stage serology is most likely to be useful. Serum may be tested by complement fixation test, and the haemagglutination test with tanned sheep red cells to which the capsular F1 antigen has been absorbed. An enzyme-linked immunosorbent assay (**ELISA**) with F1 antigen is likely to become the method of choice.

A **polymerase chain reaction** (PCR), with primers based on F1 gene sequences, offers a rapid and less hazardous means of diagnosis than culture.

33

Vibrio, Pseudomonas and Burkholderia

Vibrio cholerae

Morphology

These are short, curved or comma-shaped rods with rounded or pointed ends and 1.5×0.2–0.4 μm in size. S forms or spirals may be seen due to two or more cells lying end to end (Fig. 33.1). They show vigorous **darting motility** which is mediated by a single polar flagellum. They are Gram-negative, non-sporing, non-capsulated and non-acid-fast.

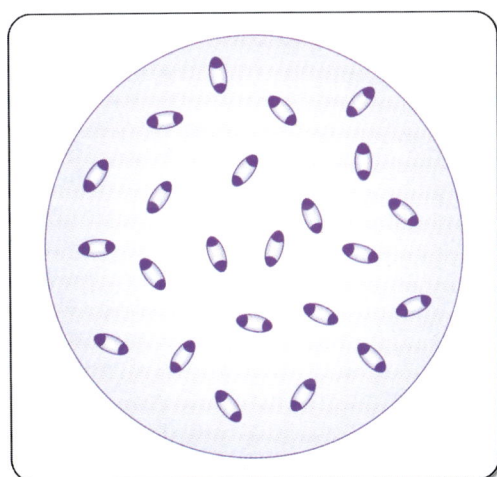

Fig. 33.1. *Vibrio cholerae.*

Cultural characteristics

V. cholerae is aerobe and facultative anaerobe, but under anaerobic conditions only scanty and slow growth is obtained. It grows within a temperature range of 16–40°C (optimum temperature 37°C). Growth occurs freely between pH 7.4 and 9.6 (optimum pH 8.2).

- **Nutrient agar:** After overnight incubation at 37°C, the colonies are glistening translucent discs, 1–2 mm in diameter with bluish or greenish tinge in transmitted light.

- **MacConkey agar:** Colonies are smaller than those on nutrient agar and are colourless, but become reddish on prolonged incubation due to the late fermentation of lactose.
- **Peptone water:** This organism grows as a surface pellicle because of its affinity for oxygen. The surface pellicle becomes visible in 6–9 hours.

Special media

A number of special culture media have been employed for the cultivation of *V. cholerae*. They may be classified as under:

Transport (holding) media

1. **Venkatraman-Ramakrishnan (VR) medium:** It is prepared by dissolving 20 g crude sea salt and 5 g peptone in 1 litre of distilled water and pH is adjusted to 8.6–8.8. It is dispensed in screw-capped bottles in 10–15 ml amounts. About 1–3 ml of stool is added to each bottle. *V. cholerae* does not multiply in this medium but remains viable for several weeks. Moreover, it prevents overgrowth by other organisms.
2. **Cary-Blair medium:** This medium is prepared by adding disodium hydrogen phosphate 1.1 g, sodium thioglycollate 1.5 g, sodium chloride 5.0 g and agar 5.0 g to 1 litre of distilled water and pH is adjusted at 8.4.
3. If a transport medium is not available, a 5 cm × 1.5 cm strip of **thick blotting paper** can be soaked in the faecal matter, then placed in a sealed plastic bag, and sent to the laboratory.

Enrichment media

1. **Alkaline peptone water (APW):** This medium contains 1% each of peptone and sodium chloride at pH 8.6. High pH of the medium suppresses the growth of many commensal intestinal bacteria while permitting uninhibited growth of *V. cholerae*. Subcultures on plating media should be done within 3–6 hours because other organisms can begin to overgrow after prolonged incubation. APW is also

an excellent transport medium. About 1 g of the stool or a rectal swab should be placed into 10 ml of APW in a screw-capped tube and transported to the laboratory.

2. **Taurocholate peptone transport and enrichment medium:** In 1 litre distilled water, dissolve peptone, sodium chloride and sodium taurocholate in amounts of 10 g, 10 g and 5 g respectively. Adjust pH at 9.2, distribute in 20 ml amounts and autoclave at 121°C for 15 minutes. To make the medium more selective for vibrios, add sterile potassium tellurite solution to the autoclaved medium to give a final concentration of 1 in 200,000. Place about 1 g stool or a rectal swab in the medium and transport to the laboratory. Subculture a loopful onto a selective plating medium within 6–8 hours at ambient temperature. Also, incubate it overnight at 37°C and subculture again on a plating medium next day.

Plating media

These include:

1. **Alkaline bile salt agar (BSA) pH 8.2:** This is modified nutrient agar medium containing 0.5% sodium tauro-cholate. The colonies on BSA are similar to those on nutrient agar medium.
2. **Monsur's gelatin taurocholate trypticase tellurite agar (GTTA) medium:** This medium is useful for the isolation of cholera and other vibrios from faeces. High (8.5) pH and potassium tellurite, in this medium, are inhibitory to most enterobacteria and Gram-positive bacteria. After 24 hours incubation, vibrios produce small (1–2 mm) translucent colonies with greyish-black centre and a turbid halo, due to hydrolysis and denaturation of gelatin. After 48 hours incubation, colonies increase in size to 3–4 mm.
3. **Thiosulphate-citrate-bile-sucrose (TCBS) agar:** This is most used selective plating medium for vibrios. This medium resembles DCA, except that it has the high pH value of 8.6 and contains sucrose instead of lactose. **Sucrose-fermenting vibrios such as V. cholerae form yellow colonies** and non-sucrose-fermenters such as V. parahaemolyticus blue green ones.

Biochemical reactions

V. cholerae is strongly indole positive and reduces nitrates to nitrites. These two properties contribute to the **'cholera red reaction'**. The development of a red colour when concentrated sulphuric acid, is added to a 4-day-old culture at 37°C in peptone water. It is due to the formation of **nitrosoindole**, which is red in colour. It ferments glucose, sucrose, mannitol, maltose and mannose with the production of acid, but no gas and ferments lactose only after several days **(late lactose fermenter)**. Arabinose and dulcitol are not fermented.

It is catalase and oxidase-positive, methyl red and urease negative and liquefies gelatin. It decarboxylates lysine and ornithine but not arginine. Voges-Proskauer reaction and

haemolysis of sheep RBCs are positive in El Tor biotype and both these reactions are negative in classical biotype. The differences between classical and El Tor biotypes of V. cholerae are given in Table 33.1.

Table 33.1. Differences between classical and El Tor biotypes of Vibrio cholerae

Property	Biotype	
	Classical	El Tor
Voges-Proskauer test	–	+
Agglutination of fowl RBCs	–	+
Haemolysis of sheep RBCs	–	+
Sensitivity to:		
• Polymyxin B	+	–
• Mukerjee's group IV phage	+	–
• Basu and Mukerjee's group V phage	–	+

Antigenic structure

V. cholerae possesses at least 139 different O antigens on the basis of which it has been divided into corresponding number of serogroups or serovars. All strains share a common, heat-labile flagellar (H) antigen. **Epidemic cholera is caused by V. cholerae serogroup O1 and V. cholerae O139 Bengal.** Both classical and El Tor biotypes, belong to serogroup O1. They are agglutinated by V. cholerae O1 antiserum.

Two recognized serogroups of V. cholerae which are choleragenic are serogroups O1 and O139. The serogroups O2–O138 are known as **non-O1 vibrios, non-cholera vibrios (NCV) or non-agglutinable (NAG) vibrios** because they are not agglutinated by O1 antiserum. However, they are readily agglutinated by their own antisera. From time to time, they have been associated with outbreaks of diarrhoeal or choleraic disease. Both V. cholerae O1 and O139 produce **enterotoxin (cholera toxin)**. Some strains of NCV also produce an entero-toxin similar to the cholera toxin.

O1 serogroup can be further subdivided into three sub-types, Ogawa, Inaba and Hikojima. This is on the basis of differences in minor O antigens (A, B and C). Antigen A is present in all the three subtypes. O antigens present in Ogawa, Inaba and Hikojima are A and B, A and C, and A, B and C respectively (Table 33.2). Ogawa and Inaba strains agglutinate with their specific absorbed antisera, while Hikojima strains which are rare are agglutinated by both Ogawa and Inaba antisera.

Table 33.2. Subtypes of Vibrio cholerae O1

Subtypes	Antigens
Ogawa	A and B
Inaba	A and C
Hikojima	A, B and C

Phage typing

Strains of the classical biotype of *V. cholerae* O1 can be divided into 5 types by means of 3 phages (I–III) and a fourth phage (IV) lyses all classical but not El Tor strains (Table 33.3). On the basis of lysis by 4 phages, El Tor strains can be divided into 6 types. All these strains are lysed by a fifth phage (V) (Table 33.4).

Table 33.3. Phage types of strains of classical biotype of *Vibrio cholerae* O1 (Mukerjee et al., 1957)

Phage type	Sensitivity to phage group			
	I	II	III	IV
1	+	+	+	+
2	–	+	+	+
3	+	–	+	+
4	–	–	+	+
5	+	+	–	+

Table 33.4. Phage types of strains of El Tor biotype of *Vibrio cholerae* O1 (Basu and Mukerjee, 1968)

Phage type	Sensitivity to phage group				
	I	II	III	IV	V
1	+	+	+	+	+
2	+	+	+	–	+
3	+	+	–	+	+
4	+	+	–	–	+
5	+	–	–	–	+
6	–	+	–	–	+

Pathogenesis

V. cholerae O1 causes an acute diarrhoeal disease known as **cholera**. It occurs only in man. The vibrios enter orally by the ingestion of faecally contaminated food or drink. Infective dose of *V. cholerae* is 10^8 organisms. After passing the acid barrier of the stomach, they multiply in the alkaline contents of the small intestine and produce a potent toxin known as **cholera toxin (CT), cholera enterotoxin or choleragen**. This leads to an outpouring of fluid that is isotonic and contains flakes of mucus and little protein and results in vomiting and profuse watery diarrhoea (*rice water stool*). This results in varying degrees of dehydration and electrolyte imbalance that can lead to metabolic acidosis, hypokalaemia, shock and death in extreme cases.

Laboratory diagnosis

Specimens

- Watery stool
- Rectal swab
- Vomitus

Collection of specimens

- Fresh faecal material should be collected as early in the disease process as possible, before the administration of antibiotics. It is best collected by inserting a sterile soft rubber catheter (No. 24–26) and letting the liquid stool flow directly into a sterile screw-capped container.
- A rectal swab may also be collected. It is particularly useful for collecting specimen from a convalescent who no longer has watery diarrhoea. Collection of stool from a bedpan should be avoided because of the risk of contamination or the presence of disinfectants.
- Culture of vomitus may yield the growth of the organisms particularly in the early stages of disease.

Transportation and enrichment

The cultures should be put up immediately. If it is not possible, then the specimen should be preserved in a suitable transport (holding) medium such as VR medium or Cary-Blair medium for long periods. If the specimen can reach the laboratory within a few hours, it may be transported in enrichment media such as APW or Monsur's taurocholate tellurite peptone water, thus saving the time required for isolation. As discussed above, if transport media are not available, a 5 cm × 1.5 cm strip of thick blotting paper can be soaked in the watery stool and sent to the laboratory packed in a plastic envelope.

Culture

In the laboratory, the sample should be plated both directly and after enrichment, onto suitable solid media. Early in the choleraic infection, *V. cholerae* are present in very large numbers (10^7–10^9/ml) in the diarrhoeal stool, so direct plating on non-selective media might well be sufficient for the isolation of these organisms. At later stage of infection, and if antibiotics have been given, the number of *V. cholerae* in the stools will be relatively less, therefore, both enrichment and selective plating media should be used to prevent overgrowth by other intestinal bacteria.

1. Inoculate 2 ml faeces in 20 ml APW. Also inoculate non-selective culture media like 5% sheep blood agar and MacConkey agar and a selective medium like TCBS or GTTA. Incubate these media at 37°C.
2. After 3–6 hours incubation, subculture a loopful from the surface of the APW onto a second plate of selective medium. The inoculated plates are examined after overnight incubation at 37°C. On **MacConkey medium**, they form translucent colonies, on **GTTA medium** they form translucent colonies with greyish-black centre and a turbid halo, and on **TCBS**, they form yellow colonies. Do the Gram staining from the suspected colonies and look for Gram-negative curved or comma-shaped rods. Perform motility and oxidase tests. Cholera vibrios show characteristic motility and are oxidase-positive.
3. Pick up oxidase-positive colonies with a straight wire and test by slide agglutination with *V. cholerae* O1 antiserum.

If positive, the test is repeated using monospecific Ogawa and Inaba antisera. Hikojima strains will agglutinate well with both Ogawa and Inaba antisera. If agglutination is negative with one colony, repeat the test with at least five more colonies as O1 and non-O1 vibrios may co-exist in the same specimen. When the isolated strain is not agglutinated by *V. cholerae* O1 antiserum, it should be tested for agglutination with *V. cholerae* H antiserum. Any vibrio which is agglutinated by H antiserum and not by O1 antiserum is considered to be serogroup O2–O138, because H antigen is shared by all serogroups of *V. cholerae*. It should then be tested with other O antisera to establish their identity as belonging to one of O2–O138 serogroups.

4. For determination of the biotype of the O1 isolate, do VP test, agglutination of fowl RBCs, haemolysis of sheep RBCs, and sensitivity to polymyxin B, Mukerjee phages IV and V (Table 33.1).

Rapid diagnosis

For rapid diagnosis, the characteristic motility of the *Vibrio* and its inhibition by antiserum can be demonstrated under the dark-field or phase-contrast microscope, using stool from acute cases or more reliably after enrichment for 6 hours.

V. cholerae non-O1

V. cholerae serogroups O2–O138 are known as *V. cholerae* non-O1, NCV or NAG vibrios. They resemble *V. cholerae* O1 biochemically and genetically. They occur widely in aquatic environments. They may produce enterotoxins, cytotoxins, haemolysins and colonizing factors. Exposure to saline environments or consumption of seafoods may lead to infection with these organisms. They may cause mild to severe diarrhoeal disease resembling cholera. Occasionally, they may lead to bloody diarrhoea, accompanied by abdominal cramps. In addition, they may cause extraintestinal infections such as wound infections, septicaemia and meningitis.

Pseudomonas aeruginosa

Morphology

It is a slender, Gram-negative bacillus, 1.5–3.0 μm × 0.5 μm, actively motile by a polar flagellum. Occasional strains have two or three flagella. Clinical isolates often possess pili. It is non-capsulated but many strains have a mucoid slime layer. Mucoid strains, particularly isolated from cystic fibrosis patients, have an abundance of polysaccharide composed of alginate polymer. This forms a loose capsule in which microcolonies of the bacillus are enmeshed and protected from host defences.

Cultural characteristics

It is a strict aerobe and grows well on ordinary media. It can grow over a temperature range of 5–42°C, the optimum temperature being 37°C.

Nutrient agar

After aerobic incubation on nutrient agar at 37°C for 24 hours, the colonies are large, 2–3 mm in diameter, smooth, translucent, irregularly round and emit a characteristic fruity odour. This is due to the production of aminoacetophenone from tryptophan. Mucoid strains often produce copious amounts of an extracellular polysaccharide on agar culture. These strains are particularly common in the sputum of patients with cystic fibrosis.

MacConkey medium

It forms non-lactose fermenting colonies.

Blood agar

Many strains are haemolytic on blood agar medium.

Nutrient broth

It produces a dense turbidity and surface pellicle.

Pigment production

P. aeruginosa produces at least 4 distinct pigments:

1. Pyocyanin

It is a bluish-green phenazine pigment soluble in chloroform and water. It diffuses into the surrounding medium. This pigment is not produced by other species of this genus, therefore, its detection is diagnostic of *P. aeruginosa*.

2. Pyoverdin (fluorescein)

It is insoluble in chloroform but soluble in water. It imparts a yellowish tinge to cultures but this is sometimes not easy to detect unless cultures are examined under ultraviolet light.

3. Pyorubrin

It is a bright red water soluble pigment. It is a phenazine pigment that is insoluble in chloroform.

4. Pyomelanin

It is a brown to black pigment and its production is uncommon. It is chemically unrelated to animal melanin.

Bacteriocin (pyocin) typing

Typing of *P. aeruginosa* based on pyocin production is the most popular method for typing *P. aeruginosa*. The most widely used method is the one described by Gillies and Govan (1966) and later modified by Govan and Gillies (1969). The test strain is inoculated as a one cm wide band across the tryptone soya blood agar plate, incubated overnight at 32°C for pyocin production. The resultant growth is removed by scraping with a sterile glass slide. The residual growth is killed by exposure to chloroform vapours and eight indicator strains (Nos. 1–8) are cross-streaked in parallel lines at right angles to the original inoculum followed by incubation at 37°C for 24 hours.

The pattern of inhibition of the indicator strains determines the type of the strain. Further discrimination among the members of the more frequent types (1, 3, 5, 10 and untypable) can be obtained by subtyping with five additional indicator (A–E) strains. Pyocin typing is easy to perform, results are available by the third day and has a reasonable reproducibility and good discrimination.

Pathogenesis

P. aeruginosa causes:

- Urinary tract infection, when it is mechanically placed into the urinary tract during catheterization.
- Acute purulent meningitis, when it is mechanically placed into the meninges during a lumbar puncture or after cranial injury.
- It is able to multiply on respiratory ventilators and deliver large numbers of organisms directly into the lungs of an already debilitated person leading to respiratory infections like necrotizing pneumonia.
- Septicaemia may develop in persons with leukaemia or persons receiving immunosuppressive drugs and in newborn babies and old debilitated persons.
- In drug addicts, it may cause endocarditis and septic arthritis.
- In addition, it may cause wound and burn infection, chronic otitis media and otitis externa, eye infection and acute necrotizing vasculitis which leads to haemorrhagic infarction of skin and internal organs.

Laboratory diagnosis

Specimens

Specimens to be collected include pus, wound swab, urine, sputum, CSF or blood.

Culture

The specimens may be inoculated on MacConkey agar and blood agar. It may be necessary to use selective media such as cetrimide agar for isolation of *P. aeruginosa* from faeces or other samples with mixed flora such as wound swab. The isolates are identified by their colonial morphology and biochemical characters. The typing of the organisms may be carried out by serotyping and pyocin typing.

Burkholderia mallei

Morphology

It is a small, 2.5 μm × 0.5 μm, non-motile, Gram-negative rod.

Cultural characteristics

It is an aerobe and facultative anaerobe and can grow on ordinary culture media under a wide range of temperature. Colonies are small and translucent initially but become yellowish and opaque on ageing.

Pathogenicity

It is an obligate animal parasite occasionally transmitted to man. In susceptible animals like horses, mules and asses, *B. mallei* produces two types of lesions:

1. *Glanders:* In glanders, respiratory system is affected. The infected animal develops profuse catarrhal discharge from the nose, and the nasal septum shows nodule formation. Later the nodules break down with the production of irregular ulcers.
2. *Farcy:* This follows infection through skin with involvement of superficial lymph vessels and lymph nodes. The lymph vessels are thickened and stand out as hard cords under the skin which are called '**farcy pipes**'.

Guinea-pigs are susceptible. Intraperitoneal inoculation of small amounts of a pure culture in male guinea-pig causes testicular swelling in 2–3 days due to bacillary invasion of the tunica vaginalis. This is known as **Strauss reaction**. This may be followed by death of the animal.

Humans may become infected via skin abrasions or wounds which come into contact with the discharges of a sick animal. Human disease may take the form of an acute fulminant febrile illness or a chronic indolent infection producing abscesses in respiratory tract or skin.

Burkholderia pseudomallei

Morphology and biochemical reactions

B. pseudomallei resembles *B. mallei* but differs in being motile, hydrolyzing aesculin and oxidizing lactose oxidatively.

Pathogenesis

It is found in soil and water particularly in Southeast Asia, the Philippines, Northern Australia, parts of Africa and Central America. Melioidosis occurs in rats, guinea-pigs and rabbits. **Human** infection may occur through inhalation, inoculation or perhaps even by ingestion of foodstuffs contaminated with excreta of infected animals. It may also get transmitted from the animals by the bite of haematophagous insects. Agriculture workers, especially those who work in moist soil (e.g., paddy fields), are particularly prone to infection.

In humans, the clinical manifestations consist of:

- A subclinical infection diagnosed by the presence of specific antibodies.
- Benign pulmonary infection that may resemble tuberculosis.
- Multiple abscesses in various organs and tissues such as lung, liver, spleen, bones, joints, muscles and subcutaneous tissues.
- A fulminating septicaemia with a mortality rate of 80–90%.

B. pseudomallei can survive intracellularly within the elements of the reticuloendothelial system and this ability may account for latency and the emergence of symptoms.

In India, cases of melioidosis have been reported from Maharashtra, Kerala, Tamil Nadu, Orissa, West Bengal & Tripura.

Laboratory diagnosis

The organisms may be detected in very small numbers, as small, bipolar stained, Gram-negative bacilli in exudates and may be isolated from sputum, urine, pus or blood. **IgG and IgM antibody** to *B. pseudomallei* may be detected in patient serum by **ELISA and indirect haemagglutination test**. A **PCR** test has also been developed to detect *B. pseudomallei* genome in pus, sputum and other specimens.

Burkholderia cepacia

Morphology

B. cepacia (previously *P. cepacia*) is a slender, motile, Gram-negative rod. The bacillus accumulates poly-β-hydroxybutyrate as granules, so stains irregularly.

Cultural characteristics

It is aerobic and grows well on nutrient agar optimally at 25–30°C. Most strains do not grow on DCA and cultures on blood agar die in 3–4 days. On prolonged incubation, colonies become reddish-purple due to the formation of a non-diffusible phenazine. It can grow in many common disinfectants and can even use penicillin G as a sole source of carbon.

Pathogenicity

B. cepacia is a plant pathogen causing onion rot. It is a low grade human pathogen and is an important cause of noso-comial infection. It has most often been associated with pneumonia in patients with cystic fibrosis. It has also been reported to cause endocarditis, especially in drug addicts, pneumonitis, urinary tract infections, osteomyelitis, dermatitis and wound infections.

Campylobacter and Helicobacter

CAMPYLOBACTER

The generic name Campylobacter is derived from the Greek word *Kampylos* meaning curved rod. The campylobacters are slender, spirally curved (comma-shaped), Gram-negative rods measuring 0.5–5.0 µm in length and 0.2–0.5 µm in width. They are non-sporing and in old cultures, they form coccal forms. They are motile by means of a single unsheathed polar flagellum at one or both poles. They spin rapidly around their long axes in corkscrew fashion. *C. jejuni* and *C. coli* are among the most rapidly motile bacteria encountered. The campylobacters resemble vibrios in their morphology, polar flagellation and oxidase-positive character, but differ in being microaerophilic, not fermenting sugars and having a lower G + C content of DNA (29–38 mol % as against 39–51 mol % in vibrios).

Genus *Campylobacter* possesses 32 species out of which *C. jejuni, C. coli, C. concisus, C. fetus, C. hyointestinalis, C. lari* and *C. sputorum* are of medical importance. Differential characteristics of these species are given in Table 34.1.

Cultural characteristics

Growth of campylobacters occurs under strict microaerophilic conditions, 5% oxygen concentration being optimal. Under ideal conditions, *C. fetus* and most other campylobacters produce visible growth after 24 hours at 37°C, but well-formed colonies are seen only after 48 hours. *C. jejuni, C. coli, C. concisus, C. lari* and *C. hyointestinalis* grow optimally at 42–43°C. They are, therefore, referred to as the thermophilic group. Colonies of most species are circular and convex but those of thermophilic group, particularly *C. jejuni*, are flat and tend to swarm on moist agar.

Table 34.1. Differential characteristics of medically important species of *Campylobacter* and *Helicobacter*

Property	C. jejuni 1	C. jejuni 2	C. coli	C. concisus	C. fetus* 3	C. fetus* 4	C. hyo-intestinalis	C. lari	C. sputorum 5	C. sputorum 6	C. sputorum 7	H. pylori	H. cinaedi	H. fenne-lliae
Growth at 42–43°C	+	–	+	+	–	–	+	+	v	v	v	–	–	–
Flagellar arrangement	a	m/a	a	m	m	m	m	a	m	m	m	l	a	a
Catalase	+/w	v	+	–	+	+	+	+	+	–	–	+	+	+
Nitrate reduction	+	–	+	+	+	+	+	+	+	+	+	–	+	+
Hippurate hydrolysis	+	+	–	–	–	–	–	–	–	–	–	–	–	–
Urease	–	–	–	–	–	–	–	–	–	–	–	+	–	–
H$_2$S (TSI)	v	–	–	+	–	–	+	–	+	+	+	–	–	–
Susceptibility to														
• Nalidixic acid	S	S	S	R	R	R	R	R	R	R	v	R	S	S
• Cephalothin	R	S	R	R	S	S	S	R	S	S	S	S	S	S

1, *C. jejuni* subsp. *jejuni*; 2, *C. jejuni* subsp. *doylei*; 3, *C. fetus* subsp. *fetus*; 4, *C. fetus* subsp. *venerealis*; 5, *C. sputorum* biovar *faecalis*; 6, *C. sputorum* biovar *bubulus*; 7, *C. sputorum* biovar *sputorum*.

a, amphitrichate; m, monotrichate; l, lophotrichate; S, sensitive; R, resistant; v, variable; w, weak reaction.

* Subsp. *venerealis* can be distinguished from subsp. *fetus* by its failure to grow in the presence of 1% glycine or to produce H$_2$S from cysteine.

Biochemical reactions

The main biochemical activities are shown in Table 34.1. In comparison with other bacteria, campylobacters are biochemically inactive. They do not produce indole and are non-saccharolytic. All species produce oxidase, most species produce catalase and with the exception of *C. jejuni* subsp. *doylei* reduce nitrate to nitrite. Of all the species of *Campylobacter*, only *C. jejuni* has the ability to hydrolyze sodium hippurate.

Pathogenesis

C. jejuni subsp. *jejuni* is the most important human pathogen among the campylobacters. This, along with enterotoxigenic *Escherichia coli* and rotaviruses, ranks as the major cause of **diarrhoeal disease** in the world, particularly in developing countries. All the campylobacters appear to be inhabitants of the gastrointestinal tract of wild and domestic animals, including house pets. Majority of chickens and turkeys are also colonized. Man acquires infection by faecal-oral route. Ingestion of raw milk, partially cooked poultry or contaminated water are common sources of human infections. The infective dose is not known but in volunteer studies, infection has been established with as few as 500–800 bacteria.

The organisms that escape killing by gastric acid colonize near neutral, microaerophilic environment of jejunum and ileum. The infection extends distally to affect the terminal ileum, colon and rectum. *C. jejuni* can produce diarrhoea by following mechanisms:

- It produces a **heat-labile enterotoxin** resembling CT that raises intracellular levels of cAMP leading to watery diarrhoea. The activity of this enterotoxin is neutralized by antiserum against *E. coli* LT and CT.
- Like *Shigella* and *Salmonella*, it **penetrates gut epithelium** leading to oedematous exudative enteritis of jejunum, ileum and colon, with infiltration by polymorphonuclear leucocytes and ulceration of the mucosa. In well-developed infections, mesenteric lymph nodes are enlarged, fleshy and inflamed. There may be a transient bacteraemia. *Heat-labile enterotoxin along with the invasive property of this organism may contribute to the production of the damage.*

The common clinical manifestations are crampy abdominal pain, bloody diarrhoea, chills and fever. The infection is usually self-limited and resolves in 3–7 days. In cases of severe disease, the patient may be treated with oral erythromycin. The convalescing patients may continue to excrete organisms for up to one month.

Laboratory diagnosis

Gram staining

Gram-stained smear of diarrhoeal stool may show characteristic, Gram-negative, curved, S-shaped or long spiral forms and polymorphonuclear leucocytes.

Dark ground or phase contrast microscopy

Wet preparations viewed by dark-ground or phase-contrast illumination may reveal **darting motility**. Stool specimen for *Campylobacter* species may not be processed further unless polymorphonuclear leucocytes are present.

Culture

Faeces or rectal swabs are inoculated on selective media. Selective media for *Campylobacter* species are blood-based and contain antibiotics. In case of delay in inoculation on selective media, a transport medium should be employed. Campylobacters survive for 1–2 weeks at 4°C in Cary-Blair transport medium. Selective media for isolation of *C. jejuni* are Butzler's selective medium, Skirrow's *Campylobacter* selective medium, Preston *Campylobacter* selective medium and Blaser's medium.

Fresh specimens of faeces should be plated directly on the selective medium, but older specimens should first be enriched in an enrichment medium such as the Preston *Campylobacter* enrichment broth, for 24 hours, before plating on selective media. Inoculated plates are incubated at 42°C to favour growth of the thermophilic campylobacters (*C. jejuni, C. coli, C. concisus, C. lari* and *C. hyointestinalis*) over that of other faecal bacteria. If, however, the presence of *C. fetus* is suspected, additional plates should be incubated at 37°C to allow growth of this non-thermophile. Incubation must be done in an atmosphere of 5% O_2, 10% CO_2 and 85% N_2. Well-formed colonies are seen after 48 hours incubation. The growth is identified by Gram staining, motility, oxidase test and biochemical reactions.

HELICOBACTER

These are strict microaerophiles with a spiral or helical morphology. They possess sheathed flagella. Various species included in this genus are – *H. pylori, H. cinaedi, H. fennelliae, H. felis, H. mustelae* and *H. nemestrinae*. Of these, first three (Table 34.1) are medically important.

Helicobacter pylori

Morphology

It is a curved, short, spiral or S-shaped Gram-negative bacterium measuring 3 μm in length and 0.5–0.9 μm in width. **It is motile by means of a tuft of up to 7 sheathed flagella at one pole (lophotrichate)**, while campylobacters have a single unsheathed flagellum. It is non-sporing and on exposure to air it transforms to coccal form.

Cultural characteristics

Like campylobacters, *H. pylori* is microaerophilic. It can grow in an atmosphere of 5% O_2, 10% CO_2 and 85% N_2. It does not grow anaerobically or in air, although many strains can also grow in humidified air with increased (10%) CO_2 content. High humidity is essential for growth, therefore, culture plates should not be dried off after pouring. The optimum temperature for its growth is 35–37°C, some grow poorly at 42°C but none grows at 25°C. It can be grown on moist freshly prepared heated blood (chocolate) agar and Skirrow's *Campylobacter* selective medium. After incubation at 35–37°C in a microaerophilic atmosphere for 3–5 days, *H. pylori* produces circular, convex and translucent colonies.

Biochemical reactions

H. pylori is biochemically inactive in most conventional tests. Notable exceptions are the production of urease, catalase and oxidase. **The urease enzyme produced by *H. pylori* is almost 100 times more active than that of *Proteus vulgaris*.**

Pathogenicity

H. pylori colonizes the surface of the gastric mucosa, especially of the antrum but any part of the stomach may be colonized. The bacteria are present in large numbers in the mucus overlying mucosa where the pH is about 7.0. Colonization extends into gastric glands. It has been isolated from gastric biopsy specimens and occasionally from gastric juices, saliva and bile. **Urease released by *H. pylori* produces ammonia ions that neutralize gastric acid in the vicinity of the organism, thus favouring bacterial multiplication.** Thus, the enzyme urease is important for the colonization of the stomach by this organism.

The pathogenic role of *H. pylori* in peptic ulcer disease, both duodenal and gastric, is well recognized. Up to 95% of patients with duodenal ulcer, and 80% of patients with gastric ulcer are infected with *H. pylori*. Eradication of the organism leads to ulcer healing and a markedly lower incidence of recurrence. *H. pylori* has been classified by the International Agency for Research in Cancer as a **group I carcinogen and definite cause of gastric cancer** and **gastric lymphoma in humans**.

Laboratory diagnosis

Specimen

Biopsy of gastric mucosa is collected.

Microscopy and culture

Biopsy is subjected to Gram staining and culture on chocolate agar and Skirrow's *Campylobacter* selective medium followed by incubation as above. The organism is identified on the basis of its colonial morphology, Gram staining and biochemical characters.

Histopathology

In histological sections stained with haematoxylin and eosin, the bacteria are barely visible. However, Warthin-Starry silver staining shows the organisms most clearly.

Biopsy urease test

Since *H. pylori* produces abundant urease, therefore, it can be detected in biopsy material without having to grow the organism. Biopsy tissue is crushed into 0.5 ml urea solution with an indicator and incubated at 37°C. If *H. pylori* is present, the pH changes within a few minutes to 2 hours due to the production of ammonia.

Urea breath test

Urea tagged with an isotope of carbon is fed to the patient. If the patient's stomach is colonized with *H. pylori*, urea is converted into ammonia and tagged CO_2. The latter appears in the breath where it can be measured.

Serological test

Antibodies to *H. pylori* or its urease can be detected in the patient serum by ELISA test. The titre of antibodies falls after several months if infection is eradicated.

Faecal antigen test

Polyclonal antibodies are used to detect *H. pylori* antigen in faeces.

Polymerase chain reaction

Various DNA probes have been developed for the direct detection of *H. pylori* by PCR in gastric juice, and faeces.

Helicobacter cinaedi

H. cinaedi (formerly known as *Campylobacter cinaedi*) has been isolated from rectal swabs of homosexual men with symptoms of proctitis. It has also been described as a cause of bacteraemia in homosexual men with concurrent tuberculosis, and in HIV-positive individuals and AIDS cases.

Helicobacter fennelliae

H. fennelliae (formerly known as *Campylobacter fennelliae*) like *H. cinaedi* has been isolated from rectal swabs taken from symptomatic and asymptomatic homosexual men. It has also been isolated from an HIV-positive bisexual man with history of intravenous-drug abuse.

35

Legionella Pneumophila

Morphology

L. pneumophila is a Gram-negative, pleomorphic rod. In infected lung or animal tissues, it appears as short rods or coccobacilli measuring $2-5\ \mu m \times 0.3-0.9\ \mu m$ with pointed ends and a tendency to filament formation on solid culture medium. It is non-sporing, non-acid-fast, motile with one or more polar or subpolar flagella, pilated and non-capsulated.

It is Gram-negative but stains less well than most other Gram-negative genera. It may be demonstrated in the tissues by silver impregnation method, immunofluorescence, immunoelectron microscopy or immunoperoxidase staining.

Culture characteristics

L. pneumophila is a strict aerobe with optimum pH and temperature of 6.9 and 35°C respectively. However, it can grow in a temperature range of 29–40°C. It does not grow on ordinary nutrient media but requires the presence of cysteine and iron for primary isolation. It can be grown on buffered charcoal yeast extract (BCYE) agar and Mueller-Hinton medium containing 1% haemoglobin (source of iron) and 1% Isovitalex (source of cysteine).

On BCYE agar, colonies of *L. pneumophila* appear in 2–3 days at 35°C in the presence of 5% CO_2, but with some species primary culture may take up to 10 days and with agar-adapted strains, growth occurs more rapidly. On primary isolation, colonies of *L. pneumophila* reach 1–2 mm in diameter after 2–3 days incubation. They are circular, grey or grey-blue and low convex with a slightly irregular edge. Under the plate microscope, the colonies show 'cut glass' appearance.

Biochemical reactions

L. pneumophila is catalase-positive and oxidase-variable. Sugar fermentation, urease and nitrate tests are negative. It hydrolyzes starch, hippurate and gelatin.

Serogrouping

L. pneumophila possesses both flagellar and somatic antigens. On the basis of direct or indirect immunofluorescence with specific antisera and by slide agglutination, it can be divided into 15 (1–15) serogroups. All these serogroups have been associated with human disease but most infections are due to serogroup 1.

Pathogenesis

The natural habitat of *L. pneumophila* is water. The organisms have been isolated from a number of air-conditioning cooling towers, cooling water systems, domestic hot-water systems in hotels and hospitals, whirlpool spa baths and showers, shower heads, industrial coolants and respiratory ventilators. Contaminated water is believed to be a source of infection for those inhaling mist from such sources. Following entry into the alveoli through aerosols, legionellae multiply inside the monocytes and macrophages. Dissemination occurs by endobronchial, haematogenous, lymphatic and contiguous spread.

Outbreaks have also occurred in areas where excavation has taken place. It is, therefore, believed that the organisms may reside in soil and may be transmitted to man by contaminated dust. It has also been shown that *L. pneumophila* may be engulfed by, and survive within, free-living amoebae. When these amoebae form cysts, then the organisms are protected from drying and disinfectants. Person to person spread has not been demonstrated.

Legionella infection may occur in two main forms:

1. **Legionnaires' disease:** It is a pneumonia which may also progress to involve virtually every system of the body including the kidney, heart and central nervous system. After an incubation period of 2–10 days, patient develops malaise, fever, myalgia, headache, confusion, respiratory distress and non-productive cough. Reported death rate

varies from 20% to more than 50% in immunologically deficient patients.

Incidence of Legionnaires' disease is more in diabetics, alcoholics, smokers, patients with pre-existing lung disease and patients receiving steroid or immunosuppressive therapy. **Pneumonia is the predominant manifestation of *Legionella* disease and places the organism among the top four causes of community-acquired bacterial pneumonia (along with *Streptococcus pneumoniae*, *Mycoplasma pneumoniae*, and *Chlamydia pneumoniae*).**

2. **Pontiac fever:** It is a self-limiting, brief febrile influenza-like illness. The disease affects previously healthy people.

Laboratory diagnosis

The tests employed in diagnosis of *Legionella* infection include the following:

1. Microscopy

Legionellae can be detected in the clinical specimens such as sputum, bronchial aspirate or washings, pleural fluid and lung biopsy or autopsy material, by fluorescent antibody technique, with labelled specific monoclonal or polyclonal antisera. Gram-stained films are of little value because legionellae stain poorly. However, the presence of poorly staining Gram-negative rods in a normally sterile site may suggest the presence of legionellae.

2. Culture

The clinical specimen is inoculated on BCYE agar and BCYE agar containing selective agents – vancomycin, polymyxin B and an antifungal agent such as anisomycin. Contaminated materials such as sputum or postmortem material may be heated at 50°C for 30 minutes in order to diminish growth of other less heat-stable respiratory tract organisms which may inhibit the growth of legionellae. The culture plates are incubated at 35°C in the presence of 5% CO_2 for up to 10 days. The cultures are identified by colonial morphology and by fluorescent antibody technique as above.

3. Detection of Legionella antigen

Legionella antigen in the urine can be detected by enzyme-linked immunosorbent assay (ELISA). This is a rapid and specific test for the identification of *L. pneumophila* as the likely cause of pneumonia. This antigen can also be detected by latex agglutination test.

4. Detection of Legionella antibodies

Antibodies of *L. pneumophila* develop 6–8 days after the clinical onset of the illness, and can be detected by ELISA and indirect fluorescent antibody test with heat-fixed or formalin-fixed antigens. A four-fold or greater rise in antibody titre or a high titre (>256) of antibody in a sample taken late in the illness may be considered diagnostic.

36

Haemophilus and Bordetella

Haemophilus influenzae

Morphology

H. influenzae is a slender, short (1.5 μm × 0.3 μm), non-motile, non-sporing, Gram-negative rod or coccobacillus. It exhibits considerable pleomorphism. In sputum, it usually occurs as clusters of coccobacillary forms, while in the CSF from meningitis cases, long bacillary and filamentous forms predominate. Cells from young cultures are usually cocco-bacillary, while older cultures are distinctly pleomorphic. The organisms are somewhat difficult to stain. Staining for 5–15 minutes with dilute carbol fuchsin or Loeffler's methylene blue often gives satisfactory results. Strains isolated from acute infections are often capsulated. Capsule can be demonstrated by **India ink wet films** and by **Quellung reaction** with type-specific antiserum. In Gram-stained direct smear the capsule appears as clear, **nonstaining area (halo) surrounding the organism** in purulent secretions.

Cultural characteristics

H. influenzae has fastidious growth requirements. Accessory growth factors known as X and V, present in blood, are essential for its growth. Therefore, it can grow on blood agar or chocolate agar and not on nutrient agar, which lacks sufficient amount of them. It grows better in aerobic than in anaerobic conditions. Some strains require extra (5–10%) CO_2. The temperature range for growth is 20–42°C, the optimum temperature being 35–37°C.

X factor

It is a heat-stable protoporphyrin IX, haemin or other iron-containing porphyrin. It is necessary for the synthesis of cytochrome and other haem enzymes such as catalase and peroxidase involved in aerobic respiration.

V factor

V factor is a heat-labile (destroyed at 121°C for 30 minutes) factor present in red blood cells and in many other animal and plant cells. It is synthesized by most bacterial species other than *H. influenzae*. It is either nicotinamide adenine dinucleotide (NAD, coenzyme I) or NAD phosphate (NADP, coenzyme II). It is essential for the oxidation-reduction processes in the growing bacterial cell.

Both X and V factors are found within red blood cells including the sheep erythrocytes in sheep blood agar used in clinical laboratories. Sheep blood also contains NADase activity that slowly hydrolyzes V factor. Therefore, ordinary blood agar is not suitable for the growth of *H. influenzae* where it forms only pin-point colonies. Heating blood agar at 80–90°C until it acquires a chocolate colour, results in lysis of erythrocytes, liberation of both X and V factors and inactivation of NADase enzyme that hydrolyzes V factor. Most laboratories rely on chocolate agar for the recovery of *Haemophilus* species from clinical specimens.

When an organism, such as *Staphylococcus aureus* is streaked across a plate of blood agar on which a specimen containing *H. influenzae* has been inoculated, after overnight incubation, the colonies of *H. influenzae* will be large and well developed alongside the streak of *S. aureus*, and smaller farther away (Fig. 36.1). This phenomenon is known as **satellitism**. The lysed erythrocytes in the agar surrounding the *S. aureus* streak provide X factor, and staphylococcal cells themselves secrete V factor during logarithmic growth. The '*Staphylococcus* streak' technique can be used to recover *Haemophilus* species from clinical specimens.

After 24 hour incubation at 35–37°C on chocolate agar, the colonies of non-capsulate strains are usually 0.5–1 mm in diameter, circular, low convex, smooth, pale grey and transparent. They have a characteristic fishy, seminal smell. The colonies of capsulate strains are larger (1–3 mm in diameter), high convex in shape and mucoid.

Good growth is also obtained on certain transparent media where red blood cells have been disrupted and NADase

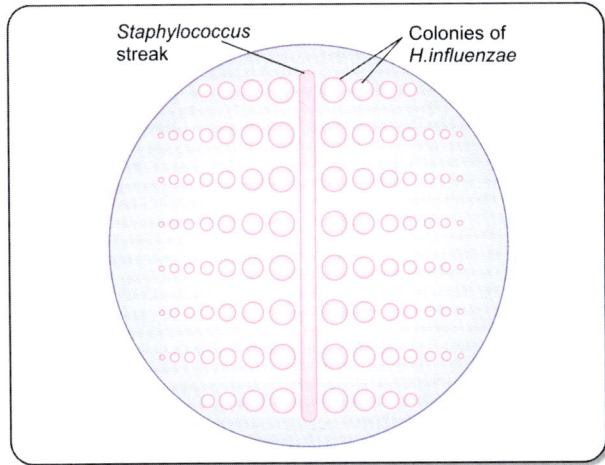

Fig. 36.1. Satellite growth of *Haemophilus influenzae*.

enzyme inactivated either by peptic digest (Fildes agar) or heat (Levinthal's agar). These media are useful for demonstrating capsulate strains, colonies of which are iridescent when viewed obliquely with transmitted light. Type b capsulate strains can also be detected by the presence of precipitin haloes on transparent media containing hyper-immune *H. influenzae* type b antiserum.

Biochemical reactions

H. influenzae is catalase-positive, oxidase-positive, reduces nitrate to nitrite and ferments glucose and galactose. It does not ferment sucrose, lactose and mannitol. On the basis of production of indole and urease, and ornithine decarboxylase activity, *H. influenzae* is divided into 8 (I–VIII) biotypes (Table 36.1). Majority of clinical isolates belong to biotype I to III, and the majority of invasive type b organisms belong to biotype I.

Antigenic structure

Three major surface antigens are present in *H. influenzae* – capsular polysaccharide, outer membrane protein (OMP) and lipooligosaccharide (LOS). Capsular polysaccharide antigen is the major antigenic determinant of capsulated *H. influenzae*,

Table 36.1. Biotypes of *Haemophilus influenzae*

Biotype	Production of		Ornithine decarboxylase activity
	Indole	Urease	
I	+	+	+
II	+	+	–
III	–	+	–
IV	–	+	+
V	+	–	+
VI	–	–	+
VII	–	–	–
VIII	–	–	–

on the basis of which strains of *H. influenzae* have been classified by Pittman into six capsular types – a to f. *Most infections are caused by H. influenzae strains belonging to capsular serotype b* (Hib). These strains are associated with rapidly progressive and even life-threatening infections.

Serotyping of *H. influenzae* is done by **agglutination** or **Quellung reaction** (swelling of the capsule) with type-specific antisera. Non-capsulated strains of *H. influenzae* are antigenically heterogeneous.

Pathogenesis

H. influenzae is an **obligate human parasite**. Twenty five to eighty per cent of healthy adults harbour non-capsulate organisms in the nasopharynx and oropharynx. Colonization by capsulate strains is seen in 5–10%, of which capsular type b strains are found in 1–5%. *H. influenzae* causes invasive and non-invasive infections. The former are caused by capsulate strains, **type b accounting for 95% cases**, and the latter by non-capsulate strains.

I. Invasive infections

Meningitis is the most common invasive infection, followed by epiglottitis, bacteraemia, pneumonia, septic arthritis and cellulitis. These infections occur in children of 2 months to 2 years of age but epiglottitis tends to occur in slightly older children, having a peak incidence between 2 and 4 years of age. Immunity in the neonate is probably acquired by transplacental antibodies that are lost within the first few months of life. Therefore, these infections are unusual in the first 2 months of life and common thereafter up to 2–4 years of age. Antibodies generally reappear later, following exposure to type b and other organisms and these infections become less common.

II. Non-invasive infections

H. influenzae produces a number of local infections. These include otitis media, sinusitis, chronic bronchitis and bronchiectasis. Acute sinusitis and otitis media are usually initiated by viral infections. These predispose to secondary infection with potential pathogenic resident microbial flora. Non-invasive infections are caused by non-capsulate strains of *H. influenzae*.

Laboratory diagnosis

Specimen collection and transportation

Depending upon the type of lesion, *H. influenzae* can be detected in cerebrospinal fluid (CSF), blood, throat swab, sputum, pus, and aspirates from joints, middle ears or sinuses, etc. In cases with epiglottitis, otitis media and pneumonia, it is often difficult to obtain a specimen from the local site of infection. In such cases blood culture should always be done and type b capsular antigen may be detected in body fluids. *As haemophili are poorly viable in clinical specimens particularly at 4°C, therefore, the specimens should never be refrigerated. For optimal yield, specimens should be transported to the laboratory and seeded onto appropriate culture media without delay.*

Direct examination

1. **Gram-stained smear** of clinical material showing poorly stained Gram-negative coccobacilli and occasionally slender filamentous forms should arouse the suspicion of *H. influenzae* infection.
2. **Immunofluorescence** and **Quellung reaction** can be employed for direct demonstration of *H. influenzae* after mixing with specific rabbit antiserum type b.
3. **Type b capsular antigen** can be detected in patient serum, urine, CSF or pus by:
   - **Agglutination of latex particles** (LA) coated with rabbit antibody to type b antigen.
   - **Coagglutination (COA) of *S. aureus* coated with antibody** to type b antigen.
   - **Counterimmunoelectrophoresis** (CIE) with specific antiserum.

Culture

- **CSF culture:** CSF should be promptly plated on blood agar or chocolate agar. A strain of *S. aureus* should be streaked across the plate. It is then incubated at 35–37°C in air with 5–10% CO_2, overnight. The isolate is identified by its colonial morphology, phenomenon of satellitism, Gram staining, biochemical reactions and serotyping. Culture may also be done on Levinthal's medium and Fildes' agar.
- **Blood culture:** Blood culture is usually positive in cases of epiglottitis and pneumonia. Culture may be done in nutrient broth, as it will be enriched with X and V factors from the blood sample itself. For early results culture may be examined after 4–5 hours by Quellung reaction. After overnight incubation, subculture is made on chocolate agar and processed further as above.
- **Throat swab and sputum culture:** For the isolation of *H. influenzae* from throat swab and sputum, antibiotics like penicillin, bacitracin and cloxacillin may be added to the medium to inhibit the growth of normal respiratory tract flora. Sputum should be homogenized by treatment with pancreatin or by shaking with sterile water and glass beads for 10–15 minutes.

Haemophilus ducreyi

Morphology

In the purulent discharge from the ulcerated surface of chancroid or in the pus from lymph node aspirate, *H. ducreyi* appear as bipolar or evenly stained Gram-negative coccobacilli, $1–1.5 \times 0.6$ µm often arranged in groups, whorls or in parallel chains. They may be found inside and outside polymorphonuclear leucocytes. It is not found as a commensal in healthy persons.

Cultural characteristics

H. ducreyi grows poorly on most media. It requires X but not V factor for growth. Several other media have been devised to improve the isolation of *H. ducreyi*. These include 30% rabbit-blood agar, fresh clotted rabbit blood, heated blood agar with 1% IsoVitalex and vancomycin 3 mg/l. The latter is added to inhibit Gram-positive organisms (e.g., staphylococci and streptococci) that may be present as contaminants or superinfecting bacteria in the chancroid lesion. A humid atmosphere and increased CO_2 concentration improve the growth of *H. ducreyi* on primary isolation. Laboratory strains do not require CO_2 for growth. Optimum temperature for growth is 33–36°C. It may also be grown on chorioallantoic membrane of the chick embryo.

After 24 hours incubation, the colonies of *H. ducreyi* are small, pin-point to 0.5 mm in diameter, nonmucoid, grey, yellow or tan, translucent or semiopaque. After 48–72 hours, the colonies are 1–2 mm in diameter and semiopaque.

Biochemical reactions

With the exception of positive nitrate reduction test, *H. ducreyi* is biochemically inert.

Pathogenicity

H. ducreyi is the aetiologic agent of **chancroid, a highly communicable sexually transmitted disease**. It is most prevalent in Africa and Southeast Asia. After incubation period of approximately 4–14 days, a nonindurated, painful lesion with an irregular edge develops, generally, on the genitalia or perianal area. Inguinal lymphadenitis, either unilateral or bilateral, is common and unless treated, often results in inguinal abscess called **bubo**. Genital lesions caused by this organism are also known as **soft chancres** or **soft sores** because they are characterized by nonindurated irregular ulcers whereas primary lesion of syphilis (hard chancre) is sharply demarcated and indurated. In males, the lesions are generally on the penis (Fig. 36.2) and in females they may be present on the labia and within the vagina. **It is likely that the lesions of chancroid facilitate the transmission of human immunodeficiency viruses (HIV-1 and HIV-2).** Chancroid may also spread to other anatomical sites by auto-inoculation.

Laboratory diagnosis

1. Scrape edge of the ulcer or aspirate material from bubo.
2. Prepare the smear, do the Gram staining and look for characteristic Gram-negative coccobacilli.
3. Inoculate heated blood agar with 1% IsoVitalex. To make the medium selective, vancomycin 3 mg/l may be added. Incubate the medium at 33–36°C in a humid atmosphere and 5–10% CO_2 for 2–3 days and look for characteristic colonies.

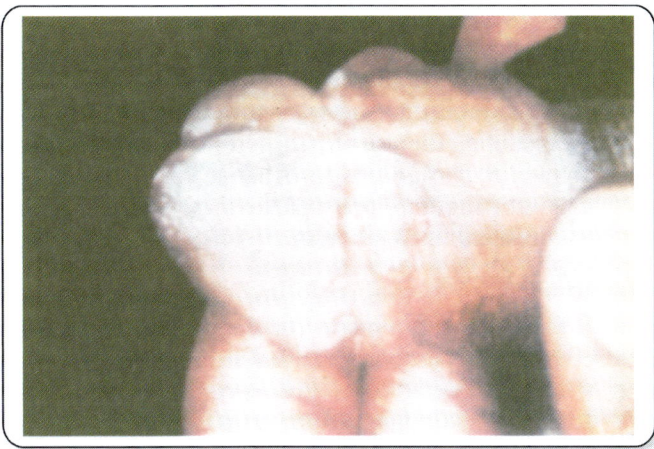

Fig. 36.2. Chancroid caused by *Haemophilus ducreyi* on the penis.

Bordetella pertussis

Morphology

B. pertussis is a small, Gram-negative, coccobacillus, measuring 0.5–2.0 μm × 0.3–0.5 μm, arranged singly, in pairs or in small groups. On subculture, it tends to become pleomorphic. It is non-motile and non-sporing. When freshly isolated it may possess a poorly defined capsule. Fimbriae may be present in freshly isolated strains of *B. pertussis*.

Cultural characteristics

It is an **obligate aerobe**. No growth occurs anaerobically. The optimum temperature for growth is 35–36°C. It **does not require X and V factors** for its growth. However, primary isolation of *B. pertussis* requires the addition of charcoal, ion exchange resins, or 15–20% blood to neutralize growth-inhibiting effects of such substances as unsaturated fatty acids, sulphides and peroxides.

The preferred medium used for the isolation of *B. pertussis* is **charcoal blood agar** to which cephalexin has been added; the antibiotic inhibits other organisms commonly found in specimens and only minimally restricts the growth of *Bordetella* species. This medium is superior to Bordet-Gengou medium in that it supports a heavier growth of the organism on primary isolation, and the colonies are larger. The inoculated medium is incubated at 35–36°C in a humidified incubator. If it is not available, a bowl of water should be placed on the floor of the incubator to provide humidity by evaporation.

Growth of *B. pertussis* is slow. After 3–5 days incubation at 35–36°C, the colonies are small (0.5 mm in diameter), dome-shaped, smooth, opaque, greyish-white with a shiny surface resembling **'bisected pearls'** or **'mercury drops'**.

Pathogenesis

B. pertussis causes the syndrome called **pertussis** or **'whooping cough'**. All age groups are susceptible but 80% of clinical cases occur in children under the age of ten. **B. pertussis is an obligate human parasite** involving primarily the ciliated epithelial cells of bronchi and trachea. They cause damage to cilia and, consequently, initiate the irritation that induces increased secretion of mucus which acts as a stimulus for **paroxysmal cough and bronchospasm**. The source of infection is the patient in the early stage. There is no healthy carrier. The organism is acquired through **droplet infection and is highly contagious**, with an attack rate of more than 90% in nonimmunized individuals. The clinical illness can be divided into three stages:

1. Prodromal or catarrhal stage

Infection is initiated 7–10 days after infectious aerosols are inhaled and the bacteria become attached to and proliferate on ciliated epithelial cells. It is characterized by sneezing, mild but irritating cough and little fever. The disease is **highly communicable** at this stage since a large number of organisms are present in the upper respiratory tract. Cultures collected at this time are more likely to be positive.

2. Paroxysmal stage

After 1–2 weeks, the disease enters the paroxysmal stage, in which the cough becomes very violent. During the paroxysm, the patient gets **violent spasms of continuous coughing, followed by a long inrush of air into the almost empty lungs** with a characteristic 'whoop' that gives the disease its name. The paroxysms of coughing may be so severe that cyanosis, vomiting and convulsions follow, completely exhausting the patient. This stage usually lasts 6–8 weeks, though in some cases it may be very protracted.

3. Convalescent stage

Paroxysmal stage is followed by a convalescent stage that lasts an additional 2–4 weeks. During this period, there is a decrease in the frequency and severity of coughing spells.

Laboratory diagnosis

The bacilli are present in the upper respiratory tract most abundantly in the early stage of the disease. In the paroxysmal stage, the bacilli are scanty and during convalescence they are not demonstrable. Antibodies develop late and help only in retrospective diagnosis. Nasopharyngeal aspirate, cough plate, pernasal swab and postnasal swab may be collected.

Nasopharyngeal aspirate

Nasopharyngeal aspirate collected through a soft catheter is the optimal diagnostic specimen.

Cough plate method

A culture plate is held about 10–15 cm in front of the patient's mouth during a bout of spontaneous or induced coughing. During the process of coughing, droplets of respiratory exudates are directly deposited on the medium.

Pernasal swab

B. pertussis can be recovered readily from the nasopharynx by pernasal swab. A calcium alginate swab on a flexible nichrome wire is passed gently along the floor of the nasal cavity until stopped by the posterior wall of the nasopharynx. The swab is left in place for 30 seconds to one minute to allow organisms to adsorb onto the swab. Cotton-tipped swab should not be used because cotton is inhibitory to the organisms. Pernasal swab has replaced 'cough plates' and postnasal swabs because of overgrowth by commensal bacteria. A pernasal swab acquires fewer commensals which can be suppressed by incorporation of methicillin or cephalexin in the medium.

Postnasal swab

A calcium alginate swab on a bent wire is employed to collect posterior pharyngeal wall secretions through oral cavity. West's postnasal swab may be conveniently employed. Contamination with saliva should be avoided for better results.

The specimen is inoculated immediately on charcoal blood agar to which cephalexin has been added and incubated in high humidity at 35–36°C for at least seven days before being discarded as negative. If cough plate has been collected, it should also be incubated in high humidity at 35–36°C. The colonies are identified by microscopy, biochemical characters and slide agglutination. If delay in transport is unavoidable, then the specimen may be transported in Regan-Lowe transport medium. The use of transport medium reduces the isolation rate. *B. pertussis* in nasopharyngeal secretions and organisms growing on culture plates may be identified by **direct fluorescent antibody test**.

Polymerase chain reaction (PCR)

PCR is the preferred method for the direct detection of *B. pertussis* from a nasopharyngeal swab or a nasopharyngeal aspirate.

Serology

Bordetella antibody can be detected in the patient serum by direct agglutination, indirect haemagglutination, complement fixation test and ELISA. However, a negative result does not exclude pertussis because the serological response is often slow and weak especially in very young children. False positive results may occur because of serological cross reactions with organisms such as staphylococci, haemophili, moraxellae and yeasts. For accurate results, paired sera should be examined.

37

Brucella

Brucellae are small, non-motile, Gram-negative, intracellular, coccobacilli that are essentially pathogens of goats, sheep, cattle and pigs. Currently, there are 10 species of *Brucella*, with 4 species most commonly associated with human disease:

1. *B. melitensis* is the classical species of the genus and is usually pathogenic for sheep and goats but other animals like cattle may also be infected. Man is also susceptible to infection with this organism.
2. *B. abortus* infects cattle, usually causing abortions. It may also infect other animals including sheep, goats, horses and dogs. It can also cause brucellosis in man.
3. *B. suis* is a natural parasite of pigs but other animals and man may also be infected.
4. *B. canis* causes abortion in dogs. Occasional cases of infection, with mild pyrexial illness, have also been reported in man.

Morphology

Brucellae are small, Gram-negative, coccobacilli measuring 0.6–1.5 μm in length and 0.5–0.7 μm in width. They are arranged singly, sometimes in end to end pairs, small clusters or short chains of 4–6 bacteria. They are non-motile, non-sporing, non-capsulated and non-acid-fast.

Cultural characteristics

Brucellae are strict aerobes and **many strains of B. abortus are capnophilic, requiring 5–10% CO_2 for growth**. The optimum temperature for growth is 37°C (range 20–40°C). The optimum pH for growth is 6.6–7.4. They may grow on nutrient agar, though the growth tends to be slow and colony size small. Growth is improved by the addition of blood, serum and tissue extracts. Trypticase soy agar, serum dextrose agar, serum potato infusion agar and tryptose agar are employed for cultivation of brucellae. **Addition of bacitracin, polymyxin and cycloheximide to the above media makes them selective.** These can be used for isolation of brucellae from contaminated material. **Erythritol has a stimulatory effect on the growth of brucellae.**

On solid media, after incubation at 37°C for 48 hours, they produce small, low convex, circular, smooth, transparent colonies 0.5–1 mm in diameter. Less fastidious strains, especially of *B. melitensis* and *B. suis* can grow on bile salt media producing non-lactose-fermenting colonies. In liquid media, growth is uniform. A powdery or viscous deposit is formed in old cultures.

Classification

On the basis of CO_2 requirement, H_2S production, urease production, growth in the presence of 20 μg/ml of basic fuchsin and thionin, and agglutination by monospecific sera, human pathogenic brucellae can be divided into four species (Table 37.1).

Biochemical reactions

Brucellae are catalase-positive, urease positive (variable in *B. melitensis*) and usually oxidase-positive but some strains of *B. abortus* are oxidase-negative. Many strains of *B. abortus* produce H_2S from sulphur-containing amino acids. Other species produce it in small quantities or not at all.

Pathogenesis

Brucellae show distinct host preferences. However, they are capable of causing infection in a wide range of host species, including man. *B. melitensis* is the most pathogenic species for man followed by *B. suis*, *B. abortus* and *B. canis*.

Brucellosis is a **zoonosis**. Man acquires infection by:

1. Direct contact with animal tissues. Therefore, farmers, dairy workers, abattoir workers, butchers, live stock producers and veterinarians are particularly at risk.
2. Ingestion of contaminated meat, raw infected milk or milk products.

Table 37.1. Differential characteristics of *Brucella* species and biotypes

Species		CO₂ requirement	H₂S production	Urease production	Growth in the presence of 20 µg/ml of		Agglutination by mono-specific sera against			Common reservoir hosts
					Basic fuchsin	Thionin	A	M	R	
B. melitensis	1	–	–	Variable	+	+	–	+	–	Sheep, goat
	2	–	–	Variable	+	+	+	–	–	Sheep, goat
	3	–	–	Variable	+	+	+	+	–	Sheep, goat
B. abortus	1	+(–)	+	1–2 h	+	+	+	–	–	Cattle
	2	+(–)	+	1–2 h	–	–	+	–	–	Cattle
	3	+(–)	+	1–2 h	+	+	+	–	–	Cattle
	4	+(–)	+	1–2 h	–(+)	+	–	+	–	Cattle
	5	–	–	1–2 h	+	+	–	+	–	Cattle
	6	–	+(–)	1–2 h	+	+	+	–	–	Cattle
	9	–	+	1–2 h	+	+	–	+	–	Cattle
B. suis	1	–	+	0–30 min	–(+)	+	+	–	–	Pig
	2	–	–	0–30 min	–	+	+	–	–	Pig, hare
	3	–	–	0–30 min	+	+	+	–	–	Pig
	4	–	–	0–30 min	–(+)	+	+	+	–	Reindeer
	5	–	–	0–30 min	–	+	–	+	–	Rodents
B. canis		–	–	0–30 min	–	+	–	–	+	Dog

+(–), variable but most strains positive; –(+), variable but most strains negative; h, hours; min, minutes; A, *B. abortus*; M, *B. melitensis*; R, rough *Brucella*.

3. Inhalation of aerosolized organisms.
4. In the laboratory, brucellae may be acquired as a result of accidental ingestion, inhalation, injection, and mucosal and skin contamination.
5. Rarely, the disease may be transmitted from person to person by sexual contact and by the transfer of tissues including blood and bone marrow.

After entering into the body, brucellae enter into the lymphatics and lymph nodes, leading to **lymphadenopathy** and subsequent blood stream invasion. From the blood, the organisms are localized in the reticuloendothelial system particularly in liver sinusoids, spleen and bone marrow. However, they may also localize in many other sites like joints, heart, kidneys, central nervous system and genital tract.

Laboratory diagnosis

I. Culture of brucellae

Blood culture is the most definitive method for the diagnosis of brucellosis. Chances of getting positive blood culture are more if the blood is collected during the pyrexial phase, preferably when the temperature is rising. Because the organisms may be scanty, at least 5–10 ml should be inoculated into a bottle of **trypticase soy broth or serum dextrose broth** and incubated at 37°C in an atmosphere containing 5–10% carbon dioxide. Other materials such as **bone marrow, solid tissue samples or exudates** are also suitable for culture. Bone marrow cultures yield a higher rate of isolation and remain positive long after the blood culture has become negative.

The intracellular localization of *Brucella* within reticulo-endothelial cells may account for the positive cultures from bone marrow aspirates at a time when blood culture from the same patient is negative. Blood culture should be repeated on three successive days. **Subcultures are made every 3–5 days for eight weeks on trypticase soy agar or serum dextrose agar before being discarded as negative.** *B. melitensis* and *B. suis* are more frequently isolated from blood than are *B. abortus* or *B. canis*.

The need for frequent subculture can be avoided by use of a two-phase system or **Castaneda method** of blood culture. In this method, both liquid and solid media are contained within the same bottle (Fig. 37.1). The blood is inoculated into the broth and the bottle incubated in the upright position.

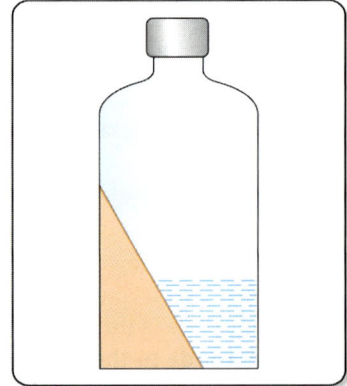

Fig. 37.1. Castaneda blood culture medium.

For subculture, the bottle is tilted, so that the broth flows over the surface of the agar slant. It is again incubated in upright position. In positive cases, colonies appear on the slant. This technique reduces the chances of contamination and risk of infection to laboratory personnel.

II. Serological tests

Blood cultures are positive only in about 30–50% of cases, even when repeated samples are tested. Therefore, serological investigation of the patient is of paramount importance for the diagnosis of the disease. Antibodies appear within 7–10 days of onset of the disease. IgM antibodies appear first. They are rapidly followed and superseded by IgG and to a lesser extent IgA antibodies. These antibodies reach their maximum titres in the third or fourth week of disease and then slowly decline, but they usually persist throughout the active phase of the disease and in some cases long thereafter.

Agglutination test identifies mainly the IgM antibody, while both IgM and IgG can fix complement. During the acute phase of illness when IgM agglutinating antibodies predominate, it is easy to detect agglutination. However, as IgG and IgA antibodies are formed during the course of the infection some of them bind with antigen, thus preventing its agglutination by larger IgM molecule. These IgG and IgA antibodies are known as **blocking** or **non-agglutinating antibodies**.

Brucella antibodies can be detected by a variety of serological tests. The most useful are:

- standard tube agglutination test (SAT),
- 2-mercaptoethanol (2ME) agglutination test,
- Rose Bengal plate test,
- complement fixation test,
- anti-human globulin (Coombs') test,
- enzyme-linked immunosorbent assay (ELISA), and
- radioimmunoassay (RIA).

Standard tube agglutination test (SAT)

The most widely used procedure is SAT. This is a tube agglutination test in which equal volumes of serial two-fold dilutions of (uninactivated) patient serum from 1 in 20 to 1 in 640 and the standardised antigen (heat-killed smooth *Brucella* cells in saline containing phenol 0.5%) are mixed, and incubated at 37°C for 24 hours.

Most patients with acute brucellosis develop agglutinin titres of 640 or more by the end of the third or fourth week of illness. Thereafter, the titre falls. In normal individuals agglutinin titres vary with geographic location and exposure to the organisms, but it is usually less than 1 in 100. A single titre greater than 1 in 160 by SAT is presumptive evidence of recent *Brucella* infection.

Prozone phenomenon is sometimes observed in the agglutination test. This may be due to the antibody excess (therefore, a range of serial dilutions of patient serum should be tested) or due to the presence of blocking or non-agglutinating antibodies. **Blocking antibodies can be detected by anti-human globulin (Coombs') test.** Organisms are exposed to patient serum, incubated for half an hour and then centrifuged, washed and resuspended in normal saline. Washed cells are treated with anti-human globulin which will cause agglutination if blocking antibodies are present in the patient serum.

Agglutination test is usually positive in acute infection, as it mainly detects IgM antibodies, but may only be weakly positive or even be negative in chronic cases. The complement fixation test is more useful in chronic cases as it detects both IgG and IgM. 2ME agglutination test has been reliably used to demonstrate IgG (2ME-resistant) agglutinins. 2ME reduces the disulphide bonds that link IgM molecules to release the subunits.

ELISA and RIA

These tests are very sensitive tests and can distinguish IgM, IgG and IgA *Brucella* antibodies. Therefore, these tests are helpful to distinguish acute and chronic brucellosis.

Rose Bengal plate test

It is a rapid slide agglutination test with a buffered stained antigen. It is widely used as a screening test in farm animals, but also gives good results in human brucellosis. It is not affected by prozones or immunoglobulin switching.

Immunofluorescence

Brucellae may be demonstrated microscopically in pathological specimens by immunofluorescence.

III. Polymerase chain reaction

Polymerase chain reaction with primers specific for the *omp 2*, *omp 25* and *rss-rrl* genes can detect *Brucella* specifically and also give an indication of species and biovar. Promising results have been obtained in clinical studies.

IV. Brucellin test (skin test)

This test, similar to tuberculin test, is no longer recommended as it does not differentiate active from past or subclinical infection. Moreover, intradermal antigen preparations are not readily available and some interfere with serological response to infection.

38

Mycoplasma and Ureaplasma

Morphology and general characters

1. Mycoplasmas and ureaplasmas are smallest free-living bacteria. They range in size for coccoid forms from approximately 0.2–0.3 μm in diameter to tapered rods approximately 1–2 μm in length and 0.2–0.3 μm in diameter. Therefore, they can pass through the bacterial filters.

2. Mycoplasma cell contains minimum set of organelles essential for growth and replication – a plasma membrane, ribosomes, and a genome consisting of a double-stranded circular DNA molecule.

3. They differ from other bacteria, in that they **lack a rigid cell wall** and their cell membrane contains sterols. They are not, however, classified as L forms, which are bacteria that have temporarily lost their cell walls as a result of environmental conditions. L forms do not have sterols in their cell membrane and can form cell walls under appropriate growth conditions.

4. *Mycoplasma, Ureaplasma, Spiroplasma* and *Anaeroplasma* **cannot synthesize their own cholesterol** and require it as a growth factor in the culture medium. However, *Acholeplasma* synthesizes carotenol as a substitute for cholesterol, but will incorporate cholesterol if it is provided.

5. Because they lack a rigid cell wall, they are **extremely pleomorphic** varying in shape from coccoid to filamentous and other bizarre forms.

6. Also, because of the lack of bacterial cell wall containing peptidoglycan, these organisms are **insensitive to cell wall-active antibiotics** such as penicillins and cephalosporins. The mycoplasmas are susceptible to antibiotics, such as tetracyclines and chloramphenicol, that inhibit protein synthesis on prokaryotic ribosomes.

7. They possess a **small genome** (molecular weight $5-10 \times 10^8$ daltons). Therefore, these organisms have limited biosynthetic capabilities. Hence for their cultivation, media enriched with precursors for nucleic acid, protein and lipid biosynthesis, and with the exception of *Acholeplasma*, a sterol component are required.

8. They **multiply by binary fission** (typical of all bacteria), grow on artificial cell-free media and contain both RNA and DNA. Cytoplasmic division may lag behind genome replication. This results in the formation of multinucleate filaments and other shapes.

9. They **do not possess flagella or pili**, but some mycoplasmas including *M. pneumoniae*, exhibit gliding motility on liquid-covered surfaces. This is attributed to specialized tip structures that also help the organisms in the attachment to the host cell.

10. They stain poorly by Gram stain and are Gram-negative. They stain well with Giemsa and Dienes' stain.

11. The organisms of the genus *Ureaplasma* can hydrolyze urea while other genera cannot do so.

12. Most species, on solid media, form characteristic small **'fried egg'** colonies.

Cultural characteristics

Mycoplasmas are aerobes and facultative anaerobes. However, for primary isolation, an atmosphere of 95% N_2 and 5% CO_2 is preferred. They can grow within a temperature range of 22–41°C, the parasitic species growing optimally at 35–37°C. For fermentative organisms, the initial pH of the medium should be adjusted to 7.3–7.8, for arginine-metabolizing organisms it should be about 7 and for ureaplasmas, range of pH should be 6.0–6.5.

A medium widely used for the isolation of mycoplasmas consists of bovine heart infusion broth (PPLO broth) to which are added 20% horse serum and 10% fresh yeast extract along with glucose and phenol red as a pH indicator. High concentration of serum is necessary as a source of cholesterol and other lipids. Growth of *M. pneumoniae* is detected by turbidity and colour change (red to yellow) of phenol red indicator due to fermentation of glucose.

Ureaplasma and other mycoplasmas which do not ferment glucose show only turbidity. This medium can be solidified by the addition of agar. Penicillin and polymyxin B may be added to the medium to inhibit contaminating bacteria and amphotericin B to inhibit contaminating fungi. Since thallium acetate is inhibitory for *U. urealyticum* and *M. genitalium*, and highly poisonous for humans, therefore, it should not be added to the medium. A diphasic medium in screw-capped bottle containing an agar phase that is overlain with broth medium of similar composition may also be used.

Colonies usually appear after incubation for 2–3 days. However, media for isolation of genital mycoplasmas and *M. pneumoniae* should be incubated for 1 and 4 weeks respectively, before a final culture report is made. Initially, the mycoplasma cells multiply within the agar to form an opaque ball-shaped colony that grows up to the surface of the agar and spreads around it forming a translucent peripheral zone. Such a colony presents a **'fried egg'** appearance (Fig. 38.1). Colony size varies from 200–500 μm for 'large colony' mycoplasmas to 15–60 μm for the ureaplasmas. The small colonies of the latter usually lack the peripheral zone.

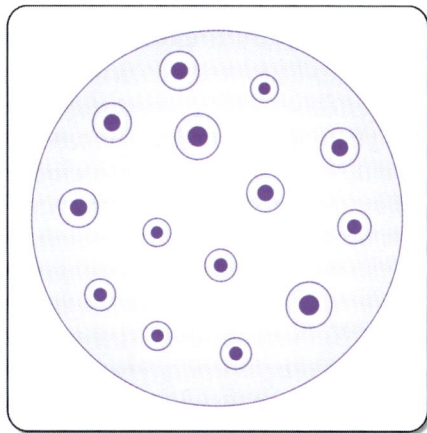

Fig. 38.1. Colonies of *Mycoplasma* on agar, showing 'fried egg' appearance.

Colonies may be seen with a hand lens. However, visualization of colonial morphology is facilitated by application of **Dienes' stain** directly to the agar surface. For this a block of agar containing the colony is cut and placed on a slide. It is covered with a cover slip on which an alcoholic solution of methylene blue azure has been dried.

Mycoplasmas with the fried egg colony morphology appear highly granular and stain with a dark blue centre and a light blue periphery. The agar background appears clear or slightly violet. Mycoplasmas other than *M. pneumoniae* remain stained, but *M. pneumoniae* reduces the methylene blue after a period of time and becomes colourless.

Pathogenicity

Mycoplasmas are **opportunistic infectious agents**. Therefore, the infections caused by these organisms occur more frequently in patients with hypogammaglobulinaemia, Hodgkin's disease, lymphoma, leukaemia, organ transplant and AIDS.

Mycoplasma pneumoniae

1. *M. pneumoniae* (also called **Eaton agent** after the investigator who originally isolated it) commonly causes tracheobronchitis, pharyngitis, sinusitis and **primary atypical pneumonia (PAP)** accompanied by formation of (i) cold haemagglutinins that agglutinate human red cells in cold, (ii) *Streptococcus* MG agglutinins, and (iii) antibodies giving biological false positive Wasserman reaction. Penicillin has no effect on PAP which has served to differentiate PAP from typical pneumonias.

2. *M. pneumoniae* has been shown to produce an exotoxin that is believed to play a major role in the damage to the respiratory epithelium that occurs during acute infection. This toxin, named the **community acquired respiratory disease (CARD) toxin**, is an ADP-ribosylating and vacuolating cytotoxin similar to pertussis toxin. The organism also has the ability to exist and possibly replicate intracellularly, which may contribute to chronicity of illness and difficult eradication.

3. In addition, *M. pneumoniae* may also cause extra-pulmonary lesions such as arthritis, hepatitis, meningo-encephalitis, cerebral ataxia, transverse myelitis, Guillain-Barré syndrome, haemolytic anaemia, myocarditis and pericarditis.

M. pneumoniae is transmitted from person-to-person through airborne transfer of droplets containing the organisms. They attach to epithelial cells in the respiratory tract and multiply. *M. pneumoniae* possesses a membrane-associated 169 kDa protein called PI, which is known to mediate the adherence of this organism to the host cell. It is a surface parasite. **It does not penetrate the epithelial cells of the respiratory tract but remains localized and invasion of blood stream is very rare.**

Incubation period is 1–3 weeks. The onset is gradual. Patient develops fever with chills, malaise, headache, sore throat, nasal congestion and nonproductive cough. The disease is self-limited, recovery occurring in 3–10 days without antimicrobial therapy.

Ureaplasma urealyticum

1. *U. urealyticum* may cause nonchlamydial, non-gonococcal urethritis (NGU), epididymitis, vaginitis and cervicitis. However, *Chlamydia trachomatis* appears to be responsible for 30–50% cases of NGU and cervicitis.

2. Ureaplasmas may cause prematurity, postpartum endometritis, chronic lung disease of the premature infant and infection of wounds and soft tissues.

3. Ureaplasmas are the commonest organisms isolated from the CNS or lower respiratory tract of sick premature or newborn infants.

4. Ureaplasmas have also been blamed to cause male and female infertility and low birth weight but there are conflicting reports.

Mycoplasma hominis

1. *M. hominis* may cause salpingitis, tubo-ovarian abscess, pelvic abscess, septic abortion, puerperal infection, septic arthritis, septic thrombophlebitis, peritonitis and brain abscess.
2. It may cause PAP similar to that caused by *M. pneumoniae* and meningitis in newborn.

Mycoplasma genitalium

M. genitalium has been associated with some cases of non-gonococcal urethritis, cervicitis, endometriosis and pelvic inflammatory disease. Its prevalence is not known, but it may be primarily a resident of the gastrointestinal tract that occurs secondarily in the genitourinary or respiratory tract. It is very difficult to recover from culture and may require 2–3 months of incubation.

Laboratory diagnosis

Laboratory diagnosis of *Mycoplasma* and *Ureaplasma* infections may be carried out by (i) culture and (ii) serological tests.

I. Culture

M. pneumoniae may be recovered from throat swabs, nasopharyngeal swabs, sputum, throat washings, bronchoalveolar lavage, tracheal aspirate and lung tissue specimens. Genital mycoplasmas may be isolated from urethral, vaginal and cervical swabs, semen, prostatic secretions, urine, blood, CSF, amniotic fluid, respiratory tract secretions, synovial fluid, pericardial fluid, and biopsy specimens from endometrium, fallopian tubes, placenta and aborted foetus.

Because of the fastidious nature of these bacteria, the culture media should be inoculated as soon after collection as possible. Standard *Mycoplasma* broth medium dispensed into small vials may be used for transport of swab specimens, while other specimens may be transported in sterile screw-capped containers. In the laboratory, if inoculation is not possible immediately, then the specimen may be held up to 24 hours at 4°C. If delay more than 24 hours is expected, then the specimen should be frozen at –70°C. Urine specimen should be centrifuged and deposit inoculated into the culture medium. If inoculation is not immediately possible, then urine deposit should be diluted with equal volume of transport medium and frozen.

Mycoplasma broth medium, containing penicillin, polymyxin B, amphotericin B, glucose and phenol red as a pH indicator is inoculated with the specimen and incubated at 37°C preferably in an atmosphere of 95% N_2 and 5% CO_2. If specimen contains *M. pneumoniae*, its growth is revealed by turbidity and a colour change (red to yellow) of phenol red, due to fermentation of glucose. It usually occurs in 4–28 days.

Ureaplasmas and other mycoplasmas which do not ferment glucose will show only turbidity. It is then subcultured on agar medium and incubated in air for 5–7 days. *M. pneumoniae* form large (200–500 μm) colonies with a characteristic 'fried egg' appearance, while colonies of ureaplasmas are small, 15–60 μm in diameter and usually lack peripheral zone. Colonies of *M. pneumoniae* may be identified by:

1. **Haemadsorption test:** Colonies growing on the surface of the agar are flooded with 2 ml of 0.2–0.4% suspension of washed guinea-pig erythrocytes suspended in *Mycoplasma* broth medium. The plate is then incubated at 35°C for 30 minutes. It is occasionally rotated during this time. It is then washed with 3 ml of *Mycoplasma* broth medium by gently rotating the plate. Wash fluid is removed by aspiration with a pipette and colonies examined under 50× to 100× magnification. Colonies of *M. pneumoniae* adsorb the erythrocytes to their surface. This is due to binding of the *Mycoplasma* to sialic acid-containing oligosaccharides present on the surface of erythrocytes. However, colonies of *M. genitalium* also share this property.
2. **Tetrazolium reduction test:** Colonies of *M. pneumoniae* appear red when these are flooded with solution of tetrazolium compound which is colourless. *M. pneumoniae* reduces tetrazolium (colourless) to red-coloured compound.
3. **Serological techniques:** These include inhibition of colony development around discs impregnated with specific antiserum, or the fluorescence of colonies treated with such antiserum labelled with a fluorochrome.

II. Serological tests

These are of two types: (a) detection of antigen, and (b) detection of antibody.

(a) **Detection of antigen:** Detection of antigen in respiratory exudates by direct immunofluorescence and counter-immunoelectrophoresis techniques, immunoblotting with monoclonal antibodies and enzyme immunoassay.

(b) **Detection of antibody:**
1. **Cold agglutinins:** Cold agglutinins (IgM antibodies that bind the I antigen on the surface of human erythrocytes at 4°C) can be detected by agglutination of O Rh-negative erythrocytes at 4°C. Cold agglutinins appear about one week after infection with a peak at 4–5 weeks. Thereafter, titre declines rapidly and the test becomes negative after about 5 months. A four-fold rise in cold agglutinin titres or a single titre of 64 or more is suggestive of *M. pneumoniae* infection. However, demonstrable cold agglutinin titres develop in 50% of patients only. Moreover, cold agglutinins are occasionally induced in other diseases such as infectious mononucleosis, rubella, adenovirus infections, psittacosis, tropical eosinophilia, trypanosomiasis, cirrhosis of liver, paroxysmal haemoglobinuria and haemolytic anaemia.

2. *Streptococcus* **MG agglutination test:** In this test, a heat-killed suspension of *Streptococcus* MG is mixed with serial dilutions of patient's unheated serum. The agglutination is observed after overnight incubation at 37°C. An antibody titre of 1 : 20 or more is suggestive of *M. pneumoniae* infection.

3. **Complement fixation test:** This is the most widely used serological test for diagnosis of *M. pneumoniae* infection. The antigen used is a glycolipid from the organism that is extracted by chloroform-methanol. A recent infection is indicated by four-fold or more rise in antibody titre or a single titre of 64 or more.

Complement fixing antibodies appear 7–10 days after infection with the organism and reach peak titre after 4–6 weeks. Such results are obtained in about 80% of cases.

4. **Enzyme immunoassay:** This is more sensitive test than complement fixation test. It can be used to detect specific IgM, IgG and IgA antibodies against *M. pneumoniae*.

III. Detection of specific DNA

Detection of specific DNA by dot blot hybridization and PCR in respiratory exudate.

39

Rickettsia and Orientia

RICKETTSIACEAE

Family Rickettsiaceae has two genera – *Rickettsia* and *Orientia* (Table 39.1).

Table 39.1. Organisms of the family Rickettsiaceae causing human infections

Genus	Species
Rickettsia	• *R. prowazekii*
	• *R. typhi*
	• *R. rickettsii*
	• *R. conorii*
	• *R. australis*
	• *R. sibirica*
	• *R. akari*
Orientia	• *O. tsutsugamushi*

Morphology and general characters of Rickettsia and Orientia

1. The organisms of these genera are small (0.3–0.5 × 0.8–2.0 μm) Gram-negative bacilli. They are non-motile and non-capsulated. The stains commonly used for staining these organisms are Gimenez, Macchiavello and Giemsa. They appear deep red with Gimenez and Macchiavello, and purple with Giemsa stain.
2. They are **obligate intracellular parasites**.
3. They require an arthropod vector as part of their natural cycle and are **transmitted to man by blood sucking arthropods**. They are found in the alimentary canal of arthropods. The species that are pathogenic for humans parasitize endothelial cells almost exclusively.
4. They multiply by binary fission.
5. They possess a trilaminar cytoplasmic membrane and cell wall of bacterial type.
6. They are sensitive to lysozyme and antibiotics.
7. They possess both RNA and DNA.
8. They are large enough to be seen under the light microscope and are held back by bacterial filters.
9. Scrub typhus rickettsiae appear to be fundamentally different and have been placed in a separate genus as *Orientia tsutsugamushi*.

Cultural characteristics

Rickettsiae are **unable to grow on cell free media**. Growth, generally, takes place in the cytoplasm of infected cells, but in the case of spotted fever rickettsiae, growth may take place in the nucleus as well. **Embryonated hens' eggs, inoculated in the yolk sac** during the 5th or 6th day of development, are highly susceptible to infection. Rickettsiae grow in the cells of the membrane surrounding the yolk.

The inoculated eggs are incubated for eight days. Optimum temperature of incubation for most rickettsiae is 35°C and for those of the spotted fever group is 33°C. After incubation, the eggs are harvested and the yolk sac membrane is removed. It serves as an excellent source of organisms for diagnostic antigens and vaccines. Limited growth occurs on the chorio-allantoic membrane also.

They can also grow on **mouse fibroblasts, HeLa, HEp-2, Detroit 6 and other continuous cell lines**, but tissue cultures are not satisfactory for primary isolation of rickettsiae from the patient. They may also be propagated in **arthropods**. **Guinea pig and mice** are commonly used laboratory animals for isolation of *Rickettsia* from patients.

Pathogenesis

Rickettsiae are transmitted to man by the bite or faeces of an infected arthropod vector. On entry into human body, they multiply locally and enter the blood stream followed by multiplication of the organisms in the endothelial cells lining the small blood vessels. This leads to endothelial proliferation and perivascular infiltration which results in thrombosis of the vessel leading to rupture and necrosis.

Diseases caused by various species of *Rickettsia* include typhus fevers, spotted fevers and scrub typhus (Table 39.2).

Table 39.2. Rickettsial diseases of man

Group	Disease	Causative agent	Insect vector	Mode of transmission
1. Typhus fevers	• Epidemic typhus	*R. prowazekii*	Human body louse	Louse faeces scratched into skin
	• Recrudescent typhus (Brill-Zinsser disease)	*R. prowazekii*	—	—
	• Murine typhus	*R. typhi* (syn. *R. mooseri*)	Rat flea	Rat flea faeces scratched into skin
2. Spotted fevers	• Rocky mountain spotted fever	*R. rickettsii*	Ixodid ticks	Tick bite
	• Boutonneuse fever	*R. conorii*	Ixodid ticks	Tick bite
	• Australian tick typhus	*R. australis*	Ixodid ticks	Tick bite
	• Siberian tick typhus	*R. sibirica*	Ixodid ticks	Tick bite
	• Rickettsialpox	*R. akari*	Mites	Mite bite
3. Scrub typhus	• Scrub typhus	*O. tsutsugamushi*	Trombiculid mites	Mite bite

Typhus fevers

This group consists of epidemic (classical) typhus and its recrudescent infection (Brill-Zinsser disease), and endemic (murine) typhus.

Epidemic (classical) typhus

R. prowazekii infects both the human body louse (*Pediculus humanus corporis*) and the head louse (*Pediculus humanus capitis*). Lice become infected by ingesting the blood from a rickettsiaemic human. The rickettsiae multiply in the gut of lice and appear in the faeces after about a week. Lice do not transmit *R. prowazekii* to their progeny but succumb to the infection within 2–4 weeks, remaining infective till they die. Lice are sensitive to temperature. They abandon a host with a body temperature of 40°C or more or the cooling carcass and parasitize other persons.

Lice defaecate while feeding. The feeding process is irritating and scratching by the host produces minute abrasions that function as portal of entry for the rickettsiae in the louse faeces. Occasionally, infection may also be transmitted by inhalation of dried louse faeces containing viable rickettsiae or through the conjunctiva.

After an **incubation period of 10–14 days**, patient develops severe headache, chills, generalized myalgia, high fever (39–41°C) and vomiting. Four to seven days after the onset of illness, a macular rash appears first on the trunk and then spreads to the limbs but sparing face, palms and soles. In the second and third weeks, the patient may become comatosed or delirious. Patient may also develop patchy pneumonia and gangrene of toes, feet, tips of fingers, ear lobes, nose, penis, scrotum or vulva. Mortality rate varies from 10–40% and increases with age.

Brill-Zinsser disease (Recrudescent typhus)

In some individuals who recover from epidemic typhus, **the rickettsiae may remain latent in the lymphoid tissues or organs for years**. Such latent infection may be reactivated, many years later, leading to recrudescent typhus. Lice that feed on a patient with recrudescent typhus can become infected and if conditions are favourable for louse-human-louse transmission, an outbreak of epidemic typhus may result. Therefore, latent human infections, act as a reservoir of *R. prowazekii*.

Brill-Zinsser disease is a milder illness. The duration of disease is shorter (less than two weeks), skin rash is rare, fever is erratic and case fatality rate is lower. Patient develops severe headache, malaise and myalgia.

Endemic (murine) typhus

It is a milder disease than epidemic typhus. It is caused by *R. typhi* (syn. *R. mooseri*). Rat acts as a reservoir and the rickettsiae are passed from rat-to-rat by two of its ecto-parasites, the rat flea (*Xenopsylla cheopis*) and the rat louse (*Polypax spinulosa*), the former is also the vector for man. Rat flea acquires infection by feeding upon a rickettsiaemic rat. The rickettsiae multiply in the gut of the flea. It may infect other susceptible rats and, thus, a natural cycle of flea-rat-flea infection may become established. The flea is not incapacitated and goes on excreting rickettsiae in its faeces for long periods. Infection in flea is not transmitted transovarially.

Man acquires the infection usually through the bite of infected fleas. When infected flea takes a blood meal, it defaecates on the host. The latter rubs the infected faeces into minute abrasions (produced by scratching) that function as portal of entry for rickettsiae in the infected faeces. Infection may also be transmitted by:

1. ingestion of food contaminated with infected rat urine or flea faeces,
2. inhalation of dried flea faeces, and
3. contamination of respiratory tract or conjunctiva, with infective flea faeces.

Man-to-man transmission does not occur. *R. typhi* can be differentiated from *R. prowazekii* by the following tests:

1. *Neil-Mooser or tunica reaction:* When a male guinea-pig is inoculated intraperitoneally with blood from a case of

endemic typhus or with a culture of *R. typhi*, it develops fever and a characteristic scrotal inflammation. The scrotum becomes enlarged and the testes cannot be pushed back into the abdomen because of inflammatory adhesions between the layers of the tunica vaginalis. This is known as Neil-Mooser or tunica reaction. This reaction is negative with *R. prowazekii*.

2. Partial sequence homology with *R. prowazekii*.
3. The two rickettsiae can also be differentiated by IFA, ELISA and PCR-based DNA tests.

Clinically, endemic typhus resembles epidemic typhus but it is usually a mild illness of shorter duration, has fewer complications and has a case fatality rate of less than 1%. Patient develops fever, headache, malaise and myalgia. Macular rash appears on third to fifth day on trunk and spreads to the extremities. As in epidemic typhus, the involvement of palms, soles and face is rare. Untreated, the illness may last up to two weeks.

Spotted fevers

Rickettsiae of spotted fevers possess a common soluble group antigen and grow in both the nucleus and the cytoplasm of infected cells. These diseases include Rocky Mountain spotted fever (RMSF), boutonneuse fever, Australian tick typhus, Siberian tick typhus and rickettsialpox. The infection is transmitted by ticks except in case of rickettsialpox, in which mite is the vector (Table 39.2). *Rickettsiae are transmitted transovarially in ticks and mites which act both as vectors and reservoirs.* Human infection occurs by the bite of an infected tick or mite or by ingestion of food contaminated with their faeces. Rickettsiae do not harm ticks and mites. An eschar frequently develops at the site of tick bite in spotted fevers except RMSF.

Rocky Mountain spotted fever (RMSF)

RMSF is the most serious type of spotted fevers. It is caused by *R. rickettsii*. After an incubation period of about one week, the patient develops fever (39.4–40°C), severe headache, myalgia, anorexia, vomiting, abdominal pain, diarrhoea, photophobia and cough. The rash usually appears on the fourth day of fever, initially on wrists, ankles, palms and soles and then becomes generalized. The rash is maculopapular early in the disease but may later become petechial, and in grave cases, haemorrhagic. In addition to haemorrhagic rash, vascular damage may lead to hypovolaemia, hypotensive shock, hemiplegia and other neurological signs and symptoms, and the patient may die within five days of onset of symptoms. Average mortality in untreated cases of RMSF varies from 6–70%.

Other tick-borne diseases

Other tick-borne diseases, i.e., Boutonneuse fever, Australian tick typhus (North Queensland tick typhus) and Siberian tick typhus (North Asian tick-borne spotted fever) caused by *R.*

conorii, *R. australis* and *R. sibirica* respectively (Table 39.2), resemble RMSF in many respects. All these three rickettsiae are maintained in nature in ixodid ticks and wild animals. Humans only accidentally enter their natural cycle of infection. Diseases produced by these rickettsiae resemble RMSF but are milder. A black spot having a necrotic centre (eschar) is normally present at the site of tick bite in the early stage of disease.

Rickettsialpox

This is a benign febrile disease with a papulovesicular rash resembling that of chickenpox. It is caused by *R. akari* (*akari* means mite). Common house mouse (*Mus musculus*) acts as a reservoir and the rickettsiae are passed from mouse-to-mouse by its ectoparasite, the mite (*Liponyssoides sanguineus*). **The mite infects its progeny transovarially.** As in case of several other rickettsial diseases, humans enter this cycle of infection only accidentally. When murine hosts are scarce, the mite readily attacks humans.

Clinically, patient develops a papulovesicular lesion at the site of bite and the enlargement of regional lymph nodes. This is followed in 3–10 days by fever, chills, headache, malaise and myalgia. About 3–4 days after the appearance of fever, a generalized papulovesicular rash, not unlike the rash in chickenpox appears. The illness lasts for 10–14 days, after which recovery occurs.

Scrub typhus

It is caused by *O. tsutsugamushi*. Scrub typhus normally occurs in a range of mammals, particularly field mice and rats and also birds including migratory birds, all of which can act as host reservoirs. Migratory birds may act as transporters of the disease agent over long distances. The rickettsiae are transmitted from animal-to-animal by trombiculid mites.

In scrub typhus, as in rickettsialpox, RMSF and murine typhus, humans only accidentally enter a natural cycle of rickettsial infection. Trombiculid mites have four-stage life cycles (egg, larva, nymph and adult). The larva (chigger) is the only stage that feeds on vertebrates. Mites lay their eggs in the soil and the larvae hatch later and feed on animals, including humans. After feeding, larvae drop off and metamorphose into nymphs and, subsequently, into adults. The latter two stages are free living in the soil. However, transmission of *O. tsutsugamushi* occurs from larva to nymph to adult and transovarially from adult to egg. Thus, the mite can act both as a vector and as a reservoir for scrub typhus.

After 1–3 weeks of chigger bite, patient abruptly develops severe headache, chills, fever, conjunctivitis, deafness and a characteristic eschar at the site of chigger bite. Spleen, and lymph nodes proximal to eschar enlarge. About one week after the onset of fever, a maculopapular rash appears on the trunk which later becomes generalized. This may be accompanied by stupor and prostration. Case fatality rate varies from 10–60%.

Laboratory diagnosis

It may be carried out by:

1. Isolation of rickettsiae in laboratory animals, embryonated hen's eggs and cell cultures.
2. Direct detection of the organisms and their antigens in clinical specimens.
3. Serology.

1. Isolation of rickettsiae

As rickettsiae are highly infectious, **isolation should be attempted only in laboratories equipped with appropriate safety provisions**. Blood clot ground in skimmed milk or brain heart infusion broth is inoculated intraperitoneally in male guinea-pigs or mice. The inoculated animals are observed for 3–4 weeks. The response of animals to different rickettsial infections vary:

- In RMSF, guinea-pigs develop fever, scrotal necrosis and may even die due to overwhelming infection of *R. rickettsii*.
- In *R. typhi*, *R. conorii* and *R. akari* infection, guinea-pigs develop fever and tunica reaction.
- In *R. prowazekii* infection, the animals develop fever without any testicular inflammation.
- For isolation of *O. tsutsugamushi*, mice are preferred over guinea-pigs. The infected animals become ill and develop ascites.
- Smears from peritoneum, tunica and spleen of infected animals may be stained by Giemsa or Gimenez methods to demonstrate the rickettsiae.
- Rickettsiae can also be grown in the yolk sac of embryonated hens' eggs and cell cultures.

2. Direct detection of the organisms and their antigens

Biopsy specimens from the rash of spotted fever, and chronic hepatitis, impression smears from the organs of infected animals, and endolymph from ticks may be stained with Giemsa, Macchiavello or Gimenez stains and with direct and indirect immunofluorescence techniques. In tissue smears, rickettsiae are usually seen as bipolar rods occurring near cells or free in the cytoplasm. *R. rickettsii* may also be seen within the nuclei of infected cells.

Immunofluorescence technique has the benefits of greater sensitivity and specificity as compared with classical staining methods. The sensitivity of the procedure in the detection of antigens of *R. rickettsii* is approximately 70% and the specificity approaches 100%. By immunofluorescence technique, antigens can also be demonstrated in paraffin-embedded, formalin fixed specimens, if the section is treated first with trypsin to unmask antigens.

Molecular methods

Primers and probes for unique sequences in the genome of the rickettsiae or its plasmids have been synthesized and the sequences amplified by PCR.

3. Serological diagnosis of rickettsial diseases

Serological diagnosis of rickettsial diseases may be done by Weil-Felix (WF) reaction or by specific tests using rickettsial antigens. The latter include:

- Complement fixation test with purified antigens.
- Immunofluorescence on microdots of purified rickettsiae.
- Enzyme immunoassay with particulate or extracted antigens.
- Latex agglutination test.

Complement fixation test is very specific but relatively insensitive for the diagnosis of rickettsial infections. Latex agglutination test is commercially available for the diagnosis of RMSF. It is positive only during an acute infection, so a single positive test is diagnostic.

Weil-Felix reaction

It is an agglutination test which detects anti-rickettsial antibodies that cross react with certain strains of *Proteus*. The basis of this test is the sharing of an **alkali-stable carbohydrate antigen** of some rickettsiae with O antigen of certain non-motile strains of *Proteus* – *P. vulgaris* OX19 and OX2, and *P. mirabilis* OXK. The test may be performed as a microagglutination reaction in microtitre plates with round bottomed wells with haematoxylin-stained antigen or as a tube agglutination test.

Sera from patients with epidemic and endemic typhus strongly agglutinate OX19 and weakly agglutinate OX2. In Brill-Zinsser disease, the test is negative or weakly reactive. In spotted fevers both OX19 and OX2 are agglutinated. OXK agglutinins are present only in scrub typhus (Table 39.3). However, this test is both insensitive and nonspecific. The agglutinins usually appear as early as 5–7 days and reach peak titres of up to 1 : 1,000 or 1 : 5,000 by the end of second week and decline rapidly during convalescence.

Table 39.3. Weil-Felix reaction in rickettsial disease

Disease	Agglutination with		
	OX19	OX2	OXK
Epidemic typhus	+++	+	–
Brill-Zinsser disease	±/–	–	–
Endemic typhus	+++	±	–
Spotted typhus	++	++	–
Scrub typhus	–	–	+++

40

Chlamydia and Chlamydophila

Family Chlamydiaceae consists of two genera – *Chlamydia* and *Chlamydophila*. The genus *Chlamydia* has one species – *C. trachomatis* and the genus *Chlamydophila* has three species – *C. psittaci*, *C. pneumoniae* and *C. picorum* (Table 40.1).

Table 40.1. Classification of Chlamydiaceae

Order	Family	Genera	Species
Chlamydiales	Chlamydiaceae	*Chlamydia*	*C. trachomatis*
		Chlamydophila	*C. psittaci*
			C. pneumoniae
			C. picorum

General characters of Chlamydiaceae

1. They are small, **obligate intracellular**, **Gram-negative bacteria**.
2. They possess both RNA and DNA, ribosomes and cell wall similar to that of Gram-negative bacteria. However, they differ from most true bacteria, in that they do not have peptidoglycan.
3. They lack the ability to produce their own ATP, therefore, they use host's ATP (**energy parasites**).
4. They multiply by binary fission.
5. They are non-motile and stain poorly with Gram, but readily with Giemsa, Castaneda, Gimenez and Macchiavello methods. They stain blue by Castaneda, and red by Macchiavello and Gimenez techniques. Giemsa staining is preferable for staining inclusions in cell culture. Inclusion bodies of Chlamydiaceae are basophilic in nature. Mature inclusions of *C. trachomatis* possess glycogen matrix, therefore, iodine stains them coppery brown. Inclusions of *C. psittaci* do not possess glycogen matrix, therefore, they do not stain with iodine.
6. They can also be demonstrated by direct immunofluorescence staining.

7. They multiply in the cytoplasm of the host cell forming microcolonies or inclusion bodies which drape around the nucleus like a cloak or mantle (*chlamys* means mantle).
8. Most strains of *C. trachomatis* and *C. psittaci* possess plasmid DNA of 7.3 and 6.2 kilobase pairs respectively. However, *C. pneumoniae* does not appear to have plasmid DNA.
9. Like Gram-negative bacteria, the outer membrane of various Chlamydiaceae possess several proteins of which major outer membrane protein (MOMP) has species-specific epitopes.
10. They possess a genus-specific lipopolysaccharide-protein complex antigen.
11. They infect a wide spectrum of vertebrate hosts including birds, mammals and humans.
12. They are susceptible to a wide range of antibiotics such as tetracyclines, erythromycin, macrolides and rifampicin. *C. trachomatis* is sensitive to sulphonamides, but *C. psittaci* and *C. pneumoniae* are not.

Morphology

There are two morphologically distinct forms of Chlamydiaceae, namely **elementary body (EB)** and **reticulate body (RB)**.

- The EB is the extracellular infectious particle. It is a small (200–300 nm in diameter), spherical body in case of *C. trachomatis* and *C. psittaci* and pear-shaped in case of *C. pneumoniae*. It has an irregular electron dense central nucleoid and a rigid trilaminar cell wall similar to the cell walls of Gram-negative bacteria.
- The RB is the intracellular, metabolically active form that divides by binary fission to form EBs. It is 500–1000 nm in diameter and its cell wall is fragile and pliable, leading to pleomorphism.

Developmental cycle

1. Infection is initiated by the attachment of infectious EB to the susceptible host cell (Fig. 40.1). The type and range of susceptible host cells vary with the species and biovar. For example, biovars trachoma and lymphogranuloma venereum (LGV) of *C. trachomatis* infect squamo-columnar epithelial cells and lymphoid cells respectively, while *C. psittaci* infects a wide range of host cells. Specific adhesin and receptors have yet to be identified. It is presumed that epitopes in variable domains of MOMP on the surface of the EB may act as adhesin and a trypsin-sensitive protein on the surface of the susceptible host cell as a specific cell receptor.

2. After attachment, organism enters the host cell within a vesicle. Chlamydiaceae-dependent modification of the endocytic membrane prevents lysosomal fusion and, thus, escapes degradation.

3. By 9 hours after infection, the EB within the vesicle loses its dense DNA core, its cell wall becomes less rigid due to breaking of the disulphide bonds, increases in size and differentiates into RB. It does not possess cytochrome and lacks the ability to produce ATP, therefore, they use host's ATP.

4. By 18 hours, within the enlarging vesicle, the RB divides by binary fission to yield pleomorphic organisms, and genus-specific antigens become associated with the host cell surface.

5. By 24 hours, there is condensation of DNA within the RB, disulphide bonds are formed in the outer membrane proteins and new EBs develop within the vesicle. The developing chlamydiaceal microcolony, within the vesicle, is termed as **inclusion body** which is typically perinuclear and may contain 100–500 EBs.

6. By 40–70 hours, infectious EBs are released from the cell by rupture of the inclusion which may infect new cells.

Susceptibility to physical and chemical agents

Chlamydiaceae lose infectivity within hours at 35–37°C and are inactivated within minutes at 56°C. They are susceptible to alcohols, ether, iodine, potassium permanganate, sodium hypochlorite and silver nitrate at concentrations used for disinfection. They can be preserved at –70°C or liquid nitrogen for months or years.

Antigenic structure

Chlamydiaceae possess the following antigens:

1. Genus-specific antigen

It is heat-stable, complement fixing, genus-specific antigen common to all Chlamydiaceae. It is a lipopolysaccharide resembling the LPS of enteric Gram-negative bacilli.

2. Species-specific protein antigens

These are present at the envelope surface. They help in classifying Chlamydiaceae into different species.

3. Serotype-specific antigens

These are found only in some members of a species. They are located on the major outer membrane proteins and can be demonstrated by microimmunofluorescence. Within each species, particularly in *C. trachomatis*, a number of serotypes (serovars) can be defined. *C. trachomatis* possesses three biovars – (1) those causing trachoma and inclusion

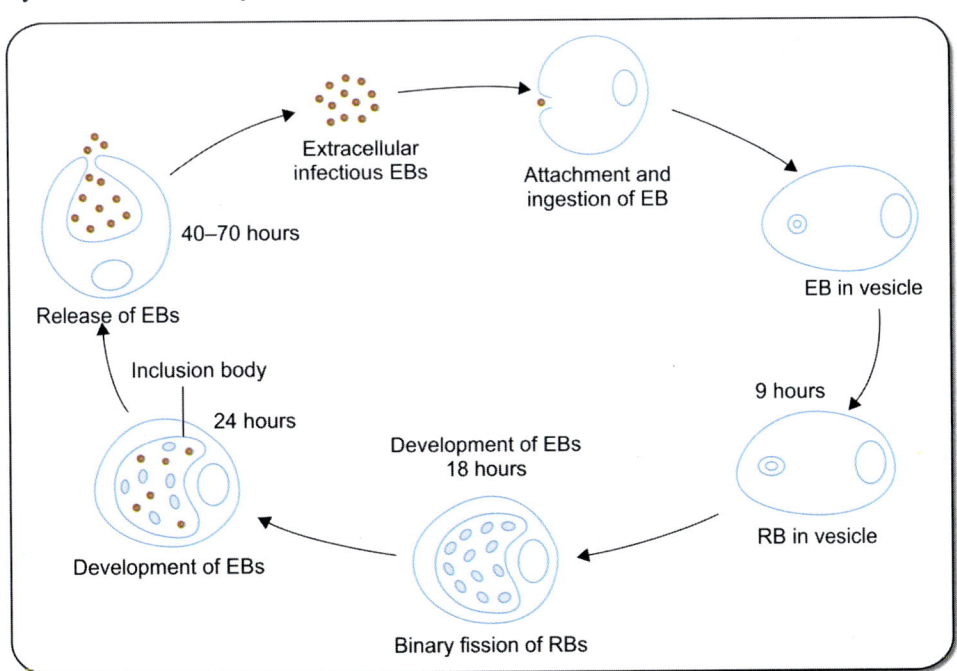

Fig. 40.1. The developmental cycle of Chlamydiaceae.

conjunctivitis (TRIC), (2) those causing lymphogranuloma venereum (LGV), and (3) the one causing mouse pneumonitis (MoPn). Both TRIC and LGV biovars which infect humans can be subdivided into 15 serovars. *C. trachomatis* biovar TRIC has 12 serovars (A, B, Ba, C, D, E, F, G, H, I, J and K) and biovar LGV has three serovars (L1, L2 and L3).

Cultural characteristics

Chlamydiaceae can be isolated (1) by intranasal, intraperitoneal or intracerebral inoculation into mice, (2) in the yolk sac of 6–8-days-old chick embryo, and (3) in cell cultures.

1. Mice

The mice die within 10 days and smears of the lung, peritoneal exudate, spleen or brain show the EBs.

2. Yolk sac

In the yolk sac, the organisms multiply in the endothelial cells and can be detected in impression smears stained by the Giemsa, Macchiavello or Gimenez methods. For the growth of *C. trachomatis* and *C. psittaci*, the inoculated embryonated eggs should be incubated at 35°C and 39°C respectively.

3. Cell culture

Cells that have been irradiated or treated with a metabolic inhibitor are used for isolation of Chlamydiaceae. Cyclo-heximide-treated McCoy cells are the most commonly used cell line, although, *C. pneumoniae* grows better in HeLa or monkey kidney cells. Mouse fibroblast cell lines can also be used for isolation of Chlamydiaceae. *C. psittaci* can even be propagated in fish and lizard cells. The presence of the organism, in the cell culture, is detected by staining for inclusions or elementary bodies.

Pathogenicity

Chlamydiaceae produces infections of eye, and genital and respiratory tracts of man (Table 40.2).

Infections of eye

Trachoma

It is a communicable chronic keratoconjunctivitis characterized by follicles, papillary hyperplasia, pannus formation and in late stages, cicatrization. It occurs only in humans. It is endemic in the Middle East, Africa, India and the Far East. In endemic areas, the prevalence of trachoma is maximum in children below 9 years of age. It is caused by *C. trachomatis* biovar TRIC and serovars A, B, Ba and C. The infection is transmitted from eye to eye by direct contact with fingers or contaminated towels and clothing. Flies may also transmit the infection mechanically. Incubation period of the disease appears to be 7–14 days.

Inclusion conjunctivitis

It is caused by *C. trachomatis* biovar TRIC serovars D–K, natural habitat of which is genital tract of both sexes. It is most prevalent in sexually active young people and is spread from genitalia to eye. The incubation period is 1–2 weeks. The onset is acute, with intense hyperaemia, mucopurulent discharge and follicular hyperplasia. Unlike trachoma, lesions are most pronounced in the lower than in the upper lid. Some patients may develop scarring, corneal lesions or pannus formation. Genital symptoms are minimal or absent particularly in women. Disease is usually self-limiting and does not lead to blindness.

Ophthalmia neonatorum (Inclusion blennorrhoea)

It is the neonatal form of inclusion conjunctivitis. It develops when the infant acquires infection from the birth canal. About 5–12% of all pregnant women have a chlamydiaceal infection of the cervix and 50% of infants born to such mothers develop conjunctivitis. Five to 12 days after birth the neonate develops swelling of the eyelids, hyperaemia and a purulent infiltration of the conjunctiva. A proportion of untreated neonates develop pneumonia.

Table 40.2. Chlamydiaceal infections of man

Site of infection	Disease	Organism	Biovar	Serovar
Eye	• Trachoma	*C. trachomatis*	TRIC	A, B, Ba, C
	• Inclusion conjunctivitis	*C. trachomatis*	TRIC	D–K
	• Ophthalmia neonatorum	*C. trachomatis*	TRIC	D–K
Genital tract				
Male	• Urethritis, epididymitis, proctitis	*C. trachomatis*	TRIC	D–K
Female	• Urethritis, cervicitis, salpingitis, infertility, perihepatitis, periappendicitis, proctitis	*C. trachomatis*	TRIC	D–K
	• Abortion, stillbirth (ovine strains)	*C. psittaci*	—	—
Male and female	• Lymphogranuloma venereum	*C. trachomatis*	LGV	L1–L3
Respiratory tract	• Pneumonitis of infant	*C. trachomatis*	TRIC	D–K
	• Pharyngitis, pneumonia	*C. pneumoniae*	—	—
	• Psittacosis	*C. psittaci*	—	—

Genital infections

Genital infection due to *C. trachomatis* is the most prevalent among the bacterial sexually transmitted diseases. *C. trachomatis* infection, if undiagnosed and untreated, can result in pelvic inflammatory disease, epididymitis, etc., finally damaging the human reproductive tract irreversibly. Further to this, growing evidence indicates that active *C. trachomatis* infection is an important risk factor facilitating sexual transmission of HIV infection. Thus, early diagnosis and treatment of chlamydial infection is important to prevent HIV risk and devastating clinical consequences.

Males

C. trachomatis biovar TRIC serovars D–K account for at least 30% of cases of non-gonococcal urethritis (NGU). This condition develops 7–14 days after sexual intercourse. A minority of cases of NGU are caused by *Ureaplasma urealyticum*. *C. trachomatis* is also responsible for 50% cases of epididymitis in men under 35 years and 15% in men above this age. It may also cause proctitis in homosexual males.

Females

C. trachomatis biovar TRIC serovars D–K may cause urethritis, mucopurulent cervicitis, vaginitis and vaginal discharge, endometritis, salpingitis, infertility, perihepatitis and periappendicitis. Endometritis and salpingitis, singly or together may be referred to as **pelvic inflammatory disease**. Ovine strains of *C. psittaci* can cause abortion and stillbirth.

Lymphogranuloma venereum

C. trachomatis biovar TRIC serovars L1–L3 can cause lymphogranuloma venereum in both males and females. Usually, 1–3 weeks after sexual contact, male patient develops a small (5–8 mm) painless papule or ulcer on the penis. Rectal infections occur in homosexuals. In women, the commonest site is the fourchette. In both sexes, the primary lesions may pass unnoticed. Primary lesions may occasionally occur on extragenital sites such as fingers or tongue. The primary lesion soon heals but after 1–2 months, the regional lymph nodes (inguinal in males and intrapelvic and pararectal in females) become enlarged and tender, and may break open with the formation of sinuses. These enlarged lymph nodes are called **bubos**.

Respiratory tract

Chlamydophila pneumoniae was first isolated in 1965 from a Taiwanese (TW) child thought to have trachoma and later from a case of acute respiratory (AR) infection. It was originally named TWAR and thought to be a variant of *C. psittaci* but later classified as a separate species – *C. pneumoniae*. It appears to be the **third most common cause of pneumonia** following *Streptococcus pneumoniae* and *Haemophilus influenzae*. It causes an acute infection of lower respiratory tract in man. Infection seems to spread from person-to-person without the intervention of an avian host.

Psittacosis is a disease of the birds of the psittacine (parrot) family, transmissible to man. Similar organisms are also present in a great variety of non-psittacine birds including pigeons, ducks and domestic fowl. The disease acquired by contact with non-psittacine birds is known as **ornithosis**. Infection in birds exists as an asymptomatic, latent infection that can become overt following stresses such as caging and overcrowding leading to diarrhoea, mucopurulent respiratory discharge and emaciation. Faecal excretions and nasal discharge contain many organisms and provide the source of infection for other birds and humans.

C. pneumoniae has been implicated as an important factor in **asthma and cardiovascular disease**, where it has been isolated from atherosclerotic tissue. Infection with *C. pneumoniae* has also been established as a risk factor for **Guillain-Barré syndrome**.

Man acquires infection by the inhalation of dried infected faeces of birds. After an incubation period of 1–2 weeks, patient develops clinical disease which may vary from a mild 'influenza-like' syndrome with general malaise, fever, anorexia, rigors, sore throat, headache and photophobia to severe illness with pneumonia, septicaemia, meningo-encephalitis, pericarditis, myocarditis, endocarditis, arthritis or a typhoid-like syndrome with enlarged liver and spleen, and a rash.

Laboratory diagnosis of chlamydiaceal infections

Collection of specimens

For the diagnosis of chlamydiaceal infections ocular, urethral, vaginal and cervical specimens are best collected by scraping the mucosa. In addition, depending upon the site of involvement, blood, respiratory secretions, sputum, lung and other tissues can be collected. In case of LGV, pus from the bubo should be collected. These specimens are processed as under:

I. **Direct detection of chlamydiaceal antigens:**
   1. *Light microscopy:* *C. trachomatis* infection of conjunctiva, urethra and cervix may be diagnosed by demonstrating typical **reniform inclusion bodies** surrounding the nucleus (Fig. 40.2), in the conjunctival, urethral and cervical smears stained with Giemsa, Castaneda or Macchiavello methods and seen under light microscope. Because the inclusion bodies possess a glycogen matrix, therefore, they may be stained with iodine solution also. This method has a low sensitivity.
   2. *Immunofluorescence (IF):* Staining of smears is done with FITC-labelled antibodies (usually monoclonal) against either the species-specific or genus-specific antigen of *C. trachomatis*. The use of the latter will also detect *C. psittaci* and *C. pneumoniae* (Fig. 40.3). It has a sensitivity and specificity of 90% and 95% respectively and it can be done rapidly in less than one hour.

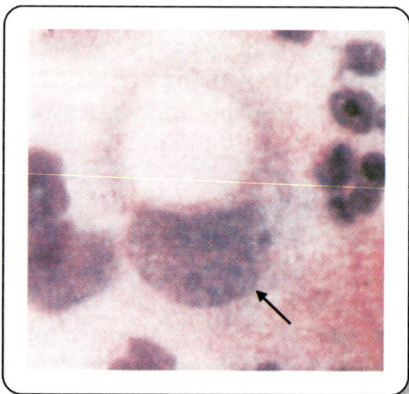

Fig. 40.2. Perinuclear inclusion body of *Chlamydia trachomatis* (Giemsa stain, ×400).

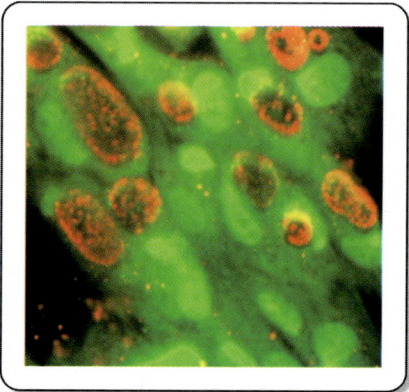

Fig. 40.3. Inclusion body of *Chlamydia trachomatis* under fluorescence microscope (×400).

3. ***ELISA for detection of chlamydiaceal antigens:*** This test is based on detection of soluble genus-specific antigen captured by antibody attached to a solid surface such as plastic bead or microtitre well and then detected with an enzyme-labelled detector system and a chromogenic substrate. The sensitivity and specificity of ELISA is similar to that of IF.

4. ***DNA probes:*** DNA hybridization can be used for detection of *C. trachomatis* DNA in conjunctival and cervical smears.

5. ***Chemiluminescence assay:*** It uses an acridium-ester-labelled single stranded DNA probe, which is complementary to RNA of *C. trachomatis*. The labelled DNA-RNA hybrid is detected in a luminometer which measures light emitted by the acridium ester label. Sensitivity and specificity of this method are 95% each.

6. ***Polymerase chain reaction (PCR):*** Common endogenous plasmid DNA, the *omp1* gene which codes for MOMP and the 16S rRNA gene can be amplified and detected by PCR. This method is more sensitive than culture.

II. **Isolation of Chlamydiaceae:** Chlamydiaceae may be isolated in mice, yolk sac of 6–8 days old chick embryo and in cell cultures.

III. **Detection of chlamydiaceal antibody:**

1. Antibodies against *C. psittaci* and serovars L1–L3 of *C. trachomatis* can be detected by complement fixation test.

2. Antibodies against *C. trachomatis* and *C. pneumoniae* can be detected by microimmunofluorescence, using elementary bodies of standard serovars, immuno-peroxidase and ELISA test.

A high level (> 64) of IgM and a rising titre of IgG are taken as diagnostic. In neonatal chlamydiaceal pneumonia, detection of IgM is diagnostic. Detection of IgG cannot distinguish maternal from neonatal infection. High titres of antibodies against *C. trachomatis* may be seen in acute salpingitis and infertility.

IV. **Skin test:** A skin test (**Frei's test**) is available for the diagnosis of LGV. A heat-inactivated *C. trachomatis* biovar LGV (0.1 ml) grown in yolk sac of embryonated egg is injected intradermally on the forearm and a control prepared from uninfected yolk sac on the other forearm. A positive reaction is indicated by an inflammatory nodule appearing on the test arm in 2 days and reaching a maximum in 4–5 days, measuring at least 7 mm in diameter. This test becomes positive 2–6 weeks after infection and remains positive for several years. Because of the availability of sensitive and rapid tests, it is now discarded.

41

Actinomyces and Nocardia

ACTINOMYCES

Morphology

Actinomyces are Gram-positive, non-motile, non-sporing, non-acid-fast, 0.5–1 μm in diameter. They often grow in mycelial forms and break up into coccoid and bacillary forms. Most show true branching.

Cultural characteristics

They are facultative anaerobes. They grow best under anaerobic or microaerophilic conditions with the addition of 5–10% CO_2. The optimum temperature for growth is 35–37°C. They can be grown on brain heart infusion agar, heart infusion agar supplemented with 5% defibrinated horse, rabbit or sheep blood. Suitable liquid media include brain heart infusion broth and thioglycollate broth which may be supplemented with 0.1–0.2% sterile rabbit serum. Most species show good growth after 3–4 days' incubation, however, A. israelii may take 7–14 days.

Pathogenesis

The Actinomyces causes the disease known as actinomycosis. In man, it is usually caused by A. israelii. The other species – A. naeslundii, A. meyeri, A. odontolyticus and A. viscosus, are very rare cause of actinomycosis. All these species are commensals of the mouth, therefore, endogenous cause of disease. In addition, A. naeslundii, A. odontolyticus and A. viscosus may cause dental plaque and caries.

Actinomycosis is a chronic suppurative disease characterized by peripheral spread to contiguous tissues, rare haematogenous spread, formation of sinus tracts which drain suppurative lesions and presence in the pus of colonies of Actinomyces. These colonies are 0.25–2 mm in diameter, white to yellowish and are known as 'sulphur granules'. There are four important sites of primary infection in actinomycosis:

1. Cervicofacial

About two-thirds of cases of actinomycosis, in man, occur in the cervicofacial region. The primary lesion is usually in the mandible or maxilla and probably occurs by direct extension from a periodontal abscess, a traumatic lesion resulting from neglected carious or broken teeth, dental extraction or accidental fracture of jaw. Maxillary lesions may extend to the orbit, the cranial bones, the meninges and brain.

2. Thoracic

Thoracic actinomycosis commences in the lung probably as a result of aspiration of hyphal fragments of Actinomyces from tooth surfaces or dental caries or of Actinomyces-containing granules which commonly grow in tonsillar crypts without invading tonsillar tissue. The lesions in the lung may involve pleura and pericardium and spread outwards through the chest wall producing multiple draining sinuses.

3. Abdominal

Abdominal actinomycosis begins most often in appendix or rarely as a complication of perforating gastric ulcer or penetration of the mucosa of the colon by an object such as fish bone.

4. Pelvic

Pelvic actinomycosis occasionally occurs in women fitted with plastic intrauterine contraceptive devices.

Actinomycotic cholecystitis and actinomycosis of breast have also been reported by the author.

Laboratory diagnosis

Specimens

Pus, sinus discharge, bronchial secretions, sputum or infected tissues are collected aseptically. These specimens may contain innumerable 'sulphur granules'. The granules may also be present on dressings removed from a draining sinus tract.

A. Microscopy

Pus from suspected cases is shaken with sterile water in a tube. **'Sulphur granules'** settle to the bottom. These are removed with a pasteur pipette. Granules are crushed between two slides and stained with Gram, and Ziehl-Neelsen staining using 1% sulphuric acid for decolourization. The granules are seen to consist of **Gram-positive hyphal fragments** 0.5–1 μm in diameter, sometimes remaining as intact hyphae several micrometers long and rarely with branches, surrounded by a peripheral zone of swollen radiating club-shaped structures presenting a **sun ray appearance**. These clubs are Gram-negative, and are believed to be antigen-antibody complexes. Acid-fast staining shows central part as non-acid-fast and acid-fast clubs.

'Sulphur granules' and mycelia in tissue sections can also be identified by direct **fluorescence microscopy**.

B. Culture

'Sulphur granules' are washed thoroughly in sterile normal saline in a petri dish or tube and crushed in a drop of saline with a glass rod. It is then inoculated on brain heart infusion agar, blood agar and in thioglycollate broth, and incubated both anaerobically and aerobically with 5–10% CO_2 at 35–37°C for up to 14 days. The colonies of *A. israelii* are 0.5–2 mm in diameter, white to grey-white, smooth, entire or lobulated resembling molar teeth (Fig. 41.1). The identity of the isolate may be confirmed by direct fluorescence microscopy and biochemical tests.

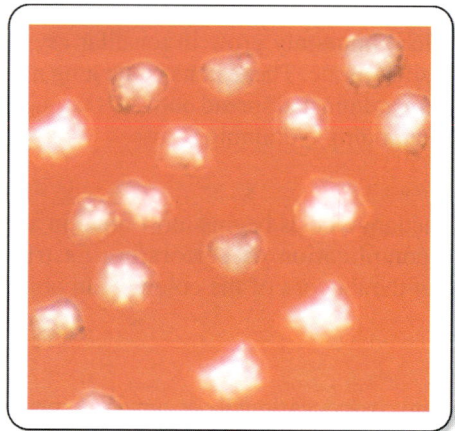

Fig. 41.1. Colonies of *Actinomyces israelii* on blood agar medium. These resemble molar teeth.

C. Biopsy

In haematoxylin and eosin stained sections, the 'sulphur granules' are deeply stained with haematoxylin except in the periphery which is stained with eosin, which shows short, radiate, club-like structures (Fig. 41.2). On Gram staining, the filaments are Gram-positive and periphery Gram-negative. The tissue reaction is a chronic suppurative, fibrosing, inflammatory process.

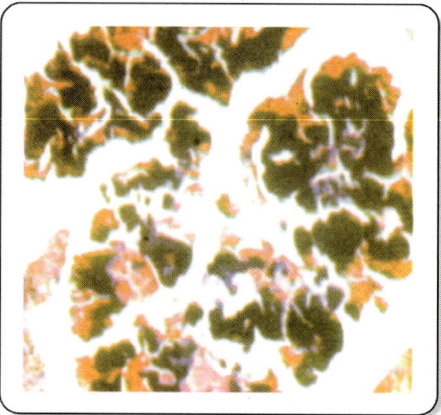

Fig. 41.2. Actinomycosis showing a grain of *Actinomyces israelii*. It is deeply stained with haematoxylin except in the periphery which is stained with eosin (H&E, ×400).

NOCARDIA

Morphology

Nocardiae are strictly aerobic, non-motile, Gram-positive bacteria (Fig. 41.3). They form hyphae that often fragment *in situ* or on mechanical disruption into rod-shaped or coccoid elements. They are acid-fast when decolourized with 1% sulphuric acid (Fig. 41.4).

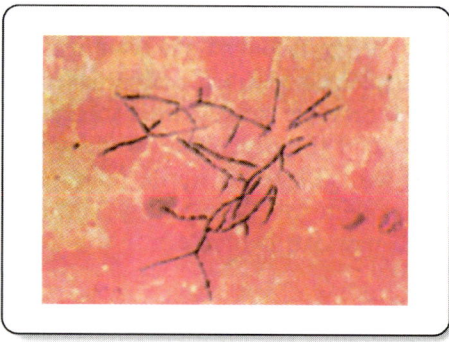

Fig. 41.3. Gram-stained sputum smear showing Gram-positive branched mycelia from a patient suffering from pulmonary nocardiosis (×1000).

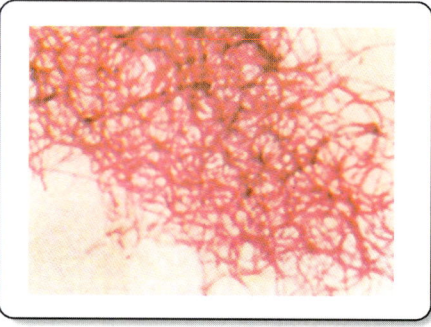

Fig. 41.4. Modified Ziehl-Neelsen staining showing acid-fast filaments of *Nocardia* (×1000).

Cultural characteristics

Nocardiae readily grow on nutrient agar, Sabouraud dextrose agar, brain heart infusion agar and yeast extract-malt extract agar. The inoculated plates should be incubated at 36°C for up to 3 weeks and examined both macroscopically and microscopically for growth every few days. Nocardiae form white, yellow, pink or brown colonies. *A. madurae* produces waxy, heaped, folded, membranous and tough colony. It may be white, tan, pale orange, pink or red in colour.

Pathogenicity

N. asteroides and sometimes *N. farcinica*, *N. nova*, *N. brasiliensis* and *N. otitidiscaviarum* produce opportunistic pulmonary disease known as nocardiosis. It is a systemic bacterial disease. It, generally, originates as a pulmonary infection, varying in its course from mild and slowly progressive to fulminant and fatal. It may be characterized by single or multiple nodules, miliary pattern, scattered infiltrations, bronchopneumonia, abscesses, masses with central cavitation, pleural effusions and empyema. Dissemination from the primary focus of infection may occur through pleural extension, lymphohaematogenous spread or invasion of blood vessels with bacteraemia.

Although, every organ of the body may be affected, involvement of brain, meninges and spinal cord is said to be commoner than that of other parts such as skin, subcutaneous tissues, eye, liver, lymph node, etc. Infection with *Nocardia* organisms is serious. Approximately 40% of the diagnoses are made at autopsy. The mortality rate is high, and those who survive often suffer significant tissue damage.

Localized cutaneous and subcutaneous nocardiosis is encountered less frequently. Infection may occur through contaminated wound and by traumatic implantation. It usually involves feet and hands. The infection begins as a localized subcutaneous abscess that is invasive and quite destructive of the tissues and underlying bone. This lesion is known as **mycetoma**. It is characterized by swelling, draining sinuses, and granules. About half of the mycetomas are caused by actinomycetes and the remaining half are caused by fungi. As the infection progresses, burrowing sinuses open to the skin surface and drain pus. The pus may contain 'sulphur granules' which are masses of filamentous organisms bound together by calcium phosphate. The granules of *Nocardia* species are soft, white to cream coloured, and 0.5–1.0 mm in size.

Laboratory diagnosis

Microscopy

Pus or purulent blood-flecked sputum is spread on a slide by crushing between two slides. The smears are stained by Gram and Ziehl-Neelsen techniques and examined under oil-immersion lens. Granules may be seen in specimens from cutaneous infection. Sampled tissue and pus from the draining sinuses are the specimens of choice for direct examination. The granules may be visualized by separating them from the pus with an inoculating needle and then washing in sterile saline. These may be crushed between two glass slides which are then used for Gram and Ziehl-Neelsen staining.

Culture

Pus, sputum or the granules are inoculated on nutrient agar, Sabouraud dextrose agar and brain heart infusion agar, and incubated at 36°C for 3 weeks. Culture media are examined both macroscopically and microscopically every few days for identification of the isolate.

Nocardia can be isolated from sputum by **paraffin bait technique** by incubating paraffin coated glass rod in sputum for one to six weeks and subculturing the actinomycete from the rod.

Animal inoculation

The mouse, guinea-pig and rabbit are susceptible to experimental nocardiosis and injection of sputum or pus into the peritoneal cavity of mouse may help in the diagnosis.

42

Gardnerella, Erysipelothrix and Streptobacillus

Gardnerella vaginalis

Morphology

G. vaginalis is small (1.5–2.5 μm × 0.5 μm), non-motile, non-sporing coccobacillus. It is Gram-variable, but because the cell wall contains lipopolysaccharide it appears to be Gram-negative. The G+C content of the DNA is 42–44 mol%. Clusters of cells may palisade, giving the appearance of Chinese letters as is seen in case of *Corynebacterium diphtheriae*. Metachromatic granules are produced when the organism is grown in the presence of a fermentable compound or sodium phosphate. The granules appear positive by Gram stain or metachromatic with alkaline methylene blue stain. It is non-motile, non-capsulated and non-sporing.

Cultural characteristics

It is facultative anaerobe; growth occurs in air but is stimulated by 5–10% CO_2. Optimum temperature and pH for its growth are 35–37°C and 6.0–6.5 respectively. It grows on enriched media such as blood agar or chocolate agar. Colonies are β-haemolytic on human and rabbit but not on sheep blood agar.

Pathogenesis

G. vaginalis is a member of the endogenous vaginal flora in up to 69% of women. However, it is present in large numbers in the vaginal secretions of the majority of women with bacterial vaginosis. This condition presents with an increased vaginal discharge with a characteristic 'rotten fish' odour. This becomes more pronounced on alkalization, and can be evoked by placing a drop of potassium hydroxide solution on the fresh exudate on a slide or the speculum used for the vaginal examination. The discharge adheres to the vaginal wall in a thin film that varies from white to grey in colour.

The pH of the vaginal secretions is over 4.5 (normal pH is <4.5). It contains many anaerobes in addition to *G. vaginalis*. There is an absence of other common causes of vaginitis such as *Trichomonas vaginalis* or yeasts.

Laboratory diagnosis

In wet smears bacterial vaginosis yields **'clue cells'** which are vaginal epithelial cells with their surface studded with numerous small bacteria.

Bacterial associates

Bacterial vaginosis is associated with a mixed bacterial flora consisting of *G. vaginalis*, *Mobiluncus mulieris*, *M. curtisii*, *Bacteroides bivius*, *B. disiens*, *Porphyromonas* spp., *Prevotella* spp. and *Mycoplasma hominis*. *Mobiluncus* spp. have been found in the vaginal secretions of over 80% of women with vaginosis but rarely in women without vaginosis. It appears that both the combination of species and their relative numbers are of importance in the development of the syndrome.

Treatment

Oral metronidazole is generally curative.

Erysipelothrix rhusiopathiae

Morphology

The genus *Erysipelothrix* consists of three species, of which *E. rhusiopathiae* is responsible for human disease. It is a slender, non-motile, non-sporing, non-capsulated, straight or slightly curved, Gram-positive rod, measuring 0.8–2.5 × 0.2–0.5 μm with tendency towards formation of long filaments as long as 60 μm.

Cultural characteristics

It is aerobe and facultative anaerobe but growth is improved by 5–10% CO_2. It can grow in the temperature range of 15–44°C, optimum temperature for growth being 30–37°C. It can grow on nutrient agar but the growth is improved by added glucose, serum or blood. On blood agar after 24–48 hours incubation both smooth and rough colonies develop. Smooth colonies are 0.5–1 mm in diameter, circular, convex, translucent and surrounded by a variable zone of α-haemolysis. On tellurite media it produces black colonies.

Biochemical reactions

It is Voges-Proskauer, methyl red, indole production, urease, nitrate reduction and catalase negative. It produces H_2S in Kligler iron agar or triple sugar iron agar and ferments glucose, lactose, fructose, maltose and galactose with the production of acid without gas.

Pathogenicity

In humans, it produces three types of disease – **septicaemia**, **endocarditis**, and **erysipeloid**. **Systemic infection** is very uncommon and rarely develops from localized infection. **Endocarditis** has been seen in patients who have had valve replacement but also in individuals with apparently normal heart valve. **Erysipeloid** is a localized skin infection that resembles streptococcal erysipelas. It usually occurs in persons handling raw meat, fish, animals, birds and crustaceans. The organisms are believed to enter the skin through minor abrasions. The lesions are painful, oedematous and erythematous, usually accompanied by local arthritis, lymphangitis or lymphadenitis.

Laboratory diagnosis

Specimen

A full-thickness skin biopsy from the advancing margin of the lesion.

Culture

It is inoculated into glucose or serum broth and incubated aerobically under 5–10% CO_2 at 35°C. Subcultures are made on blood agar medium at 24 hours intervals. Blood culture should be done in suspected cases of septicaemia and endocarditis.

Streptobacillus moniliformis

Morphology

S. moniliformis is a fastidious, Gram-negative, non-motile, non-capsulate and highly pleomorphic bacillus measuring 1–5 × 0.1–0.5 μm forming chains appearing as filaments with club-shaped swellings (moniiform), giving rise to a 'string of beads' appearance, hence the species name 'moniliformis'. It may lose its cell wall and exist as an L-form.

Cultural characteristics

S. moniliformis is a nutritionally exacting aerobe and facultative anaerobe. Growth is improved by addition of 5–10% CO_2 and a moist atmosphere. Optimum pH and tempe-

rature for growth are 7.6 and 37°C respectively. Growth ceases at 22°C. It can grow on culture media containing blood, serum or ascitic fluid. It grows well on moist Loeffler's serum slope or moist plate of nutrient agar containing 20% horse serum and in 20% serum broth.

After incubation for 2 days, discrete, granular, greyish yellow colonies 1–5 mm in diameter are visible on the surface, while minute **'fried egg'** colonies appear in the depth of the medium. The latter are L-phase variants that have little or no virulence for laboratory animals.

Biochemical characteristics

It is catalase, oxidase, indole production, urease and nitrate reduction negative. It attacks sugars fermentatively and produces acid without gas from glucose, galactose, dextrin, raffinose and starch.

Pathogenicity

S. moniliformis is a normal inhabitant of the nasopharynx of wild and laboratory rats, in which it may cause respiratory, ear or conjunctival infection. It sometimes causes a disease in mice resulting in multiple arthritis and swelling of feet and legs. In humans, it causes streptobacillary **rat-bite fever**. It occurs worldwide and follows the bite of a rat or occasionally a mouse, squirrel, dog or cat. Another type of clinically indistinguishable, rat-bite fever is caused by *Spirillum minus*. In man, the organisms enter the body through the wound caused by the bite of rat or other animals. When the organisms are acquired by ingestion of food, milk or water contaminated by rat excrement it is known as **Haverhill fever**.

After an incubation period of 1–10 days, there is an abrupt onset of chills, fever, headache, muscle aches and vomiting. After about 2 days, fever subsides and an erythematous or petechial rash appears on the extremities mainly on the hands and feet. This is followed by a secondary rise in temperature. During the course of illness, patient may also develop arthritis, endocarditis, pneumonia and brain abscess.

Laboratory diagnosis

Diagnosis of streptobacillary rat-bite fever or Haverhill fever may be made by the isolation of *S. moniliformis* from blood, joint fluid or pus. Mice are highly susceptible to intraperitoneal inoculation of infected material. The animals develop a rapidly fatal generalized condition or a more progressive disease with swelling of feet and legs.

Specific agglutinins may be detected in patient's serum as early as 10 days or as late as several weeks after the rat-bite. As they can also occur in healthy individuals, at least a four-fold rise in titre is needed for diagnosis. ELISA is the method of choice for detecting antibodies.

43

Antimicrobial Sensitivity Testing

Kirby-Bauer disc diffusion test is most widely used and is satisfactory for pathogenic aerobes and facultative as well as rapidly growing anaerobes. These methods have, however, been found to be unsuitable for slow growing microbes.

Medium

The medium must support good overnight growth of test and control organisms. Mueller-Hinton broth and agar may be used for testing aerobic and facultative anaerobic isolates.

Inoculum

The ideal inoculum after overnight incubation gives even semi-confluent growth. Too heavy an inoculum reduces the size of inhibition zones produced by many antibiotics. Isolation of organisms in pure culture is of utmost importance. Using a straight wire, touch the tops of 5–10 similar appearing well isolated colonies on an agar plate. Inoculate them in a suitable broth medium. Incubate at 35–37°C for 4–6 hours when the growth is considered to be in logarithmic phase. Five to ten colonies rather than a single colony, are selected to minimize the possibility of testing a colony that might have been derived from a suspected mutant.

The density of the organisms is adjusted to approximately 10^8 colony-forming units (cfu)/ml by comparing its turbidity with that of 0.5 McFarland opacity standard. McFarland 0.5 standard contains 9.95 ml of 1% sulphuric acid and 0.05 ml of 1% barium chloride. This solution is dispensed into a tube comparable to that used for inoculum preparation. It is sealed tightly and stored in the dark at room temperature. The McFarland 0.5 standard provides a turbidity comparable to that of a bacterial suspension containing 1.5×10^8 cfu/ml.

Control strains

Control strains for Kirby-Bauer disc diffusion method are given in Table 43.1.

Table 43.1. Control strains for Kirby-Bauer disc diffusion method

Test bacteria	Control strain
Coliform organisms	*E. coli* ATCC 25922
Pseudomonas	*P. aeruginosa* ATCC 27853
Haemophilus spp.	*H. influenzae* ATCC 49247
Gonococci	*N. gonorrhoeae* ATCC 49226
Enterococci	*E. faecalis* ATCC 29212
Other organisms that can grow aerobically	*S. aureus* ATCC 25923

Antibiotic discs

Commercially prepared discs 6 mm in diameter may be used. Manufacturers produce discs with accurate antibiotic content. If discs are prepared locally in the laboratory, then pure antimicrobial agents obtained from the manufacturers and not the ones for clinical use should be used. Proper diluents should be used. Disc contents of antimicrobial agents are given in Table 43.2. Discs and disc dispensers should be stored in sealed container with a desiccant. Bulk stock should be stored at –20°C and working ones at <8°C. These should be warmed slowly to room temperature to overcome hydrolysis. Therefore, they should be taken out from refrigerator 1–2 hours before applying on the culture medium.

Drugs to be tested against each species of bacteria should be grouped in sets of seven, the maximum number that can be accommodated on a single 100 mm diameter plate by Kirby-Bauer method. First line tests include those antibiotics that are locally available and commonly prescribed, and reserve for second line tests those antibiotics for which prescription is restricted to special circumstances.

Kirby-Bauer disc diffusion method

Within 15 minutes after adjusting the turbidity of the inoculum suspension to that of standard, dip a sterile nontoxic cotton

Table 43.2. Disc contents of various antimicrobial agents

Antimicrobial agent	Disc content
Benzyl penicillin	
– Staphylococci	1.2 μg
– Pneumococci and meningococci	0.15 μg
Ampicillin	
– Enterobacteriaceae and enterococci	10 μg
– *Haemophilus* and *Moraxella* spp.	2 μg
Amoxicillin/clavulanic acid	
– Enterobacteriaceae and enterococci	20 μg/10 μg
– *Haemophilus* spp., *Moraxella* spp. and staphylococci	2 μg/1 μg
Piperacillin	100 μg
Mezlocillin	30 μg
Azlocillin	30 μg
Cephalothin	30 μg
Cephalexin	30 μg
Cephadroxil	30 μg
Cephradine	30 μg
Cefuroxime	30 μg
Ceftazidime	10 μg
Cefotaxime	10 μg
Cefsulodin	30 μg
Methicillin	5 μg
Carbenicillin	100 μg
Ticarcillin	75 μg
Imipenem	10 μg
Gentamicin	10 μg
Amikacin	30 μg
Tobramycin	10 μg
Neomycin	30 μg
Netilmicin	10 μg
Erythromycin	15 μg
Clindamycin	2 μg
Tetracycline	30 μg
Fusidic acid	30 μg
Chloramphenicol	
– Enterobacteriaceae	30 μg
– Haemophili, pneumococci and meningococci	10 μg
Colistin	10 μg
Nalidixic acid	30 μg
Nitrofurantoin	300 μg
Trimethoprim	5 μg
Trimethoprim/sulphamethoxazole	1.2 μg/23.8 μg
Vancomycin	30 μg
Rifampicin	5 μg
Ciprofloxacin	1 μg

than 15 minutes for surface of the agar to dry before applying the antibiotic discs.

Place the appropriate antimicrobial-impregnated discs on the surface of the agar, using either sterile forceps or multidisc dispenser. After placement, press the disc on the surface of the medium to provide uniform contact. Do not move the disc once it has contacted the agar, because some of the drug diffuses almost immediately. The discs must be evenly distributed on the agar, so that they are not closer than 24 mm centre to centre. On a plate of 100 mm diameter, seven discs may be placed one in the centre and six in the periphery (Fig. 43.1).

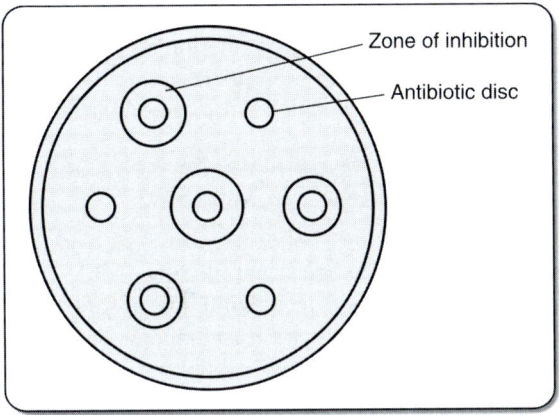

Fig. 43.1. Kirby-Bauer disc diffusion method.

As soon as the antibiotic impregnated disc comes in contact with the moist agar surface, it absorbs moisture from the agar and the antibiotic diffuses into the surrounding medium (Fig. 43.2). The rate of extraction of the antibiotic out of the disc is greater than outward diffusion into the medium, so that the concentration immediately adjacent to the disc may exceed that in the disc itself. However, as the distance from the disc increases, there is logarithmic reduction in the antibiotic concentration. The extent of antibiotic diffusion is also affected by the depth of the agar. The plates are then incubated at 35–37°C for 16–18 hours.

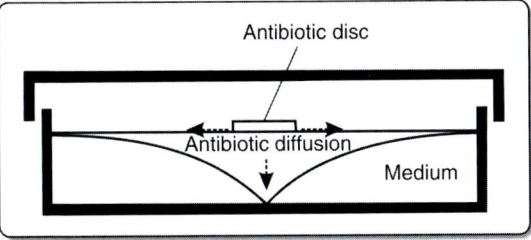

Fig. 43.2. The principle of antibiotic diffusion in agar. The concentration of antibiotic decreases as the distance from the disc increases.

Visible growth of the bacteria occurs on the surface of the agar where the concentration of the antibiotic has fallen below

swab into the inoculum and rotate the swab several times with firm pressure on the inside wall of the tube to remove excess fluid. Inoculate the dried surface of Mueller-Hinton agar plate that has been brought to room temperature by streaking the swab three times over the entire agar surface. Replace the lid of the dish. Allow 3–5 minutes but no longer its inhibitory level for the test strain. Bacterial growth occurs in the form of a circle with middle of the disc forming the centre of the circle. The concentration of diffused antibiotic at the interface of growing and inhibited bacteria approximates to the minimum inhibitory concentration (MIC) obtained in dilution tests.

By using caliper or a transparent plastic ruler, the zones of complete growth inhibition around each of the discs are carefully measured. The diameter of the disc is included in this measurement. The zone size that is observed in a disc diffusion test has no meaning by itself. The interpretation of zone size into susceptible (infection treatable with normal dosage), moderately susceptible (infection that may respond to therapy with higher dosage) or resistant (not treatable with this agent) is based on the interpretation chart (Table 43.3). Reference strains of *S. aureus, E. coli, P. aeruginosa*, etc. should be tested each time a new batch of discs or agar is used.

Determination of minimum inhibitory and minimum bactericidal concentrations

The minimum inhibitory concentration (MIC) is the least amount of antimicrobial agent that inhibits visible growth of an organism after overnight incubation. The minimum bactericidal concentration (MBC) is the least amount of antimicrobial agent that prevents growth after subculture of the organism in antimicrobial-free medium. The uses of determination of MIC are:

1. When equivocal results are obtained with disc diffusion tests.
2. In patients with serious infections, e.g., infective endocarditis.

MIC of an antimicrobial agent may be determined in liquid (Mueller-Hinton broth) or solid medium (Mueller-Hinton agar). Antimicrobial agent is incorporated into the culture medium in the concentrations of 0.25, 0.5, 1, 2, 4, 8, 16, 32, 64, 128 µg/ml, etc. The inoculum is prepared as in case of disc diffusion methods by comparing with 0.5 McFarland opacity standard. For broth dilution, the final inoculum should be 10^5 cfu/ml and for agar dilution method, 1–2 µl of the inoculum is applied on the agar surface. It delivers approximately 10^4 cfu/spot. An organism of known sensitivity should also be titrated. Incubate at 35–37°C for 16–18 hours and read the results. For determination of MIC of methicillin, incubate at 30°C.

MIC is the lowest concentration of antimicrobial agent at which there is no visible growth. For determination of MBC,

Table 43.3. Interpretation chart of zone size in Kirby-Bauer disc diffusion method

Antimicrobial agent	Diameter of zone of inhibition (mm)		
	Resistant	Moderately susceptible	Susceptible
Benzyl penicillin	≤ 28	—	≥ 29
Ampicillin			
– Enterobacteriaceae	≤ 13	14–16	≥ 17
– Enterococci	≤ 16	—	≥ 17
– *Haemophilus* and *Moraxella* spp.	≤ 19	—	≥ 20
Cephalothin	≤ 14	15–17	≥ 18
Cefuroxime	≤ 14	15–17	≥ 18
Ceftazidime	≤ 14	15–17	≥ 18
Cefotaxime	≤ 14	15–22	≥ 23
Methicillin	≤ 9	10–13	≥ 14
Carbenicillin			
– *E. coli* and *Proteus* spp.	≤ 17	18–22	≥ 23
– *P. aeruginosa*	≤ 13	14–17	≥ 18
Gentamicin	≤ 12	–	≥ 13
Amikacin	≤ 14	15–16	≥ 17
Tobramycin	≤ 12	13–14	≥ 15
Erythromycin	≤ 13	14–17	≥ 18
Clindamycin	≤ 14	15–20	≥ 21
Tetracycline	≤ 14	15–18	≥ 19
Fusidic acid	≤ 14	15–18	≥ 19
Chloramphenicol	≤ 12	13–17	≥ 18
Colistin	≤ 8	9–10	≥ 11
Nalidixic acid	≤ 13	14–18	≥ 19
Nitrofurantoin	≤ 14	15–16	≥ 17
Trimethoprim	≤ 10	11–15	≥ 16
Trimethoprim/ sulphamethoxazole	≤ 10	11–15	≥16
Ciprofloxacin	≤ 15	16–20	≥ 21
Piperacillin			
– Enterobacteriaceae	≤ 17	18–20	≥ 21
– *Pseudomonas*	≤ 14	15–17	≥ 18

subculture from each tube showing no growth over a quarter of a nutrient medium free from antimicrobial agent. Incubate and examine them for growth. The tube containing lowest concentration of the antimicrobial agent that fails to yield growth, on subculture, is the MBC of the antimicrobial agent for the test strain.

Bacteriology of Water, Milk and Air

BACTERIOLOGY OF WATER

Water is one of the chief vehicles of gastrointestinal disease. Therefore, water for human consumption must be free from chemical substances and microorganisms which may cause disease in man.

Bacterial flora in water

It can be divided into three groups (Table 44.1):

1. *Natural water bacteria:* This group includes those organisms that are commonly found in water free from gross pollution.
2. *Soil bacteria:* These organisms are not normal inhabitants of water, but are frequently washed into it during heavy rains.
3. *Sewage bacteria:* Many of the bacteria in this group are normal inhabitants of the intestine of man and animals. Others live mainly on decomposing organic matter of either animal or vegetable origin.

Table 44.1. Bacterial flora in water

Natural water bacteria	*Micrococcus, Pseudomonas, Serratia, Flavobacterium, Chromobacterium, Acinetobacter* and *Alcaligenes*
Soil bacteria	*Bacillus subtilis, B. megaterium, B. mycoides, Enterobacter aerogenes* and *E. cloacae*
Sewage bacteria	
• Intestinal bacteria	*Escherichia coli, Enterococcus faecalis, Clostridium perfringens, Salmonella* Typhi and *Vibrio cholerae*
• Sewage bacteria proper	*Proteus vulgaris, Clostridium sporogenes, Zoogloea ramigera, Sphaerotilus natans, Haliscomenobacter hydrossis, Nostocoida limicola, Microthrix parvicella, Flexibacter, Microscilla* and *Nocardia*

Water-borne pathogens

Faecal pollution of drinking water may introduce a variety of intestinal viral, bacterial, protozoal and helminthic pathogens (Table 44.2).

Table 44.2. Water-borne pathogens

Viruses	Hepatitis A virus, hepatitis E virus, poliovirus, rotavirus.
Bacteria	*Vibrio cholerae, Salmonella* Typhi, *S.* Paratyphi A, B and C, *Escherichia coli, Shigella* spp., *Yersinia enterocolitica, Campylobacter jejuni* and *C. coli*
Protozoa	*Entamoeba histolytica, Giardia lamblia, Balantidium coli, Cryptosporidium parvum, Isospora belli*
Helminths	*Ascaris lumbricoides, Enterobius vermicularis, Trichuris trichiura, Echinococcus granulosus*
Pathogens borne by aquatic hosts	*Dracunculus medinensis* and *Diphylobothrium latum* through cyclops and schistosomes through snail

Indicator organisms

The aim of microbiological examination of water is to detect whether pollution by pathogenic organisms has taken place or not. It is impracticable to attempt directly to detect the presence of all the different kinds of water-borne pathogens, any of which may be present only intermittently. Therefore, indicator organisms of human/animal faecal pollution are used.

These organisms should be present in faeces in large number. They should be unable to grow in water. They should be more resistant than pathogens to the stresses of the aquatic environment and disinfection process (chlorination). Various indicator organisms include coliforms (presumptive coliforms), faecal or thermotolerant coliforms, faecal *Escherichia coli*, faecal streptococci (enterococci), sulphite-reducing clostridia, *Pseudomonas aeruginosa* and bacteriophages.

Collection of water samples

Water sample should be collected in heat-sterilized glass bottle of 230 ml with ground glass stopper. To neutralize the bactericidal effect of chlorine in water, it should contain 0.23 ml of a fresh 1.8% aqueous solution of sodium thiosulphate.

1. Sampling from a tap or pump outlet

Clean the tap or pump outlet from outside. Turn on the tap at maximum flow rate and let the water flow for 2–3 minutes. Then open the stopper, fill the bottle, replace the stopper and wrap the bottle in a kraft paper.

2. Sampling from reservoir (streams, rivers, lakes and tanks)

Fill the bottle by holding it at its lower part, submerge it to a depth of about 30 cm below the surface of water. The bottle is then turned, so that the mouth is directed to the current and water flows into the bottle without coming in contact with the hand. If there is no current the bottle should be moved horizontally, the mouth foremost, so that water flows into it. Thereafter, stopper the bottle and wrap it in a kraft paper.

3. Sampling from a dug well

A stone of suitable size is tied with the bottle. Then a clean cord of suitable length is tied with the bottle and lowered into the well. Immerse the bottle completely in the water. When the bottle is filled, pull it out, stopper it and wrap it in a kraft paper. The bottle should not touch the sides of the well any time.

The water sample should be properly labelled with full details of the source, time and date of collection and it should be delivered to the laboratory as quickly as possible, at least within 6 hours, in a cool container and protected from light.

Bacteriological examination

The standard tests usually employed for water bacteriology are given in Table 44.3.

Table 44.3. Standard tests usually employed for water bacteriology

MULTIPLE TUBE TEST
- Total coliform (presumptive coliform) count
- Faecal coliform and confirmed *Escherichia coli* count: Eijkman test
- Count of faecal streptococci
- Count of *Clostridium perfringens*

MEMBRANE FILTRATION TESTS

Total coliform (presumptive coliform) count

This test is called presumptive coliform count because the reaction observed may occasionally be due to the presence of some other organisms. Double strength and single strength MacConkey broth containing bromocresol purple indicator in bottles or tubes containing inverted Durham tubes for indication of gas production is used. Measured amount of water sample is added by sterile graduated pipettes as under:

1. One, 50 ml volume of water to 50 ml double strength medium.
2. Five, 10 ml volumes of water each to 10 ml double strength medium.
3. Five, 1 ml volumes of water each to 5 ml single strength medium.
4. Five, 0.1 ml volumes of water each to 5 ml single strength medium.

The inoculated tubes/bottles are incubated at 37°C for 48 hours. The presumptive coliform count per 100 ml is determined from the tubes/bottles showing acid and gas production using the probability table. The probability table with one 50 ml and five each of 10 ml and 1 ml of water is given in Table 44.4. The presumptive coliform count of water 0, 1–3, 4–10 and more than 10 per 100 ml is interpreted as excellent, satisfactory, suspicious and unsatisfactory for human consumption respectively.

Faecal coliform and confirmed *Escherichia coli* count

Eijkman test

Some spore-bearing bacteria give false positive reactions in the presumptive coliform test. Therefore, it is necessary to confirm the presence of true (faecal) coliform bacilli. After the usual presumptive test, subcultures are made from all the tubes/bottles showing acid and gas to fresh tubes of single strength MacConkey broth warmed to 44°C. These are incubated at 44°C in thermostatically controlled water bath and examined after 24 hours. Those tubes showing gas in Durham tube contain *E. coli*. It can be further confirmed by plating on solid media and testing for indole production and citrate utilization.

Count of faecal streptococci (enterococci)

Subcultures are made from all positive tubes/bottles in the presumptive coliform count into the tube containing 5 ml glucose azide broth. The presence of *Enterococcus faecalis* is indicated by the production of acid in the medium within 18 hours at 45°C. Further confirmation can be done by plating on to MacConkey agar medium. Alternatively, the membrane filtration method may be used, the membranes being cultured on well dried plates of glucose azide agar.

Count of Clostridium perfringens

Varying quantities of water sample are inoculated in litmus milk medium, and incubated at 37°C for 5 days. A typical stormy clot reaction together with acidity confirms the presence of *C. perfringens*. Further confirmation may be made by motility and nitrate reduction test.

Table 44.4. McCrady probability table

Quantity of water	50 ml	10 ml	1 ml	
No. of samples of each quantity tested	1	5	5	
	0	0	0	0
	0	0	1	1
	0	0	2	2
	0	1	0	1
	0	1	1	2
	0	1	2	3
	0	2	0	2
	0	2	1	3
	0	2	2	4
	0	3	0	3
	0	3	1	5
	0	4	0	5
	1	0	0	1
	1	0	1	3
	1	0	2	4
	1	0	3	6
	1	1	0	3
	1	1	1	5
	1	1	2	7
	1	1	3	9
	1	2	0	5
	1	2	1	7
	1	2	2	10
	1	2	3	12
	1	3	0	8
	1	3	1	11
	1	3	2	14
	1	3	3	18
	1	3	4	20
	1	4	0	13
	1	4	1	17
	1	4	2	20
	1	4	3	30
	1	4	4	35
	1	4	5	40
	1	5	0	25
	1	5	1	35
	1	5	2	50
	1	5	3	90
	1	5	4	160
	1	5	5	180 +

(Left column label: Number giving positive reaction (acid and gas). Right column label: Probable number of coliform bacilli in 100 ml of water)

Membrane filtration tests

In this method, a measured volume of water is filtered through a membrane which retains the bacteria on its surface. The membrane is then placed and incubated on a selective indicator medium, so that the indicator bacteria grow into colonies on its upper surface. The number of the colonies is counted and the bacteriological content of water calculated.

Examination for specific pathogens

Specific pathogens such as *Salmonella* Typhi and *Vibrio cholerae* may be isolated from water by employing enrichment and selective media. For isolation of *S.* Typhi, equal volume of water is added to double strength selenite broth followed by incubation and subculture on Wilson and Blair's medium. For isolation of *V. cholerae*, alkaline peptone water (10X) is mixed with nine times its volume of water, incubated and subcultured on bile salt agar. Pathogenic organisms may also be isolated by membrane filtration method already described.

BACTERIOLOGY OF MILK

Milk contains bacteria of different types (Table 44.5) derived from various sources, including the commensal and pathogenic flora of the udder, teat canals and skin, faecal contamination, milkers' hands or milking equipment, storage vessels and water supply particularly when used for adulteration. Bacterial spores, some preformed bacterial or fungal toxins and thermoduric bacteria are not destroyed by pasteurization temperatures. Thermoduric bacteria which survive pasteurization belong to the genera *Bacillus*,

Table 44.5. Microorganisms likely to be present in milk

Microorganisms likely to be present in hygienically produced raw milk
- Coagulase-negative staphylococci
- Micrococci
- Streptococci

Microorganisms likely to be present in milk if the cow has mastitis
- *Staphylococcus aureus*
- *Streptococcus agalactiae* (Lancefield group B)
- *S. dysgalactiae* (Lancefield group C)
- *S. uberis*
- *S. pyogenes* (Lancefield group A)
- *Mycobacterium bovis*
- *Escherichia coli*
- *Leptospira interrogans* serovar *hardjo*
- *S. zooepidemicus* (Lancefield group C)
- *Listeria monocytogenes*
- *Bacillus cereus*
- *Pasteurella multocida*
- *Clostridium perfringens*
- *Nocardia* spp.
- *Actinomyces* spp.
- *Corynebacterium ulcerans*
- *Salmonella* spp.
- *Campylobacter jejuni*
- *Cryptococcus neoformans*

Clostridium, Microbacterium, Micrococcus, Streptococcus and *Lactobacillus*. Therefore, these organisms may be present in pasteurized milk.

Bacteriological examination

Bacteriological examination of milk can be carried out by following methods:

1. Viable count

This is done by plate dilution method. Raw milk may contain 500 to several million bacteria per ml.

2. Coliform count

Varying dilutions of milk are inoculated into 3 tubes of MacConkey broth with Durham tube and incubated at 37°C for 48 hours. Look for the production of acid and gas as the evidence of presence of coliform bacilli. All coliforms are killed by adequate pasteurization and their presence in pasteurized milk indicates faults in pasteurizer or postpasteurization contamination.

3. Methylene blue test

This test is a simple substitute for the viable count. It depends on the reduction of methylene blue by bacteria in milk when incubated at 37°C in complete darkness. The rate of reduction is related to the degree of bacterial contamination. The test is performed by adding 1 ml of standard methylene blue solution to 10 ml of milk in a test tube. The tube is closed with a sterile rubber stopper, inverted twice and incubated in the dark at 37–38°C. The milk is considered satisfactory, if it fails to reduce the dye in 30 minutes.

4. Phosphatase test

Alkaline phosphatase is a normal constituent of raw milk and is inactivated if pasteurization has been carried out properly. The test depends upon the ability of the enzyme to liberate *p*-nitrophenol from disodium *p*-nitrophenyl phosphate and thereby produce a yellow colour that can be quantitated by a colorimeter.

5. Turbidity test

This is a check on the sterilization of milk. If milk has been boiled, all heat coagulable proteins are precipitated. If ammonium sulphate is then added to the milk, filtered and boiled for 5 minutes, no turbidity results. Absence of turbidity indicates that the milk has been heated to at least 100°C for at least 5 minutes.

6. Examination for specific pathogens

(a) **Tubercle bacilli:** Centrifuge 100 ml of milk at 3,000 rpm for 30 minutes and inoculate two guinea-pigs and two slants of Lowenstein-Jensen medium.

   If the milk contains tubercle bacilli, growth of these organisms, in the animals and culture media, can be seen (see Chapter 25).

(b) **Brucella:** *Brucella* may be isolated by inoculating cream from the milk sample on serum dextrose agar. It may also be injected intramuscularly into guinea-pigs. The animals are sacrificed after six weeks and serum is tested for agglutinins and spleen is used for culture of brucellae. Brucellosis in animals can also be detected by demonstrating antibodies against brucellae, by milk ring test and whey agglutination test.

BACTERIOLOGY OF AIR

Since a man respires about 15 metre^3 of air in a day, therefore, the bacterial content of air he breathes, is important, particularly so when the air contains pathogenic organisms. Ventilated rooms commonly show contamination levels between 150–4000 per metre^3. The higher levels are observed when there are many occupants, much bodily movements or dust raising activities. Bacterial content of outdoor air depends on a variety of factors such as density of human and animal population, nature of soil, amount of vegetation, atmospheric conditions such as humidity, temperature, wind conditions, rainfall, and sunlight. Most of the bacteria in the open air are non-pathogenic. On the other hand, indoor air may have pathogenic bacteria distributed in droplet nuclei from nose and mouth.

Bacteriological examination of air is essential in following conditions:

- In hospital wards in which there is an outbreak of cross-infection.
- Surgical operation theatre.
- Premises where food articles are prepared and packed.
- Premises where pharmaceutical preparations are made.

The methods for bacteriological examination of air are of two types:

1. Those that measure the rate at which bacteria-carrying particles, chiefly the larger particles, settle by gravity from the air on to exposed surface, e.g., the settle plate method.
2. Those that count the number of bacteria-carrying particles contained in a given volume of the air, e.g., the slit sampler method.

Each bacteria-carrying particle or droplet nucleus may contain from 1 to 100 or more bacteria.

Settle plate method

Petri dishes containing an agar medium of known surface area are left open for a measured period of time. Large bacteria-carrying dust particles settle onto the medium. The plates are incubated at 37°C for 24 hours and a count of the colonies formed shows the number of settled particles. Blood agar medium may be used for the count of the pathogenic, commensal and saprophytic bacteria in the air and is used for testing air in surgical operation theatres and hospital wards. However, this method measures only the rate of deposition of large particles from air and not the total number of large and small bacteria-carrying dust particles suspended in it.

Slit sampler method

By this method, the number of bacteria in a measured volume of air is determined. One foot^3 of air is directed onto a plate of culture medium through a slit 0.25 mm wide. The plate is rotated mechanically so as to allow the organisms to spread out on the medium. The culture medium is incubated and colonies counted which gives the number of bacteria present in the air.

Bacterial count should not exceed 50 per foot^3 in factories, offices and homes, 10 per foot^3 in general operation theatre and 1 per foot^3 in theatre for neurosurgery.

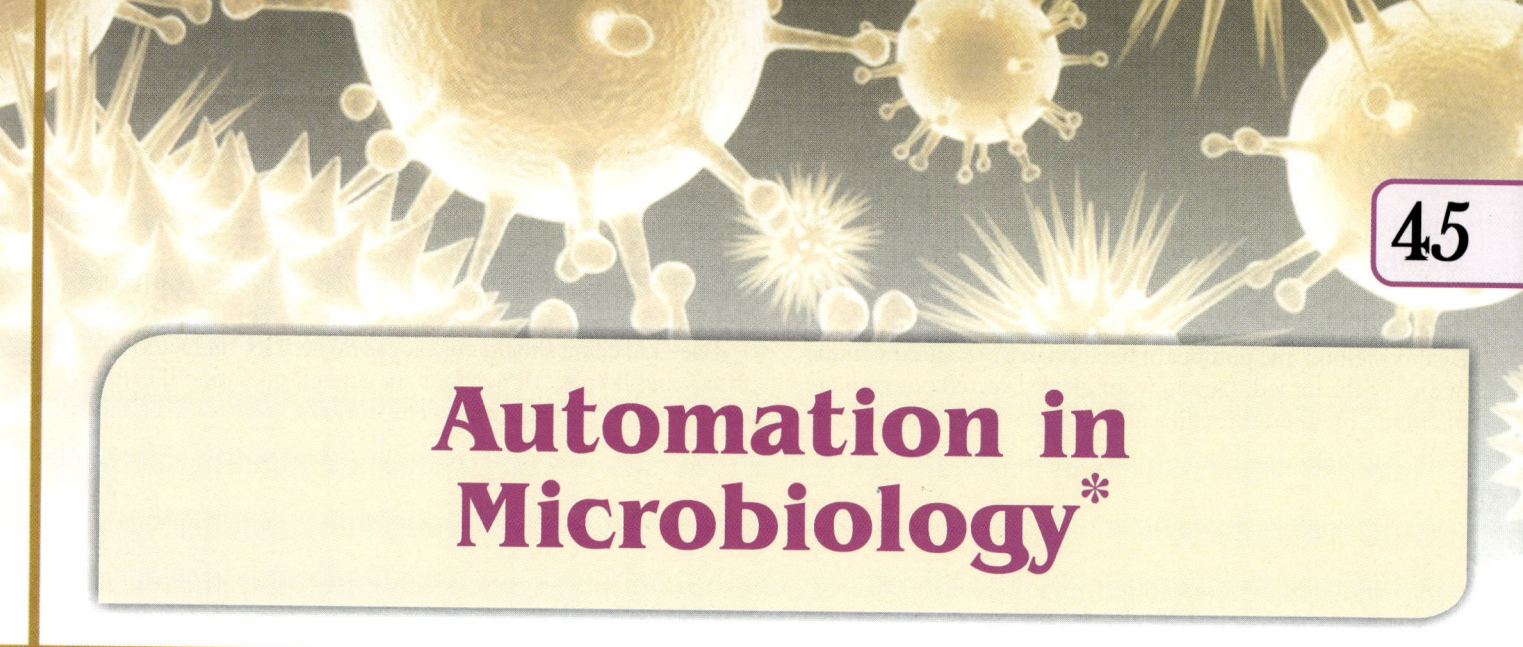

Automation in Microbiology*

Traditionally, the identification of bacteria and fungi has been based on conventional procedures which often yield poor results because of low microbial load and increased chances of contamination. Due to the need for simpler and faster methods with better outcomes, automated systems have been introduced.

Automation in microbiology was first introduced in the early 1970s with the launch of semi-automated blood culture systems. Then followed the systems for identification and antimicrobial susceptibility testing of bacteria. The earliest automated blood culture system i.e. Bactec 460 was based on radiometric detection of ^{14}C-labelled CO_2 production by microorganisms but the disposal of radiometric material was always a concern. These were followed by Continuous Monitoring Blood Culture Systems (CMBCS) in late 1980s namely BacT/Alert, BACTEC 9000 series and VersaTREK systems. The CMBCS get their name by the fact that they monitor CO_2 production more frequently, virtually every 10–15 minutes, than previous systems. These are non radiometric based assays, therefore, disposal of radiolabelled waste is not a concern.

The first automated system for identification (ID) of microorganisms was introduced just after the first automated blood culture system. It was Vitek system which was developed by National Aeronautics and Space Administration (NASA) to test astronauts for unusual organisms acquired during their space visit. It was a colorimetric system i.e. colour change due to carbohydrate utilization which results in pH change. The current versions i.e. Vitek 2 systems, Phoenix, MicroScan and Trek diagnostic systems are based on this system and the difference is that these utilize preformed enzymes in addition to carbohydrates as substrate. The detection relies on colour change which is produced when an enzyme hydrolyzes a colourless complex resulting in release of a colour producing compound (chromogen) or fluorescence emitting compound (fluorogen). These systems can also perform antimicrobial susceptibility testing (AST) as minimum inhibitory concentration (MIC) values based on similar principle as for identification.

Although many systems are available but still they are not adopted by most of the microbiology laboratories. A number of factors have contributed to the delay in automating the clinical microbiology laboratory. These are:

1. The complexity of the microbiological specimens.
2. The nature of diagnosing infectious disease is complicated by nonspecific clinical manifestations.
3. The cost of automation is also a significant barrier.

However, the high volume centralized laboratory model is becoming common and may be an attractive setting for automation in microbiology laboratory over the coming years. Current systems for microbiology laboratory automation are given in Table 45.1.

1. AUTOMATED SPECIMEN PROCESSING

The manual specimen processing has many disadvantages which include cross-contamination, increased processing time and cumulative cost. The automated processing systems promise to improve the quality of the streaking process, and overcome the above mentioned disadvantages. The streaking process is reproducible and reliably yield isolated colonies. Another advantage of these systems is that, they reduce the number of subcultures required for identification and susceptibility testing. The systems usually process liquid-based specimen.

---

* This chapter has been contributed by Dr Ashima Katyal, Senior Resident, Dr Deepinder Singh, Resident, and Dr Paramjeet Singh Gill, Professor, Department of Microbiology, Postgraduate Institute of Medical Sciences, Rohtak.

Table 45.1. Current systems for microbiology laboratory automation

1. **Automated specimen processing**
   - Automated loop (BD diagnostics)
   - Magnetic bead (BD-Kiestra, Netherlands)
   - Comb applicator (bioMérieux)
2. **Automated identification and susceptibility testing systems**
   - Radiometric detection of blood culture
   - Continuous monitoring blood culture systems (CMBCS)
   - Automated ID and AST systems for bacteria and yeasts
   - Automated system for identification of *Mycobacterium* spp.
3. **Molecular automation**
4. **Total laboratory automation (TLA)**
5. **Proteomic based automated identification system**
   - **M**atrix-**A**ssisted **L**aser **D**esorption **I**onization-**T**ime **O**f **F**light **M**ass **S**pectrometry (**MALDI-TOF MS**)

The available devices are classified according to different inoculation techniques using
- automated loop (BD diagnostics),
- magnetic bead (BD-Kiestra, Netherlands), or
- comb applicator (bioMérieux).

The systems automatically agitate, decap and recap the specimens followed by inoculation on whole agar plates or biplates as required for the specimen type. All of these systems are equipped with high efficiency particulate air (HEPA) filters.

2. AUTOMATED IDENTIFICATION AND ANTI-MICROBIAL SUSCEPTIBILITY TESTING SYSTEMS

The conventional methods for ID and AST are labour-intensive, have long turnaround time, poor reliability and reproducibility, and are prone to higher chances of cross-contamination. The newer automated systems overcome all the disadvantages of conventional procedures (Fig. 45.1). The currently available automated ID and AST systems are:

Radiometric detection of blood culture

This was the first automated system for blood culture introduced in 1970s. It is based on the principle that the microbial growth can be detected by monitoring CO_2 production by growing organisms. This system uses radiometric detection of ^{14}C-labelled CO_2. The two major drawbacks of this system are very less frequency of monitoring of blood culture bottle i.e. once or twice daily, and concern regarding disposal of radiolabelled waste.

Continuous monitoring blood culture systems (CMBCS)

There are three CMBCS available currently viz. BacT/Alert 3D, BD BACTEC system and VersaTREK blood culture system. These alert the microbiologist that a culture is positive, after which relevant bottles can be removed for Gram stain and subculture. Also, these systems being non radiometric, disposal of waste is not a concern.

These systems work on two principles:

1. Detection of CO_2 (BacT/Alert 3D, BD BACTEC system)

In CO_2 detection systems, as the microorganisms grow in the blood-broth mixture, CO_2 is liberated. A CO_2 sensitive sensor is present at the bottom of each bottle separated from broth by CO_2-permeable membrane.

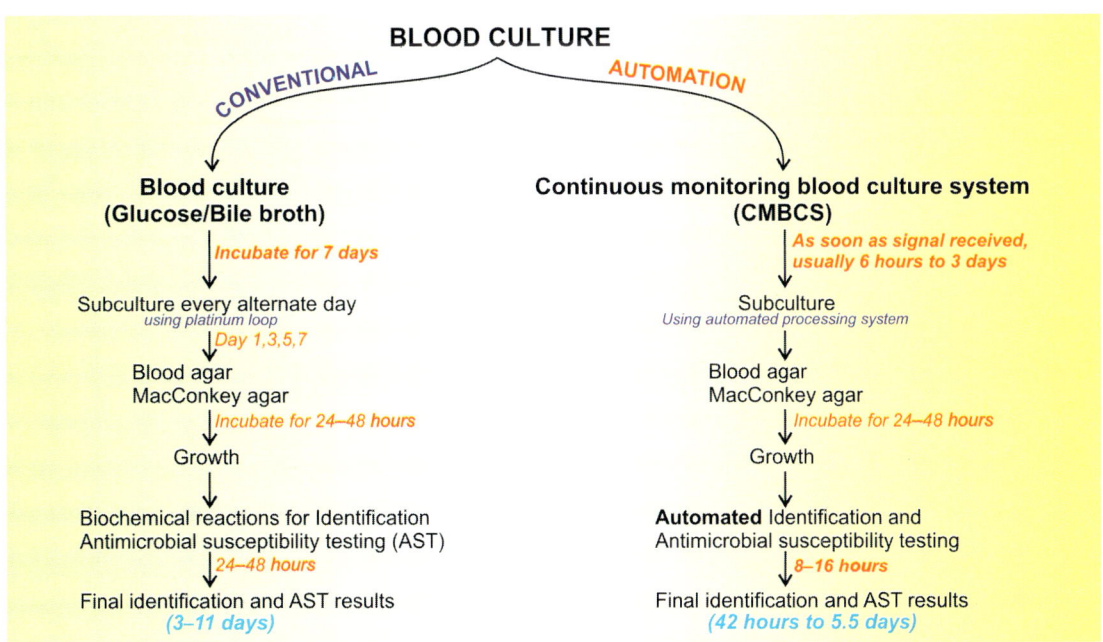

Fig. 45.1. Comparison of blood culture by conventional and automated systems.

- In BacT/Alert 3D system, detection is colorimetric and pH sensitive sensor turns green to yellow in the presence of CO_2, produced by actively multiplying microorganisms which leads to pH change of the medium (Fig. 45.2A).
- BD BACTEC system, has fluorescent based detection system. In uninoculated broth, large amount of dissolved oxygen quenches the fluorescent dye but the multiplying bacteria in inoculated broth consume oxygen and liberate CO_2 removing the quenching effect and emit a fluorescent light which is detected by the sensor (Fig. 45.2B).

2. Pressure change in the head of the bottle (VersaTREK blood culture system)

The VersaTREK blood culture system differs in a way that it detects changes in concentration of H_2 and O_2 in addition to CO_2 manometrically. Also, both production as well as consumption of gas is detected in this system.

Media

These CMBCS require specialized blood culture bottles which are available with these automated systems. As is the case with conventional blood culture technique, different broths are used for Gram-positive and Gram-negative microorganisms i.e. glucose and bile broth respectively. Similarly, various media are used in the blood culture bottles of these CMBCS. These are:

BacT/Alert 3D system

Tryptic soy broth with brain heart infusion (BHI) solids and activated charcoal.

BD BACTEC system

Soy casein digest broth with added resins in plus medium, and lytic agents in lysis medium.

VersaTREK system

Redox 1: soy casein peptone broth and Redox 2: modified protease peptone broth.

Automated ID and AST systems for bacteria and yeasts

The last five decades have witnessed an evolution of sophisticated automated identification of microorganisms and antimicrobial susceptibility testing systems. The first automated identification system to become available for clinical laboratories more than 40 years ago was the Vitek system (bioMerieux). Since then many advances have been achieved in the field of automation and more research has led to development of newer systems like Vitek 2 series, MicroScan WalkAway, BD Phoenix, Omnilog and Sherlocks MIDI. All these systems have panels or cards with dried analytes for identification of organisms and dried antimicrobials for detection of minimum inhibitory concentration. The panels are charged with the help of ID and AST broth available with system after inoculation with microorganism. Currently, the

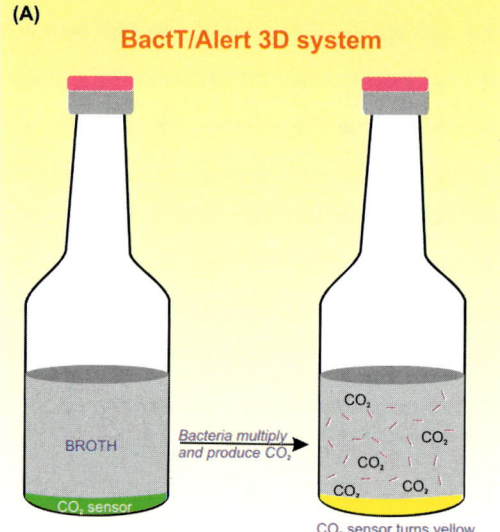

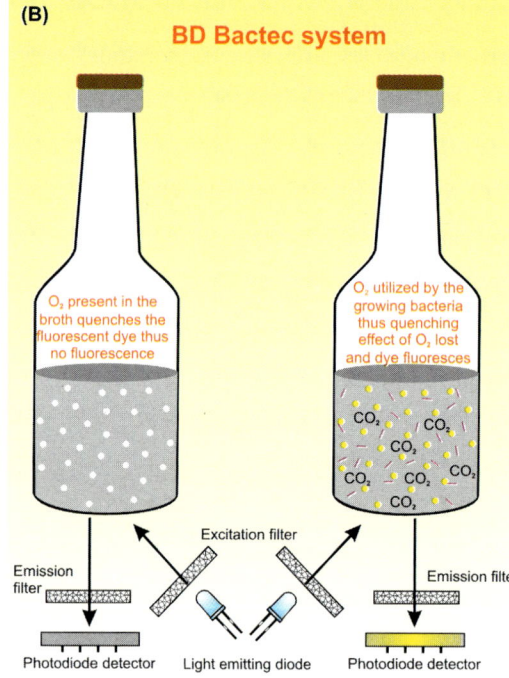

Fig. 45.2. Diagrammatic representation showing working principle of (A) BacT/Alert 3D system and (B) BD Bactec system.

identification of microorganism by automated systems is based on four principles:

1. pH-based reactions (15–24 hours)

- The analytes in these reactions are carbohydrates which when utilized by microorganism produce acidic pH, and colour changes due to pH indicator.
- There is a need for growth prior to charging the panels in these systems. Direct samples cannot be put up in these panels.
- The examples include Phoenix panels, Vitek cards.

2. Enzyme profile (mostly 2–4 hours)

- The analytes in these reactions are preformed enzymes which produce colour change due to chromogen or fluorogen release when colourless complex is hydrolyzed by an appropriate enzyme.
- There is a need of prior growth.
- The examples include MicroScan rapid panels, Vitek cards, and Phoenix panels.

3. Carbon source utilization

- The analytes are organic products that produce colour change as a result of metabolic activity of transferring electrons to colourless tetrazolium-labelled carbon sources and converting the dye to purple.
- There is a need for prior growth.
- The example includes OmniLog.

4. Volatile or nonvolatile compound detection

- The cellular fatty acids (analytes) are degraded to their end products that are detected by chromatographic tracing, which are then compared to a library of known patterns.
- They also require prior growth of microorganisms.
- The examples include Sherlock microbial ID.

The comparison of currently available automated systems of bacteria and yeasts is given in Table 45.2.

Automated system for identification of *Mycobacterium* spp.

Automated system for identification of *Mycobacterium* spp. is given in Table 45.3. For details refer to Chapter 25.

3. MOLECULAR AUTOMATION

Traditional molecular biology is a tedious and labour-intensive process. The future of molecular biology is going to be very different as these processes are being automated and consolidated into single system. The systems are commonly referred to as being "sample-to-answer" or "walk-away". Nucleic acid amplification techniques are now commonly used to diagnose and manage patients with infectious diseases. The growth in the number of FDA approved tests have facilitated the use of this technology in clinical laboratories. Simple, automated sample-in, answer-out molecular test systems are now available that can be deployed in clinical microbiology laboratories.

4. TOTAL LABORATORY AUTOMATION (TLA)

TLA in microbiology aims to improve quality, reduce time to result, better manage an increasing number of specimens, compensate for reduction in skilled staff, and be more economically effective. The field is evolving quickly. More methods are expected to be automated in near future like automated colony picking for charging of panels and preparation of dilutions for susceptibility testing. The TLA in microbiology is currently provided by bioMerieux, BD-Kiestra and Copan.

Advantages and limitations of automated systems

Advantages

- Labour saving
- Reproducibility
- Expert analysis

Table 45.2. Comparison of currently available automated systems of bacteria and yeasts

Manufacturer	Instruments	Principles	Panels	Incubation (hours)	AST
bioMérieux	Vitek 2 XL Vitek 2 60 Vitek 2 Compact 60/30/15 Vitek 2	Colorimetric carbon source utilization; enzymatic activity	Gram-positive, Gram-negative *Nesseria*, *Haemophilus*, anaerobes, yeasts	8	Yes
Siemens	MicroScan WalkAway plus	Overnight panels: turbidimetric detection of carbon source utilization; enzymatic activity Rapid panels: fluorometric detection of preformed enzymes	Gram-positive, Gram-negative *Nesseria*, *Haemophilus*, anaerobes, yeasts	16–18	Yes
BD Diagnostics	BD Phoenix	Colorimetric and fluorometric detection	Gram-positive, Gram-negative *Streptococcus*, yeast ID	8–16	Yes
TREK Diagnostics	ARIS	Fluorometric detection	Gram-positive, Gram-negative	5–18	Yes
Biolog	OmniLog	Reduction of tetrazolium violet	Gram-positive, Gram-negative	4–24	No
MIDI, Inc.	Sherlock microbial ID	Cellular fatty acid by gas chromatography	Gram-positive, Gram-negative, yeasts	24	No

Table 45.3. Automated system for identification of *Mycobacterium* spp.

System	Constituents	Principle	Detection time
BACTEC 460 TB	Middlebrook 7H9 broth or 7H12 broth + bovine serum albumin + PANTA* + catalase	**Radiometric:** detection of radioactive CO_2 ($^{14}CO_2$) liberated in the head space of vial by growing mycobacteria	14.8 days, 87% yield, 4% contamination
MGIT and MGIT 960	7H9 broth base + ODAC** + PANTA	**Fluorescent** compound embedded in silicone base, at the bottom of tube, sensitive to oxygen	13.3 days, 82% yield, 10% contamination
MB BacT/Alert	Middle brook 7H9 broth in CO_2, O_2 and N_2 under vacuum + PANTA	**Colorimetry:** green to yellow detection of change in CO_2 concentration by a pH sensitive sensor at the base of bottle	16 days, 85% yield
BACTEC Myco/F lytic	Lytic agents to release mycobacteria phagocytosed by white blood cells	**Fluorescence based:** detects decreasing O_2 concentration due to consumption by growing mycobacteria	12.8 days, 81% yield
GeneXpert system	Cartridge containing freeze dried primers and molecular beacons for detection of *rpoB* gene	Cartridge-based nucleic acid amplification testing (**CBNAAT**)	2 hours Detects *M. tuberculosis* along with rifampicin resistance

* PANTA= Polymyxin B, amphotericin B, nalidixic acid, trimethoprim and azlocillin
** ODAC= oleic acid, dextrose, albumin and catalase

- Rapid results
- Susceptibility can be performed

Limitations

- High cost
- Predetermined susceptibility panels
- Pure growth required
- Inability to test all clinically relevant organisms
- Not able to detect resistant phenotypes

5. PROTEOMIC BASED AUTOMATED IDENTIFICATION SYSTEM

Matrix-**A**ssisted **L**aser **D**esorption **I**onization-**T**ime **O**f **F**light **M**ass **S**pectrometry (**MALDI-TOF MS**)

MALDI stands for matrix assisted desorption and ionization of highly abundant bacterial and fungal proteins through energy from a laser. In this system, isolated colonies are charged to a "spot" on MALDI target plate which is then overlaid with matrix and air dried. A laser energy is passed through the target plate enabling desorption of target proteins with the help of matrix molecules and gets converted to an ionized state. These ionized molecules are then passed through a positively charged electrostatic field into a time of flight (TOF) tube. In this vacuum tube, ions are separated according to their mass charge ratio with small analytes travelling fastest. These ions are detected by ion detector on the other end of the tube and for each ion a peak is generated in the computer. The peaks generated in the computer together produce a profile which is unique to an organism which is then compared to the database of reference spectra, and the organism is identified at the family, genus or species level. Commercially this system is available from bioMerieux, Inc. and Bruker Daltonics, Inc.

Advantages of MALDI-TOF MS

- Minimal sample preparation
- Cost effective: low consumable cost
- Powerful bioinformatic approaches
- Species to strain resolution
- Non-expert identification possible
- Dedicated databases continue to expand
- Rapid turnaround time, high throughput: impact on appropriate empiric therapy
- Single colony requirement: direct from blood culture
- Low exposure risk: sample inactivation
- Broad applicability (all types of microorganisms including anaerobes, yeasts, filamentous fungi)

Limitations of MALDI-TOF MS

- Cannot resolve polymicrobial cultures
- Some organisms require extraction
- Pure culture is required, cannot be done directly from sample
- Databases: still in their infancy
- High initial capital expenditure
- New approaches (business models)

CRITERIA FOR EVALUATION AND SELECTION OF AUTOMATED SYSTEM

Prior to choosing an automated system, the daily routine in the laboratory like specimen volume, arrival time of specimen, and workflow should be evaluated. Factors to consider when selecting an automated system are as follows:

1. **Productivity:** It depends upon the number of specimens processed and the turnaround time for the entire processing. It is affected by specimen type, the choice of streaking pattern and number of plates per sample.

2. **Reliability, stability and durability:** These indicators are directly proportional to the malfunction of a system. Plans for possible failures of the system should be planned in advance.

3. **Technical aspects:** Survey of the building should be done to determine the infrastructure of the rooms. Required space, power supply and dimensions of the devices should be calculated before finalizing the infrastructure.

4. **Software applications:** The required system software should be installed and updated regularly by the manufacturer.

5. **Safety and hygiene:** Occupational health and safety measures should be taken into consideration. There are no regulations regarding the issue of safety in laboratory automation. The exposures generated during errors in automatic incubation are of great concern. The systems should be disinfected and cleaned after every run to avoid cross-contamination.

6. **Quality control and scientific aspects:** The entire system should be integrated into the quality management programme. The individual work steps must be monitored in compliance with the laboratory regulations and standard operating procedures.

7. **Costs:** It is one of the major barriers especially in the resource poor settings. The cost of devices, consumable supplies and media required should be calculated as per requirement and budget.

8. **The final decision:** The choice of the type and extent of laboratory automation is dependent upon the individual circumstances and the financial resources available.

SECTION 3

VIROLOGY

Chapter 46   General Properties of Viruses
Chapter 47   Bacteriophage
Chapter 48   Poxviruses and Herpesviruses
Chapter 49   Adenoviruses, Papillomaviruses and Rotaviruses
Chapter 50   Polioviruses and Rabies Virus
Chapter 51   Influenza, Parainfluenza, Mumps, and Measles Viruses
Chapter 52   Chikungunya, Rubella, Dengue, Japanese Encephalitis and Kyasanur Forest Disease
Chapter 53   Human Immunodeficiency Viruses: AIDS
Chapter 54   Hepatitis Viruses

General Properties of Viruses

Viruses are the **smallest infective agents**. They are **obligate intracellular parasites**. Three main properties distinguish viruses from other microorganisms:

1. Small size

Viruses are smaller than other organisms. **They vary in size from 10 to 300 nm.** Therefore, they can pass through bacterial filters and they cannot be seen by light microscope. However, the poxviruses which are the largest members of the virus family and are very similar in size to the smallest bacteria, are close to the resolution of light microscope. For visualization of all other viruses an electron microscope is necessary.

2. Genome

A virus carries its own genetic information in the form of either RNA or DNA, but not both. The genome may be single-stranded or double-stranded, circular or linear, and segmented or unsegmented.

3. Metabolically inert

Viruses have no metabolic activity outside susceptible host cells. They do not possess ribosomes or protein-synthesizing apparatus, although, some viruses contain one or more enzymes within their particles. Viruses, therefore, cannot multiply in inanimate media but only inside living cells.

STRUCTURE OF THE VIRUSES

Viruses consist of nucleic acid core surrounded by a protein coat called **capsid**. The capsid is composed of repeating protein units called **capsomers**. The capsid with the enclosed nucleic acid is known as **nucleocapsid**.

Virus symmetry

Capsid of the virus particles shows three types of symmetry. It is determined by the arrangement of the capsomers around the nucleic acid.

1. *Icosahedral symmetry:* The capsomers are arranged as if they lay on the faces of an icosahedron which has 20 equilateral triangular faces and 12 corners or apices (Fig. 46.1).
2. *Helical symmetry:* The nucleic acid and the capsomers are wound together in the form of a helix or spiral.
3. *Complex symmetry:* Viruses (e.g., poxviruses) which do not show either icosahedral or helical symmetry due to complexity of their structure are referred to have complex symmetry.

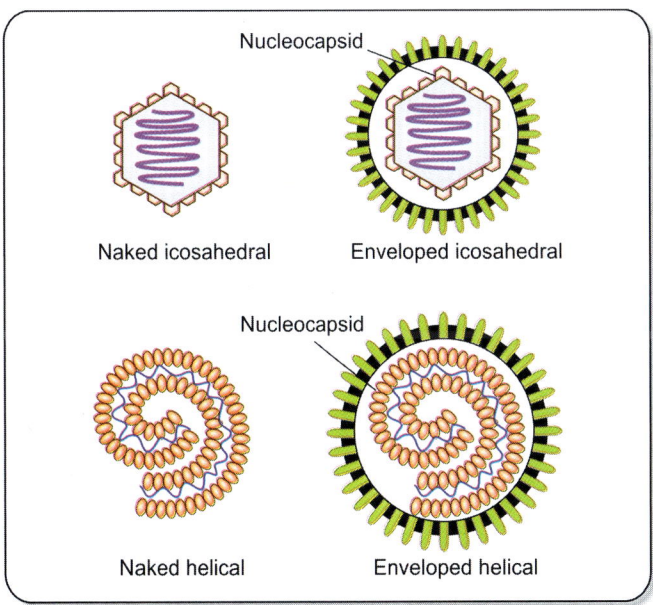

Fig. 46.1. Symmetry of viruses.

Envelope

Generally, DNA viruses replicate and are assembled in the nucleus, and RNA viruses are assembled in the cytoplasm. The final assembly of some viruses occurs at the nuclear or cytoplasmic membrane. As the virus particle moves from the nucleus to the cytoplasm or passes from the cytoplasm to the extracellular space, an external lipid-containing envelope (host origin) with virus-coded polypeptides or virus-specified glyco-proteins is added to the nucleocapsid. In mature virus particle the glycoproteins often appear as projecting spikes on the outer surface of the envelope. These are known as **peplomers**.

SHAPE

The overall shape of the virus particle varies in different groups of viruses. Most of the animal viruses are roughly spherical, some are irregular and pleomorphic. Poxviruses are *brick-shaped*, rabies virus is *bullet-shaped*, tobacco mosaic virus is *rod-shaped* and bacteriophages have a *complex morphology*. The extracellular infectious virus particle is known as **virion**.

REPLICATION OF VIRUSES

The genetic information necessary for viral multiplication is contained in the viral nucleic acid but the biosynthetic enzymes are lacking. They replicate by taking over the biochemical machinery of the host cell and redirecting it to the manufacture of virus components. The viral replication is divided into six stages.

1. Adsorption

The first event in the infection of a cell by a virus is the attachment of the virus particle to the cell surface.

2. Entry into the host cells

Viruses enter the cells by the following mechanism:

- After attachment nonenveloped viruses are engulfed by a mechanism resembling phagocytosis, a process known as viropexis. In case of enveloped viruses, the envelope fuses with the plasma membrane of the host cell and releases the nucleocapsid into the cytoplasm.
- Bacteria possess rigid cell walls. Bacteriophages, therefore, cannot penetrate into bacterial cells and only nucleic acid is introduced intracellularly by a complex mechanism.

3. Uncoating

This is the process of stripping the virus of its outer layers and capsid, so that nucleic acid is released into the cell. With most viruses, uncoating is effected by the action of lysosomal enzymes of the host cells when the phagosome and lysosome fuse together.

4. Biosynthesis

This phase includes synthesis of:
- The viral nucleic acid.
- Capsid protein.
- Enzymes necessary in the various stages of viral synthesis, assembly and release.

- Certain regulatory proteins which serve to shut down the normal cellular metabolism and direct the sequential production of viral components.

    Biosynthesis consists of following steps:

- Transcription of messenger RNA (mRNA) from viral nucleic acid.
- Translation of mRNA into '**early proteins**' or '**non-structural proteins**'. These are enzymes and factors which initiate and maintain synthesis of virus components and induce shutdown of host protein and nucleic acid synthesis.
- Replication of viral nucleic acid.
- Synthesis of **late** or **structural proteins** which constitute daughter virion capsids.

5. Virion assembly

Assembly of the various viral components into virions occurs shortly after the replication of the viral nucleic acid and may take place in either the nucleus (herpes and adenoviruses) or cytoplasm (picorna and poxviruses). In case of enveloped viruses, the envelope is derived from the nuclear membrane, if they assemble in the nucleus (herpesviruses), and from plasma membrane, if they assemble in the cytoplasm of the host cell (orthomyxoviruses, paramyxoviruses and retro-viruses). However, in this envelope virus encoded peplomers are also embedded.

6. Release

Release of completed viruses is the final step in virus multiplication. Viruses that exist as naked nucleocapsids may be released by:

- The lysis of the host cell (polioviruses) or they may be extruded by a process which may be called **reverse phago-cytosis**.
- Enveloped viruses are released by a process of **budding** through special areas of host cell membrane (cytoplasmic or nuclear), where virus-specified transmembrane glyco-proteins (peplomers) have been embedded.
- In case of bacterial viruses, the release of progeny virions takes place by **the lysis of the infected bacterium**.

VIRUS ISOLATION

Viruses can replicate only in living cells, therefore, they cannot be grown on any of the inanimate culture media. Most of the viruses can be cultivated in laboratory animals, chick embryos or cell cultures.

Laboratory animals

These animals have now almost disappeared from virus diagnostic laboratories, because simpler methods such as tissue cultures are available. However, suckling mice, less than 24 hours old, are still used for the isolation of arboviruses, rabies virus, and some of the group A coxsackieviruses. These are inoculated intracerebrally and/or intraperitoneally, then observed for up to 2 weeks for the development of pathognomic signs before sacrificing for histologic examination of affected organs.

Chick embryos

Embryonated eggs offer several sites for the cultivation of viruses. Chorioallantoic membrane (CAM), allantoic cavity, amniotic cavity and yolk sac (Fig. 46.2) of 8–11 day old eggs are inoculated and incubated for 2–9 days. The duration of incubation depends on the virus type and route of inoculation. Viruses may kill the embryo or may produce visible lesions like pocks on CAM, and haemagglutinating activity in the harvested amniotic and allantoic fluid. These effects help in the identification of the virus. Many viruses can be grown in eggs.

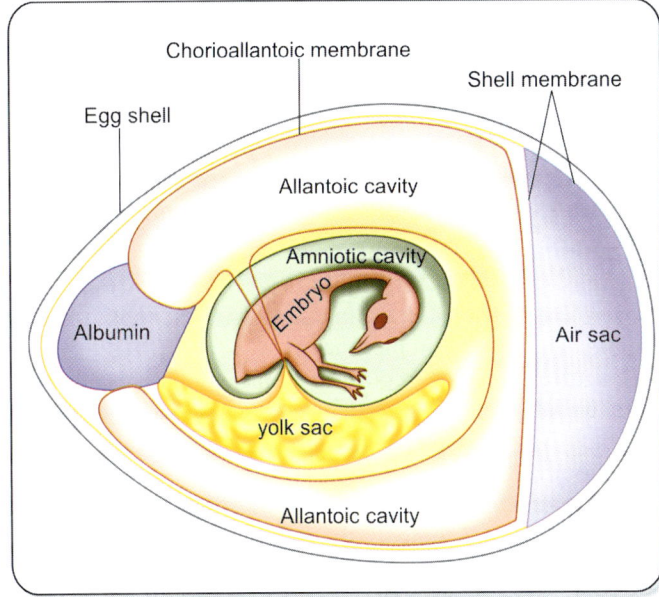

Fig. 46.2. Cross-section of an embryonated hen's egg.

1. Chorioallantoic membrane (CAM)

Inoculation of CAM produces visible lesions (pocks). Pocks produced by different viruses have different morphology. Each infectious virus particle forms one pock. Pock counting, therefore, can be used for the assay of pock-forming viruses such as variola and vaccinia.

2. Amniotic cavity

Inoculation of amniotic cavity is used for primary isolation of the influenza virus.

3. Allantoic cavity

Inoculation of allantoic cavity provides a rich yield of influenza and some parainfluenza viruses. Allantoic inoculation is used for growing influenza virus for vaccine production. Other chick embryo vaccines are yellow fever

(**17D strain**) and rabies (**Flury strain**) vaccines. Duck eggs are bigger than hen's eggs. Therefore, duck eggs provide a better yield of rabies virus and are used for the preparation of the inactivated nonneural rabies vaccines.

4. Yolk sac inoculation

Inoculation of yolk sac is used for the cultivation of some viruses, chlamydiae and rickettsiae.

Cell culture

The term cell culture is used to indicate culture of cells *in vitro*; the cells are not organized into a tissue. The term tissue culture or organ culture is used to denote the growth of tissues or an organ so that the architecture or function of the tissue or organ is preserved. Both these terms are used interchangeably, however, cell culture is technically more correct.

Organ culture

Small bits of organs are maintained in tissue culture growth medium. Organ cultures are useful for the isolation of highly specialised viruses of certain organs. For example, the tracheal ring organ culture is employed for the isolation of coronavirus, a respiratory pathogen.

Explant culture

Fragments of minced tissue can be grown as 'explants' embedded in plasma clots. This method is now seldom employed in virology.

Cell culture

This is the type of culture routinely employed for diagnostic virology and for studying virus-cell interactions. Tissues are dissociated into component cells by the action of proteolytic enzymes such as trypsin or collagenase and mechanical shaking. The cells are washed, counted and suspended in a growth medium. The cell suspension is dispensed in glass or plastic bottles, tubes or petri dishes. The cells adhere to glass or plastic surface and on incubation, if culture conditions are suitable, they divide to form a confluent monolayer sheet of cells covering the surface within about a week. At this stage, cell division ceases due to contact inhibition. Cell culture is of three types (Table 46.1):

1. Primary cell cultures

These are normal cells freshly taken from the body and cultured. They are capable of very limited growth *in vitro* perhaps 5–10 divisions at the most. These cells have a normal diploid chromosome complement, meaning that they contain two copies of each chromosome. Diploid is the normal genetic make up of eukaryotic cells. Therefore, primary cell cultures are preferred for cultivating viruses meant for vaccine production. Important examples of primary cell cultures are rhesus monkey kidney cell culture, human amnion cell culture and chick embryo fibroblast cell culture.

Table 46.1. Cell cultures in common use

1. Primary cell cultures
   • Rhesus monkey kidney cell culture
   • Human amnion cell culture
   • Chick embryo fibroblast cell culture
2. Finite (diploid) cell cultures
   • WI-38 Human embryonic lung cell strain
3. Continuous cell cultures
   • HeLa (Human carcinoma of cervix cell line)
   • HEp-2 (Human epithelioma of larynx cell line)
   • KB (Human carcinoma of nasopharynx cell line)
   • McCoy (Human synovial carcinoma cell line)
   • Detroit 6 (Sternal marrow cell line)
   • Chang C/I/L/K (Human conjunctiva, intestine, liver and kidney cell line)
   • Vero (African monkey kidney cell line)
   • BHK-21 (Baby hamster kidney cell line)

2. Finite (diploid) cell cultures

These are cells of a single type, usually fibroblasts, that retain their original diploid chromosome number and karyotype. They can be subcultured for about 50 passages (serial subcultures) before the cells die off. Diploid cells developed from human fibroblasts are susceptible to a wide range of human viruses. They are useful for isolation of some fastidious pathogens and for the production of viral vaccines, e.g., rabies vaccine is produced by cultivation of the fixed rabies virus in WI-38 human embryonic lung cell strain.

3. Continuous cell cultures

These are cells of a single type that are capable of indefinite propagation *in vitro*. Therefore, they are known as continuous cell cultures. They have been derived from diploid cell lines or from malignant tissues. These cells are heteroploid meaning that they have abnormal and variable number of chromosomes that are not a multiple of normal haploid number. Often they no longer bear any close resemblance to their cells of origin because of numerous sequential mutations during their long history in culture. Continuous cell lines such as HeLa, HEp-2 and KB derived from human carcinoma of cervix, human epithelioma of larynx, and human carcinoma of nasopharynx respectively, support the growth of a number of viruses. These cell lines have been used in the virus laboratories throughout the world for many years.

These cell lines may be maintained by serial subcultivation or stored at –70°C for use when necessary. Other cell lines (and their sources) in common use are McCoy (human synovial carcinoma cell line), Detroit 6 (sternal marrow cell line), Chang C/I/L/K (human conjunctiva, intestine, liver and kidney cell lines), Vero (African green monkey kidney cell line) and BHK-21 (baby hamster kidney cell line). The type of cell culture used for viral cultivation depends on the sensitivity of the cells to a particular virus.

Growth media

Cells are grown *in vitro* in chemically defined media which are made up of balanced isotonic salt solutions that contain essential amino acids, fatty acids, vitamins, carbohydrates and sometimes nucleic acid precursors. Newborn or foetal calf serum, generally 10%, is always added to provide a number of unidentified growth factors. The media are buffered with bicarbonate to give a pH of 7.2–7.4 and phenol red is added as a pH indicator. Penicillin, streptomycin and amphotericin B or nystatin are sometimes added to prevent bacterial and fungal contamination. CO_2 is either provided by cultured cells as a metabolic by-product (necessitating stoppered test tubes or screw-capped bottles) or by enrichment of the atmosphere using a CO_2 incubator.

Detection of virus growth in cell culture

Virus growth in cell culture can be detected by the following methods:

1. Cytopathic effect

Many viruses produce morphological changes in the cultured cells in which they grow. These changes are known as **cytopathic effects (CPE)** and viruses causing CPE are known as **cytopathogenic viruses**. Following are the main types of CPE:

• **Rounding of cells:** Viral replication may lead to nuclear pyknosis, rounding, refractility, degeneration and eventually complete or partial detachment of infected cells from the glass. This is seen in picornaviruses.
• **Rounding and aggregation:** Some viruses may lead to cell rounding and aggregation into grape-like clusters which detach from the glass, leaving clear areas. It is seen in adenoviruses.
• **Syncytium formation:** Some viruses (measles, syncytial virus and HIV) lead to syncytium formation in which infected cells fuse with neighbouring infected or uninfected cells to form giant cells containing several (up to 100) nuclei.
• **Inclusion bodies:** These are intranuclear or cytoplasmic aggregates of products of viral replication such as virus particles ready for release, overproduction of a particular viral protein or proteins or some aberrant cellular structure such as clumped chromatin. They can be seen in stained preparations under a light microscope. They may be present in the cytoplasm or in the nucleus, or both, of infected cells and may be acidophilic or basophilic, single or multiple, large or small, and round or irregular. Vaccinia and rabies viruses produce intracytoplasmic inclusion bodies, and adenoviruses and herpesviruses produce intranuclear inclusions. Inclusion bodies of measles virus are seen in both the locations.

2. Haemadsorption

Orthomyxoviruses (influenza) and paramyxoviruses (para-influenza, measles and mumps) code for red cell agglutinins which are incorporated into the cell membrane during infection, so that guinea-pig erythrocytes adhere to the infected cells. This adherence of erythrocytes to the infected cells is known as haemadsorption.

3. Interference

The multiplication of one virus in a cell usually inhibits the multiplication of a second virus, called **the challenge virus**, when it is added to the culture. This is because the first virus interferes with the replicative process of the challenge virus and is known as **interference challenge test**. This can be used for the detection of the growth of a non-cytopathogenic virus in cell culture.

4. Transformation

Tumour-forming (oncogenic) viruses induce cell transformation and loss of normal contact inhibition, so that growth appears in a piled-up fashion producing **microtumours**.

5. Fluorescent antibody testing

Cells from virus infected cultures can be stained with fluorescein-conjugated antiserum and seen under fluorescence microscope for virus antigens.

6. Detection of enzymes

The virus isolate can be identified by detection of viral enzymes, such as reverse transcriptase in retroviruses, in the culture fluid.

7. Electron microscopy

Viruses have distinctive appearances and can be detected by electron microscopy of ultra thin sections of infected cells.

NOMENCLATURE OF VIRUSES

The orders, families, subfamilies and genera of viruses are named with the suffix *virales*, *viridae*, *virinae* and *virus* respectively. For example, names of order, family, subfamily and genus of measles virus are *Mononegavirales*, *Paramyxoviridae*, *Paramyxovirinae* and *Marbillivirus* respectively. Viral species are designated by vernacular terms, for example, measles virus.

CLASSIFICATION OF VIRUSES

Viruses are classified into DNA and RNA viruses (Tables 46.2 and 46.3).

Viroids

Viroids are very simple structures consisting of uncapsidated RNA of only a few hundred (246–399) nucleotides length, i.e., a size significantly smaller than the genome of even smallest virus. They lack a protein coat. Since they do not code for any protein, viroids rely on host enzymes for their replication. Despite their simplicity, viroids induce pathogenic effects in their plant hosts by direct interaction between the viroid RNA (or viroid-specific RNAs generated in course of an infection) and one or more cellular targets. The molecular biology of these fascinating RNA molecules is beginning to be understood. As yet there are no known viroids of animals and humans. Viroids differ from viruses in the following ways:

1. Each viroid consists of a single circular RNA molecule of low molecular weight.
2. Viroids exist inside cells as particles of RNA without capsids or envelops.

Table 46.2. DNA viruses infecting humans

Family	Subfamily	Genus	Common members (species)
Poxviridae	Chordopoxvirinae	*Orthopoxvirus*	Variola, vaccinia, cowpox, monkeypox, ectromelia (mousepox) and rabbitpox viruses
		Parapoxvirus	Contagious pustular dermatitis virus of sheep (orf virus) and pseudocowpox (milker's node) virus
		Molluscipoxvirus	Molluscum contagiosum virus
		Yatapoxvirus	Yabapox, tanapox
Herpesviridae	Alphaherpesvirinae	*Simplexvirus*	Herpes simplex virus types 1 and 2
		Varicellovirus	Varicella-zoster virus
	Betaherpesvirinae	*Cytomegalovirus*	Human cytomegalovirus
		Roseolovirus	Human herpesvirus 6
	Gammaherpesvirinae	*Lymphocryptovirus*	Epstein-Barr virus
Adenoviridae	—	*Mastadenovirus*	47 serotypes of human adenovirus
Papovaviridae	—	*Papillomavirus*	Wart viruses
		Polyomavirus	Human polyomaviruses, murine polyoma virus and simian virus 40
Hepadnaviridae	—	*Orthohepadnavirus*	Hepatitis B virus of man, woodchuck and other animal hepatitis viruses
Parvoviridae	—	*Dependovirus*	Adeno-associated viruses (AAV)
		Erythrovirus	Parvovirus B19

Table 46.3. RNA viruses infecting humans

Family	Subfamily	Genus	Common members (species)
Orthomyxoviridae	—	*Influenzavirus A, Influenzavirus B* and *Influenzavirus C*	Influenza A virus, Influenza B virus and Influenza C virus
Paramyxoviridae	Paramyxovirinae	*Paramyxovirus*	Human parainfluenza virus types 1 and 3
		Rubulavirus	Human parainfluenza virus types 2, 4a and 4b, and mumps virus
		Morbillivirus	Measles virus
	Pneumovirinae	*Pneumovirus*	Human respiratory syncytial virus
Rhabdoviridae	—	*Vesiculovirus*	Vesicular stomatitis virus
		Lyssavirus	Rabies virus
Filoviridae		*Filovirus*	Marburg, Ebola and Reston viruses
Picornaviridae	—	*Enterovirus*	Polioviruses (3), human echoviruses (32), coxsackieviruses (29) and a few other human enteroviruses
		Hepatovirus	Human hepatitis A virus
		Rhinovirus	Common cold rhinoviruses (over 100 serotypes)
Caliciviridae		*Calicivirus*	Human caliciviruses and hepatitis E virus
		Orthoreovirus	Human and animal reoviruses
		Rotavirus	Rotaviruses of man and animals
		Orbivirus	Tick-borne Kemerovo viruses of Siberia
		Coltivirus	Tick-borne agent causing Colorado tick fever in North America
Togaviridae	—	*Alphavirus*	Eastern, Western and Venezuelan Equine encephalitis viruses, Ross River virus and Chikungunya virus
		Rubivirus	Rubella virus
Flaviviridae	—	*Flavivirus*	Yellow fever, dengue, and St. Louis, Japanese, Murray Valley and Russian tick-borne encephalitis
		Hepatitis C	Hepatitis C virus
Coronaviridae	—	*Coronavirus*	Coronaviruses of mammals and birds
Arenaviridae	—	*Arenavirus*	Lymphocytic choriomeningitis virus, Lassa, Machupo, Junin and Guanarito viruses
Bunyaviridae	—	*Phlebovirus*	Sandfly fever virus and Rift Valley fever virus
		Bunyavirus	La Crosse and Oropouche viruses
		Nairovirus	Crimean-Congo haemorrhagic fever virus
		Hantavirus	Hantaan, Puumala, Belgrade, Seoul and Muerto Canyon viruses
Astroviridae	—	*Astrovirus*	Astroviruses
Retroviridae	Oncovirinae	BLV-HTLV retrovirus	HTLV-1 and HTLV-2
	Lentivirinae	*Lentivirus*	HIV-1 and HIV-2
	Spumavirinae	*Spumavirus*	Human foamy virus
—	—	*Deltavirus*	Hepatitis D virus

3. Viroid RNA does not produce proteins.
4. Unlike virus RNA, which may be copied in the host cells' cytoplasm or nucleus, viroid RNA is always copied in the host cell nucleus.
5. Viroid particles are not apparent in the infected tissues without the use of special techniques to identify nucleotide sequences in the RNA.

Prions

Prions (proteinaceous infectious particles) are composed largely of a protein without any detectable nucleic acid. They are highly resistant to inactivation by physical and chemical agents. They produce slow infections (**subacute spongiform encephalopathy**) with long incubation period (in years), followed by progressive disease, which leads to death from a degenerative condition of the brain characterized by a spongiform appearance. Diseases caused by them include scrapie of sheep and goats, bovine spongiform encephalopathy, mink and feline encephalopathy, wasting disease of deer and elk, Creutzfeldt-Jakob disease, Gerstmann-Sträussler-Scheinker syndrome and fatal familial insomnia in humans.

LABORATORY DIAGNOSIS OF VIRAL INFECTIONS

Laboratory diagnosis of viral infections can be carried out by the following methods:

I. Direct detection of virus, viral antigen or viral genome.
II. Virus isolation.
III. Detection of specific antiviral antibodies.
IV. Cytological or histological examination of cells from the site of infection.

I. Direct detection of virus, viral antigen or viral genome

1. Electron microscopy

Electron microscopy (EM) is one of the most useful tools for the direct demonstration of viruses in clinical specimens. On the basis of their distinctive appearances, most of the viruses can be assigned to the correct family. Viruses that are difficult to culture (*Rotavirus*, astroviruses) can be recognized by electron microscopy. The clinical material can be negatively stained with potassium phosphotungstate or uranyl acetate and scanned by EM. Clinical applications of electron microscopy include detection of *Rotavirus* and hepatitis A virus in faecal specimens, poxviruses in vesicle fluid and herpesvirus in brain biopsy tissue. This method can also be used for the identification of virus isolates in cell culture.

2. Immunoelectron microscopy

EM as a diagnostic tool has low sensitivity. For satisfactory results, the specimen should contain 10^7 virions per ml. The sensitivity of electron microscopy can be increased by mixing specific antibody with the specimen to aggregate the virus particles. These aggregates can be sedimented by centrifugation, negatively stained and observed under EM.

3. Fluorescence microscopy

Virions or viral antigens can be detected in frozen tissue sections, acetone-fixed cell smears, cells from virus infected cultures or vesicle fluid by direct or indirect fluorescent antibody technique. Fluorescence microscopy of brain biopsy can be used for the diagnosis of herpes simplex encephalitis and subacute sclerosing panencephalitis (a late sequelae of measles) and for the verification of rabies in the brain of animals suspected to be rabid. This method is also useful for the rapid diagnosis of respiratory infections caused by paramyxoviruses, orthomyxoviruses, adenoviruses and herpesviruses.

4. Light microscopy

Viral antigens in infected cells can be detected by immunoperoxidase staining. Tissue section or smear of infected cells is stained with antibody coupled to horseradish peroxidase. Hydrogen peroxide together with a benzidine derivative is then added. It forms a coloured insoluble precipitate which can be seen under ordinary light microscope (LM).

5. Viral antigens

These may be detected by direct and indirect ELISA, radioimmunoassay and latex agglutination.

6. Nucleic acid probes

- Enzyme-labelled or radiolabelled nucleic acid (DNA or RNA) sequences complementary to unique regions in nucleic acid sequences of most viruses are now manufactured commercially. These labelled complementary sequences are known as nucleic acid probes. Two strands of the target DNA molecule in the clinical specimens are first separated by boiling, then, following cooling, allowed to hybridize with a labelled single-stranded DNA or RNA probe present in excess. Depending on the type of label attached to the probe, hybridized-labelled probe can be detected by radiography, gamma-counting or by a simple colourimetric evaluation (dot-blot hybridization).
- By use of nucleic acid probes cytomegalovirus, papillomavirus and Epstein-Barr virus have been identified.
- *In situ* **hybridization** may be used to detect integrated or nonintegrated copies of viral genome in persistent infections or viral cancers.
- **Southern blot hybridization and northern blot hybridization** can be used for detection of DNA and RNA respectively.

7. Polymerase chain reaction (PCR)

It is a DNA amplification system that allows molecular biologists to produce microgram quantities of DNA from picogram amounts of starting material. It is based on repeated cycles of high temperature template denaturation, oligonucleotide primer annealing and polymerase mediated extension. With the revolutionary PCR technique, a target DNA sequence can be amplified at least 100,000 folds in just a few hours, a sharp contrast to the days required for conventional amplification method (culture). Thus, viral DNA extracted from a very small number of virions or infected cells can be amplified to the point, where it can readily be identified using labelled probes in a hybridization assay. For the detection of viral RNA, it is first converted into DNA by reverse transcriptase.

PCR can be used for the diagnosis of infections caused by HIV-1, HIV-2, HTLV-1, cytomegalovirus, human *Papillomavirus*, herpes simplex viruses, HBV, HCV, HDV, HEV, rubella virus, Epstein-Barr virus, varicella-zoster virus, human herpesvirus 6 and 7, *Parvovirus* B19, enteroviruses, coxsackieviruses, echoviruses, rhinoviruses, measles virus and *Rotavirus* (Table 7.5).

II. Virus isolation

Most of the viruses can be cultivated in laboratory animals, chick embryos and cell cultures.

III. Detection of specific antiviral antibodies

Using panels of known antigens, a number of serological techniques may be used to detect specific viral antibodies. Paired sera should be collected from the patient, the 'acute-phase' serum sample collected as early as possible in the illness and the 'convalescent-phase' sample collected at least 2 weeks later. Antibodies in the serum samples can be detected by ELISA, RIA, western blot, latex agglutination, virus neutralization, haemagglutination inhibition, immunofluorescence, immunodiffusion and complement fixation tests.

IV. Cytological or histological examination of cells from the site of infection

Virus-induced histopathology (multinucleate giant cells and inclusion bodies) may be recognized by light microscopy. For example, demonstration of Negri bodies in the brain cells of animals is a useful method for presumptive diagnosis of rabies.

47

Bacteriophage

Bacteriophages or simply phages are viruses that infect bacteria.

Morphology

Bacteriophages that infect *Escherichia coli*, called the T-even phages (T2, T4, T6), have been studied in great detail. They serve as the prototypes in describing the properties of bacteriophages. They are tadpole shaped with a hexagonal head and a cylindrical tail (Fig. 47.1).

- **Head:** It consists of a tightly packed core of nucleic acid (double-stranded DNA) surrounded by a protein coat or capsid. The size of the head varies from 28–100 nm.
- **Tail:** It consists of a long hollow core surrounded by a contractile sheath and a terminal base plate. Attached to the base plate of the tail are six tail fibres and six tail pins. The virus uses the tail fibres to find a bacterium to infect and the tail pins on the base plate anchor the virus to the host cell during infection.

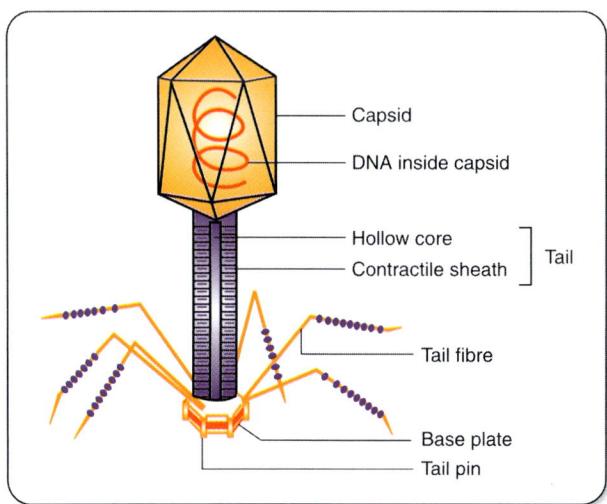

Fig. 47.1. Morphology of T4 phage particle.

Most of the phages possess double-stranded DNA, but single-stranded RNA or DNA and double-stranded RNA is present in some other phages.

Life cycle

Phages exhibit two different types of life cycle. In virulent or lytic cycle, there is intracellular multiplication of phages followed by lysis and release of progeny virions. In temperate or lysogenic cycle, the phage DNA becomes integrated with the bacterial genome replicating synchronously with it, causing no harm to the host cell.

1. Lytic cycle

The events between infection of a cell by a phage and its subsequent lysis to release daughter phage particles are similar for most phages. The lytic cycle of T-even phages is described below.

1. **Adsorption:** With the help of tail fibres and tail pins, phage particles attach to virus-specific receptors on the host cell. Adsorption is a specific process and depends on the presence of complementary chemical groups on the receptor sites on the bacterial surface and on the terminal base plate of the phage. Infection cannot occur in the absence of adsorption. Therefore, most phages are highly specific for a limited number of bacterial hosts and this constitutes the basis of bacteriophage typing of bacteria. Experimental infection by direct injection of phage DNA can be achieved even in bacterial strains that are insusceptible to infection by the whole phage. The infection of a bacterium by the naked phage nucleic acid is known as **transfection**.
2. **Penetration:** Following adsorption, six tail pins make contact with the host cell surface and firmly attach the phage plate to it. The contractile tail sheath then contracts forcing the hollow interior tail tube about 12 nm into the bacterial cell wall. The phage DNA then passes through

In the figure, labels read: Capsid; DNA inside capsid; Hollow core; Contractile sheath (Tail); Tail fibre; Base plate; Tail pin.

the hollow interior tail tube. Penetration may be facilitated by the presence on the phage tail of lysozyme, which produces a hole on the bacterial cell wall for the entry of phage core. After penetration, phages leave their empty capsids and tails outside the bacteria.

When the bacteria are mixed with very large number of phages per bacterial cell, multiple holes are produced on the cell with the consequent leakage of the cell contents. Bacterial lysis occurs without viral multiplication. This is known as **lysis from without**.

3. **Synthesis:** Immediately after penetration of the phage nucleic acid, synthesis of phage components is initiated. The first products to be synthesized are **early proteins**. These are enzymes necessary for synthesis of phage components. Subsequently, **late proteins** appear, which are the protein subunits of the phage head and tail. During this period, the synthesis of bacterial protein, DNA and RNA ceases.

4. **Maturation:** Phage DNA, head protein and tail protein are synthesized separately in the bacterial cell. The DNA is condensed into a compact polyhedron and packaged into the head and, finally, the tail structures are added. This assembly of phage components into the mature infective phage particles is known as maturation.

5. **Release:** The release of mature progeny phage particles occurs by lysis of the bacterial cell. During replication of the phage, the bacterial cell wall is weakened and assumes a spherical shape. Phage enzymes act on the weakened cell wall causing it to burst or lyse, resulting in the release of mature daughter phages.

Eclipse phase: The interval between entry of the phage nucleic acid into the bacterial cell and the appearance of the first infectious intracellular phage particles is known as the eclipse phase. It represents the time required for the synthesis of the phage components and their assembly into mature phage particles. The duration of eclipse phase is 15–30 minutes.

Latent period: The interval between the infection of a bacterial cell and the first release of infectious phage particles is known as latent phase.

2. Lysogenic cycle

Not all phage infections result in immediate progeny production and lysis of the host cell. There are many phages that, upon entering a sensitive cell, either undergo a lytic cycle like that described above or alternatively enter into a benign relationship with their hosts, called **lysogeny**. The phages that can develop both lytically and lysogenically are said to be **temperate phages**. In lysogenic state, the bacteriophage nucleic acid becomes integrated into the bacterial chromosome. The phage genome in this state is known as **prophage**. It replicates along with the bacterial chromosome. A bacterium that carries a prophage is known as a **lysogenic bacterium** or **lysogen**.

The prophage confers certain new properties on the lysogenic bacterium. This is known as **lysogenic** or **phage conversion**. Following are the examples of lysogenic conversion:

- **Toxin production** in *Corynebacterium diphtheriae* is determined by the presence in it of the prophage β. The elimination of this prophage abolishes the toxigenicity of the bacillus and nontoxigenic strains can be made toxigenic by lysogenization.

- *Clostridium botulinum* types C and D produce toxin only if these are infected with phage CE β and DE β respectively.

- A wide variety of temperate phages of *Salmonella* can **modify the antigenic properties** of somatic O antigen. The antigenic formula of *S.* Anatum is 3, 10:e, h:1, 6 but when it is lysogenised by a temperate phage its antigenic formula becomes 3, 15:e, h:1, 6 (*S.* Newington).

Occasionally, integrated prophage is excised from bacterial DNA, and phage multiplication and subsequent cell lysis ensues. This is known as **spontaneous induction of prophage**. It is a rare event, but all lysogenic bacteria can be induced to shift to the lytic cycle by certain physical (UV rays) and chemical (nitrogen mustard) agents. A lysogenic bacterium is resistant to reinfection by the same or related phages. This is known as **superinfection immunity**.

Bacteriophages may act as **carriers of genes** from one bacterium to another. This is known as **transduction**. It has been discussed in the chapter on bacterial genetics.

Phage typing

The limited host range of many phages enables them to be used as an epidemiological marker to discriminate between bacterial strains that are biochemically or serologically indistinguishable. This method has been used to trace outbreaks of infection caused by *Staphylococcus aureus*, *S.* Typhi and *Vibrio cholerae*. The strain to be typed is inoculated on a plate of nutrient agar to produce a lawn culture. After drying, the phages are applied over marked squares in a fixed dose (**routine test dose**). Routine test dose is the highest dilution of the phage preparation that produces confluent lysis. After overnight incubation, the culture will be observed to be lysed by some phages but not by others. The phage type of the strain is expressed by the designation of the phage/phages that lyse it. For example, if a strain of *S. aureus* is lysed by phages 50, 52A and 80, then the phage type is expressed as 50/52A/80.

Phage assay

When a phage is applied on the lawn culture of a susceptible bacterium, areas of clearing or lysis occur after incubation. Area of lysis caused by phage is known as **plaque**. Since a single phage particle is capable of producing one plaque, **plaque assay** can be employed for titrating the number of viable phages in a preparation.

48

Poxviruses and Herpesviruses

POXVIRUSES

Morphology

Poxviruses are the largest animal viruses. They are large enough to be seen by light microscopy after special staining procedures. In most genera, the virions are **brick-shaped** with rounded corners, measuring 300 × 200 × 100 nm in size (Fig. 48.1). Nucleocapsids of these viruses do not conform to either of two types of symmetry found in most other viruses, hence, they are known as **complex viruses**. Poxviruses have a biconcave dumb-bell-shaped DNA core and two lateral bodies

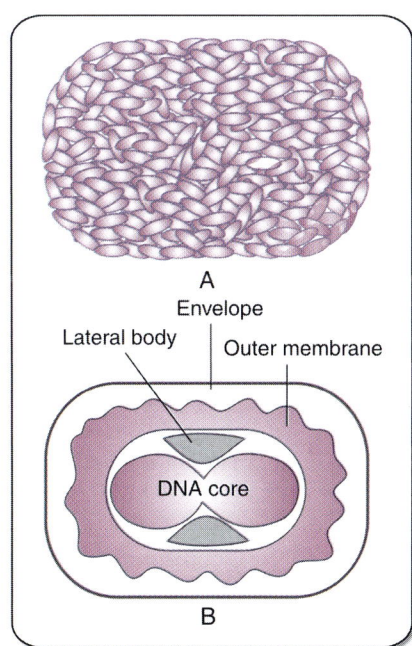

Fig. 48.1. The structure of vaccinia virion. (A) Surface structure of nonenveloped virus particle showing surface tubules; (B) Section of enveloped virion.

enclosed in a protein shell about 12 nm thick. It is known as outer membrane, surface of which consists of irregularly arranged tubules. Virions released from the cell are enclosed within an envelope which consists of host cell lipids and several virus-specified polypeptides, including the haem-agglutinin.

Cultivation

Chick embryo

Variola and vaccinia viruses grow on chorioallantoic membrane of 11–13-day-old chick embryo, producing pocks in 48–72 hours. Variola pocks are small, shiny, white, convex, non-necrotic and non-haemorrhagic. In contrast, vaccinia pocks are larger, irregular, greyish, flat, necrotic and some of these are haemorrhagic.

Tissue culture

Variola and vaccinia viruses can be grown in monkey kidney, HeLa and chick embryo cells. Cytopathic effects are produced by vaccinia in 48–72 hours but variola takes longer to produce these changes. Intracytoplasmic, eosinophilic inclusion bodies – **Guarnieri bodies** – can be demonstrated in the stained preparation. Vaccinia, but not variola, produces plaques in chick embryo tissue culture.

Smallpox (variola)

The virus causing classical smallpox was called variola major (fatal disease) and that causing alastrium (non-fatal disease) variola minor. On May 8, 1980, the WHO formally announced the **global eradication of smallpox**.

Vaccinia

Origin of vaccinia virus is not known. It may have evolved from cowpox or smallpox virus. In the past, this virus was used for smallpox vaccination.

Molluscum contagiosum

Molluscum contagiosum is a common, self-limiting viral disease of skin caused by *Molluscipoxvirus*. Lesions are characterized by multiple discrete umbilicated nodules 2–5 mm in diameter, limited to the epidermis and occurring anywhere on the body except on soles and palms. Lesions are more commonly seen on the trunk and anogenital areas. Nodules are dome-shaped, waxy, pearly white or pink in colour and are painless (Fig. 48.2). A white caseous material can be squeezed from them. Lesions can persist for months and usually regress spontaneously.

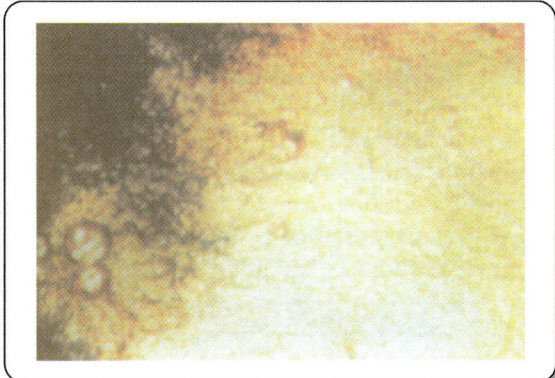

Fig. 48.2. Multiple lesions of molluscum contagiosum in the pubic area.

The virus is transmitted by direct contact, perhaps through minor abrasions and sexually in adults. Extensive skin involvement is seen in AIDS patients. The cells in the nodules are greatly hypertrophied and contain large (up to 35 μm) hyaline acidophilic intracytoplasmic inclusion bodies which displace the nuclei to the margin. These are known as **molluscum bodies** (Fig. 48.3). These can be seen in cells of the stratum granulosum and the stratum corneum. Molluscum contagiosum virus has not so far been cultured.

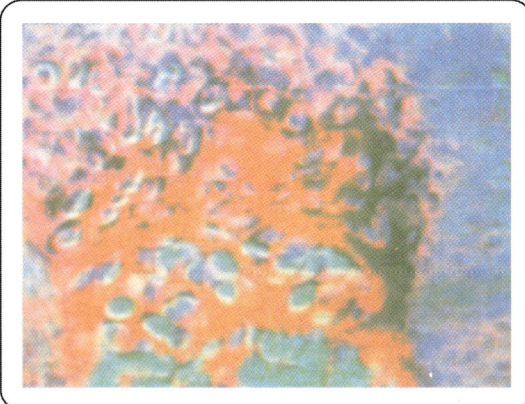

Fig. 48.3. Molluscum contagiosum. Horny layer shows numerous large, hyaline, acidophilic, intracytoplasmic inclusion bodies called molluscum bodies (H&E stain, ×400).

HERPESVIRUSES

Morphology

Herpesviruses are 120–200 nm in diameter. They comprise of four distinct structural elements – envelope, tegument, capsid and core (Fig. 48.4). Envelope is the outermost, it is composed of lipid with numerous small glycoprotein peplomers. Tegument is the electron-dense material present between envelope and capsid. It contains several proteins. Inner to the tegument is icosahedral capsid of 100 nm diameter. It has a total of 162 capsomers. Core, inside the capsid, consists of double-stranded, 124–235 kb DNA. With the exception of Epstein-Barr virus, members of the family Herpesviridae can be cultivated in cell cultures and produce giant cells and Cowdry type A intranuclear inclusion bodies in infected cells.

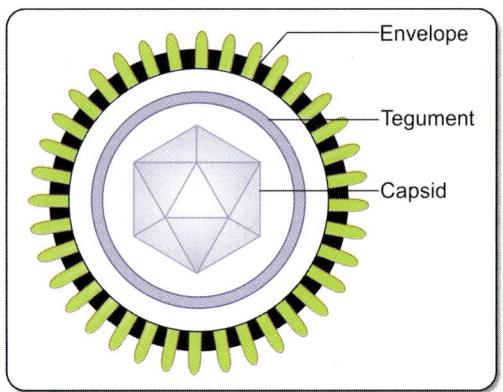

Fig. 48.4. Herpesvirus.

HERPES SIMPLEX VIRUS (HSV)

There are two types of herpes simplex virus – type 1 virus (HSV-1) and type 2 virus (HSV-2).

Pathogenesis

HSV-1 infects primarily the mouth, the eye and the central nervous system (regions of the body above the waist), but it is also responsible for a proportion of cases of genital herpes. HSV-2 infects genital and anal regions. The infections caused by herpes simplex viruses can be divided into primary infection, latent infection, reactivation and recrudescence.

Primary infection

HSV is transmitted only by contact. The portal of entry in primary infection is the damaged skin or mucosa and the classic lesion is a vesicle beneath the keratinized squamous epithelial cells.

Infections caused by HSV-1

1. Acute gingivostomatitis.
2. Herpetic whitlow.
3. Keratoconjunctivitis.

4. Eczema herpeticum.
5. Encephalitis.
6. Generalized infection.

Infections caused by HSV-2

1. Genital herpes.
2. Aseptic meningitis.
3. Neonatal infection.

Latent infection

During primary infection, the virus travels from the site of infection in the mouth to the trigeminal and probably other cranial and cervical ganglia. In genital herpes, HSV-2 travels to sacral ganglia. Within the sensory ganglia, viral DNA exists as a free circular episome perhaps about 20 copies per infected cells.

Reactivation and recrudescence

Reactivation of the virus is provoked by various stimuli such as common cold, fever, pneumonia, menstruation, exposure to sunlight, stress, etc. Infectious virions migrate along the nerve axon back to the nerve endings, where infection of epithelial cells may result in cluster of vesicles at the muco-cutaneous junctions of the lips, in the nose, or eyes or on areas of skin that have experienced a primary infection. Reactivation recurs sporadically, sometimes often, throughout life.

Laboratory diagnosis

1. Specimens

Vesicle fluid, skin swab, saliva, conjunctival fluid, corneal scrapings, brain biopsy and CSF.

2. Microscopy

Diagnosis of HSV infection can be made by direct examination of clinical specimens by electron microscopy (EM), fluorescence microscopy (FM) and light microscopy (LM). Herpes virions may be demonstrated in the negatively stained smear of the specimen by EM. Viral antigens can be detected by FM in the cells scraped from the base of the lesions and tissue preparations stained by immunofluorescent staining. By LM, infected cell may be identified by characteristic changes, which include ballooning of cells, ground glass nuclei, **eosinophilic intranuclear inclusions and multinucleated giant cells** (Fig. 48.5).

3. Virus isolation

HSV can be isolated on human fibroblast or Vero cells, although, other mammalian cells also support its growth. Within 1–5 days distinctive foci of swollen, rounded cells appear. Some virus strains (particularly HSV-2 strains) may give rise to fusion of infected cells leading to **syncytium formation**. Diagnosis can be confirmed within 24 hours by **immunofluorescent staining** of infected cell culture.

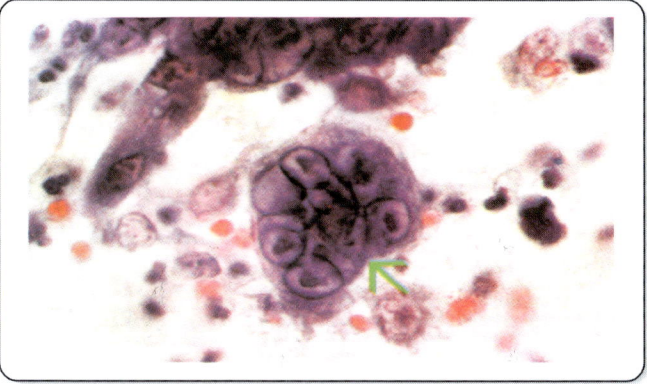

Fig. 48.5. Multinucleated giant cells with intranuclear inclusion bodies of herpes simplex virus (H&E stain, ×400).

4. Serology

Primary infections can be diagnosed serologically by detection of virus-specific IgM or of a rising IgG titre by complement fixation, neutralization, immunofluorescence, ELISA or RIA. However, serology is not widely used.

5. Polymerase chain reaction

Polymerase chain reaction may be used for detection of HSV DNA in CSF.

VARICELLA-ZOSTER VIRUS (VZV)

VZV causes varicella (chickenpox) in children and herpes zoster (shingles) in adults and immunocompromised patients. **Varicella follows primary infection in a nonimmune individual while herpes zoster is a reactivation of latent virus when immunity has fallen to ineffective levels.** A child can catch varicella from an elderly patient with herpes zoster, but the latter occurs only if the elderly or immuno-compromised person had suffered from varicella in early part of his life.

Varicella

It is one of the common childhood exanthemata. Portal of entry of the virus is respiratory tract. Incubation period is about 2 weeks. The earliest manifestation is a **maculopapular rash** that progresses within a few hours to the vesicular stage. Vesicles characteristically are surrounded by a red rim. The lesions then rupture and crust or may become secondarily infected and pustular before healing.

Herpes zoster

Herpes zoster or shingles is an **endogenous reactivation of virus** which has remained latent in one or more sensory ganglia following primary varicella many years earlier. Virus travels down the sensory nerves to produce painful vesicles in the area of skin (dermatome) enervated from the affected ganglion (Fig. 48.6). Thoracic nerves supplying the chest wall are most often affected. When the ophthalmic nerve of

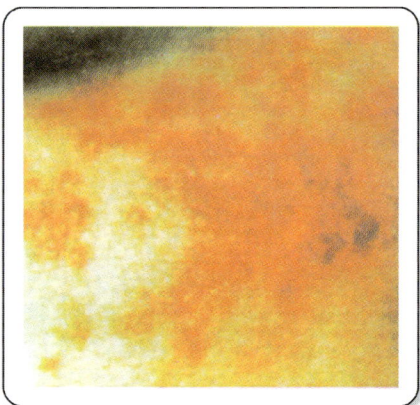

Fig. 48.6. Vesicles of varicella zoster infection on the left shoulder and neck.

trigeminal ganglion is affected, the rash is distributed on the scalp and forehead. In about half of the patients, the eye is affected leading to corneal ulceration, stromal keratitis and anterior uveitis.

Laboratory diagnosis

1. Direct examination of vesicle fluid by **electron microscopy** may reveal herpes virus particles.
2. Stained smears from the base of the lesion or sections from biopsy tissue show **multinucleated giant cells containing acidophilic intranuclear inclusion bodies**.
3. Rapid diagnosis is possible by using **monoclonal fluorescent antibody technique**.
4. VZV antigens can be detected in vesicle fluid by **ELISA**.
5. DNA can be extracted from virions in vesicle fluid, CSF, aqueous humour, and amplified by **PCR** and detected by nucleic acid hybridization.
6. The virus can be **isolated** from vesicle fluid in human embryonic lung fibroblasts, human amnion, HeLa or Vero cells. Cytopathic effect is focal with refractile ballooned cells. It develops slowly over a period of 2 or more weeks. However, VZV antigen can be demonstrated in nuclear inclusions by immunofluorescence with monoclonal antibody before the end of first week.
7. Recent infection can be diagnosed by **ELISA test** for varicella-zoster specific IgM antibody in patient serum.

EPSTEIN-BARR VIRUS (EBV)

EBV replicates in epithelial cells of nasopharynx and salivary glands, especially the parotid, lysing them and releasing infectious virions into saliva. It causes:

1. Infectious mononucleosis (Glandular fever)

After an incubation period of 4–7 weeks, patient presents with sore throat due to exudative tonsillitis, generalized lymphadenopathy, fever, malaise, headache, sweating, fatigue and gastrointestinal discomfort. In some cases spleen and liver

are often enlarged. A faint transient morbilliform rash may be seen.

2. Burkitt's lymphoma

This lymphoma is a **malignant B cell lymphoma** (a tumour of the jaw).

3. B cell lymphoma

Immunodeficient patients, e.g., recipients of transplants and HIV-infected patients may develop EBV associated B cell lymphoma.

4. Nasopharyngeal carcinoma

It is also associated with EBV and viral DNA is regularly present in the malignant epithelial cells of the tumour.

5. Oral hairy leukoplakia

This lesion is a wart-like growth that develops on the tongue in some HIV-infected patients and recipients of transplant (Fig. 48.7). It is an epithelial focus of EBV replication.

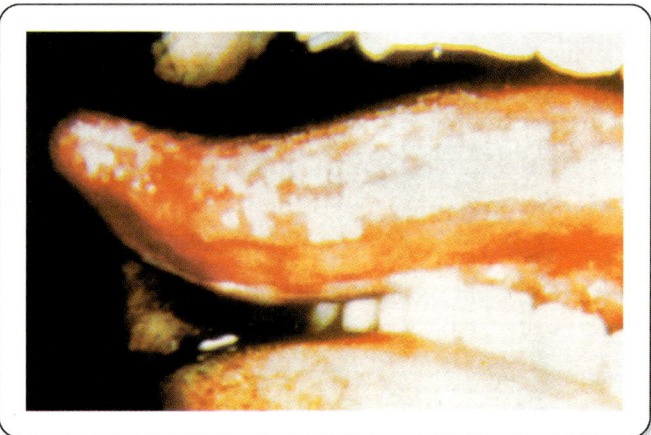

Fig. 48.7. Oral hairy leukoplakia in an AIDS patient.

Laboratory diagnosis of infectious mononucleosis

1. Differential white blood cell count

By the second week of the illness patient develops leucocytosis (10,000–20,000/µl or more). Lymphocytes and monocytes account for 60–80%. Of these, 20% or more are **'atypical lymphocytes'**. The latter are large pleomorphic blasts with deeply basophilic vacuolated cytoplasm and lobulated nuclei. They persist for 2 weeks to several months.

2. Paul-Bunnell heterophile antibodies

Infectious mononucleosis is accompanied by production of **heterophile agglutinins**. These are heterophile IgM antibodies elicited by EBV infection. These antibodies appear in 85–90% of patients' sera during the acute phase of illness, reaching peak levels 2 weeks after the onset. Their titre decreases rapidly after fourth week and are not detectable after 3 months. Heterophile antibodies may be readily detected by a rapid slide agglutination test or Paul-Bunnell test. Agglutination of sheep or horse red cells by patient serum, adsorbed with guinea-pig kidney cells, to remove Forssman antibody, is the basis of this test.

3. EBV-specific antibodies

More reliable indicator of EBV infection is the demonstration of IgM antibody to the EBV viral capsid antigen by ELISA or indirect immunofluorescence. This antibody becomes detectable within 4 weeks and declines rapidly over the next 3 months or so.

4. Virus isolation

Saliva or throat washing and peripheral blood leucocytes can be inoculated onto umbilical cord lymphocytes. If the specimen contains EBV, it leads to immortalization of the cells to produce a lymphoblastoid cell line.

5. PCR and DNA hybridization

EBV can also be detected by PCR and DNA hybridization.

CYTOMEGALOVIRUS (CMV)

CMV is the largest virus in the family Herpesviridae, being 150–200 nm in size. It may be acquired at any time, i.e. prenatal, perinatal and postnatal.

Prenatal (intrauterine) infection

CMV is the most common agent to cause intrauterine infection and prenatal damage to foetus leading to congenital abnormalities.

Perinatal infection

This is acquired from infected maternal genital secretions or from breast feeding.

Postnatal infection

This may be acquired by kissing (from saliva), sexual intercourse or artificial insemination (from semen), blood transfusion and organ transplantation.

Infections acquired after birth are generally subclinical. However, it may cause hepatitis in young children. In adults and older children, it may cause a syndrome resembling EBV infectious mononucleosis, but with a negative Paul-Bunnell test and no pharyngitis or lymphadenopathy.

Laboratory diagnosis

1. Specimens

CMV can be isolated from urine, saliva, stool, breast milk, semen, cervical secretions and blood leucocytes.

2. Demonstration of cytomegalic cells

Cytomegalic cells can be demonstrated in centrifuged deposits of urine or saliva.

3. Isolation of virus

The specimens are inoculated on cultured human fibroblasts. The virus replicates very slowly, therefore, characteristic CPE of foci of swollen refractile cells with cytoplasmic granules may take 2–3 weeks to appear. When stained, these cells are **multinucleated giant cells containing acidophilic inclusions with perinuclear halo (owl's eye appearance) in the nuclei and cytoplasm** (Fig. 48.8).

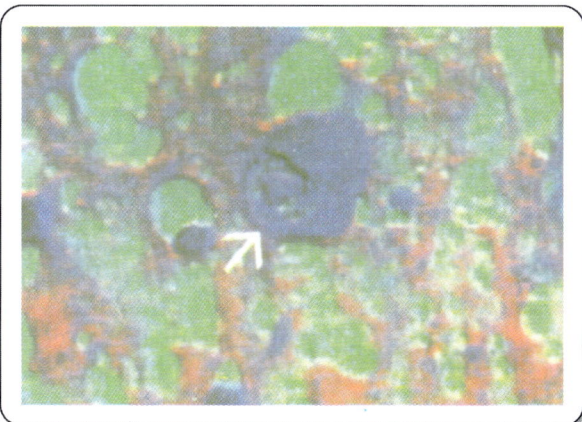

Fig. 48.8. Cytomegalovirus infection showing intranuclear inclusion bodies with perinuclear halo (owl's eye appearance) (H&E stain, ×400).

4. Polymerase chain reaction (PCR)

CMV DNA, in the specimen, can be amplified by PCR.

5. Serology

CMV-specific IgM can be detected in the patient serum by ELISA.

49

Adenoviruses, Papillomaviruses and Rotaviruses

ADENOVIRUSES

Adenoviruses belong to the family Adenoviridae. They are nonenveloped, icosahedral viruses containing linear double-stranded DNA that replicate in the nucleus of infected cells.

Classification

The family comprises of two distinct genera – *Mastadenovirus* and *Aviadenovirus*. They possess mammalian and avian adenoviruses respectively. The genus *Mastadenovirus* comprises at least 52 serotypes which infect humans.

Morphology

Adenoviruses are icosahedral virions containing a single linear, double-stranded DNA. They measure 70–75 nm in diameter. Each capsid is composed of 252 capsomers – 240 hexons make up the 20 triangular faces of icosahedron and 12 pentons form the vertices. From each penton projects an apical fibre, 9–31 nm in length that serves to bind specifically to receptor sites on the host cell (Fig. 49.1).

Cultivation

Human adenoviruses can be grown in monolayers of HeLa, HEp-2, KB and human embryo kidney cells. Cytopathic effects may take several days to develop and consist of **cell rounding and aggregation in grape-like clusters**. Infected cells swell and become ballooned and show characteristic **basophilic intranuclear inclusions** in stained preparation.

Pathogenesis

Adenoviruses may infect via the conjunctiva or the nasal mucosa. Faecal-oral spread, particularly among children can also occur. They multiply initially in the conjunctiva, pharynx or small intestine and spread to preauricular, cervical and mesenteric lymph nodes. Most of the enteric and some of the respiratory infections are subclinical.

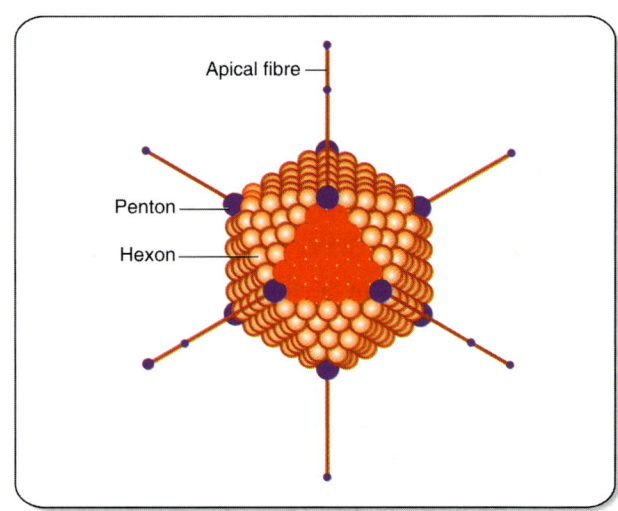

Fig. 49.1. Morphology of adenovirus.

Clinical syndromes

Incubation period is 5–8 days after which it may lead to:

I. Respiratory infections

- Pharyngitis
- Pneumonia
- Acute respiratory disease

II. Ocular infections

- Pharyngoconjunctival fever
- Epidemic keratoconjunctivitis

III. Genitourinary infections

- Cervicitis and urethritis
- Acute haemorrhagic cystitis

IV. Enteric infections

- Infantile gastroenteritis

Laboratory diagnosis

1. Specimens

Throat swab, nasopharyngeal aspirate, transtracheal aspirate, bronchial lavage, conjunctival swab, corneal scraping, urine, anal swab, faecal swab, genital secretions, and biopsy and autopsy materials.

2. Light microscopy

Adenovirus-infected cells can be visualized by light microscopy as 'smudge cells' in hematoxylin and eosin or Wright-Giemsa-stained tissues, fluid sediments, or cultures. Smudge cells are large, late-stage-infected cells containing solitary, central, intranuclear, basophilic inclusions composed of adenoviral particles.

3. Electron microscopy

Virus particles may be seen directly in stool extracts by **electron microscopy** and **immunoelectron microscopy**.

4. Immunofluorescence

Viral antigens in the cells from respiratory tract, eye, urine, biopsy or autopsy material and infected cell cultures may be demonstrated by **immunofluorescence** using polyclonal or monoclonal antibodies.

5. Detection of enteric adenoviruses

Enteric adenoviruses may be detected by **latex agglutination** method using latex particles coated with specific antibody to each virus.

6. Detection of antigen

Viral antigens in faeces and nasopharyngeal secretions may be detected by **ELISA** using monoclonal or polyclonal antibodies.

7. Detection of viral DNA

Viral DNA in the faeces may be detected by **polyacrylamide gel electrophoresis**.

8. Virus isolation

Virus from the clinical specimens, may be isolated on HeLa, HEp-2, KB and human embryo kidney cells.

9. DNA probes and polymerase chain reaction

DNA probe and polymerase chain reaction are used to identify enteric adenoviruses.

10. Serology

For serological diagnosis, rise in titre of antibodies should be demonstrated in paired sera. Examination of a single sample of serum is inconclusive as adenovirus antibodies are so common in the population.

PAPILLOMAVIRUSES

Papillomaviruses are small (55 nm in diameter), nonenveloped and have an icosahedral capsid composed of 72 capsomers.

The genome is a supercoiled dsDNA molecule of 7.2–8 kilobase pairs. They are host species-specific and infect the squamous epithelia and mucous membranes of higher vertebrates, including man. There are over 100 types of human papillomaviruses (HPV). **Papillomaviruses cannot be grown in cell cultures.**

Pathogenesis

HPV are not only host species-specific but also display a predilection for the skin and certain mucous membranes. They cause cutaneous warts, genital warts, recurrent respiratory papillomatosis, oral papillomatosis and cancer. The infection is transmitted by indirect or direct contact including sexual contact.

Laboratory diagnosis

It can be carried out by:

1. Histopathology and cytopathology

These reveal hypertrophy of all layers of the dermis and hyperkeratosis of the horny layer.

2. Electron microscopy

Papillomavirus particles can be readily seen by electron microscopy in most warts but are less in number in genital warts.

3. Immunocytochemistry

The HPV capsid antigen in paraffin sections of tissues or in cell smears can be detected by an immunoperoxidase test using a commercially available antiserum prepared by immunization of rabbits with bovine *Papillomavirus* particles disrupted with sodium dodecyl sulphate.

4. Detection of viral nucleic acid

Viral DNA in fresh tissues, fixed tissues and exfoliated cells can be detected by DNA hybridization and polymerase chain reaction.

POLYOMA VIRUSES

1. JC polyomavirus

It causes infection in man. It was first isolated from the brain of a male patient with Hodgkin's disease who developed progressive multifocal leukoencephalopathy (PML). It was designated by the initials of the person from whom it was isolated. The virus persists for life in the kidneys and is shed in urine sporadically and more frequently during pregnancy and immunosuppression.

2. BK polyomavirus

It was isolated from the urine of a renal transplant recipient and was named after his initials. It causes subclinical infection of children before the age of 10. It may, however, cause upper respiratory symptoms. The virus persists for life in kidneys. Reactivation may occur during last trimester of pregnancy and following immunosuppression for organ transplantation leading to asymptomatic shedding of virus in urine.

ROTAVIRUSES

Rotavirus (*rota*, meaning wheel) has two concentric icosahedral shells, resembling a wheel with short spokes radiating from a wide hub to a clearly defined outer rim. The genome consists of double-stranded segmented RNA.

Rotaviruses have been found to be the main aetiological agents of gastroenteritis in infants and young children worldwide. Mature rotavirus particles are about 70 nm in diameter and are nonenveloped. They are classified into seven serogroups, (A–G). Groups A to C rotaviruses infect both humans and animals, with the group A rotaviruses infecting humans most frequently and causing disease mainly in children. Group D to G rotaviruses are mainly animal pathogens.

Rotaviruses infect epithelial cells at the tips of the villi of small intestine. As a result of infection, the cells are destroyed and virus is released in large numbers in the intestinal lumen which may involve the entire length of small intestine and sometimes colon. Cellular damage leads to malabsorption resulting in fluid accumulation in the lumen of the gut, vomiting and diarrhoea which may lead to severe dehydration. **Incubation period is 1–2 days and illness lasts for 4–5 days.**

Laboratory diagnosis

During acute stage of the disease, 10^{11} virus particles are present in the faeces. These can be detected by:

- Latex agglutination test, using latex particles coated with rotavirus-specific antibody.
- Reverse passive haemagglutination.
- ELISA.
- Electron microscopy.
- Immunoelectron microscopy.

50

Polioviruses and Rabies Virus

POLIOVIRUSES

Morphology

The virion is 27–30 nm in diameter. Capsid is composed of 60 capsomers arranged in icosahedral symmetry. The genome is a single strand of positive sense RNA.

Antigenic properties

On the basis of neutralization tests, polioviruses can be divided into three serotypes. Type 1 is the common epidemic type, type 2 is usually associated with endemic infections and type 3 occasionally causes epidemics.

Pathogenesis

Polioviruses have affinity for nervous tissue and narrow host range. Only man and some primates like cynomolgous and rhesus monkeys are susceptible. These monkeys can be infected by the oral route and develop paralysis.

Natural infection occurs only in man. The virus is spread from man to man by faecal-oral route and because early multiplication occurs in both the oropharynx and the intestinal mucosa, therefore, the virus is also spread by pharyngeal secretions (droplet infection) during first week of illness. No intermediate host is known.

On entering the body of a new host the virus multiplies in the tonsils and Peyer's patches of the ileum. Spread to regional lymph nodes (cervical and mesenteric) leads to a viraemia, enabling the virus to become disseminated throughout the body including spinal cord and brain.

In the central nervous system, the virus multiplies selectively in the neurons and destroys them. The lesions are mostly in the anterior horns of the spinal cord, causing flaccid paralysis, but posterior horns and intermediate columns may also be involved to some extent. In some cases encephalitis occurs, primarily involving the brain stem but extending upto the motor and premotor areas of the cerebral cortex.

Clinical features

There are four types of poliovirus infection:

1. **Asymptomatic illness:** Patient does not have any symptom but the virus may be isolated from stool or throat or both. This is seen in 90–95% individuals.
2. **Minor illness:** Patient develops mild, transient 'influenza-like' illness. This is seen in 4–8% cases.
3. **Non-paralytic poliomyelitis or aseptic meningitis:** In addition to 'influenza-like' illness patient also develops headache, neck stiffness and back pain that may indicate some degree of aseptic meningitis. The illness lasts 2–10 days with rapid and complete recovery. This is seen in 1–2% individuals.
4. **Paralytic poliomyelitis or the major illness:** Patient develops paralysis during the course of the illness. It is uncommon, occurring in 0.1–2% poliovirus infections.

Laboratory diagnosis

Specimens

Virus can be isolated from blood, faeces and throat swab taken early in the disease. It can seldom be isolated from CSF but can be obtained from the spinal cord and brain, postmortem.

Virus isolation

It can be cultivated on monkey kidney, human amnion, HeLa, HEp-2 and other cell cultures. A cytopathic effect is usually seen in the cells within 48 hours. It consists of cell retraction, increased refractivity, cytoplasmic granularity and nuclear pyknosis. The identification of the serotype is carried out by neutralization tests. A wild virulent virus can be differentiated from an attenuated vaccine strain in the following ways:

1. Virulence tests in the monkeys.
2. Because the nucleotide sequences of all vaccine strains and prevalent wild strains are now known, the two can be readily distinguished by nucleic acid hybridization.

Prophylaxis

Two effective vaccines are available:

- Inactivated polio vaccine (Salk vaccine), and
- Live attenuated oral polio vaccine (Sabin vaccine).

Inactivated polio vaccine (IPV)

This vaccine contains formalin inactivated strains of the three serotypes of virus grown in monkey kidney cell culture. The vaccine is given by deep subcutaneous or intramuscular injection. Three injections are given with intervals of 6–8 weeks between the first and second doses and 4–6 months between the second and third doses. IPV produces long-lasting immunity to all three poliovirus types.

Live attenuated oral polio vaccine (OPV)

It contains live attenuated strains of the three serotypes of poliovirus grown either in cultures of monkey kidney cells or human diploid cells. At the age of 1½ months first dose of OPV is given along with DPT. Second, third and fourth doses of these vaccines are given at the ages of 2½, 3½ and 16–24 months, respectively.

With the programme of pulse polio, it has now been eradicated from India. It was declared on 11-02-2014. Since 11-02-2011, no case of poliomyelitis has ben reported from India.

RABIES VIRUS

Morphology

Rabies virus is **bullet-shaped** 180 × 75 nm, with one end rounded or conical and the other plane or concave (Fig. 50.1). **The core of the virion consists of a negative sense 11–12 kilobase, single-stranded RNA enclosed in a helically wound nucleocapsid.** RNA-dependent RNA polymerase enzyme, which is essential for the initiation of replication of the virus, is enclosed within the virion in association with the ribonucleoprotein core. The latter is surrounded by **matrix protein** (viral membrane) which may be invaginated at the plane end. The matrix protein, in turn, is surrounded by a **lipoprotein envelope**, which carries glycoprotein peplomers (spikes). The spikes do not cover the plane end of the virion.

Pathogenesis

Rabies is the classic zoonotic infection. It is a natural infection of dogs, foxes, wolves, skunks, cats and bats. Rabies virus is excreted in the saliva of affected animals. Man acquires infection by the bite of rabid dog or other animals. Rarely, infection can occur following licks on abraded skin and intact mucosa. Infection has occurred through the inhalation of massive virus aerosols generated in bat caves and in laboratory accidents.

Infection by bite of rabid animal results in deposition of rabies-infected saliva in the wound (Fig. 50.2). The virus replicates in the muscles, connective tissue or nerves at the site of deposition. After it reaches a sufficient concentration, it infects peripheral nerves in the muscle or skin. Once within the nerve fibres, it is out of reach of any circulating antibody and it travels along the axon towards the central nervous

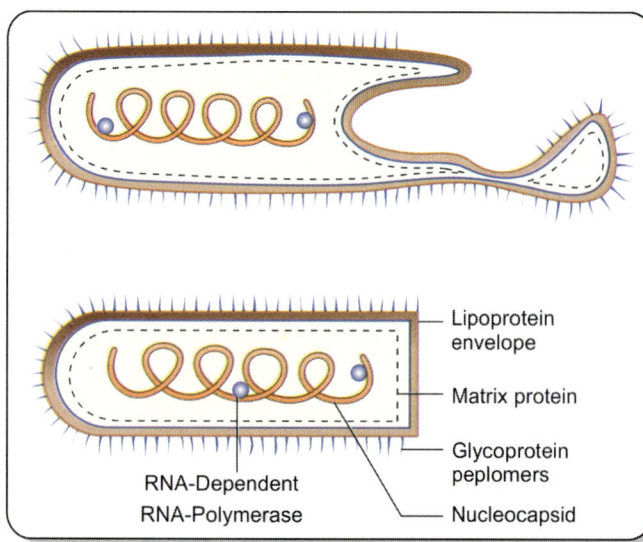

Fig. 50.1. Rabies virus.

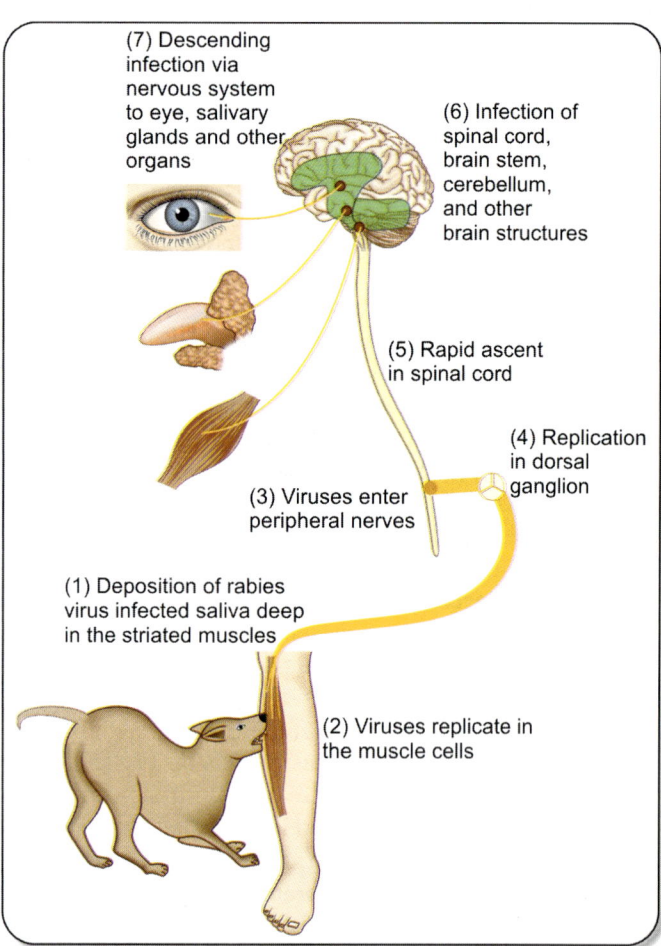

Fig. 50.2. Pathogenesis of rabies virus.

system **at a speed of 3 mm per hour**. In the central nervous system, it multiplies and produces encephalitis. The virus then spreads outwards along the nerve trunks to various parts of the body including the salivary glands. **It multiplies in the salivary glands and is shed in the saliva.** There is little evidence that haematogenous or other modes of spread are involved.

The presence of virus in the saliva, and the irritability and aggression brought on by the encephalitis ensure the transmission and survival of the virus in nature. The virus ultimately reaches virtually every tissue in the body and is almost invariably present in the cornea and the skin of face and nape of the neck of the patient because of their proximity to the brain. This provides a method for the antemortem diagnosis of rabies. The virus may also be shed in the milk and urine.

Clinical features

Following the bite of a rabid animal, the **incubation period** is usually between 1–2 months. However, it may be as short as 9 days and rarely as long as a year or more. It is shorter in children than in adults and shorter in persons bitten on the face or head and longer in those bitten on the legs. This is related to the distance the virus has to travel to reach the brain.

After a prodromal phase of malaise, headache, fever and paraesthesia at and around the site of bite, muscles become hypertonic and the patient becomes anxious, with episodes of hyperactivity, aggression and convulsions. **Patient develops difficulty in drinking, together with intense thirst. Patient may be able to swallow dry solids but not liquids.** Attempts to drink bring on painful spasm of pharynx and larynx producing choking and gagging. Thereafter, mere sight or sound of water precipitates distressing muscular spasm leading to **hydrophobia** (fear of water). **The rabies in animals does not have this peculiar feature.** The furious form of rabies gradually subsides into delirium, convulsions, coma and death.

Laboratory diagnosis

1. Demonstration of Negri bodies

Sections or impression smears of brain stained by Seller's technique may reveal inclusion bodies, known as **Negri bodies**. These are intracytoplasmic, round or oval, eosinophilic with basophilic inner granules (Fig. 50.3). Negri bodies vary in size, from 3–27 μm in diameter and are seen mainly in the pyramidal cells of Ammon's horn, in Purkinje cells of hippocampus, brain stem and cerebellum. Negri bodies may be absent in about 20% of the cases.

2. Demonstration of rabies antigen by direct immunofluorescence

(a) Antemortem

In salivary, corneal or conjunctival smears or skin biopsy from the nape of the neck by direct immunofluorescence using antirabies serum tagged with fluorescein isothiocyanate.

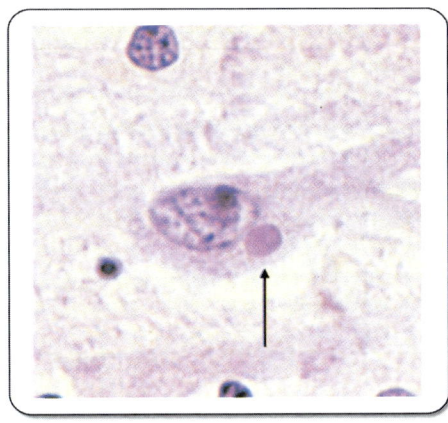

Fig. 50.3. Intracytoplasmic eosinophilic inclusion body in cells infected with rabies virus (Negri body) (Seller's stain, ×400).

(b) Postmortem

In impression smears of the cut surface of the salivary gland, hippocampus, brain stem or cerebellum by direct immunofluorescence using antirabies serum tagged with fluorescein isothiocyanate.

3. Detection of genomic RNA and viral mRNA

It is carried out by PCR and dot-blot hybridization assay with ^{32}P-labelled cDNA probes on skin biopsy, corneal impression or saliva.

4. Virus isolation

(a) Mouse inoculation

Rabies virus can be isolated by intracerebral inoculation of saliva or cerebral fluid (antemortem) and salivary gland or brain tissue extract (postmortem) in suckling mice. The animals die in 7–21 days. However, they may be killed after five days and brain smears stained with fluorescent antibody.

(b) Isolation in cell culture

Rabies virus can be grown in baby hamster kidney, human diploid lung fibroblasts, chick embryo fibroblasts and Vero monkey kidney cells. No cytopathic changes are observed but rabies antigen can be detected by fluorescent antibody staining 18–24 hours after inoculation.

5. Detection of rabies antibodies

Rabies antibodies can be detected in the serum and CSF of the patient by ELISA. **High titre antibodies are present in the CSF in rabies but not after immunization.** Their demonstration can, therefore, be used for diagnosis.

Rabies vaccines (Table 50.1)

Rabies is the only human disease that can be prevented by active immunization after infection, because a long incubation period of the disease allows time for immunity to develop before the onset of symptoms.

Table 50.1. Rabies vaccines

I. Neural vaccines
1. Semple vaccine
2. Beta-propiolactone (BPL) vaccine
3. Suckling mouse brain vaccine

II. Non-neural vaccines
A. Duck egg vaccine
B. Cell culture vaccines
- Human diploid cell (HDC) vaccine
- Purified chick embryo cell (PCEC) vaccine
- Purified Vero cell (PVC) vaccine

I. Neural vaccines

1. Semple vaccine

It is 5% suspension of sheep brain infected with fixed virus and inactivated with phenol at 37°C, leaving residual live virus.

2. Beta-propiolactone vaccine

This is a modification of Semple vaccine in which BPL is used as the inactivating agent instead of phenol. It is believed to be more antigenic.

3. Suckling mouse brain vaccine

Since the brain tissues of newborn animals contain little myelin, therefore, a vaccine prepared from suckling mouse brain and inactivated with BPL was used, but was discontinued because of its poor immunogenicity.

II. Non-neural vaccines

A. Duck egg vaccine

Vaccine prepared from virus grown in duck embryos and inactivated with BPL was used for many years. It has poor immunogenicity and is also associated with certain neurological complications which are primarily due to myelin basic proteins in the vaccine.

B. Cell culture vaccines

(a) **Human diploid cell (HDC) vaccine:** This vaccine consists of fixed rabies virus grown on human diploid lung fibroblasts and inactivated with BPL or tris-*n*-butyl phosphate. It is highly antigenic and free from serious side effects but there may be local reaction in around 15% vaccinees. Because of the greater potency of HDC vaccine, quantity administered is much less than that of neural vaccines.

(b) **Purified chick embryo cell (PCEC) vaccine and purified Vero cell (PVC) vaccine:** Because of its high cost, HDC vaccine is not available to majority of the patients in developing countries where rabies is a major public health problem. Therefore, to reduce the cost, a number of other cell culture vaccines have been developed, using cells more easily grown in bulk than human diploid cells. This has allowed the cost of vaccine to be reduced. Rabies vaccines with a similar potency to HDC vaccine have been produced in chick embryo fibroblasts and Vero cells. The vaccines produced in these cell cultures are known as purified chick embryo cell (PCEC) vaccine and purified Vero cell (PVC) vaccine respectively.

Dosage schedule of cell culture vaccines

Only five or six doses of cell culture vaccine given intramuscularly in the **deltoid region** in 1.0 ml volumes on days 0, 3, 7, 14, 30 and 90 after exposure are recommended. The last dose is optional. *Cell culture vaccines should not be injected in gluteal region because high fat content in this region retards the absorption of vaccine.*

51

Influenza, Parainfluenza, Mumps, and Measles Viruses

INFLUENZA VIRUSES

Morphology

Influenzavirus A and *Influenzavirus B* are morphologically similar, but *Influenzavirus C* differs from them in certain respects, particularly in having **only a single type of glycoprotein spike**. The virions are spherical, 80–120 nm in diameter, but larger pleomorphic and filamentous forms 1,000 nm or more in length may be abundant. The nucleocapsid (Fig. 51.1) has helical symmetry. Influenza A and B viruses have eight RNA segments, and influenza C virus has seven segments. Gene segments range from 800–2500 nucleotides in length, and the entire genome ranges from 10–14.6 kb. The segmented genome of influenza viruses allows the exchange of one or more gene segments between two viruses when both infect a single cell. This exchange is known as **genetic reassortment** and results in the generation of new strains containing a mix of genes from both parental viruses.

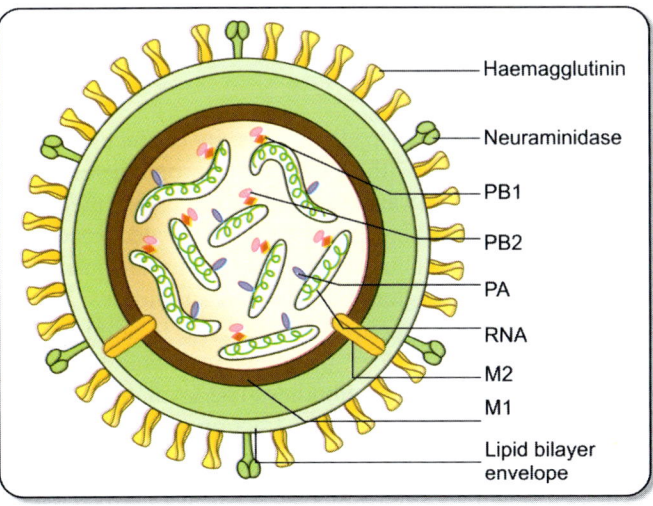

Fig. 51.1. Influenza virus.

The nucleocapsid is surrounded by a protein layer or **matrix protein (M1)**, which, in turn, is enclosed in host plasma membrane derived **lipid bilayer envelope**. Attached to the lipid envelope of *Influenzavirus A* and *B* are two types of glycoprotein peplomers or spikes, the haemagglutinin (HA) and the neuraminidase (NA). HA peplomers exist as 500 tapered projections, 10 nm in length, with their broadest (5 nm) ends outermost and their narrow ends inserted in the lipid membrane. NA peplomers are 100 mushroom-shaped projections per virion measuring 9 nm in length.

The virus particles bind to the host cell receptors (sialic acid) by haemagglutinin peplomers. The haemagglutinin activity of influenza virus results from the ability of the haemagglutinin peplomers present on the surface of the virus to attach to the sialic acid present on glycoproteins on the surface of erythrocytes causing them to agglutinate.

The **haemagglutination reaction** is important in laboratory work because it provides a simple and rapid method for detection of viruses in egg or tissue culture fluid. Influenza viruses can agglutinate erythrocytes of fowl, guinea-pig, man and others. Haemagglutination is followed after a time by the detachment of the virus from the cell surface, reversing the haemagglutination. This is known as **elution** and is caused by the enzyme neuraminidase present in the neuraminidase peplomers. The enzyme acts on the cell receptor, destroying it by splitting off *N*-acetylneuraminic acid from it. Neuraminidase peplomers are not present in *Influenzavirus C*.

Virus particles which have eluted from red cells are still capable of agglutinating fresh red cells but red cells that have been acted on by the virus are not susceptible to agglutination by the same strain of the virus. **Haemagglutination inhibition** offers a convenient method for the detection and quantitation of the antibody to the virus in patient sera.

Plasma membrane of cells in which virus is multiplying contains haemagglutinins. Therefore, RBCs get adsorbed to the surface of such cells. This is known as **haemadsorption**, a technique by which the growth of influenza virus can be identified in cell culture.

Cultivation

Animal inoculation

The virus can produce experimental infection in ferrets and mice by intranasal inoculation.

Chick embryo inoculation

Influenzavirus A, B and *C* can be isolated in the **amniotic cavity** of 11–13-day-old chick embryos incubated at 33–35°C for 2–3 days. After a few egg passages, *Influenzavirus A* and *B* grow well in allantoic cavity also, whereas *Influenzavirus C* can be grown only in amniotic cavity. Virus growth is detected by the appearance of haemagglutinin in the amniotic and allantoic fluids.

Tissue culture

Influenza virus can also be isolated on primary monkey kidney or human embryo kidney cells. Madin-Darby canine kidney (MDCK) cells, a continuous line, may also be used to isolate influenza viruses, provided trypsin (2 μg/ml) is present in the medium to cleave the haemagglutinin of progeny virions and enable spread to other cells. Cytopathic effects are not prominent and virus growth is detected by haemadsorption or demonstration of haemagglutinin in culture fluid.

Pathogenesis

Influenza viruses are transmitted from person to person primarily via droplets generated by sneezing, coughing and speaking. Direct or indirect (fomites) contact with contaminated secretions and small-particle aerosols are other potential routes of transmission.

Incubation period is short varying from 1–4 days. The illness is characterized by a sudden onset of systemic symptoms such as chills, fever, sore throat, rhinorrhoea, nasal congestion, nonproductive cough, myalgia, headache and malaise. The uncomplicated illness usually lasts for 3–7 days.

Laboratory diagnosis

Electron microscopy

Influenza viruses may be detected in clinical specimens by visualization of their typical morphological appearance by electron microscopy (EM). Immune EM is the most sensitive EM method and allows differentiation of virus type and subtype when specific hyperimmune sera are used in the assay.

Fluorescence microscopy

Smears of nasopharyngeal secretions and nasal swab or centrifuged deposit of throat garglings are stained with fluorescein-tagged influenza antiserum and seen under fluorescence microscope.

Nucleic acid analyses

Molecular methods are increasingly being used for both the detection and the characterization of influenza viruses. The most commonly used molecular method is reverse transcription PCR (RT-PCR).

Virus isolation

Influenza viruses can be isolated during first 2–3 days of illness. Throat garglings are collected using suitable buffered salt solution. The specimen should be processed immediately. If short delay is expected then store it at 4°C and if long delay is expected then store it at –70°C. The specimen is treated with antibiotics to destroy bacteria and inoculated into amniotic cavity of chick embryos, primary monkey kidney cells, human embryo kidney cells or MDCK cells.

The material is inoculated into the **amniotic cavity** of 11–13-day-old eggs, using at least six eggs per specimen. After incubation at 35°C for three days, the eggs are chilled and the amniotic and allantoic fluids harvested separately. The fluids are tested for haemagglutination using guinea pig and fowl RBCs in parallel at room temperature and at 4°C. Some strains of influenza virus type A agglutinate only guinea pig cells on initial isolation. The type B virus agglutinates both cells, while type C strains agglutinate only fowl cells.

Inoculated cell cultures are incubated at 33°C in roller drums and the virus growth can be identified by testing the culture fluid for haemagglutination or by haemadsorption.

Serological tests

- **Haemagglutination inhibition (HAI)** is a convenient and sensitive test for the serological diagnosis of influenza.
- **Complement fixation test** with the RNP antigen of influenza virus is very useful as the antibodies are formed during infection, but not following immunisation with inactivated vaccines.

Prophylaxis

1. Inactivated vaccines

Influenza virus is grown in allantoic cavity of chick embryos. These are inactivated with formalin or β-propiolactone, then purified by zonal ultracentrifugation and disrupted with detergents. The resulting polyvalent inactivated vaccine is used every autumn. This vaccine can be further purified to contain only haemagglutinins and neuraminidases. This is known as **subunit vaccine**. The vaccine is administered parenterally in a single dose. Inactivated vaccines induce the formation of circulating antibodies. The level of antibodies in the respiratory mucosa is only a fraction of the serum level.

2. Live attenuated vaccines

Temperature-sensitive (ts) mutants of influenza virus may be used as live vaccine. They can grow at lower temperature of the nasopharyngeal mucosa (32–34°C) but not in lungs (37°C). Live vaccine is administered by **aerosol spray or**

intranasally. It stimulates the production of local IgA antibodies. Circulating antibodies of IgM and IgG classes are not raised to the same extent as when killed vaccine is injected.

Avian influenza (Bird flu)

Avian influenza is a contagious disease caused by virus that normally infects only birds and less commonly pigs. First evidence of direct transmission from birds to humans was observed in 1997, when an unusual case of human respiratory illness caused by influenza A (H5N1) was identified in Hong Kong. Later that year, more cases began to be seen. Eventually, a total of 18 human illnesses, one third fatal, were found in children and young adults.

Certain water birds such as waterfowls and migratory birds act as reservoir of avian influenza viruses, and usually only get asymptomatic infection. They carry the virus in their intestines and shed it in their faeces. Avian influenza viruses are spread to susceptible birds through inhalation of influenza particles in nasal and respiratory secretions and from contact with the faeces of infected birds. The disease can spread from country to country through international trade in live poultry. Migratory birds, including waterfowl, sea birds, and shore birds can also carry the virus for long distances and have, in the past, been implicated in the international spread of highly pathogenic avian influenza.

The symptoms can vary from a mild disease with little or no mortality to a highly fatal, rapidly spreading epidemic depending on the infecting virus strain and host factors. Domestic poultry including chickens and turkeys are particularly susceptible to epidemics of rapidly fatal influenza. Decreased food consumption and drops in egg production are some of the earliest and most predictable signs of the disease. Other signs may include coughing, sneezing, ruffled feathers, swollen heads and diarrhoea. In some cases, birds die rapidly without clinical signs of disease.

Laboratory diagnosis

Specimens

A variety of specimens are suitable for the diagnosis of avian influenza. These include nasal swab, nasopharyngeal swab, nasopharyngeal aspirate, nasal wash and throat swab. In addition to swabs from upper respiratory tract, invasive procedures can be performed for the diagnosis of virus infections of lower respiratory tract where indicated. These include transtracheal aspirate, bronchoalveolar lavage and lung biopsy.

Laboratory diagnosis of avian influenza in humans can be carried out by:

1. *Detection of antigen by:*
   - Immunofluorescence test.
   - Antigen capture ELISA with monoclonal antibody to the nucleoprotein.
   - Polymerase chain reaction.

2. *Virus isolation in:*
   - Cell line Madin-Darby canine kidney cells.
   - Egg inoculation.

H1N1 (Swine flu) virus

H1N1 (Swine flu) virus is a swine origin influenza A virus. This new virus was first detected in the United States in April 2009. Other countries, including Mexico and Canada, have also reported people sick with this new virus. It spreads from person-to-person probably in much the same way that regular seasonal influenza viruses spread.

Existing vaccines against seasonal flu provide no protection. It is more contagious than seasonal flu and is believed to spread from human-to-human in much the same way as seasonal flu. The most common mechanism by which it spreads is by droplets from coughs and sneezes of infected people and also by touching a surface or the hands of a person contaminated with the virus and then touching one's eyes, nose or mouth. Unlike seasonal flu, H1N1 can infect cells deep in the lungs. Most people infected with this virus suffer a mild illness, but only a small minority are often severely ill. H1N1 destroys the lung alveoli, often causing acute respiratory distress. People at high risk for developing flu-related complications include:

- Children younger than 5, but especially younger than 2-years-old.
- Adults 65 years of age and older.
- Pregnant women.

Patient develops fever, cough, sore throat, running or stuffy nose, body aches, chills and fatigue. Some people may have vomiting and diarrhoea. Existing vaccines against seasonal flu provide no protection.

Laboratory diagnosis

Specimens

Samples should be taken from deep nostrils (nasal swab), nasopharynx (nasopharyngeal swab), nasopharyngeal aspirate, and throat or bronchial aspirates. Acute and convalescent serum specimens should be used for the detection of rising antibody titres.

Molecular diagnostics

Molecular diagnostics are currently the method of choice for pandemic (H1N1) virus. Important gene targets are – type A influenza matrix gene; haemagglutinin gene specific for pandemic (H1N1) 2009 virus; and haemagglutinin gene specific for seasonal influenza A H1/H3. Protocols currently available are – influenza A type-specific conventional and real time PCR; pandemic (H1N1) 2009 virus-specific conventional and real time PCR; CDC realtime RT-PCR (rRT-PCR) protocol for the detection and characterization of pandemic H1N1 2009; and seasonal influenza A (H1N1 and H3N2); and avian influenza A (H5, H7 and H9) realtime RT-PCR.

Virus isolation

Current protocols for virus isolation of seasonal influenza viruses using MDCK cells and egg inoculation can be used. Turkey, chicken, guinea pig and human red blood cells agglutinate with pandemic (H1N1) 2009 virus.

Immunofluorescence

Immunofluorescence tests designed for direct detection of influenza A viruses do not differentiate seasonal influenza from pandemic (H1N1) 2009 virus.

Serology

Haemagglutination inhibition and microneutralization tests using pandemic (H1N1) 2009 virus are expected to be able to detect antibody responses following infection.

Prophylaxis

- Wash your hands with soap and water. If soap and water are not available, use an alcohol-based hand rub.
- Avoid touching your eyes, nose or mouth.
- Try to avoid contact with sick people.
- If you are sick with flu-like illness, you stay home for at least 24 hours after your fever has disappeared except to get medical care.

PARAINFLUENZA, MUMPS AND MEASLES VIRUSES

Morphology

Parainfluenza, mumps and measles viruses are indistinguishable under the electron microscope. They range from 150–300 nm or more in diameter, occasionally there are filamentous forms and giant forms up to 800 nm in diameter. They are enclosed by a lipid envelope derived from plasma membrane of the host cell. The envelope of parainfluenza and mumps viruses contains HN and F glycoprotein peplomers 12–14 nm long and 2–4 nm wide. The former carries both haemagglutinating and neuraminidase functions and latter causes fusion of cell membranes leading to the formation of syncytia. The spikes on the measles virus envelope carry a haemagglutinin but not a neuraminidase. The inner surface of the envelope is lined by matrix (M) protein. Within the virion, there is a nucleocapsid of helical symmetry. It contains a single-stranded, negative sense RNA genome as a single piece, 16–20 kb in size, and an RNA-dependent RNA polymerase (Fig. 51.2).

Parainfluenza viruses

There are four types of parainfluenza viruses – types 1, 2, 3 and 4.

Pathogenesis

Parainfluenza viruses are highly transmissible and are acquired by droplets and by contact with respiratory

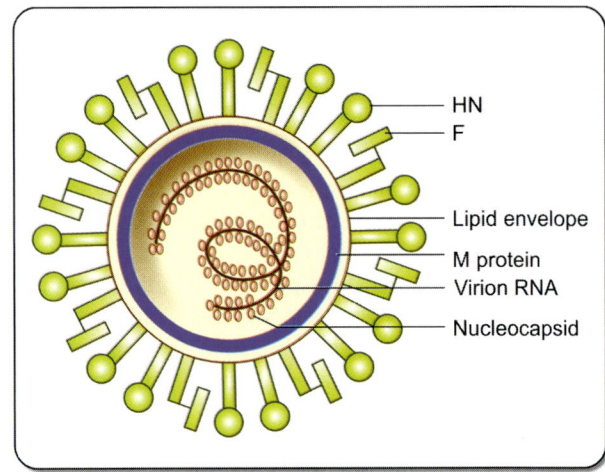

Fig. 51.2. Schematic diagram of parainfluenza and mumps viruses.

secretions. **Incubation period varies from 2–6 days.** All parainfluenza viruses produce upper respiratory tract infections. In infants and children, these viruses may invade the lower respiratory tract, causing **pneumonia**. In older children (6 months to 5 years), parainfluenza virus type 1 and to some extent, type 2 may cause **laryngotracheobronchitis or croup**. The patient presents with fever, cough and respiratory distress that may need emergency tracheostomy. Type 3 infects infants within first year or two of life. Type 4 produces only mild illness.

Laboratory diagnosis

Microscopy

Electron microscopy can easily demonstrate the presence of parainfluenza viruses, but these and other paramyxoviruses appear the same.

Immunofluorescent staining

Viral antigens can be demonstrated in exfoliated cells aspirated from respiratory tract by immunofluorescent straining using monoclonal antibodies. It is used for rapid diagnosis.

Detection of free antigen

Detection of free antigen in mucus by ELISA and RIA.

Virus isolation

Parainfluenza viruses may be isolated in primary human or monkey kidney cells or in continuous cell lines such as H292 derived from human lung mucoepidermoid carcinoma. They produce little cytopathic effect, except type 2 which induces syncytia. Viral growth can be detected by haemadsorption of guinea-pig red cells or by use of specific immunofluorescent antibody.

Serology

Type-specific antibody may be detected by neutralization,

ELISA and complement fixation test. A four-fold rise in titre is indicative of infection with a parainfluenza virus.

MUMPS VIRUS

Pathogenesis

Mumps is predominantly a disease of childhood. The mumps virus is transmitted by way of respiratory and oral secretions, and **respiratory tract is the portal of entry**. It multiplies in the upper respiratory tract and in local lymph nodes. The virus then enters the blood stream and the infection spreads to many organs of the body. The major manifestation is **painful swelling of one or both parotid glands** occurring 14–18 days after exposure. It may also cause meningoencephalitis, orchitis, oophoritis, pancreatitis, arthritis, myocarditis and renal dysfunction.

Laboratory diagnosis

Microscopy

Microscopic examination of affected salivary glands reveals an oedematous interstitium diffusely infiltrated by macrophages, lymphocytes, and plasma cells, which compress acini and ducts. Neutrophils and necrotic debris may fill the ductal lumen, causing focal damage to ductal epithelium.

Antigen detection

Mumps virus antigen may be detected by immunofluorescence staining of throat swab specimens.

Nucleic acid detection

Mumps virus RNA may be detected by RT-PCR in oral fluid, CSF, saliva, and urine.

Virus isolation

Virus can be isolated from saliva from affected gland, throat swab, CSF and urine on primary monkey kidney cells, H292 and HEp-2 cells. It produces little cytopathic effect, but virus can be detected by immunofluorescence and haemadsorption (of guinea-pig or chicken red cells) which can be inhibited by specific antiserum.

Serology

For rapid diagnosis, ELISA is useful for detecting mumps-specific IgM antibodies in the serum.

Prophylaxis

A live attenuated vaccine, derived by passage in chick fibroblasts, offers 95% protection which lasts for 12 years. It can be given by subcutaneous injection in combination with attenuated measles and rubella strains (MMR vaccine). This vaccine is administered to children of both sexes, aged 15 months.

MEASLES VIRUS

Pathogenesis

Measles is the **commonest highly contagious childhood disease** spread by respiratory secretions. Virus gains access to the human body via the respiratory tract, where it multiplies locally. The infection then spreads to the regional lymphoid tissue, where further multiplication occurs. This leads to **primary viraemia**. It disseminates the virus, which then replicates in the reticuloendothelial system, followed by **secondary viraemia**. It seeds the epithelial surfaces of the body, including skin, respiratory tract, and conjunctiva where focal replication occurs.

After an **incubation period of 10–12 days**, patient develops upper respiratory tract infection with high fever, rhinitis, cough and conjunctivitis. **Koplik's spots**, which are small, 1–3 mm in diameter, bluish white spots surrounded by erythema can be seen on the buccal mucosa during this stage and are pathognomonic of measles. After 1–2 days, the acute symptoms decline with the appearance of characteristic **maculopapular rash** which appears first on the neck and then spreads to the rest of the body.

Laboratory diagnosis

Specimen collection and transport

For successful virus isolation specimens should be collected early in the acute phase of infection, when the virus is present in high concentrations, and transported to a laboratory under conditions that maintain the infectivity of labile viruses. Suitable samples for isolation of measles virus or for detection of viral antigens are whole blood, serum, throat and naso-pharyngeal secretions, urine, and in special circumstances, brain and skin biopsy samples. Specimens should be processed as soon as possible after collection and are best kept at 4°C rather than frozen; since freezing causes significant loss of recoverable virus.

Direct microscopy

Giemsa-stained smears of nasal secretions show multi-nucleated giant cells.

Immunofluorescence

The measles virus antigen can be detected in the infected cells of nasal secretions by immunofluorescence.

Virus isolation

The measles virus can be isolated, though with some difficulty, from throat washings, blood, urinary sediment, etc. on monkey kidney, primary human embryo kidney and human amnion cells. Cytopathic changes may take 7–10 days to develop. The appearance of multinucleated giant cells containing numerous acidophilic inclusions in cytoplasm and nuclei, in the cultured cells, suggests the presence of measles virus, but earlier diagnosis is possible by immunofluorescent staining with monoclonal antibody.

Serology

Measles antibody in the patient serum can be detected by IgM capture ELISA. Complement fixation test can be carried out on acute and convalescent sera. A rise in antibody titre is diagnostic. Demonstration of high titres of measles antibody in the CSF is diagnostic of SSPE.

Polymerase chain reaction (PCR)

Reverse transcriptase PCR is a sensitive and specific method of diagnosis.

Prophylaxis

Children of the age of 15 months are given MMR vaccine, followed by a booster at the age of 4–6 years.

52

Chikungunya, Rubella, Dengue, Japanese Encephalitis and Kyasanur Forest Disease

CHIKUNGUNYA

The name 'Chikungunya' is derived from the native word for the disease in which the patient lies 'doubled up' due to severe joint pains. Chikungunya epidemics in India and Southeast Asia causing hundreds-of-thousands of cases involve *Aedes aegypti* transmission in a human-mosquito-human cycle. It has frequently been isolated from humans and mosquitoes during epidemics in India, Southeast Asia, Southeast Africa and sub-Saharan Africa.

After an **incubation period of 2–4 days**, patient develops fever, crippling joint pains, chills, flushed face, headache, myalgia, backache, photophobia, rash, anorexia and constipation with recovery in 5–7 days. Clinical picture resembles that of dengue fever, with which it is often confused.

In India and Southeast Asia, this virus has been implicated in outbreaks of haemorrhagic fever, often in association with dengue viruses. However, chikungunya is not a cause of severe haemorrhagic disease. It is transmitted by *Aedes aegypti* and *A. africanus*.

Laboratory diagnosis

- Using an IgM capture ELISA, serotype specific IgM antibody may be detected in the patient serum within 1–3 days after the onset of illness.
- The detection of a four-fold or greater rise of antibody titre by ELISA test on paired sera collected during the initial week and several days later also provides a good evidence of infection.

RUBELLA VIRUS

Morphology

Rubella virus is a pleomorphic, roughly spherical, 50–70 nm in diameter, with a single-stranded RNA genome. It is surrounded by an envelope carrying haemagglutinin peplomers.

Pathogenesis

Rubella or German measles is primarily a mild childhood fever. It may be acquired congenitally or postnatally. It is not transmitted by arthropods.

A. Postnatal rubella

Rubella virus is excreted in oropharyngeal secretions and infection is acquired by inhalation. Virus multiplies locally in the upper respiratory tract and in the cervical lymph nodes, followed by dissemination throughout the body by the way of the blood stream. After an **incubation period of 2–3 weeks**, patient develops fine, pink, discrete macules of the erythematous rash which first appear on the face, then spread to the trunk and limbs. Fever is usually inconspicuous, but a characteristic feature is that postauricular, suboccipital and posterior cervical lymph nodes are enlarged and tender from very early in the illness. The illness is of short duration and recovery is usually complete within 3–4 days after appearance of rash.

B. Congenital rubella

Rubella virus can cross the placental barrier, particularly in early pregnancy, and infect the foetus, where it disseminates and grows in every foetal organ. It may result in a large variety of **congenital abnormalities or death of the foetus**.

Laboratory diagnosis

Virus isolation

Rubella virus can be isolated from adult throat swab, and from the throat, urine, CSF or leucocytes of a newborn infant with congenital abnormalities on RK13 (rabbit kidney), SIRC (rabbit cornea) and Vero cells. CPE is inconspicuous, therefore, rubella virus, in cell culture, is detected by **interference** with the CPE of a challenge virus (coxsackievirus A9) and by **immunofluorescence** or **immunoperoxidase staining** for detection of antigen in such cells.

Serology

- Recent infection with rubella virus can be diagnosed by the demonstration of rubella IgM antibody in a single sample of blood by ELISA, radioimmunoassay and haem-adsorption inhibition test.
- In case of rubella IgG antibody, four-fold or more rise in titre in paired sera has a diagnostic value. Antibodies of IgM class, generally, do not persist beyond 4–5 weeks after onset of illness, but IgG antibodies usually persist throughout life.

In a newborn baby, demonstration of rubella IgM antibody is diagnostic of congenital rubella as IgM antibodies do not cross the placenta. However, many babies have rubella IgG antibodies, acquired transplacentally.

Prophylaxis

A live attenuated MMR vaccine is recommended for all infants in the second year of life, followed by a booster at the age of 4–6 years.

DENGUE

Dengue virus has four serotypes – dengue-1, dengue-2, dengue-3 and dengue-4. Considerable cross-reactivity is observed among the different serotypes and recovery from an infection by one type does not provide complete immunity against infection by other types. Thus, individuals can have as many as 4 dengue infections in their life, one with each serotype. The virus is transmitted from person-to-person by several species of mosquitoes of the genus *Aedes* principally *A. aegypti*. Humans and the *Aedes* mosquito are recognized reservoir and vector respectively.

Clinical features

Dengue may occur in two forms – classic dengue and dengue in more serious forms, with haemorrhagic manifestations.

Classic dengue

Classic dengue usually affects older children and adults. After an **incubation period of 5–8 days**, patient develops fever of sudden onset and often biphasic (saddle back) with severe headache, chills, retrobulbar pain, conjunctivitis and severe pain in the back, muscles and joints ('*breakbone fever*'). A **maculopapular rash**, generally, appears on the trunk in 3–5 days of illness and spreads later to the face and extremities. Petechiae may sometimes be seen on the dorsum of the feet, legs, hands, axillae and palate. **The disease lasts for about 10 days** after which recovery is generally complete.

More serious forms of dengue

Dengue may also occur in more serious forms, with haemorrhagic manifestations. These are known as **dengue haemorrhagic fever** (DHF) and **dengue shock syndrome** (DSS).

Prophylaxis

Control measures include elimination of *Aedes* mosquitoes. In order to avoid provoking or enhancing the DHF/DSS in vaccinated persons, a live attenuated vaccine containing all four dengue serotypes is undergoing clinical trials.

JAPANESE ENCEPHALITIS

Japanese encephalitis (JE) virus was first isolated from the brain of a fatal case of encephalitis in Tokyo, Japan.

Pathogenesis

The mosquito, *Culex tritaeniorhynchus*, breeding in irrigated rice fields is the main vector. It transmits the virus to man from water birds and pigs, which act as amplifying hosts. Infection in man is the dead end of the transmission. Man-to-man transmission has not been documented.

Clinical features

Incubation period varies from 5–15 days. The disease has an abrupt onset with fever, headache and vomiting. After 1–6 days, signs of encephalitis set in with neck rigidity, convulsions, altered sensorium and coma. Residual neurological damage may persist in up to 50% of survivors.

Prophylaxis

Preventive measures include mosquito control and locating piggeries away from human dwellings. Inactivated vaccines prepared in mice and hamster kidney cell cultures and a live attenuated vaccine are available.

KYASANUR FOREST DISEASE

Kyasanur Forest disease (KFD) is an Indian haemorrhagic disease. It appeared in Kyasanur Forest in Shimoga district in Karnataka, India in 1957 as a fatal epizootic affecting wild monkeys, along with a severe prostrating illness in some of the villagers in the area. The causative virus was isolated, from the patients and dead monkeys, in National Institute of Virology, Pune.

Pathogenesis

Forest birds and small mammals are believed to be the reservoirs of the virus. It is transmitted by the bite of tick (*Haemaphysalis spinigera*). As infection in monkeys leads to fatal disease, therefore, they are unlikely to be the reservoirs, but only amplifier hosts. However, ticks may act as the reservoir to some extent as transovarial transmission of the virus has been demonstrated in them.

Clinical features

After an incubation period of 3–7 days, patient develops fever of sudden onset with headache, vomiting, myalgia, conjunctivitis and severe prostration. Massive haemorrhage in alimentary canal, chest cavity and epistaxis may occur in some cases. Case fatality is about 10%. An inactivated vaccine is available.

Laboratory diagnosis of dengue, Japanese encephalitis and Kyasanur Forest disease

Virus isolation

Virus can be isolated by intracerebral inoculation of newborn mice and by inoculation of cultured mosquito or vertebrate cells, from blood. The viral isolates can be identified by immunofluorescence of the cultured cells, haemagglutination inhibition and neutralization tests.

Serology

In primary dengue infection, circulating IgM antibody to the viral coat proteins is detected 5–6 days after the onset of illness, and gradually decreases within 1–2 months of onset. IgG antibody to dengue virus is detected approximately 14 days after onset in primary infection. In secondary infection, IgM antibody may reappear, but gradually diminishes, while IgG antibody persists, often at high titre. These patterns of dengue antibody development permit serological differentiation of primary and secondary infections.

53

Human Immunodeficiency Viruses: AIDS

Morphology

Human immunodeficiency viruses are enveloped positive-stranded RNA viruses. Mature viral particles measure 80–120 nm in diameter and have a conical core. The core contains two identical copies of single-stranded RNA, 9.2 kb each associated with reverse transcriptase, which are surrounded by structural proteins that form nucleocapsid, matrix protein shell and host cell membrane derived lipid bilayer envelope from which project 72 glycoprotein peplomers (Fig. 53.1).

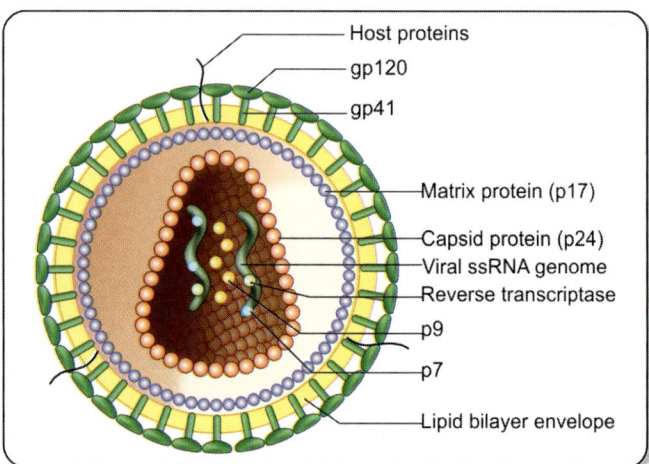

Fig. 53.1. Schematic representation of a mature HIV virion showing the localization of viral proteins.

Viral genes and antigens

The genome of HIV contains three structural genes (*gag*, *env* and *pol*):

1. The *gag* (group-specific antigen) gene encodes a precursor protein p55. It is cleaved into three proteins – p24 (core and capsid protein), p15 and p17 (matrix protein).

2. The *env* gene determines the synthesis of envelop glyco-protein (gp160) which is cleaved into the two envelope components – gp120 which forms the suface spike and gp41 which is the transmembrane anchoring protein.

3. The *pol* gene encodes polymerase reverse transcriptase and other viral enzymes, such as protease and endonuclease. It is expressed as precursor protein which is cleaved into proteins p31, p51 and p66.

The proteins (p) and glycoproteins (gp) are indicated by their molecular weight expressed in kilodaltons.

Antigenic types

Two antigenic types of HIV have been identified – HIV-1 and HIV-2.

Modes of transmission of the virus

There are three modes of transmission of HIV – **sexual**, **parenteral** and **perinatal**. Of these, unprotected, penetrative sexual mode of transmission is the most important.

Parenteral transmission may occur through blood transfusion. Therefore, each unit of blood should be tested for HIV and if found positive, it should be incinerated.

Infection can also be transmitted by blood products like plasma, serum and cells from HIV-positive individuals and AIDS cases. It can also be transmitted from the donors of bone marrow, semen and organs like cornea, kidney, heart, etc. Therefore, donors of various fluids and organs should be screened for AIDS before they donate them. AIDS can also be transmitted by sharing blood contaminated syringes. Therefore, HIV is more common in intravenous drug users who share syringes and needles. HIV can also be transmitted by the use of unsterile syringes and needles, needle-stick injury and through the barber's razor.

The third mode of transmission of infection is **perinatal, i.e., vertical transmission** from mother to the baby. Infection may be transmitted across the placenta before birth, from the genital secretions during birth and from mother's milk after birth.

Pathogenesis

I. Acute HIV infection

Two to six weeks after infection, most patients develop acute-onset fever with or without night-sweats, malaise, headache, myalgia, arthralgia, lethargy, diarrhoea, depression, sore throat, lymphadenopathy, skin rash, mucocutaneous ulcerations and sometimes meningoencephalopathy. Spontaneous resolution occurs within one month. Tests for HIV antibodies are usually negative at the onset of the illness but become positive during its course. Therefore, acute HIV infection is also known as **seroconversion illness**.

II. Asymptomatic infection

The asymptomatic period, which usually lasts several years, is the period between primary infection and the development of clinical immunodeficiency. During this period, the number of CD4+ lymphocytes declines slowly and virus continues to replicate, albeit at a relatively stable level. During this clinical latency period, high titres of virus can be found in lymphoid and other tissue compartments. The length of the clinical latency period varies considerably but is 10 years on average. They show positive HIV antibody tests during this phase and are infectious.

III. Persistent generalized lymphadenopathy (PGL)

Twenty five to thirty per cent of patients who are otherwise asymptomatic develop enlarged lymph nodes, at least 1 cm in diameter, in two or more noncontiguous extrainguinal sites, that persist for at least three months.

IV. Symptomatic HIV infection

When CD4+ T cell count falls below 400/μl, the patient may develop constitutional symptoms like fever, night sweats, diarrhoea, weight loss and opportunistic infections which generally are not life-threatening.

When CD4+ T cells drop below 200/μl, their number generally begin to decline at an accelerated rate, the titre of virus in blood increases markedly and there is irreversible breakdown of immune defence mechanisms, leaving the patient a prey to progressive opportunistic infections and malignancies. Most of the patients with HIV disease die of infections other than HIV. Tuberculosis is the commonest opportunistic infection.

Laboratory diagnosis

Serum samples are used routinely for standard HIV antibody and antigen detection, although plasma samples are also acceptable. The serum/plasma should be promptly separated from the clot/cellular elements and refrigerated at 2–8°C. If testing will not be performed within 7 days, the serum specimen should be frozen at –20°C or lower. Serum/plasma specimens can be transported either refrigerated (if transport takes place within 7 days of collection) or frozen in screw-cap plastic vials. Laboratory tests employed for the diagnosis of HIV infection may be classified into three groups (Table 53.1).

Table 53.1. Laboratory tests for the diagnosis of HIV infection

1. **Screening (E/R) tests**
   (a) ELISA
   (b) Rapid tests
      – Dot blot assays
      – Particle agglutination (gelatin, RBC, latex, microbeads)
      – Dip stick and comb tests (ELISA technology based)
      – Immunochromatography based tests
2. **Supplemental tests**
   (a) Western blot assay
   (b) Immunofluorescence test
3. **Confirmatory tests**
   (a) Virus isolation
   (b) Detection of p24 antigen
   (c) Detection of viral nucleic acid
      – In situ hybridization
      – Polymerase chain reaction

1. Screening (E/R) tests

These are serological tests which are used to screen antibodies against HIV. These tests are of two types.

(a) *ELISA:* It is a highly sensitive and specific test and a standard procedure for diagnosing HIV infection.
(b) *Rapid tests:* These tests have a total reaction time of less than 30 minutes and do not require expensive equipment.

2. Supplemental tests

These tests also detect antibodies against HIV. These tests are recommended for validation of the positive results of the screening tests. These include Western blot assay and immunofluorescence.

3. Confirmatory tests

These include:

(a) *Virus isolation:* HIV can be isolated from patient's peripheral blood lymphocytes by co-cultivation with normal healthy donor's lymphocytes in the presence of mitogens and T cell growth factor (interleukin-2).
(b) *Detection of p24 antigen:* p24 antigen can be detected in the serum by ELISA.
(c) *Detection of viral nucleic acid:* Viral nucleic acid can be detected by **in situ hybridization and polymerase chain reaction**.

54

Hepatitis Viruses

The term **'viral hepatitis'** is reserved for infection of the liver caused by a small (but growing) group of hepatotropic viruses named hepatitis A virus (HAV), hepatitis B virus (HBV), hepatitis C virus (HCV), hepatitis D virus (HDV), hepatitis E virus (HEV) and hepatitis G virus (HGV).

HEPATITIS A VIRUS (HAV)

Morphology

HAV is a nonenveloped 27 nm icosahedral virus containing linear, single-stranded RNA, 7.5 kb in length and of positive polarity. It has only one serotype.

Cultivation

HAV can be transmitted to chimpanzees and several species of mormoset monkeys and can be grown in cell cultures of primate and human cells. It is the only one of the human hepatitis viruses that can be cultivated in cell culture. It has also been cloned.

Pathogenesis

HAV is shed early in the stools of infected individuals, 1–2 weeks prior to the onset of symptoms, and persists for the first several days after the transaminase levels peak. There is very little virus in the serum and hardly any at all in other body fluids which explains the epidemiology of the disease as **faecal-oral enteric infection**.

Clinical features

Hepatitis A is an acute self-limiting disease with an incubation period of 2–6 weeks. The onset is abrupt with fever, malaise, anorexia, nausea and lethargy which comprise the prodromal (preicteric) stage. Hepatomegaly, due to cell necrosis, causes blockage of the biliary excretions resulting in jaundice. It may also produce pain in the right upper abdominal quadrant.

Laboratory diagnosis

Biochemical tests

Serum levels of both alanine and aspartate aminotransferase are markedly raised.

Immunoelectron microscopy

Virus particles can be demonstrated in faecal extracts by immunoelectron microscopy.

Serology

- Faecal HAV may be detected by **ELISA**.
- Detection of IgM anti-HAV by **ELISA or RIA** is the method of choice for the diagnosis of HAV infection.

Virus isolation

Virus, from the faeces, may be cultured on continuous cell lines of monkey kidney cells or human fibroblasts or hepatoma.

Polymerase chain reaction (PCR)

Trace amounts of HAV in food or water can be detected by PCR.

HEPATITIS B VIRUS (HBV)

Morphology

HBV or **Dane particle** is a complex 42 nm double shelled particle (Fig. 54.1). The outer surface or envelope contains **hepatitis B surface antigen (HBsAg)**. It is made up of lipid, protein and carbohydrate. It encloses an inner icosahedral 27 nm nucleocapsid (core), which contains **hepatitis B core antigen (HBcAg)**. **HBeAg** is hidden antigenic component of the core. Inside the core is the genome of HBV and a DNA-dependent DNA polymerase. The HBV genome consists of a 3.2 kilobase pair molecule of circular partially dsDNA of most unusual structure. The plus strand is incomplete leaving 15–50% of the molecule single-stranded.

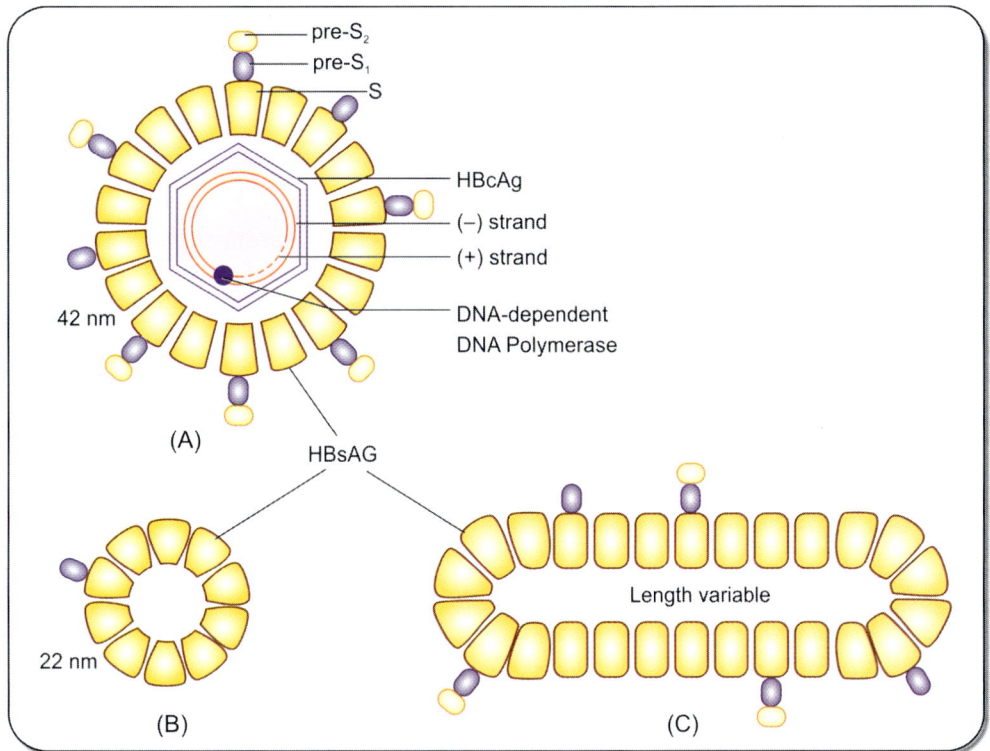

Fig. 54.1. Schematic diagram of hepatitis B virus particles: A, Dane particle; B, spherical particle; and C, tubular particle.

Pathogenesis

There are three important modes of transmission of HBV infection – parenteral, perinatal and sexual.

1. Parenteral transmission

HBV is present in the blood and in body fluids such as semen, vaginal secretions, menstrual discharge, saliva, colostrum and breast milk. Transmission of infection may result from accidental inoculation of minute amounts of blood or fluid containing HBV during medical, surgical or dental procedures. Needle-stick injuries, use of contaminated needles and syringes, intravenous and percutaneous drug abuse, ear and nose piercing, tattooing, acupuncture, sharing of shaving razor and kissing can transmit HBV infection.

2. Perinatal transmission

HBV can be transmitted from carrier mothers to their babies during the perinatal period. Transmission probably occurs when maternal blood contaminates the mucous membranes of the newborn during birth. Infection may also result from haematogenous **transplacental transmission**, **breast-feeding** and **close postnatal contact** between infant and the infected parent.

3. Sexual transmission

Since HBV is present in semen and vaginal secretions, therefore, it can be transmitted by sexual contact.

The course of acute HBV infection can be divided into three phases – preicteric, icteric and convalescent.

1. Preicteric (prodromal) phase

After an **incubation period** of 6 weeks to 6 months patient develops malaise, anorexia, weakness, myalgia, nausea, vomiting and pain in the right upper abdominal quadrant.

2. Icteric phase

Two days to two weeks following the initial symptoms patient develops jaundice, pale stools and dark urine (bilirubinuria).

3. Convalescent phase

This phase is long and drawn out with malaise and fatigue lasting for several weeks.

Hepatitis B carriers

About 5–10% of HBV infections result in chronic carrier state. The latter may be defined as **persistence of HBsAg in the circulation for more than six months**.

Laboratory diagnosis

1. Biochemical tests

Levels of serum transaminases (aminotransferases) are increased 5- to 100-fold. Both alanine aminotransferase and aspartate aminotransferase rise together late in the incubation period. Peak level is obtained about the time jaundice appears and reverts to normal in next 2 months. Serum bilirubin levels may rise up to 25-fold.

2. Detection of viral markers

Specific diagnosis of hepatitis B can be carried out by serological demonstration of the viral markers (Table 54.1).

- **HBsAg** is the first marker to appear in blood after infection. It is detectable in blood even before elevation of transaminases and onset of clinical illness. Peak levels of HBsAg are seen in the preicteric phase of disease. It remains in circulation throughout the icteric or symptomatic course of the disease. It disappears with recovery from clinical disease in most patients, but may sometimes last for six months and even beyond. Antibody to HBsAg (anti-HBs) appears after disappearance of HBsAg and persists for very long periods. Anti-HBs is the protective antibody.
- **HBcAg** is not demonstrable in serum because it is enclosed within the HBsAg coat. Anti-HBc antibody appears in serum a week or two after the appearance of HBsAg. It is the earliest antibody to appear in the blood. It persists lifelong, therefore, it serves as a useful indicator of prior infection with HBV, even after all viral markers become undetectable.
- **HBeAg** appears in blood along with HBsAg or soon afterwards. Circulating HBeAg is an indicator of active intrahepatic viral replication. **The presence in blood of DNA polymerase, HBV DNA and virions indicates high infectivity.** The disappearance of HBeAg coincides with the fall of transaminase levels in blood. It is followed by the appearance of anti-HBe.

3. Viral DNA polymerase

Viral DNA polymerase appears transiently during preicteric phase.

4. Polymerase chain reaction (PCR)

HBV DNA can be detected in serum by PCR. It is highly sensitive test.

HEPATITIS C VIRUS (HCV)

The HCV viral particle is 50–60 nm in diameter and consists of an envelope derived from host cell membrane into which are inserted the virally encoded glycoproteins (E1 and E2) surrounding a nucleocapsid and a positive-sense, single-stranded RNA genome of about 9,500 nucleotides.

Pathogenesis

HCV transmission occurs by needle-stick injuries or cuts with sharps, use of contaminated blood, and sexual intercourse. HCV can be transmitted in utero, during parturition and by breast milk.

Incubation period of hepatitis C averages 6–8 weeks, though it may range up to several months. As compared to hepatitis B, clinical infection with hepatitis C is generally less severe, has shorter preicteric period, milder symptoms, absent or less marked jaundice, and the case fatality rate from fulminant hepatitis is 1% or less.

Laboratory diagnosis

Diagnosis of HCV infection can be established by:

- detection of anti-HCV by ELISA,
- viral genome by PCR and by immunofluorescence, and
- in situ hybridization on biopsy and autopsy specimens.

HEPATITIS D VIRUS (HDV)

The HDV is a defective satellite virus requiring HBV as helper virus. It is spherical, 36–38 nm in diameter with HBsAg envelope and HDAg nucleoprotein (Fig. 54.2). The genome consists of a single small circular molecule of minus sense RNA of 1.7 kilobase pairs. It encodes its own nucleoprotein, the **delta antigen** or HDAg, but the envelope (HBsAg) of HDV virion is encoded by the genome HBV coinfecting the same cell. Replication of HDV requires the concomitant expression of HBV gene products, therefore, HBV is necessary for the production of HDV virions. It belongs to the genus *Deltavirus*.

Pathogenesis

HDV is transmitted principally by blood and blood products, but also by sexual contact. Vertical transmission is also possible.

Table 54.1. Serological markers of hepatitis B infection

Clinical condition	Serological marker						
	HBsAg	HBeAg	Anti-HBs	Anti-HBe	Anti-HBc		HBV DNA
					IgM	IgG	
Incubation period	+	+	–	–	–	–	+
Acute hepatitis	+	+	–	–	+	+	+
Chronic active hepatitis	+	+	–	–	+	+	+
Asymptomatic carrier state	+	–	–	+	–	+	–
Past infection	–	–	+	–	–	+	–
Immunization without infection	–	–	+	–	–	–	–

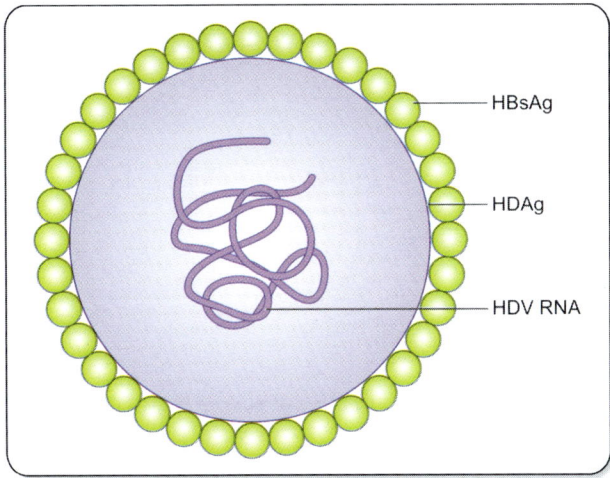

Fig. 54.2. Hepatitis D virus.

Two types of HDV infections are possible:

1. **Simultaneous coinfection with HBV and HDV in the same inoculum.** It most commonly results from parenteral transmission, for example, in intravenous drug users. The clinical and biochemical features of such infection resemble those of acute hepatitis B alone. However, coinfection with HBV and HDV may be more severe than the disease caused by HBV alone.

2. **Superinfection of an HBsAg carrier by HDV.** It is commoner and more serious because a large number of hepatocytes are already producing HBsAg, and HDV can replicate without delay with a relatively short incubation period. It leads to severe liver damage, fulminant HBsAg positive hepatitis and elevated mortality (up to 20%).

Laboratory diagnosis

The delta antigen is primarily expressed in liver cell nuclei, where it can be demonstrated by **immunofluorescence**. It is only occasionally present in serum. In patients with HBV-HDV coinfection, shortly before the end of incubation period, HBsAg appears in the serum and towards the end of incubation period HDAg appears, which can be detected by **ELISA** or **immunoblotting**, and HDV RNA can be detected by **hybridization to a radiolabelled RNA probe**. Two to three weeks after infection, anti-HD IgM appears followed by anti-HD IgG. However, in chronic infection, the IgM antibody persists for years. It can be detected by **ELISA**.

HEPATITIS E VIRUS (HEV)

Morphology

Virions of HEV are spherical, nonenveloped and 27–38 nm in diameter. They possess single-stranded positive sense RNA genome of 7.6 kb which is surrounded by icosahedral capsid with characteristic surface depressions.

Pathogenesis

Hepatitis E is primarily associated with **ingestion of faecally contaminated drinking water**.

   Incubation period of hepatitis E ranges from 2–8 weeks, with an average of 5–6 weeks. Clinically, the disease closely resembles that of hepatitis A. However, bilirubin levels tend to be higher and jaundice deeper and more prolonged.

Laboratory diagnosis

1. **Exclusion of hepatitis A** by IgM serology and hepatitis B by absence of HBsAg and IgM anti-HBc.
2. **Immunoelectron microscopic examination** of patient faeces for aggregated calicivirus-like particles using monoclonal antibodies.
3. **ELISA** tests for IgM and IgG anti-HEV.
4. A **Western blot assay** for IgM and/or IgG anti-HEV.
5. **Polymerase chain reaction (PCR) assay** for the detection of HEV RNA (as cDNA) in patient faeces or in acute-phase sera.

HEPATITIS G VIRUS (HGV)

The genome of HGV consists of 9.4 kb molecule of ssRNA of positive polarity. Its structure resembles that of HCV, but it has <25% homology with HCV. HGV replicates in peripheral blood cells, however, its replication in the liver is not known. The virus is transmitted parenterally (exposure to blood through transfusions, haemodialysis, or sharing equipment in injecting drug use), sexually, and from mother to child. More than 30% of transfusion recipients and up to 80% of injecting drug users are HGV marker positive. HGV and human immunodeficiency virus (HIV) share same infection routes, and a significant proportion of HIV-infected subjects are HGV-coinfected.

   Majority of the individuals with HGV infection have no detectable evidence of liver disease. There have been, however, cases of acute, fulminant and chronic hepatitis where HGV is presently the only explanation for their liver disease.

Laboratory diagnosis

HGV infection is mainly detected by reverse transcriptase polymerase chain reaction (RT-PCR).

SECTION 4

MYCOLOGY

Chapter 55   Mycology

Mycology

Fungi are a group of non-motile eukaryotic organisms that contain a well-defined nucleus, mitochondria, Golgi apparatus and endoplasmic reticulum. They are distinguished from other eukaryotes by a rigid cell wall composed of chitin and β-glutans, as well as other polysaccharides, proteins and lipids. In the cell membrane ergosterol is substituted for cholesterol as the major sterol component.

CLASSIFICATION OF FUNGI

On the basis of morphology, there are four groups of fungi:

1. **Yeasts:** Yeasts are round, oval or elongated unicellular fungi. These organisms remain in the yeast form at both room temperature and body temperature (37°C). Most of them reproduce by an asexual process called **budding** in which the cell develops a protuberance which enlarges and eventually separates from the parent cell (Fig. 55.1A).

2. **Yeast-like:** In some yeasts, like *Candida*, the bud remains attached to the mother cell and elongates, followed by repeated budding forming chains of elongated cells known as **pseudohyphae**. *C. albicans* and *C. stellatoidea* also produce germ tubes. Germ tubes are the beginning of true hyphae and appear as filaments that are constricted at their points of origin on the parent cell. If the filaments are constricted at their points of origin on the parent cell, they are pseudohyphae, not germ tubes (Fig. 55.1B and C). Some species like *C. albicans* also produce true hyphae.

3. **Molds:** In molds, spores germinate to produce branching filaments called **hyphae** (singular hypha). They are 2–10 µm in diameter (Fig. 55.1D and E). They may be septate or nonseptate (coenocytic). The hyphae continue to grow (Fig. 55.1F) and branch to form tangled mass of growth called **mycelium** (pl., mycelia).

4. **Dimorphic fungi:** Many fungi pathogenic to man like *Histoplasma capsulatum*, *Sporothrix schenckii*, *Blastomyces dermatitidis*, *Coccidioides immitis*, *Paracoccidioides brasiliensis*, and *Penicillium marneffei* have

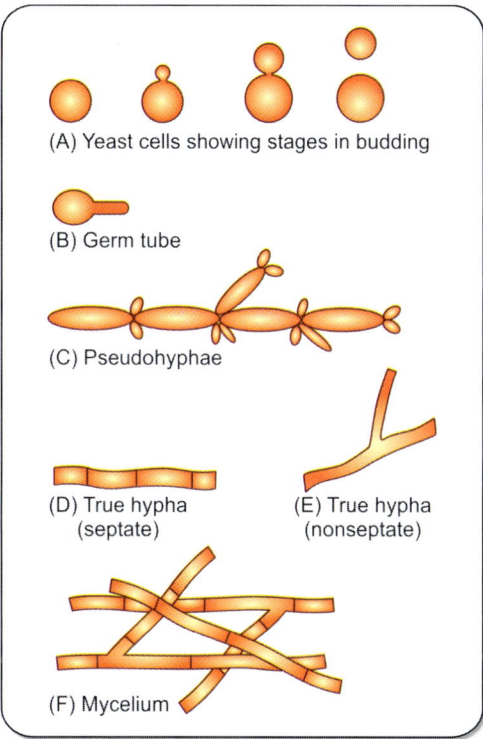

Fig. 55.1. Basic fungal morphology.

a yeast form in the host tissue and *in vitro* at 37°C on enriched media, and hyphal (mycelial) form *in vitro* at 25°C.

LABORATORY DIAGNOSIS OF MYCOSES

Laboratory diagnosis depends on:

- Recognition of the pathogen in tissue by microscopy.
- Isolation of the causal fungus in culture.
- Use of serological tests.
- Detection of fungal DNA by the polymerase chain reaction.

I. Direct microscopic examination of specimens

The direct microscopic examination of clinical specimen may be as simple as placing a drop of liquid specimen on a clean glass slide and examining it with light microscope, or it may involve more complex procedures, including staining of tissues. Although, the Gram stain performed in the routine microbiology laboratory often gives the first evidence of infection with yeast, other direct stains give more specific information concerning a mold infection. The types of direct examination used in identification of fungal infections include wet preparation such as KOH preparation, KOH with calcofluor white, India ink, and tissue stains such as periodic acid-Schiff (PAS) stain, Gomori methenamine silver (GMS) stain, Giemsa stain, and haematoxylin and eosin (H&E) stain.

KOH preparation

A 10–20% solution of KOH is useful for detecting fungal elements in skin, hair, nails, and tissue. In this procedure, KOH is mixed in equal proportions with the specimen on a slide and the specimen material is teased with two inoculating needles. A coverslip is placed over it and heated gently. Preparation with KOH clears the tissue and cellular debris from all types of clinical specimens without damaging the fungal cells. This clearing process requires only 5–10 minutes, after which one can observe the fungal morphology as well as the pigment of the fungal cell wall under a phase-contrast or bright-field microscope, using low-power followed by high-power objectives.

KOH with calcofluor white

A drop of 0.1% calcofluor white solution (fluorescent reagent) can be added to the KOH preparation prior to placing coverslip over it. Calcofluor white binds to polysaccharide present in the chitin of the fungus or to cellulose. Fungal elements fluoresce apple green or blue-white, depending on the combination of filters used. The actual fungal structure must be seen before a positive preparation is reported.

India ink

India ink preparations may be used for detecting encapsulated yeast *Cryptococcus neoformans* in cerebrospinal fluid (CSF). A drop of India ink is mixed with a drop of centrifuged deposit of CSF, and the preparation is examined under high power. With this negative stain, budding yeast surrounded by a large clear area against a dark background is presumptive evidence of *C. neoformans*.

Tissue stains

Haematoxylin and eosin (H&E) stain used routinely in the pathology laboratory is often not adequate for detecting fungal elements. Many fungi stain poorly and some fungi do not stain at all with H&E. However, with this stain the tissue response can be demonstrated better than with any special stain and the innate colour of the fungal elements, whether dematiaceous or hyaline, can be determined.

Special stains used in the histologic section for detection of fungal elements are GMS, the Gridley fungus (GF), the periodic acid-Schiff (PAS), Giemsa, Mayer's mucicarmine and alcian blue stains.

- **The GMS staining procedure** provides better contrast between the fungi and background tissue. This procedure results in the brownish black colouration of all forms of viable and non-viable fungal cells.
- **The GF stain** colours fungal cells purplish red with a yellow background. Mucin and elastic tissue are also stained purplish red. Non-viable fungi at the time of fixation may not be stained.
- **The PAS stain** is one of the most widely used stains for fungal histopathology. Aldehydes produced by the oxidation of fungal polysaccharide react with periodic acid and colour the fungi pinkish red. In old caseous foci of histoplasmosis, yeast cells may be stained **by GMS** but not by PAS.
- **Giemsa stain** is used primarily to detect *Histoplasma capsulatum* in blood or bone marrow.
- **Mayer's mucicarmine and alcian blue procedures** stain the mucopolysaccharide capsule of *Cryptococcus* species red and blue respectively.

II. Culture

Most pathogenic fungi are easy to grow in culture. **Sabouraud dextrose agar** (SDA) is most commonly used. It may be supplemented with chloramphenicol (50 mg/l) to minimize bacterial contamination and cycloheximide (500 mg/l) to reduce contamination with saprophytic fungi. Cycloheximide should not be added to all media because the growth of *Cryptococcus* spp., *Candida* spp., *Trichosporon* spp., *Aspergillus* spp., Mucorales, hyalohyphomycetes, yeast phase of *Histoplasma capsulatum*, *Blastomyces dermatitidis* and *Paracoccidioides brasiliensis* are completely or partially inhibited by it.

Many fungal pathogens have an optimum growth temperature below 37°C. With some dimorphic pathogens, enriched media such as **brain heart infusion** or **blood agar** are used to promote growth of yeast phase. Many fungi grow relatively slowly and cultures should be retained for at least 2–3 weeks (in some cases up to 6 weeks) before being discarded. Growth of *Candida*, *Aspergillus*, *Mucor* and *Rhizopus* species appears within 24–72 hours. Therefore, culture should be examined for growth daily for the first week.

Once an organism has grown, it is examined for characteristic gross and microscopic structures, so that identification can be made. Pigment on the reverse side of the colony or in aerial mycelium is noted. For microscopic examination, **slide mounts** should be made in **lactophenol cotton blue** (LCB). On occasion, a slide culture may be prepared, when the initial isolate fails to show conidial morphology. Characteristics that should be observed are septate versus nonseptate hyphae, hyaline or dematiaceous hyphae and the types, size, shape, and arrangement of conidia.

III. Serological tests

Serological tests have been developed for the diagnosis of fungal infections. Tests for antibody have an established diagnostic use in coccidioidomycosis, paracoccidioidomycosis, aspergillosis, blastomycosis, and in some patients with histoplasmosis.

IV. Molecular testing

In situ hybridization

One of the simplest approaches used has been in situ hybridization using specific nucleic acid probes for identification of organisms in patient specimens.

Polymerase chain reaction

Amplification assays using the polymerase chain reaction allow for the detection of small amounts of target DNA in clinical specimens. Specific primers with or without specific probes have been used with some success. Assays have been developed to detect DNA of *Candida, Aspergillus, Fusarium, Cryptococcus, Histoplasma, Blastomyces, Paracoccidiodes, Pneumocystis jirovecii*, and *Penicillium marneffei*.

CLASSIFICATION OF MYCOSES

Infection caused by fungus is known as mycosis (pl., mycoses). It can be divided into four categories:

I. Superficial mycoses

These are strictly surface infections involving skin, hair, nail and mucous membrane. These include:

- Infection of skin, hair and nail caused by dermatophytes.
- Infection of skin, nail and mucous membrane caused by *C. albicans*.
- Infection of skin caused by *Malassezia* spp. (pityriasis versicolor) and *Hortaea werneckii* (tinea nigra).
- Infection of hair caused by *Piedraia hortae* (black piedra) and *Trichosporon* spp. (white piedra).

II. Subcutaneous mycoses

Mycoses of the skin, subcutaneous tissues and bones result from the inoculation of saprophytic fungi of the soil or decaying vegetation leading to progressive local disease with tissue destruction and sinus formation. The lesion may spread via lymphatics. These occur mainly in the tropics and subtropics. The principal subcutaneous mycoses are mycetoma, chromoblastomycosis, sporotrichosis and rhinosporidiosis.

III. Systemic mycoses

Systemic mycoses are caused by inhalation of airborne spores/conidia produced by the fungi which are present as sapro-phytes in soil and on plant material. From the lungs the fungus may disseminate to CNS, bone and other internal organs. Systemic mycoses include blastomycosis, histoplasmosis, coccidioidomycosis and paracoccidioidomycosis.

IV. Opportunistic mycoses

The opportunistic mycoses are infections attributable to fungi, that are normally found as human commensals or in the environment. Virtually, any fungus can serve as an opportunistic pathogen, and the list of those identified as such becomes longer each year. The most common opportunistic mycoses include aspergillosis, penicilliosis, mucormycosis, candidiasis, cryptococcosis and pneumocystosis.

I. SUPERFICIAL MYCOSES

Pityriasis versicolor

It is caused by *Malassezia* spp. which are lipophilic yeast-like fungi. These are common members of the normal skin flora and most infections are thought to be endogenous. The lesions may appear hypo- or hyperpigmented, depending on the degree of pigmentation of the surrounding skin. The commonest sites involved include chest, back, abdomen, neck and upper arms.

Laboratory diagnosis

KOH preparation

Scales are scraped with a scalpel and placed in a drop of 10% KOH. It is heated gently, covered with coverslip and seen under microscope. Clusters of round or oval yeast cells 2–7 μm in diameter along with short, curved and occasionally branched hyphae 2.5–4 μm in diameter can be seen (Fig. 55.2).

Histopathology

In biopsy specimens, they can be seen with H&E stain but are best demonstrated by special stains for fungus, preferably PAS.

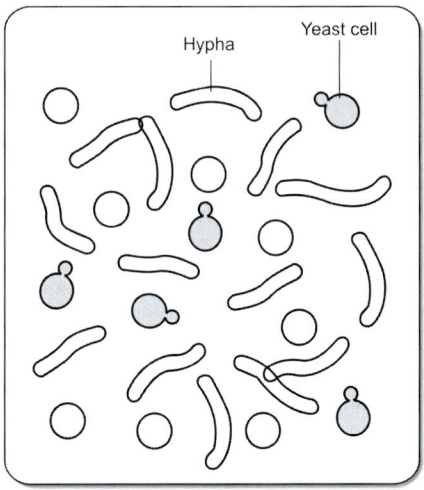

Fig. 55.2. *Malassezia* spp.

Culture

The fungus can be isolated from skin scrapings by inoculating it on SDA containing chloramphenicol and cycloheximide. The etiologic agent, *Malassezia* spp., will grow only on a medium that has been overlaid or supplemented with olive oil or another long chain fatty acid. Creamy colonies develop in 5–7 days at 30°C. LCB wet mount of the colonies shows yeast-like cells measuring 1.5–4.5 × 2–6.5 μm in diameter.

Tinea nigra

Tinea nigra is a superficial mycosis of the stratum corneum caused by traumatic inoculation from soil, wood or compost. No invasion of living tissue occurs.

It is characterized by single, discrete, painless, brown to black (due to an accumulation of melanin-like substance), non-scaly macules or patches affecting thickly keratinized sites such as palms and soles, and rarely other skin surfaces. Tinea nigra is so superficial that it can be scraped off with vigorous effort.

It is caused by melanized ascomycete, *Hortaea* (*Phaeo-annellomyces*) *werneckii*. This organism has also been described as *Exophiala werneckii*.

Laboratory diagnosis

KOH preparation

The diagnosis is made by scraping the stratum corneum and examination of 10% KOH wet mount. It shows darkly pigmented, branched, septate, narrow hyphae (1.5–3.0 μm wide) usually accompanied by elongated budding cells (1.5–5.0 μm in diameter) (Fig. 55.3).

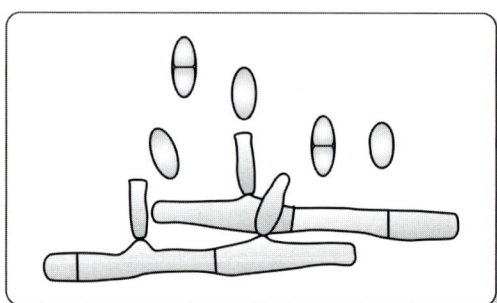

Fig. 55.3. Darkly pigmented, septate hyphae and budding cells of *Hortaea werneckii* in 10% KOH preparation.

Histopathology

A biopsy specimen can be obtained painlessly from a patient infected with tinea nigra by carefully scraping off the stratum corneum with a scalpel blade.

The organism stains well with special fungal stains, but the natural pigmentation can be best seen with H&E stain. Tissue reaction reveals mild to moderate hyperplasia and/or hyperkeratosis in the epidermis. A minimal mononuclear cell infiltrate may occur in dermis.

Fungal culture

H. werneckii can be cultured on SDA with cycloheximide. It is incubated at 25–30°C. Growth usually appears in 2–3 weeks. The colony is at first yeast-like and white to grey but quickly changes to olive or greenish-black. Microscopic examination reveals budding yeasts with 0–1 septa and hyphae. Hyphae are up to 6 μm wide, becoming thick walled, olivaceous-black, and densely septate at maturation. Conidia are produced laterally from hyphae or from the poles of budding cells by annellidic conidiogenesis. Annellated zones are conspicuous and 1–2 μm wide, with clearly visible annellations. Conidia are initially hyaline and one-celled but soon become olivaceous. After liberation they inflate and develop transverse and occasionally oblique septa. Liberated cells are converted into budding cells or chlamydoconidia-like cells.

Piedra

Piedra is an asymptomatic fungal infection of the hair shaft, resulting in the formation of **nodules** of different hardness on the infected hair. Two varieties of piedra are seen – black piedra and white piedra.

1. Black piedra

It is caused by *Piedraia hortae*. It is characterized by the presence of discrete, black, gritty, hard nodules which are composed of a mass of fungus cells on the hair shaft. The nodules vary in size from microscopic to a millimetre or more and are adherent to the hair shaft. Infection is normally restricted to scalp hair but may involve hairs of the beard, moustache and pubic hair with fungal activity limited to the cuticle.

Laboratory diagnosis

KOH preparation

Crushing the nodule in 10% KOH reveals dark septate hyphae around the surface of the hair with round or oval asci containing 2–8 hyaline, nonseptate, banana-shaped asco-spores. *P. hortae* produces sexual spores in its parasitic phase.

Fungus culture

It grows on SDA at 25°C. Growth is slow. It matures in 21 days. Colonies are small, adherent, compact, somewhat raised, and dark greenish-brown to black and may be glabrous or covered with very short aerial hyphae. Reverse is black. Microscopic examination shows closely septate, dark, and thick-walled hyphae with many intercalary chlamydo-conidium-like cells. Asci may be produced in culture. The walls of the asci readily dissolve, releasing single-celled, curved ascospores (5–10 × 30–35 μm) that taper at the ends to form whiplike extensions (Fig. 55.4).

2. White piedra

White piedra is a superficial infection of the hair shaft of the scalp, face, axillary or pubic regions. It is characterized by

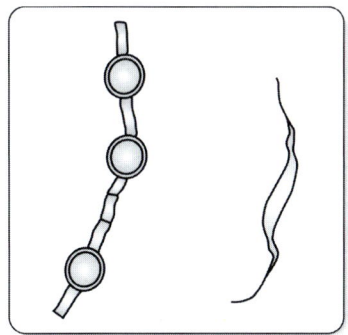

Fig. 55.4. *Piedraia hortae.*

white, yellow or green nodules composed of hyaline septate hyphae and arthroconidia.

White piedra is caused by several *Trichosporon* species. Genus *Trichosporon* is characterized by the production of true hyphae, pseudohyphae, arthroconidia and blastoconidia (budding yeast cells).

Laboratory diagnosis

KOH preparation

Hair mounted in 10% KOH mount reveal intertwined hyphae around the shaft which fragment into arthroconidia or produce blastoconidia 2–8 μm in diameter. The mycelial elements are held together in a cement-like substance.

Fungus culture

On SDA, *Trichosporon* spp. form cream-coloured, dry wrinkled colonies within 48–72 hours upon incubation at room temperature. The fungus is composed of septate hyphae that fragment into oval or rectangular arthroconidia. Blastoconidia are also produced (Fig. 55.5). Most *Trichosporon* species are inhibited by cycloheximide, therefore, this antibiotic should be excluded from the culture medium.

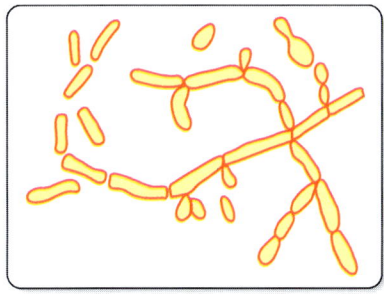

Fig. 55.5. Septate hyphae, oval or rectangular arthroconidia and blastoconidia of *Trichosporon* spp. in culture.

Dermatophytosis

Dermatophytosis, tinea or ringworm is the most common type of superficial mycosis seen in human beings. It infects keratinized tissues of the skin, hair and nails. Dermatophytosis is caused by 41 species of dermatophytes which belong to three genera (*Trichophyton*-24, *Microsporum*-16 and *Epidermophyton*-1).

The *Trichophyton* spp. usually infect skin, hair and nails, *Microsporum* spp. infect skin and hair, and *Epidermophyton* spp. infect skin and nails.

In lesions, dermatophytes appear as hyphae and arthroconidia. Three types of hair infection can be seen in 10% KOH wet mounts:

1. **Ectothrix:** In this, the fungus is present on the surface of hair shaft. It is caused by *M. audouinii*, *M. canis* and *T. mentagrophytes* (Fig. 55.6A).
2. **Endothrix:** In this, the arthroconidia are present within the hair completely filling the hair shaft without a conspicuous external sheath of arthroconidia. This is caused by *T. tonsurans* and *T. violaceum* (Fig. 55.6B).
3. **Favus:** In this, there is sparse hyphal growth and formation of air bubbles or tunnels and fat droplets within the hair shaft. This is caused by *T. schoenleinii* (Fig. 55.6C).

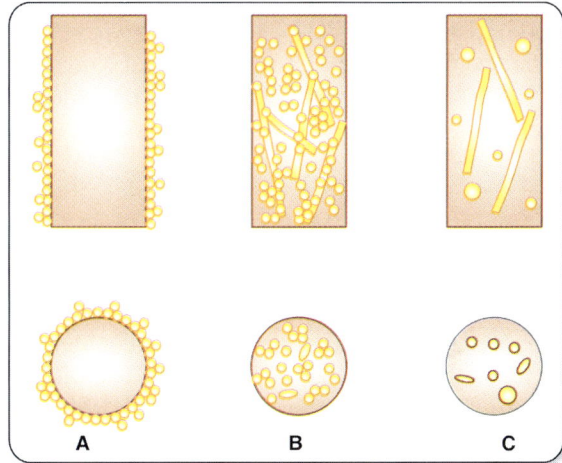

Fig. 55.6. Hair invasion of dermatophytes in longitudinal and transverse sections. (A) Ectothrix; (B) Endothrix; (C) Favus.

Laboratory diagnosis

KOH preparation

The direct microscopic examination of a properly collected specimen is one of the most rapid and effective methods of detecting dermatophytes. Skin scrapings, hair stubs, and nail clipping or scrapings are collected. A drop of 10% KOH is placed on a slide, a small amount of specimen is added to the drop, a coverslip is placed over it and the preparation is gently heated. KOH softens and clears the specimen for easier detection of hyphae by digesting any proteinaceous debris and disrupting the keratin cellular sheets, thereby rendering the more biochemically resistant fungus more visible as highly refractile, septate branched or unbranched hyphae (2–4 μm in diameter) and arthroconidia.

In hairs, fungal elements may appear as arthroconidia on the outside (ectothrix invasion) of the hair shaft, or within the hair completely filling the hair shaft (endothrix), or they may appear as hyphae co-occurring, with bubbles and channels (favic invasion).

Calcofluor white stain

Calcofluor white stain, a fluorescent dye, binds to chitin and cellulose in fungus cell wall and fluoresces on excitation by long-wave ultraviolet rays or short-wave visible light. This increases the sensitivity of the direct examination; however, this requires a fluorescence microscope. Calcofluor white stain can be combined with KOH for rapid clearance of the specimens. Although, background elements may also fluoresce, the fungal components are generally brighter and readily recognizable.

Culture method

Culture is available adjunct to direct microscopy. The clinical specimen should be inoculated on SDA with cycloheximide and chloramphenicol.

In cultures on SDA, dermatophytes form characteristic colonies consisting of septate hyphae and two types of asexual spores, microconidia and macroconidia. Sexual spores of some species have also been identified. The differentiation of the three genera is based mainly on the nature of macroconidia (Table 55.1 and Fig. 55.7).

Trichophyton

Colonies may be powdery, velvety or waxy with pigmentation characteristic of different species. Macroconidia are usually rare but microconidia are abundant. The latter are arranged in clusters along the hyphae or borne on conidiophores. Some species possess special types of hyphae, i.e., spiral hyphae,

racquet hyphae and favic chandeliers (Fig. 55.8). Fungi of this genus can infect skin, hair and nails. **_T. rubrum_ is the most common species infecting man.**

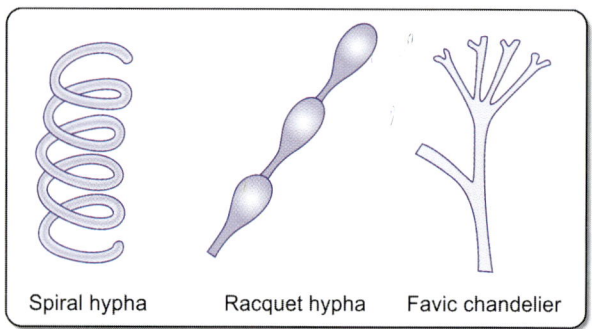

Fig. 55.8. Special types of hyphae in dermatophytes.

Microsporum

Colonies of the fungi of this genus are cottony, velvety or powdery with white to brown pigmentation. Macroconidia are very numerous and microconidia are relatively scanty. They infect skin and hair but not the nails.

Epidermophyton

Colonies are powdery and greenish-yellow. Microconidia are absent and macroconidia are club-shaped, and are arranged in groups of two or three. It infects skin and nails but not the hairs.

Colony characters and microscopic morphology of common dermatophytes are given in Table 55.2. Differential tests for dermatophytes include hair perforation test and urease test.

Table 55.1. Generic characteristics of dermatophyte macroconidia						
Genus	**Frequency**	**Size**	**Number of septations**	**Thickness of wall**	**Surface of wall**	**Manner of attachment**
Microsporum	Very numerous (except _M. audouinii_)	5–100 × 3–8 µm	3–15	Thick (except _M. gypseum_ and _M. nanum_)	Rough	Singly
Trichophyton	Usually rare	20–50 × 4–6 µm	2–8	Thin	Smooth	Singly
Epidermophyton	Numerous	20–40 × 7–12 µm	2–6	Both thin and slightly thick	Smooth	Singly or in clusters

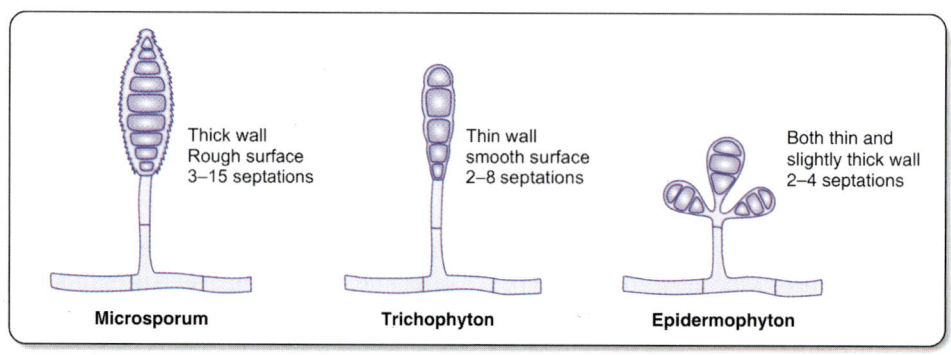

Fig. 55.7. Macroconidia in the three genera of dermatophytes.

Table 55.2. Salient characteristics of common dermatophytes

Species	Colony character	Microscopic morphology
T. mentagrophytes	Growth on SDA is relatively rapid, maturing in 3–5 days. Colony varies greatly; surface may be tan and powdery, becoming yellowish, or white and downy. Powdery form exhibits concentric and radial folds. Reverse is usually brownish tan but may be colourless, yellow, or red.	Hyphae are septate. Microconidia in powdery culture are round (4–6 μm in diameter) and clustered on branched conidiophores or, in fluffy strains, are smaller, fewer in number and tear-shaped. Macroconidia are sometimes present. They are thin-walled, club-shaped, spindle-shaped or long pencil-shaped. They are 4–8 × 20–50 μm in size, contain 1–6 cells and have narrow attachment to hyphae.
T. rubrum	Growth on SDA is relatively slow, requires 4–7 days until maturity. The surface is granular or fluffy, white to buff. The reverse is deep red or purplish or occasionally brown, yellow-orange or colourless. The pigment production is best seen on potato dextrose agar or corn dextrose agar.	Hyphae are septate. Tear-shaped microconidia (2–3.5 × 3–5.5 μm) usually form singly along the sides of the hyphae. Macroconidia (4–8 × 40–60 μm) are narrow and thin-walled with parallel sides (pencil-like), and have 4–10 cells. They may be abundant, rare or absent.
T. tonsurans	White, tan, yellow or reddish brown with radial or concentric folds. The reverse is usually reddish brown. Pigment may diffuse into the medium.	Hyphae are septate, with many teardrop or club-shaped microconidia formed along the hyphae or on short conidiophores. Intercalary and terminal chlamydoconidia are common in older cultures. Macroconidia are rare, irregularly shaped and slightly thick-walled.
T. schoenleinii	Colony is white to tan, glabrous, waxy, heaped and folded. Growth is often submerged and splits the agar medium. Reverse is colourless or pale yellowish orange to tan.	Hyphae are septate, highly irregular, and tend to become knobby and clubbed at ends (favic chandeliers). Chlamydoconidia are numerous. Microconidia and macroconidia are absent. Initial growth from clinical specimen may resemble yeast both macroscopically and microscopically.
T. violaceum	Grows slowly, producing in a typical primary culture a conical colony with irregularly folded surface, very short velvety aerial hyphae and a deep violet colour. Subcultures are more downy, and they decrease in colour. Reverse is lavender to purple.	Irregularly branched hyphae with intercalary chlamydo-conidia. Microconidia and macroconidia are not usually seen on SDA, but a few may form on thiamine-enriched media.
T. verrucosum	Growth is slow. It matures in 14–21 days. Unlike other dermatophytes, this fungus grows best at 37°C. The colony is raised, irregularly folded and (on enriched media) covered with very short aerial hyphae. Usually white, but may be gray or yellow. Reverse varies from nonpigmented to yellow.	On SDA at 37°C it forms hyphae with many chlamydo-conidia and some antler-like branches. On media, enriched with thiamine, it produces many small, delicate, single microconidia and occasional long, thin, irregular, macro-conidia.
M. audouinii	*M. audouinii* grows slowly, producing a gray colony with short aerial hyphae and usually with a radially folded surface. On the reverse side the centre of the colony is reddish brown.	Hyphae are septate with terminal chlamydoconidia that are often pointed on the end. Pectinate hyphae are commonly seen. It sporulates poorly on SDA, and the spindle-shaped macroconidia which characterize the genus may be lacking in many strains. Rate of growth and sporulation are increased by addition of yeast extract to the medium.
M. canis	Grows more rapidly, sporulates more freely and is more deeply pigmented than *M. audouinii*. The colony has abundant coarse, woolly aerial mycelium. The colour of the colony is white to bright yellow with bright yellow to orange-brown on reverse.	Hyphae are septate with abundant, thick-walled, spindle-shaped, macroconidia which usually are 15–20 × 60–125 μm in size. The macroconidium may be divided into as many as 15 cells by septa. Microconidia are clavate, sessile borne laterally directly from the hyphae and are less numerous than macroconidia.
M. gypseum	It grows rapidly. The colony is fawn brown to buff or reddish brown. The reverse of the colony may be yellow, orange-tan, brownish red, or purplish red in spots.	Septate hyphae. Macroconidia (25–60 × 7.5–16 μm) are produced in greater numbers. They are broadly spindle-shaped with moderately thick walls and 4–6 septa. Club-shaped microconidia are usually present along the hyphae.

(Contd.)

Table 55.2 (*Contd.*)

Species	Colony character	Microscopic morphology
M. gallinae	Grows slowly and produces in two weeks a conical, folded and wrinkled colony with short aerial hyphae which may be white or pink. Reverse is yellow at first and later has a red pigment that diffuses into the medium.	Hyphae are septate. Macroconidia are 15–50 × 6–8 µm with 2–10 septa. Microconidia are clavate and are usually abundant.
M. vanbreuseghemii	Surface is yellowish, cream or pink; powdery to downy. Reverse is colourless or yellow to orange-tan.	Hyphae are septate; macroconidia are long (44–87 × 11 µm); up to 12 septa, thick walls smooth to spiny; numerous microconidia.
M. ferrugineum	Grows slowly on SDA; produces an irregularly folded, glabrous, reddish-yellow to orange-yellow colony with almost waxy surface. Reverse is usually brownish tan but may be colourless, yellow or red.	Hyphae are septate; some are long and straight with prominent cross walls; these are called "bamboo" hyphae. Other hyphae are irregularly branched, clubbed, and fragmented, and may have intercalary chlamydoconidium-like cells. Macroconidia, rarely produced, resemble those of *M. canis*.
M. cookei	Moderate growth, surface yellowish, reddish or tan, powdery or granular; reverse deep wine-red.	Hyphae are septate and branched. Macroconidia are numerous, mostly ellipsoid (10–15 × 30–50 µm), thick walled, and rough, with 5–8 cells. Club-shaped microconidia are usually abundant.
M. nanum	Moderate growth; surface cream to tan, powdery or downy; reverse reddish brown.	Septate hyphae; macroconidia (12–18 × 5–7 µm) are rough, fairly thin-walled and ovate or elliptical, having 1–3 cells (usually 2). Microconidia, clavate, 2–5 µm, are rare to moderate.
M. persicolor	Flat powdery to cottony, buff to peach colony. Reverse is pink to reddish-brown.	Macroconidia are rare, clavate to fusiform and have minutely echinulate walls. Microconidia are clavate and abundant.
E. floccosum	Colonies grow rapidly, within 3–5 days. Surface of the colony is brownish-yellow to olive-gray or khaki. The centre of the colony is marked by irregular concentric and radial folds and furrows. After several weeks, fluffy white sterile mycelium covers the colony. Reverse is orange to brownish, sometimes with a thin yelllow border.	Septate hyphae; microconidia are never produced, therefore, if microconidia are observed in an unknown culture of a dermatophyte, *E. floccosum* can be excluded. Numerous macroconidia (20–40 × 7–12 µm), seen best in young cultures, are smooth, both thin and slightly thick-walled and club-shaped with round ends. They contain 2–6 septa and are found singly or in clusters.

Hair perforation test

Hair perforation test is useful in differentiating *T. rubrum* from *T. mentagrophytes*. To observe hair perforation, short (5–10 mm) strands of human hair (ideally hair from an under 18-month-old child) are placed in a petri dish with 20 ml of distilled water and autoclaved. Two to three drops of 10% sterilized yeast extract are added to the petri dish and hair strands are inoculated with small fragments of test fungus grown on SDA. It is incubated at 25–30°C and the hair strands are removed and microscopically examined in lactophenol cotton blue at weekly intervals for up to 1 month. **T. rubrum which may be morphologically similar to *T. mentagrophytes*, usually causes only surface erosion of hair shafts in this test, whereas *T. mentagrophytes* causes wedge-shaped perforation perpendicular to the hair shaft** (Fig. 55.9).

Urease test

Urease test is useful for distinguishing isolate of *T. mentagrophytes* from that of *T. rubrum*. Urease splits urea in

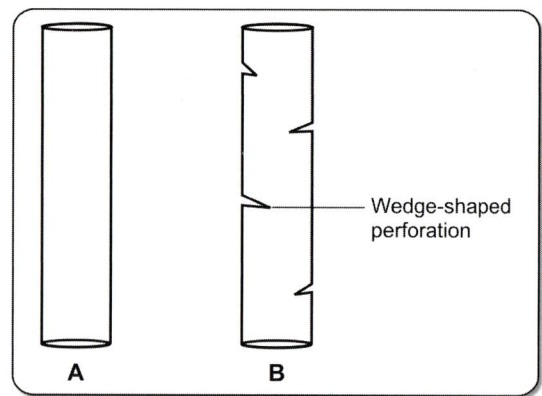

Fig. 55.9. Hair perforation test: (A) Normal hair; (B) Hair showing wedge-shaped perforations.

Christensen's medium, producing ammonia which raises the pH and causes a colour shift of the phenol red indicator from amber to bright pink. For example, *T. mentagrophytes* produces a bright pink colour (positive), while *T. rubrum* produces no colour change (negative). A tube of Christensen's urea agar is very lightly inoculated with the dermatophyte and incubated at 25–30°C for 7 days. A positive reaction is indicated by a change of the original colour to bright pink.

II. SUBCUTANEOUS MYCOSES

Mycetoma

Mycetoma is a chronic granulomatous infection usually of exposed parts of the body especially feet and hands (Figs. 55.10 and 55.11). Infection follows traumatic inoculation of the organism into the subcutaneous tissue from soil or vegetable sources, e.g., thorns or splinters and results in **tumefactions, deformities and draining sinuses discharging fungal colonies called grains or granules (triad of symptoms)**. Granules are white, yellow, pink, red or black depending upon the species of etiologic agent.

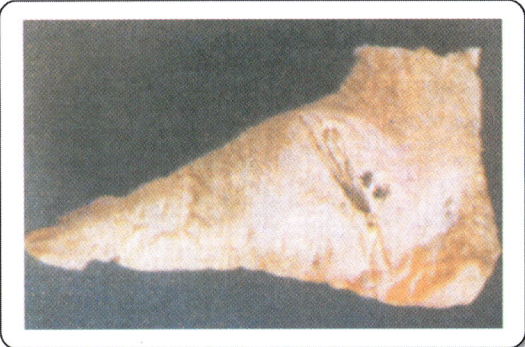

Fig. 55.10. Mycetoma foot showing black granules.

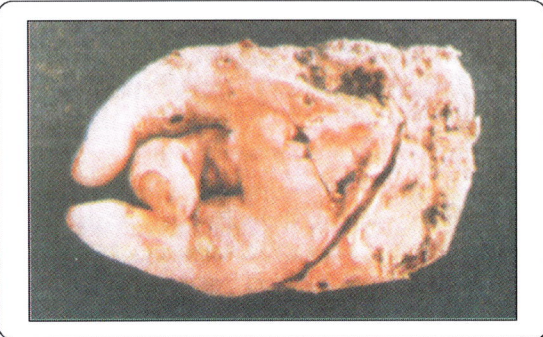

Fig. 55.11. Mycetoma hand showing black granules.

It can be divided into three types, **eumycetomas, actinomycetomas** and **botryomycosis**. Important causative agents of these are given in Table 55.3. Grains can be mounted in a drop of 10% KOH on a slide and crushed under a coverglass. Observation of the colour of the grains, and the size and septations of the hyphae allow differentiation between actinomycetoma and eumycetoma. In actinomycetoma, the grains are composed of very thin filaments (0.5–1 µm in diameter) with coccoid and bacillary elements while in eumycetoma

Table 55.3. Important causative agents and colour of the grains of various types of mycetoma

Causative agent	Colour of the grains
A. *Eumycetoma*	
• *Madurella mycetomatis*	Brown to black
• *M. grisea*	Brown to black
• *Exophiala jeanselmei*	Brown to black
• *Curvularia geniculata*	Brown to black
• *Leptosphaeria senegalensis*	Brown to black
• *Pseudallescheria boydii*	White to yellow
• *Acremonium falciforme*	White to yellow
• *Aspergillus nidulans*	White
• *Fusarium* species	White
B. *Actinomycetoma*	
• *Actinomadura madurae*	White to yellow
• *A. pellitieri*	Red to pink
• *Nocardia asteroides*	White to yellow
• *N. brasiliensis*	White
• *Nocardiopsis dassonvillei*	Cream
• *Streptomyces somaliensis*	Yellow
C. *Botryomycosis*	
• *Staphylococcus aureus*	White
• *Escherichia coli*	White
• *Proteus* species	White
• *Pseudomonas aeruginosa*	White

they are broad (2–6 µm in diameter), septate and often have large, globose swollen cells (up to 15 µm or more) at the margin. Grains are crushed between two slides and then heat fixed. Filaments of the actinomycotic grain are Gram-positive and the cement substance and peripheral fringe are Gram-negative. However, Gram stain, in general is of limited value in demonstrating the presence of eumycetes, though some eumycetes are Gram-positive. *Madurella mycetomatis* and *Actinomadura madurae* are the most common causes of eumycetoma and actinomycetoma respectively.

Chromoblastomycosis

It is a chronic, localized fungal infection of skin and subcutaneous tissue, characterized by crusted, warty lesions usually involving lower legs. It is caused by several darkly pigmented, soil inhabiting phaeoid (dematiaceous) fungi. These include *Phialophora verrucosa, Fonsecaea pedrosoi, F. compacta, Cladosporium carrionii* and *Rhinocladiella aquaspersa*. Infection occurs following a wound or slight abrasion of the skin which is contaminated with soil or vegetable matter containing any of these fungi. The disease has been reported from most parts of the world, but it is more common in tropical and subtropical regions of the Americas and Africa. The causative organisms have been isolated from soil and decaying vegetation in high-prevalence areas. It more often involves males and those who work outdoor without footwear.

Lesions develop most commonly on the distal lower extremities, a location compatible with exposure of damaged skin to soil.

- **The primary skin lesion** is a small papule that gradually enlarges over weeks to months to form a superficial nodule with an irregular, friable surface. Lesions continue to evolve over many years.
- **The verrucous lesions** are warty and hyperkeratotic.
- **Tumorous lesions** are larger than nodular lesions, with raised surface projections that may be covered by crusting and epidermal debris. These lesions can become very large, and their surface texture has been compared with that of cauliflower.
- **Plaque lesions**, the least common type, are flat, reddish and scaly.
- **Cicatricial (scarring) lesions** have irregular borders and expand at their periphery with central healing and scarring. "Black dots" may be observed on the surface of lesions. Samples of material from these areas are particularly useful for microscopic examination.

Tissue reaction in skin shows a characteristic pseudo-epitheliomatous hyperplasia with hyperkeratosis and para-keratosis. Inflammation is generally granulomatous. It is often accompanied by a suppurative reaction, possibly from a secondary reaction, causing satellite microabscesses.

Laboratory diagnosis

1. Superficial crusts scraped from the lesions, preferably from an area containing "black dots", contain long, brown, branching hyphae (3–5 μm in diameter) which are easily seen upon microscopic examination after digestion in potassium hydroxide.
2. In pus, granulation tissue obtained by curettage, or in biopsy specimens of epidermis and subcutaneous tissue, the fungus is present in the form of rounded, thick walled, brown cells with a diameter of 5–12 μm. They have horizontal and/or vertical septations. They reproduce by equatorial splitting and not by budding. They are known as **sclerotic bodies** (Fig. 55.12). Sclerotic bodies are seen within giant cells, rarely in macrophages or extracellularly in microabscesses. **The fungi typically migrate to the surface of the skin and are seen as "black dots" in the keratin scales.**
3. Because the causative agents cannot be distinguished on the basis of histologic features, culture of lesion material is necessary. Crusts, pus, and biopsy material are inoculated on culture media both with and without antibiotics because of the possibility of bacterial contamination, and inoculated plates should be incubated at both 25°C and 30°C. In most cases colonies are formed within 2 weeks; but cultures should be held for 4 weeks before being reported as negative.

Phaeohyphomycosis

It is a mycotic infection caused by phaeoid (dematiaceous, brown-pigmented) fungi where the tissue morphology of the causative organism is mycelial. This separates it from other clinical types of disease involving brown-pigmented fungi where the tissue morphology of the organism is a grain (eumycotic mycetoma) or sclerotic body (chromoblasto-mycosis). Phaeohyphomycosis may be divided into four disease categories – superficial (tinea nigra and black piedra), cutaneous and corneal, subcutaneous, and systemic.

Common causative agents of subcutaneous phaeohypho-mycosis are *Cladosporium bantiana*, *Ochroconis gallopavum*, *Wangiella dermatitidis*, *Curvularia* spp., *Bipolaris* spp., *Exophilia jeanselmei*, *Nattrasia mangiferae*, *Alternaria* spp. and *Exserohilum* spp.

Laboratory diagnosis

The diagnosis of phaeohyphomycosis is established in the laboratory by KOH mount, histopathology and culture. There are no available serologic tests to diagnose infection with these fungi.

KOH mount

The aspirates from cysts, curettings from the cutaneous and corneal lesions, and biopsy material are examined in KOH wet mount. In case of phaeohyphomycosis, the fungus is present in the form of darkly pigmented septate hyphae 2–6 μm in diameter.

Histopathology

The pathological features are similar regardless of the etiologic agent. In systemic phaeohyphomycosis lesions of a given organ may occur as single or multiple abscesses. The abscesses are usually circumscribed and encapsulated granulomas, the walls of which comprise epithelial histiocytes and giant cells surrounded by connective tissue. The centre of the granulomas contain necrotic debris, fibrin, and degenerated polymorpho-nuclear cells.

Within the necrotic debris and inflammatory infiltrates, as well as in the giant cells, fungal elements can be observed.

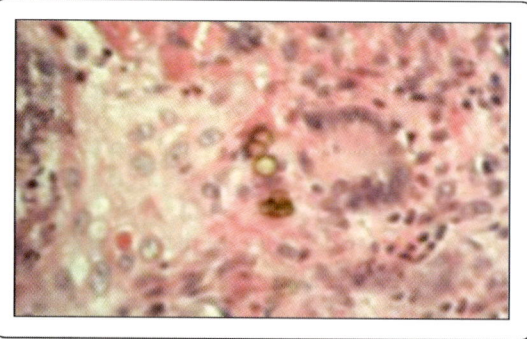

Fig. 55.12. Chromoblastomycosis showing sclerotic bodies (H&E stain, ×400).

The fungus in the tissue is present in the form of darkly pigmented, septate hyphae (2–6 µm in diameter) (Fig. 55.13) and pseudohyphae. Large, bizarre, thick-walled vesicular swellings (up to 25 µm in diameter), resembling chlamydoconidia may be seen along, or at the end of the hyphae. Yeast-like cells producing buds singly or in chains are also commonly present. **Special fungal stains such as Gomori methenamine silver and periodic acid-Schiff mask the natural colour of the hyphae, but in haematoxylin and eosin sections the brown colour may be obvious.** In some cases, however, the hyphae appear unpigmented and a specific stain for melanin, Masson Fontana stain, must be used to reveal the presence of the fungal pigment.

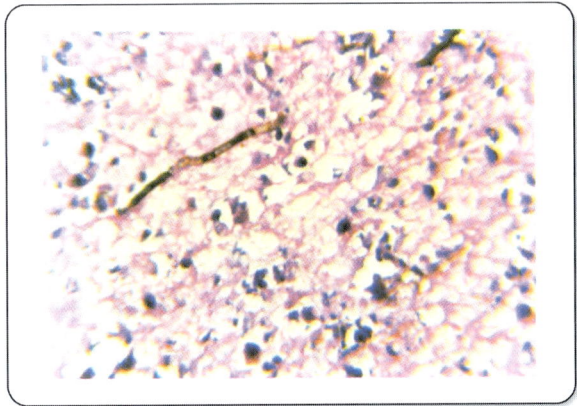

Fig. 55.13. Phaeohyphomycosis showing brown septate fungal hypha (H&E stain, ×400).

Rhinosporidiosis

Rhinosporidiosis is a chronic granulomatous disease characterized by the development of pedunculated or sessile, red, spongy, friable, polypoid, granulomatous growths in the nose, conjunctiva and occasionally in ears, larynx, bronchus, penile urethra, vagina, rectum and skin. It is caused by *Rhinosporidium seeberi*.

It has not been cultured and animal inoculation is also not successful. Nothing definite is known about the mode of transmission of infection. However, it has been suggested that the organism is transmitted in dust or water. Infection is more common in:

• Persons bathing in muddy stagnant pools of water.
• Those who dive into streams to collect sand from riverbeds.
• Paddy cultivators.
• In dry areas, after dust storm and eye injuries.

Laboratory diagnosis

The definitive diagnosis of rhinosporidiosis depends on the histopathological examination of biopsied or resected tissues. **Large numbers of sporangia at different stages of development are a main feature of the histopathologic tissue sections.**

R. seeberi can be identified in haematoxylin and eosin stained sections, but sometimes one may need special stains such as Gomori methenamine silver (GMS) and periodic acid-Schiff (PAS) stains to demonstrate the causative agent. Sporangia can be seen with the naked eye as small white dots. The mature sporangium measures 100–500 µm in diameter and contains hundreds of endoconidia 5–20 µm in diameter (Fig. 55.14).

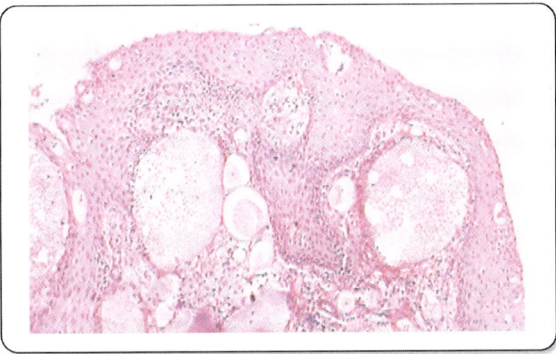

Fig. 55.14. Rhinosporidiosis showing sporangia and endoconidia (H&E stain, ×400).

Sporotrichosis

Sporotrichosis is a chronic pyogranulomatous infection of the skin and subcutaneous tissues, although it may become disseminated by lymphatic spread. It is caused by *Sporothrix schenckii*, a dimorphic fungus.

Infection with *S. schenckii* typically occurs by direct skin inoculation from contaminated soil or thorny plants. **Sporotrichosis is a recognized occupational hazard of farmers and gardeners.**

The initial lesion is a small ulcerated nodule commonly on the hand or the forearm. Nodules and abscesses occur along the draining lymphatics and the regional lymph nodes enlarge, suppurate and ulcerate. The primary lesion may remain localized or disseminate to involve the bones, joints, lungs and rarely CNS particularly in debilitated or immunosuppressed individuals.

In infected tissues, *S. schenckii* appears in the form of round, oval (4–6 µm), elongated or cigar-shaped yeast-like cells with irregular budding (Fig. 55.15A). With ordinary stains, they are difficult to find. The use of PAS or GMS stains and fluorescent antibody technique facilitates detection of these organisms. The abscesses may show the **asteroid body**. This consists of central budding yeast cell with eosinophilic Splendore-Hoeppli material (antibody complex) radiating from it (Fig. 55.16).

The diagnosis is confirmed by isolation of the causative organism by culture of swabs from the ulcerated lesions or pus aspirated from subcutaneous nodules or biopsy material. *S. schenckii* grows well on routine agar media, and at room temperature (25–30°C). The young colonies are blackish and

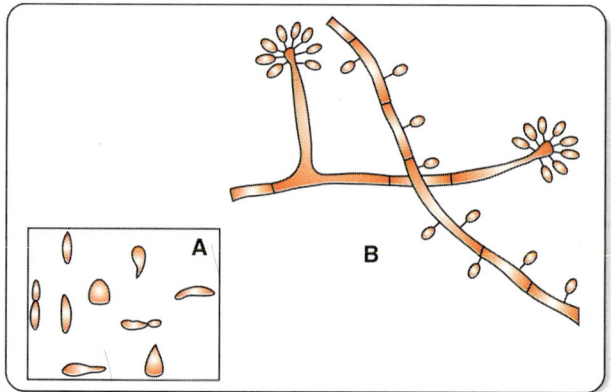

Fig. 55.15. *Sporothrix schenckii:* (A) yeast phase; and (B) mycelial phase.

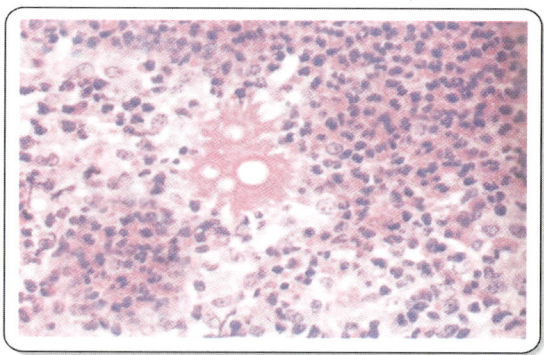

Fig. 55.16. Asteroid body in sporotrichosis. The yeast-like cells are surrounded by eosinophilic Splendore-Hoeppli material (H&E stain, ×400).

shiny, becoming wrinkled and fuzzy with age. Strains vary in pigmentation from shades of black and grey to whitish.

Microscopic examination reveals thin, delicate hyphae bearing conidia developing in a 'rosette' pattern at the ends of delicate conidiophores. Conidia are also produced along the sides of the hyphae (Fig. 55.15B).

A **latex agglutination test**, for detection of antibodies against *S. schenckii*, is available for the diagnosis of the extra-cutaneous forms of sporotrichosis.

III. SYSTEMIC MYCOSES

Histoplasmosis

Histoplasmosis is an intracellular mycosis of reticulo-endothelial system involving lymphatic tissues, lungs, spleen, liver, adrenals, kidneys, skin, central nervous system and other organs of the body. It is caused by a dimorphic fungus, *Histoplasma capsulatum.*

Pathogenicity

H. capsulatum grows in soil with high nitrogen content. Disturbances of such sites create aerosols laden with infectious propagules of *H. capsulatum.* When inhaled, these aerosols

result in infections varying in degree of severity depending on the size of the inoculum and the immunological status of the individuals involved.

Histoplasmosis is ordinarily an asymptomatic or relatively mild, self-limiting pulmonary infection, although chronic or acute disseminated disease with poor prognosis may occur. In addition, it may also involve lymph nodes, spleen, liver, adrenals, kidneys, skin, CNS and other organs of the body. Granulomatous and ulcerative lesions may develop on the skin and mucosa.

In tissues, *H. capsulatum* is present inside phagocytic cells in yeast phase. They are round or oval, yeast-like cells, 2–5 μm in diameter with budding on a narrow base at the smaller end. They reproduce within monocytes or macrophages. They fill the cytoplasm of macrophages, monocytes and occasionally polymorphonuclear leucocytes. Some organisms may be found free in the tissues also. With Giemsa or Wright stains, the cell wall and the cell protoplasm stain light blue and dark blue respectively.

With H&E staining, only a central protoplasmic mass surrounded by a halo is seen (Fig. 55.17). Only a dark staining can outline the cell wall. In the PAS stain, the wall is stained pink to purplish red with pallor coloured protoplasm filling the cell. In the GMS stain the cell wall stains intense black (Fig. 55.18).

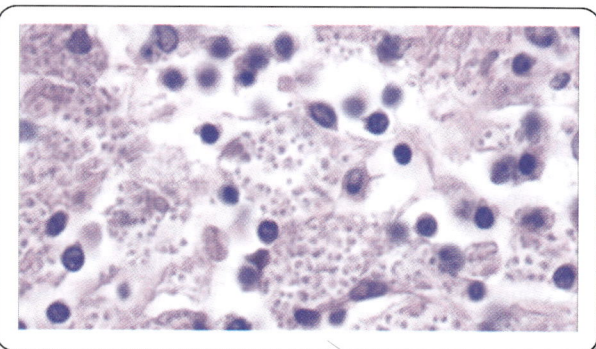

Fig. 55.17. Section of skin stained with haematoxylin and eosin showing *Histoplasma capsulatum* surrounded by clear halo filling the cytoplasm of phagocytes (H&E stain, ×400).

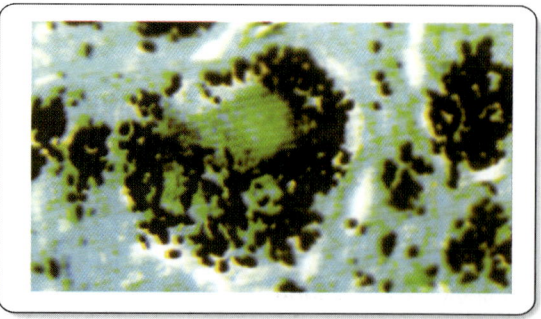

Fig. 55.18. Section stained with Gomori methenamine silver staining (×400). It shows black budding yeast cells.

Culture

On SDA, at 25–30°C, it forms white to tan fluffy colony with septate branching hyphae with two types of unicellular, asexual spores:

1. Large round, tuberculate macroconidia (8–14 μm) are most prominent and are diagnostic.
2. Small spores or microconidia usually appear first. They are sessile or stalked, smooth-walled, round to pyriform, 2–5 μm in diameter (Fig. 55.19A). The yeast phase cells (2–5 μm) can also be produced *in vitro* by culture at 35–37°C on brain heart infusion agar (Fig. 55.19B).

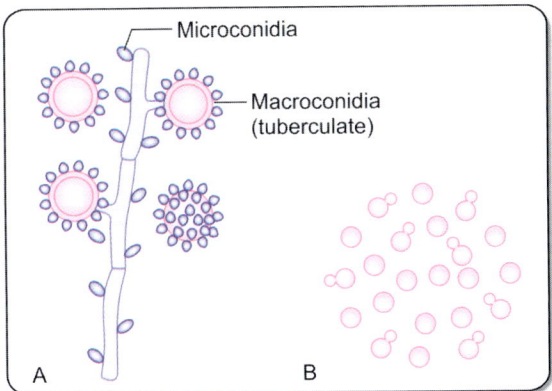

Fig. 55.19. *Histoplasma capsulatum*: (A) mycelial phase; and (B) yeast phase.

Laboratory diagnosis

Diagnosis may be made by microscopic examination of sputum or pus smear stained by Wright or Giemsa procedures. Blood smears may be positive for *H. capsulatum*, especially in patients with AIDS. Liver or lung biopsies stained with PAS or GMS may provide a rapid diagnosis of disseminated histoplasmosis in some patients. *H. capsulatum* is seen as small, oval yeast cells, typically packed within macrophages or monocytes. Specimen should be cultured on SDA at 25–30°C to obtain the mycelial phase.

Serological tests like latex agglutination, precipitation and complement fixation become positive two weeks after infection.

Blastomycosis

Blastomycosis is a chronic infection of the lungs, which may spread to other tissues, particularly skin, bone and genitourinary tract.

Pathogenesis

The infectious particles of *B. dermatitidis* are its mycelial fragments and conidia. The respiratory tract is the portal of entry for all forms of blastomycosis except direct transcutaneous inoculation. In the alveoli, the organism transforms into the yeast and induces an acute inflammatory response that includes neutrophils and macrophages, resulting in granuloma formation.

Culture

In tissue or culture on brain heart infusion agar at 37°C, *B. dermatitidis* grows as a thick-walled multinucleated spherical yeast (8–15 μm) that usually produces single buds. The bud and the parent yeast are attached with a broad base (Fig. 55.20A), and the bud often enlarges to the same size as the parent yeast before it becomes detached. The yeast colonies are wrinkled, waxy, and soft. When grown on SDA at 25°C, a white or brownish colony develops, with branching hyphae bearing spherical, ovoid, or pyriform conidia (2–10 μm in diameter) on short or long conidiophores or directly on the hyphae (Fig. 55.20B). Larger chlamydoconidia (7–18 μm) may also be produced.

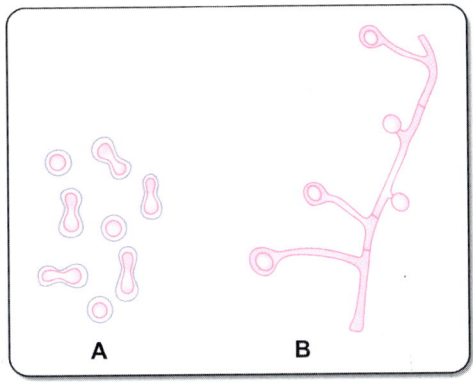

Fig. 55.20. *Blastomyces dermatitidis*: (A) yeast phase; and (B) mycelial phase.

Laboratory diagnosis

Diagnosis can be made by direct microscopy (calcofluor white, potassium hydroxide mount) and culture of sputum, pus and scrapings from skin lesions. An ELISA test that appears to be more than 90% specific has been developed.

Paracoccidioidomycosis

Paracoccidioidomycosis is a chronic progressive granulomatous infection caused by *Paracoccidioides brasiliensis*, a dimorphic fungus. It is characterized by primary pulmonary infection that spreads by haematogenous route, to mucosa of the nose, mouth and the gastrointestinal tract, skin, lymphatic system, and the internal organs producing chronic granulomatous reaction. Infection is acquired usually via respiratory route by inhalation of spores from environmental sources. The fungus has been isolated from soil.

Laboratory diagnosis

- Microscopic examination of KOH wet mount of pus, crusts, sputum and biopsies from granulomatous lesions usually shows numerous yeast cells (10–60 μm) with multiple buds.

The buds are attached to the mother cell (resembling 'pilot wheel') by very narrow necks (Fig. 55.21A).

- Tissue sections should be stained with H&E, PAS and GMS.
- The tissue form (yeast phase) may be obtained *in vitro* by inoculation of clinical material on enriched media such as brain heart infusion agar and incubating at 35–37°C.
- Mycelial (mold) phase of the fungus develops on SDA incubated at 25–30°C. It shows septate hyphae bearing intercalary and terminal chlamydoconidia. A few microconidia are sometimes observed along the hyphae (Fig. 55.21B).

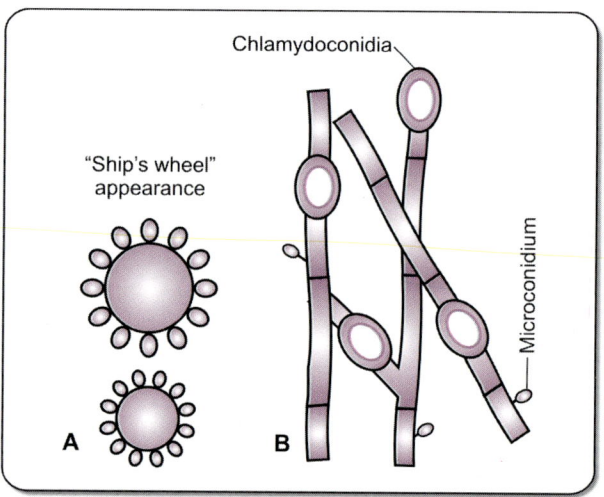

Fig. 55.21. *Paracoccidioides brasiliensis*: (A) yeast phase; and (B) mycelial phase.

The tests for antibody detection like immunodiffusion, complement fixation and ELISA are useful for diagnosis and prognosis.

Coccidioidomycosis

Coccidioidomycosis is primarily an infection of the lungs caused by *Coccidioides immitis*, a dimorphic fungus.

C. immitis differs from other dimorphic fungi because under standard laboratory conditions **it grows as a mold at 25°C as well as 37°C**. The hyphae develop barrel-shaped arthroconidia measuring 2.5–4 × 3–6 μm. They characteristically alternate with smaller intervening empty cells (Fig. 55.22A). The walls of empty cells break easily and are characteristically present on either side of the freed conidia. The latter are highly infectious and are readily airborne, therefore, the handling of a well developed culture is hazardous.

In the lungs, the arthroconidia form **spherules** (30–100 μm or more in diameter). These contain numerous **endoconidia**, 2–4 μm in diameter (Figs. 55.22B and 55.23). The mature spherules have double wall measuring 2 μm in thickness. At maturity, the spherules rupture and their endoconidia are released, which develop to form new spherules in adjacent tissue or following dissemination, in other organs of the body.

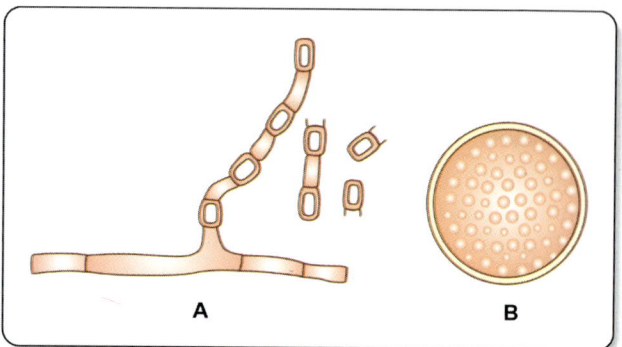

Fig. 55.22. *Coccidioides immitis*: (A) tissue phase; (B) mycelial phase.

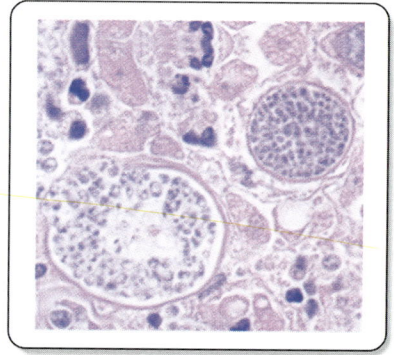

Fig. 55.23. Spherules of *Coccidioides immitis* containing endoconidia (H&E stain, ×400).

Laboratory diagnosis

Diagnosis may be made by microscopic examination of sputum, pus and biopsy material and culture on SDA incubated at 25–30°C.

IV. OPPORTUNISTIC MYCOSES

Candidiasis

The genus *Candida* comprises about 200 species, of which about 20 have been associated with pathology in humans and animals. The major pathogenic species include *C. albicans*, *C. dubliniensis*, *C. glabrata*, *C. guilliermondii*, *C. kefyr*, *C. krusei*, *C. lusitaniae*, *C. parapsilosis* and *C. tropicalis*. *C. albicans* is round to oval yeast 3–6 μm in diameter. It produces budding cells, pseudohyphae, and true hyphae.

Pathogenesis

Candida is a human commensal, so that the source of infection is mostly endogenous. *Candida* spp. reside primarily in the gastrointestinal tract, but they are also commensals in the vagina, urethra, on the skin and under fingernails. *Candida* can be introduced from exogenous sources as well. These include introduction through various catheters and lines, or other indwelling prosthetic medical devices. *C. albicans* is the species most often associated with human disease.

Clinical features

Candida species can cause a range of clinical forms, from superficial manifestations involving skin, nails, and mucosal surfaces to deep-seated infections involving various internal organs and to disseminated disease.

SUPERFICIAL INFECTIONS

Superficial infections result from invasion of the superficial layers of skin and/or mucosae by the microorganism. These infections are characterized by the formation of a grayish plaque, surrounded by edema, which on histopathological examination consists of the infecting microorganisms, neutrophils, and cell debris.

DEEP INFECTIONS

Candida spp. may cause deep infections of several parenchymatous organs. These infections are characterized by microabscesses. Microscopically, these reveal blastoconidia, pseudohyphae, true hyphae (in case of *C. albicans*), neutrophils and mononuclear cells, and a necrotic centre. In chronic infections granulomata with giant cells and lymphocytes may be formed.

Laboratory diagnosis

Specimens

Scrapings from mucosal, dermal or nail lesions, sputum, bronchial aspirate, pus, swabs, etc.

Direct examination

Place the specimen in a drop of 10% KOH, warm gently over a small flame and examine under microscope. All species of *Candida* form round to oval budding yeast cells, 3–6 µm in diameter.

They occur singly, in chains, or in small loose clusters. Most species, when invading tissue, form both pseudohyphae and true hyphae. Pseudohyphae are actually chains of blastoconidia that have elongated and have not separated from one another. They can be recognized by distinct constrictions at the septa. True hyphae have no, or only slight constrictions at the septa. Blastoconidia develop along the sides of both types of hyphae (Figs. 55.24 and 55.25).

Histopathology

In systemic infections, *Candida* spp. most commonly elicit an acute suppurative inflammation composed of polymorphonuclear as well as mononuclear cells. Granulomas only rarely occur. *Candida* spp. are also known to invade blood vessels and produce infarcts.

Culture

Candida albicans: For isolation in culture spread pathological material on slants of SDA with chloramphenicol and incubate at 30°C. It grows rapidly. Growth matures in 3 days. Colonies are cream-coloured, pasty and smooth. Lactophenol cotton

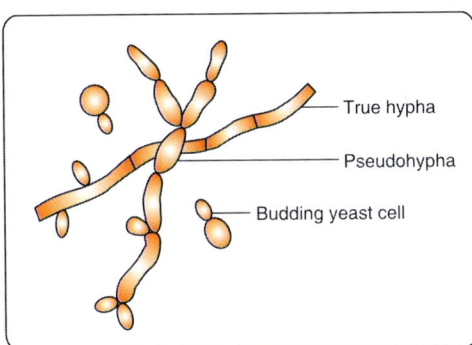

Fig. 55.24. Budding yeast cells, pseudohyphae and true hyphae of *Candida albicans*.

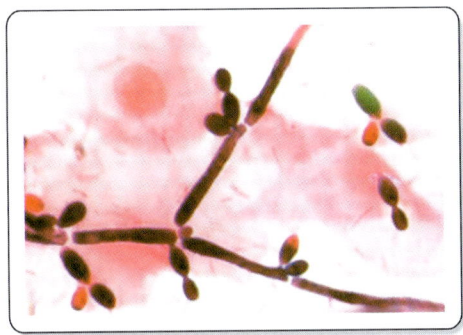

Fig. 55.25. Vaginal smear showing budding yeast cells, true hyphae and epithelial cells (PAS stain, ×400).

blue preparation and Gram-stained smears show round to oval budding yeast cells (3.5–7 × 4–8 µm) and pseudohyphae. Rarely true hyphae may also be seen. On cornmeal-Tween 80 agar at 25°C for 72 hours, pseudohyphae form with clusters of round blastoconidia at the septa. Large thick-walled, usually single terminal chlamydoconidia are characteristically formed (Fig. 55.26). Chlamydoconidia formation is inhibited at 30–37°C.

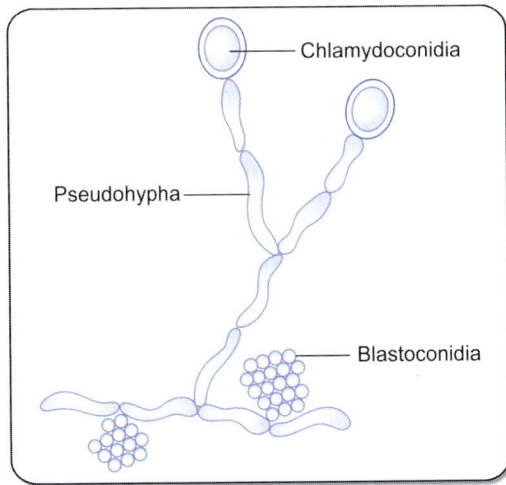

Fig. 55.26. Blastoconidia and chlamydoconidia of *Candida albicans*.

After incubation in sheep, horse or normal human serum for about 90 minutes at 37°C yeast cells of *C. albicans* begin to form germ tubes (Fig. 55.27). Germ tube test is also positive in *C. dubliniensis*. All other species are negative for this test. **Germ tubes are the beginning of true hyphae and appear as filaments that are not constricted at their points of origin on the parent cell. If the filaments are constricted at their points of origin, they are pseudohyphae, not germ tubes** (Fig. 55.27).

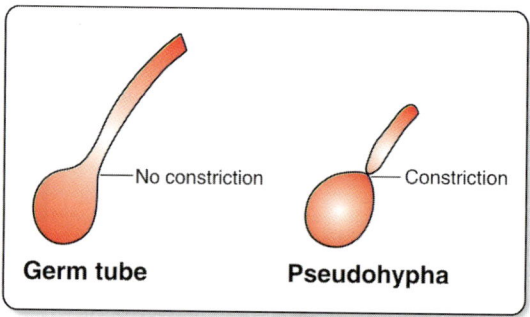

Fig. 55.27. Germ tube and pseudohypha of *Candida albicans*.

Cryptococcosis

Cryptococcosis is an acute, subacute or chronic fungal infection caused by encapsulated basidiomycetous yeast, *Cryptococcus neoformans*. It is most frequently recognized as a disease of the central nervous system, although the primary site of infection is the lungs. The disease occurs sporadically throughout the world.

Mycology

C. neoformans is a round or oval encapsulated yeast, measuring 4–10 μm in diameter in clinical specimens, and having a capsule ranging in size from 1 to > 30 μm.

Pathogenesis

Cryptococcosis is usually acquired by inhalation of aerosolized yeast cells. In the immunocompetent host, inhalation of the fungus leads to a variety of clinical features. Patient may develop asymptomatic or mildly symptomatic pulmonary disease. It may resolve spontaneously or result in an encapsulated lung nodule. Patients who develop progressive pulmonary cryptococcosis, usually present with chronic cough, low grade fever, chest pain, scant mucoid or blood-tinged sputum, malaise, and weight loss. *C. neoformans* may also involve central nervous system, eye, bone, skin, and in disseminated cryptococcus, any organ or tissue may have foci of infection.

Laboratory diagnosis

Direct microscopy

The clinical specimens are collected as per the site involved particularly CSF, sputum, pus, brain tissue, etc. Place **a drop** of India ink on a clean glass slide, add and mix with it a drop of centrifuged deposit of CSF or other body fluid and, under reduced light, look for the spherical cells of *C. neoformans* and their enveloping capsule (Fig. 55.28).

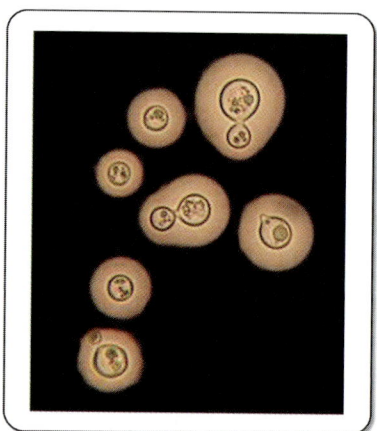

Fig. 55.28. An India ink wet mount (×400) of *Cryptococcus neoformans* showing encapsulated budding yeast cells.

The ink's carbon particles do not penetrate the capsule which appears as a clear halo surrounding the yeast cells. If fungus is not found upon immediate examination, centrifuge CSF at 3000 rpm for 10 minutes and carefully withdraw the sediment with a pipette for microscopic examination and culture. India ink examination of CSF is the most rapid test for diagnosing cryptococcal meningitis.

Sputum or pus should be mixed with **10% potassium hydroxide** before examination. In a properly prepared specimen, pus cells and partially digested cellular debris delineate the capsule which is resistant to potassium hydroxide.

Histopathology

The histopathological examination of biopsy specimen can be done **by staining with Mayer's mucicarmine, periodic acid-Schiff, Gomori methenamine silver, and haematoxylin and eosin staining**.

The yeast cells are round or oval with thin walls, 4–10 μm in diameter, vary in size within the microscopic field, bud on a narrow base and characteristically produce thick capsules. Tissue stained with Mayer's mucicarmine show the capsule as bright carmine red, often with a spiny or scalloped appearance (Fig. 55.29). Drying, fixing, and staining may cause the yeast cells to collapse or become crescent-shaped.

Culture

Cryptococci can be cultured from biologic samples on SDA. Chloramphenicol (0.05 mg/ml) can be incorporated in the medium to inhibit growth of bacterial contaminants, but do not use cycloheximide because this inhibits *C. neoformans*. As only a few yeast cells may be present at the site of infection, pellets from centrifuged CSF and other biologic fluids should be cultured.

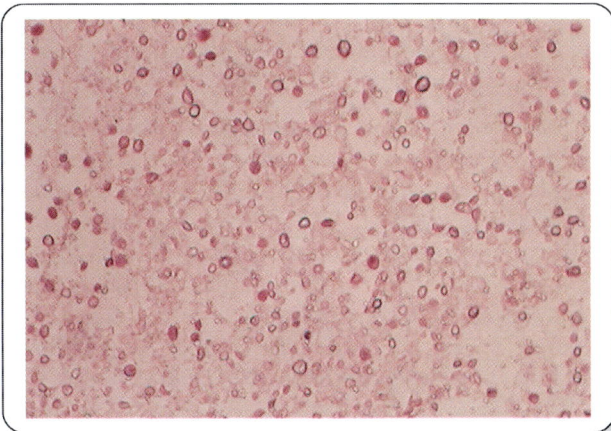

Fig. 55.29. Cryptococci stained with Mayer's mucicarmine stain (×400). The capsule is stained bright carmine red in colour.

Colonies are flat or slightly heaped, shiny, moist, and usually mucoid with smooth edges. Colour is cream at first later becoming tannish. *C. neoformans* grows equally well at 25°C and 37°C, and incubation at 37°C inhibits other species of the genus.

C. neoformans possesses the enzyme phenol oxidase, and testing for its presence is another means of accurate identification. This can be done by culturing the suspected yeasts on special agars such as niger seed agar, bird seed agar and caffeic acid agar and looking for the black colonies. *C. neoformans* breaks down caffeic acid to melanin.

Aspergillosis

There are more than 200 species of *Aspergillus* to which humans are constantly exposed. However, approximately 19 species have been implicated in human disease (aspergillosis), which is worldwide in occurrence. Of these *A. fumigatus* is most important. Other important pathogens in this group are *A. niger*, *A. flavus*, *A. terreus* and *A. nidulans*. Aspergilli are ubiquitous in nature. Aspergillosis is caused by inhalation of *Aspergillus* conidia or mycelial fragments which are present on vegetation (especially nuts and grains), decaying matter, soil and air. A high degree of natural resistance exists in healthy host, but when the host defence is compromised, as in AIDS and in patients on immunosuppressive therapy, aspergillosis may develop. It may cause:

1. Allergic bronchopulmonary aspergillosis (ABPA).
2. Intracavitary aspergilloma (fungus ball).
3. Acute invasive pulmonary aspergillosis. This occurs in severely immunocompromised individuals who are on immunosuppressive drugs, cytotoxic drugs, corticosteroids, broad spectrum antibiotics and AIDS patients. There is a widespread growth of the fungus in lung tissue that disseminates to involve other organs particularly kidneys and brain. The disease has poor prognosis.
4. Endocarditis.

5. Paranasal *Aspergillus* granuloma.
6. Cerebral aspergillosis.
7. Keratitis.
8. Otomycosis.

Laboratory diagnosis

Direct examination and histopathology

Diagnosis may be made by microscopic examination and by culture. Ten per cent KOH preparation of sputum, broncho-alveolar lavage, transbronchial biopsy and other biopsies reveal non-pigmented septate hyphae, 3–5 μm in diameter with characteristic dichotomous branching. The hyphae have a tendency to branch repeatedly. The branches arise at an angle of approximately 45 degrees. In a majority of pulmonary and disseminated lesions, only hyphal forms are seen. Histological sections can be stained with H&E and GMS and examined for characteristic hyphae (Figs. 55.30 and 55.31). In allergic aspergillosis there is usually abundant fungus in the sputum and mycelial plugs may also be present. In aspergilloma, fungus may be difficult to find in sputum smear. In invasive aspergillosis, sputum smear is often negative.

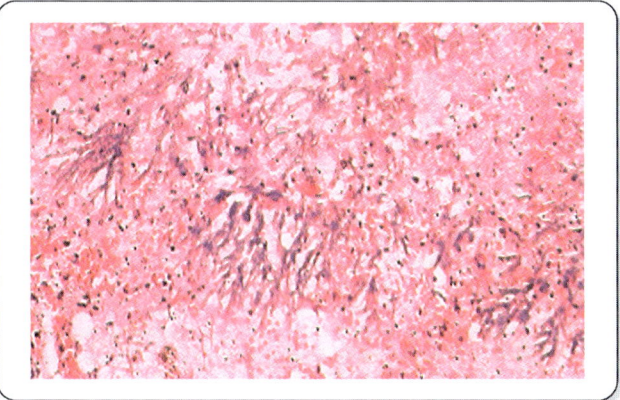

Fig. 55.30. *Aspergillus* showing septate hyphae with characteristic dichotomous branching (H&E stain, ×400).

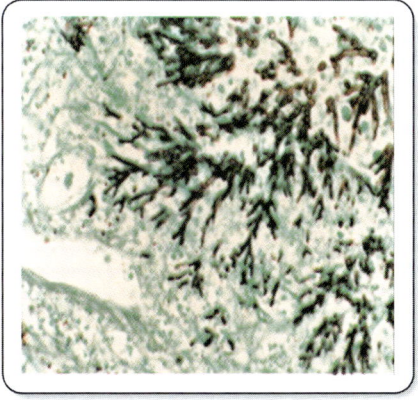

Fig. 55.31. Section stained by Gomori's methenamine silver stain (×400). The hyphae are stained black in colour.

Culture

For species identification, the clinical material is inoculated on SDA without cycloheximide and incubated at 25°C. Colonies appear after incubation for 1–2 days. The isolate is identified on the basis of growth characteristics and microscopic morphology. LCB mount shows branching and septate hyphae. From the latter arise conidiophores, the ends of which are expanded to form vesicles. The vesicle bears phialides which arise directly from the vesicle (uniseriate) or from sterile cells called metulae (biseriate).

Aspergillus fumigatus

The colonies of *A. fumigatus* are granular to cottony and usually have some shades of green, green-grey or green-brown pigmentation. Microscopically, the conidiophores are short (usually less than 300 μm long), and 5–10 μm in diameter. The vesicles are 20–30 μm in diameter. The phialides are uniseriate, compact, forming only on the upper two thirds of the vesicle, parallel to the axis of the conidiophore. Conidia

are round, smooth, or slightly rough and 2–3.5 μm in diameter. (Fig. 55.32A).

Aspergillus flavus

The colonies of *A. flavus* are granular to woolly and have some shade of yellow or yellow-brown. Microscopically, the conidiophores are long (400–800 × 8–18 μm), the vesicles are 25–45 μm in diameter. The phialides may arise directly from the vesicle from three-fourths or the entire circumference of the vesicle (uniseriate) or from sterile cells called metulae (biseriate). Both these conditions may exist in the same head. Conidia are spherical, smooth, or slightly roughened with maturity and form long chains (Fig. 55.32B).

Aspergillus niger

The surface of the colonies of *A. niger* is covered by a dense aggregate of jet black conidia. The underside of the colony is buff or yellow-grey, distinguishing *A. niger* from the dematiaceous fungi. Microscopically, the conidiophores are long (400–3000 × 12–17 μm). The vesicles are globose and

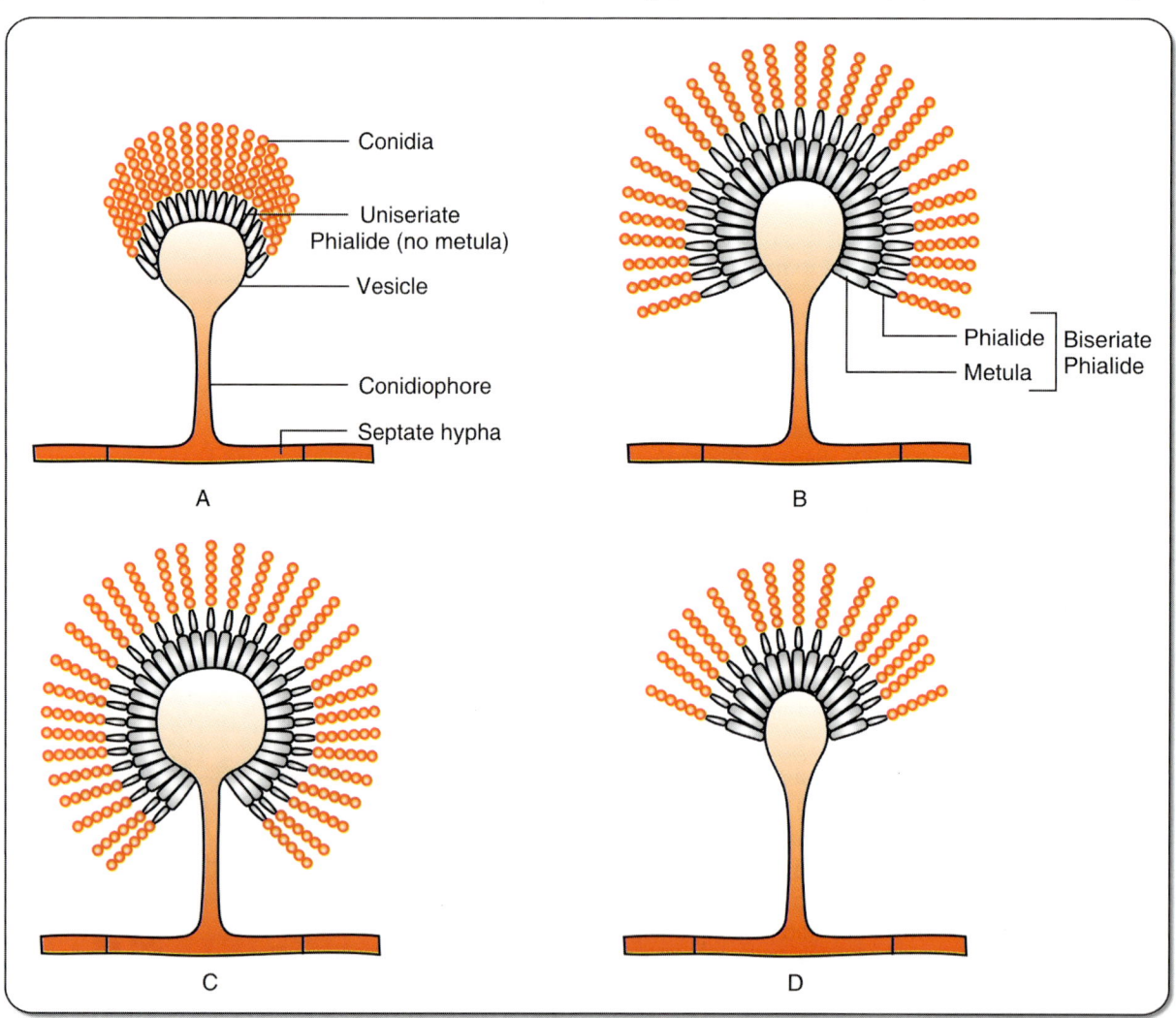

Fig. 55.32. *Aspergillus* spp.: (A) *A. fumigatus*; (B) *A. flavus*; (C) *A. niger*; (D) *A. terreus*.

measure 30–75 µm in diameter. Phialids arise from metulae (biseriate) from entire circumference of the vesicle. Conidiation is extremely profuse, to the extent that the vesicles are obscured by dense aggregates of 3–5 µm diameter, spherical, black conidia that become roughened with maturity (Fig. 55.32C).

Aspergillus terreus

The colonies of *A. terreus* are cinnamon buff, brown or orange-brown. Radial folds emanating from the centre of the colony are often observed. Microscopically, the vesicles are relatively small (10–16 µm in diameter) flask-shaped or hemispherical. Phialids arise from metulae (biseriate) on the upper half only. Conidia are smooth, elliptical, measure 2–2.5 µm in diameter (Fig. 55.32D).

Aspergillus nidulans

A. nidulans may rarely be recovered from cases of human infections. Phialids arise from metulae (biseriate) on their upper half surface. *A. nidulans* may form sexually-derived ascospores contained within sac-like structures called cleistothecia.

Mucormycosis

Mucormycosis is an opportunistic infection caused by sapro-phytic fungi, notably species of *Mucor*, *Rhizopus* and *Lichtheimia* (*Absidia*). These fungi are common saprophytes of soil, manure and decaying vegetables, and fruits. These are essentially opportunistic fungi. The major predisposing factors to mucormycosis are acute diabetes mellitus, metabolic acidosis, debilitating diseases such as leukaemia or lymphoma, immunosuppression, starvation, and widespread use of broad-spectrum antibiotics, steroids and antimetabolites. Mucor-mycosis may lead to:

1. Rhinocerebral mucormycosis.
2. Pulmonary mucormycosis.
3. Gastrointestinal mucormycosis.
4. Subcutaneous mucormycosis.
5. Disseminated mucormycosis.

The characteristic pathological changes in mucormycosis are suppuration and necrosis. Invasion of thrombosed blood vessels by the fungus is a conspicuous feature. In tissues (Figs. 55.33 and 55.34), the organisms appear as irregularly branched, nonseptate, very broad hyphae (7–15 µm in diameter), which characteristically are deeply stained with routine H&E stain. On the other hand, the coloration by special fungus stains such as Gridley, PAS and in some cases GMS may be very poor. True septa are rarely seen in the hyphae but under low magnification, cross folds in the walls of the hyphae may resemble septa.

Subcutaneous mucormycosis shows chronic inflammatory reaction in which, sparse, thin-walled, broad hyphae are seen in the centre of the granulomas. **The hyphae are surrounded by eosinophilic Splendore-Hoeppli material.**

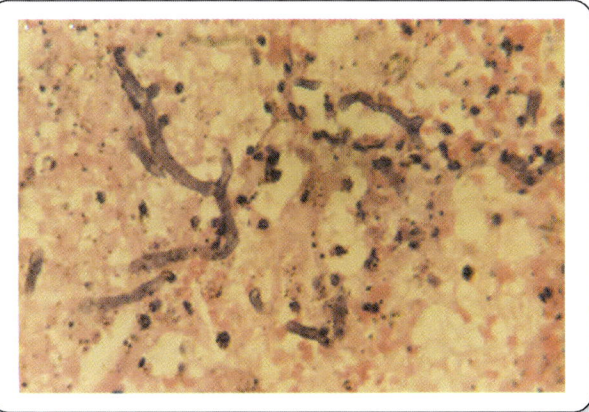

Fig. 55.33. Mucormycosis showing broad nonseptate hyphae (H&E stain, ×400).

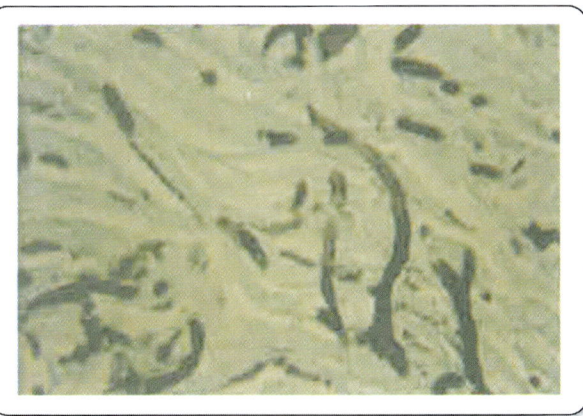

Fig. 55.34. Section stained by Gomori's methenamine silver stain (×400). The hyphae are stained black in colour.

Laboratory diagnosis

Diagnosis can be made by examination of:

- KOH wet mounts of scrapings from the lesions, pus, sputum and nasal discharge shows characteristic hyphae.
- The fungi can be readily seen by histological sections stained with routine H&E stain.
- Fungi can be readily isolated on SDA at 37°C. *Rhizopus* has rhizoids and sporangiophores that arise in groups directly above the rhizoids. *Mucor* does not possess rhizoids and shows branched sporangiophores arising randomly along aerial mycelium. *Lichtheimia* (*Absidia*) has rhizoids and sporangiophores that arise from the aerial mycelium in between the rhizoids (Fig. 55.35).

V. MISCELLANEOUS MYCOSES

Penicilliosis marneffei

There are more than 250 described species of the genus *Penicillium*. They occur as saprophytes in the soil and decomposing organic debris. ***P. marneffei* is the only species**

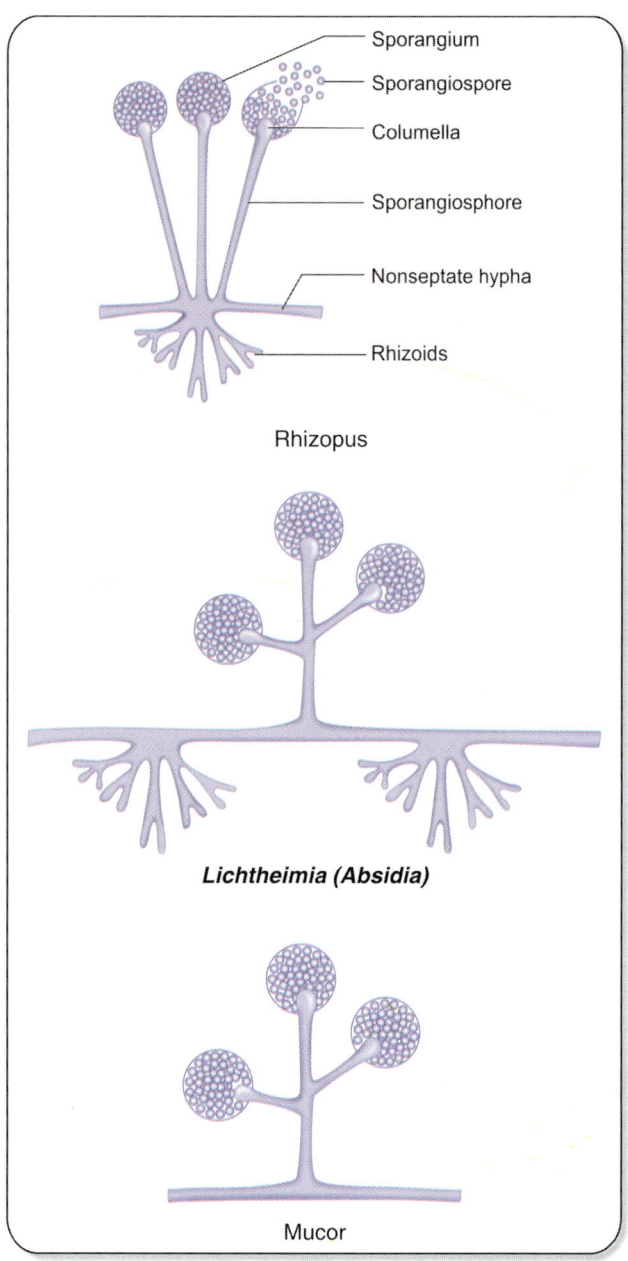

Fig. 55.35. *Rhizopus, Mucor* and *Lichtheimia.*

of genus *Penicillium* which is pathogenic dimorphic fungus.

The disease caused by *P. marneffei* is known as Penicilliosis marneffei.

The natural habitat of *P. marneffei* is probably soil. Like other dimorphic fungal pathogens that produce conidia in their saprophytic habitats in nature, the infection is thought to occur through inhalation of the conidia or through cutaneous inoculation. The organisms are engulfed by macrophages, in which they multiply intracellularly and transform into yeast.

Patient develops fever, anaemia, leucopenia, thrombocytopenia, weight loss, diarrhoea, hepatosplenomegaly, generalized lymphadenopathy, cough and pulmonary infiltrates. Skin lesions occur in over 50% of cases. They are small papules, ulcers or molluscum-like lesions. They are usually widely scattered on the face and trunk. Left untreated, this infection is fatal.

Mycology

SDA supports the growth of *P. marneffei* and demonstrates thermal dimorphism. Cycloheximide inhibits growth. At 25–30°C on SDA growth matures within 3 days. It produces rapidly growing **greenish-yellow sporulating colonies, with a pink or red centre and dark green edges**. A characteristic brick-red pigment is released into the medium.

Microscopically, at 25–30°C, structures typical of the genus *Penicillium* develop, i.e., smooth conidiophores with 4–5 terminal metulae, each metula bearing 4–6 phialides. Conidia are ellipsoidal to globose (2–3 μm), smooth walled, often with prominent disjunctors, and arranged in short chains. The terminal conidia of the conidial chains are sometimes larger than the ones beneath them, which is a characteristic of *P. marneffei* (Fig. 55.36A).

At 35–37°C on SDA or brain heart infusion agar, colony is soft, white to tan, dry and yeast-like. Conversion from mold to yeast-like form may take up to 14 days. Hyphae first become shorter, develop more septa and branches, and cease to produce conidia. They eventually fragment at the septa, producing single-celled round to oval arthroconidia (2.5–5 μm in length). This form is referred to as yeast-like cells. Buds are not produced. The arthroconidia continue to reproduce by fission and in so doing may elongate to 8–9 μm (Fig. 55.36B).

Histopathology

P. marneffei yeast-like cells are engulfed by histiocytes where they proliferate within the phagosomes. As the lesion progresses, central necrosis develops, with infiltration of neutrophils and formation of abscesses. Granulomas slowly evolve in the lung and may lead to fibrosis and cavitation.

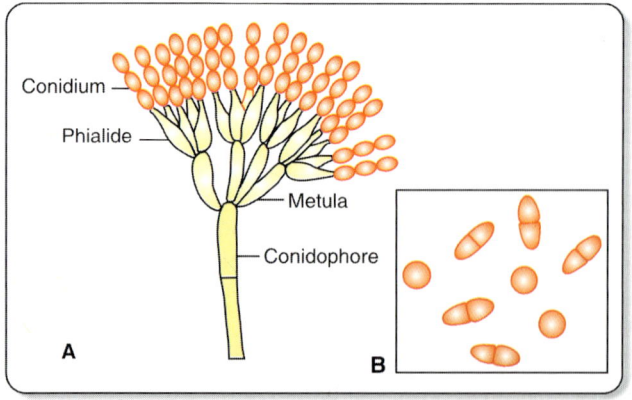

Fig. 55.36. *Penicillium marneffei*: mycelial phase (A) and yeast-like phase (B).

Laboratory diagnosis

Microscopic examination

Clinical specimens include bone marrow aspirate, buffy coat of blood, lymph node aspirate or biopsy, liver biopsy, skin biopsy, skin scrapings, sputum, bronchoalveolar lavage pellets, pleural fluid, cerebrospinal fluid, pharyngeal ulcer scrapings, palatal papule scrapings, urine and stool. Impression smears and histopathological sections are stained with H&E, PAS and GMS.

Microscopic examination reveals oval yeast-like cells, 3–6 μm in length. They multiply within histiocytes in tissue or within monocytes in blood or bone marrow. Budding does not occur. A prominent central septum forms, and reproduction is by fission. Outside the histiocytes, yeast cells are up to 8 μm in length. These may have several septa, and are often curved to be sausage-shaped.

P. marneffei gives a false impression of having a capsule when stained with H&E. Therefore, they can very closely mimic *H. capsulatum* var. *capsulatum*, especially when intracellular. However, the two organisms multiply differently. *P. marneffei* replicates by fission, instead of budding, and the considerable variation in size and shape of the extracellular yeasts makes *P. marneffei* easily distinguishable from the budding tissue-form cells of *H. capsulatum* var. *capsulatum*.

A specific indirect fluorescent antibody examination of histological sections has been described.

Culture

P. marneffei can be isolated from various clinical specimens particularly bone marrow, skin biopsy and blood (for cultural characteristics see above).

Serodiagnosis

Penicilliosis marneffei infection may be diagnosed by detection of IgG antibodies in the sera of patients by an **indirect fluorescent antibody test**, using germinating conidia and yeast cells as antigens. **Latex agglutination, ELISA and immunodiffusion tests** can be used for detection of *P. marneffei* antigens in body fluids of the patients. Antigens may be detected in urine as well as serum.

Otomycosis

Otomycosis is a subacute or chronic superficial fungal infection of external auditory canal. It is more prevalent in warm and humid climate, particularly during rainy season as compared to cold climate. It is a common disease and is usually caused by *A. niger*, *A. fumigatus*, *Penicillium*, *Candida albicans*, *C. tropicalis* and *C. krusei*. The symptoms are itching, pain and deafness. Secondary bacterial infection, caused usually by *Pseudomonas* and *Proteus*, may develop. The diagnosis can be made by demonstration of the fungi in scrapings and by culture.

Keratomycosis

Keratomycosis or mycotic or fungal keratitis is an invasive fungal infection of the cornea. It is most frequently caused by *A. fumigatus*, *A. flavus*, *A. glaucus* and *A. niger*. In addition, species of *Fusarium*, *Curvularia*, *Candida*, *Acremonium*, *Paecilomyces*, *Penicillium*, *Alternaria*, *Fonsecea*, *Pseudallescheria*, *Drechslera* and *Aureobasidium* may also cause keratomycosis. It usually follows trauma. Fungal spores colonize the injured tissue and initiate an inflammatory reaction leading to hypopyon, ulcer and endophthalmitis. If not recognized and treated early, enucleation may become necessary. Increased incidence of keratomycosis is due to widespread use of corticosteroids. Diagnosis can be made by microscopic examination and culture of scrapings taken from the base or edge of the ulcer.

Pneumocystosis

Pneumocystosis is caused by *Pneumocystis jirovecii*. Three developmental forms of *P. jirovecii* are generally recognized – trophozoite, pre-cyst and cyst.

Trophozoite

The trophozoite of *P. jirovecii* is the smallest of the life cycle stages of the organism. It ranges in size from 1–4 μm and is ellipsoidal in shape when unfixed preparations are viewed by light microscopy. After fixation it may appear amoeboid in form. It is thought to reproduce by binary fission.

Pre-cyst

The pre-cyst is recognized as an intermediate stage of the sexual phase of reproduction leading to cyst development. It is presumed that a mating event first occurs to provide a zygote that initiates sporogenesis.

Cyst

The cyst is the end product of sporogenesis. This form is spherical, 5–8 μm in diameter, and has a thick wall composed of three layers. Eight spores are commonly found within each cyst. The spores are 1–2 μm in diameter. The cysts can be stained with GMS stain, toluidine blue, Giemsa, and calcofluor white. With GMS stain the organisms appear deep blue-black (Fig. 55.37).

P. jirovecii causes *Pneumocystis* pneumonia (PCP). It is the most important opportunistic infection in HIV-infected patients.

Laboratory diagnosis

Histopathology

To establish the diagnosis of *P. jirovecii* pneumonia, specimens of bronchoalveolar lavage, lung biopsy or induced sputum (by administration of a saline mist to induce production of sputum) are stained by GMS, toluidine blue, Giemsa and

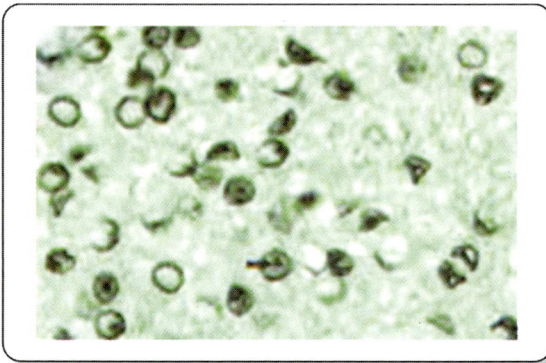

Fig. 55.37. Intra-alveolar clusters of non-budding cysts of *Pneumocystis jirovecii* stained by Gomori methanamine silver stain (×400) in an AIDS patient suffering from *Pneumocystis jirovecii* pneumonia.

calcofluor white and examined for the presence of cysts or trophozoites. The Papanicolaou stain, frequently used for staining cytopathological specimens, can demonstrate the foamy exudate surrounding the organisms, although the organisms stain poorly. With Giemsa stain, all forms of the organism are stained, which permits assessment of the total organism burden. The nuclei appear reddish-purple in contrast to the light blue cytoplasm. The cell wall excludes the dye and appears as a circumscribed clear zone around the cyst contents. Organisms can also be demonstrated by immuno-fluorescent techniques, using fluorescein-tagged monoclonal antibodies against surface antigens of both cysts and trophic forms. ***P. jirovecii* cannot be cultured.**

Polymerase chain reaction (PCR)

PCR-based detection of *P. jirovecii* DNA has been shown to have greater sensitivity and specificity for the diagnosis of PCP from respiratory specimens than conventional (Giemsa or GMS) microscopic methods.

Serology

A presumptive serodiagnosis can be made in suspected cases of *P. jirovecii* infections. Complement fixation titres of 1 : 4 or higher usually indicate active disease. Latex agglutination tests for *P. jirovecii* are positive in only about one third of patients with known disease.

Mycotoxicosis

Many fungi produce poisonous substances called myco-toxins that can cause acute or chronic intoxication and damage. The mycotoxins are secondary metabolites and their effects are not dependent on fungal infection or viability. The diseases that result from ingestion of food that contains mycotoxins are known as mycotoxicoses. Mycotoxins produced by various species of fungi are aflatoxin, ergot alkaloids, ochratoxin, fumonisins, gliotoxin, zearalenone and trichothecenes. Cooking has little effect on the potency of these toxins, which may cause severe or fatal damage to the liver and kidney.

Classic examples of human diseases caused by *Fusarium* mycotoxins include alimentary toxic aleukia, Urov or Kashin-Beck disease and Akakabi-byo (scabby grain intoxication). *Fusarium germinearum*, *F. poae* and *F. sporotrichoides* have been linked to human mycotoxicosis. T-2 toxin is produced by these fungi. T-2 toxin is a potent inhibitor of eukaryotic protein synthesis and inhibits platelet aggregation. It increases prothrombin time and causes cardiomyopathy.

Some fungi produce mutagenic and carcinogenic compounds that can be extremely toxic for experimental animals. One of the most potent is **aflatoxin** which is elaborated by *Aspergillus flavus* and related molds and is a frequent contaminant of peanuts, corn, grains, and other foods.

SECTION 5

PARASITOLOGY

Chapter 56   Parasitology
Chapter 57   Parasitic Diagnostic Procedures

Parasitology

Parasitology is the area of biology concerned with the phenomenon of dependance of one living organism on another. Medical parasitology is the science that deals with organisms living in the human body (the host) and the medical significance of the host-parasite relationship.

Parasite

It is defined as an animal or plant which lives in or upon another organism and derives its nutrient directly from it.

Host

It is defined as an organism which harbours the parasite and provides the nourishment and shelter to the latter. It is of following types:

1. Definitive host

The host which harbours the adult parasite, the most highly developed form of a parasite or where the parasite replicates sexually. When the most highly developed form is not obvious, the definitive host is the mammalian host.

2. Intermediate host

This is the host which alternates with the definitive host and harbours the larval or asexual stages of a parasite. Some parasites require two intermediate hosts for completion of their life cycle.

3. Reservoir host

It is the host that harbours the parasite and serves as an important source of infection to other susceptible hosts.

4. Vector

It is the insect host which transmits parasites to man and animals.

HOST-PARASITE RELATIONSHIPS

Host-parasite relationship is of following types:

1. Symbiosis

An association in which both host and parasite are so dependent upon each other that one cannot live without the help of the other. Neither of the partners suffers from any harm from this association.

2. Commensalism

An association in which only parasite derives benefit without causing any injury to the host. A commensal lives on food residues or waste products of the body and is capable of leading an independent life.

3. Parasitism

An association in which the parasite derives benefit and host gets nothing in return and always suffers from some injury. The parasite is so adapted to this association that it cannot live an independent life.

CLASSIFICATION OF PARASITES

Parasites are classified into protozoa (unicellular organisms) and helminths (multicellular organisms).

PROTOZOA

Principal protozoan pathogens of man are given in Table 56.1.

ENTAMOEBA HISTOLYTICA

Morphology

The parasite exists in three morphological forms – trophozoite, precyst and cyst (Fig. 56.1).

1. Trophozoite

It measures 10–60 μm (average 20–30 μm) in diameter.

Cytoplasm

The cytoplasm of the trophozoite can be divided into a **clear outer ectoplasm and an inner finely granular endoplasm**

Table 56.1. Principal protozoan pathogens of man	
Group	**Species**
1. Amoebae	*Entamoeba histolytica, Acanthamoeba* spp., *Balamuthia mandrillaris*
2. Flagellates	*Giardia lamblia, Trichomonas vaginalis, Trypanosoma brucei gambiense, T. brucei rhodesiense, T. cruzi, Leishmania* spp., *Naegleria fowleri*
3. Sporozoa	*Plasmodium falciparum, P. vivax, P. malariae, P. ovale, P. knowlesi, Toxoplasma gondii, Cryptosporidium parvum, Isospora belli*
4. Others	*Balantidium coli, Babesia microti, B. divergens*

in which red blood cells, leucocytes and tissue debris are found within the food vacuoles. Trophozoites are motile with active, unidirectional and purposeful motility. Movement results from long finger-like pseudopodial extensions of ectoplasm into which endoplasm flows.

Nucleus

It is spherical in shape varying in size from 4–6 µm in diameter. In stained preparations it shows **a central dot-like karyosome which is surrounded by a clear halo**. The nuclear membrane is delicate and is lined by a single layer of **fine chromatin granules**. The space between the karyosome and the nuclear membrane is traversed by linin network (achromatic fibrils) having spoke-like radial arrangement.

2. Precyst

It is smaller in size, varying from 10–20 µm in diameter. It is oval with a blunt pseudopodium projecting from the periphery. Food vacuoles disappear. There is no change in the nucleus which shows characteristics of that of the trophozoite.

3. Cyst

It is spherical, 10–15 µm in diameter. It is surrounded by a thick chitinous wall. It starts as a uninucleate body, but later the nucleus divides to form two and then four nuclei. Uninucleate and binucleate cysts in addition also possess a glycogen mass, which stains brown with iodine, and 1–4 chromidial or chromatoid bars. These do not stain with iodine but appear as refractile oblong bars with rounded ends in normal saline preparations. With iron-haematoxylin stain they stain black in colour.

Life cycle

It passes its life cycle in only one host (Fig. 56.2). Man acquires the infection by ingestion of water or food contaminated with mature quadrinucleate cysts. In the small intestine the cyst wall is lysed by trypsin and a single tetranucleate amoeba (**metacyst**) is liberated. Each nucleus divides by binary fission giving rise to eight nuclei. Almost immediately the cytoplasm becomes separated into as many parts as there are nuclei, thus from each mature cyst eight small amoebulae (**metacystic trophozoites**) are produced. This process is known as **excystation**. Metacystic trophozoites are carried in the faecal stream into the caecum. They invade the mucosa and ultimately lodge in the submucous tissue of large intestine. Here they grow and multiply by binary fission.

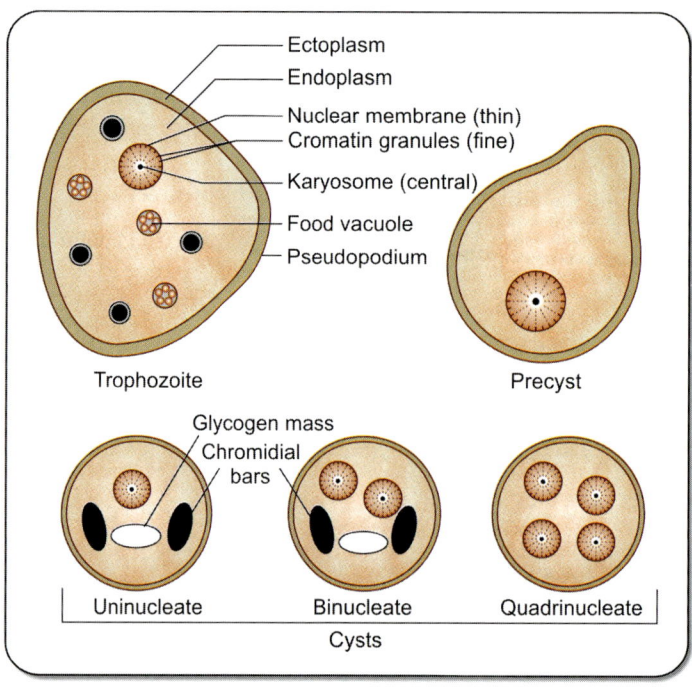

Fig. 56.1. Various morphological forms of *Entamoeba histolytica*.

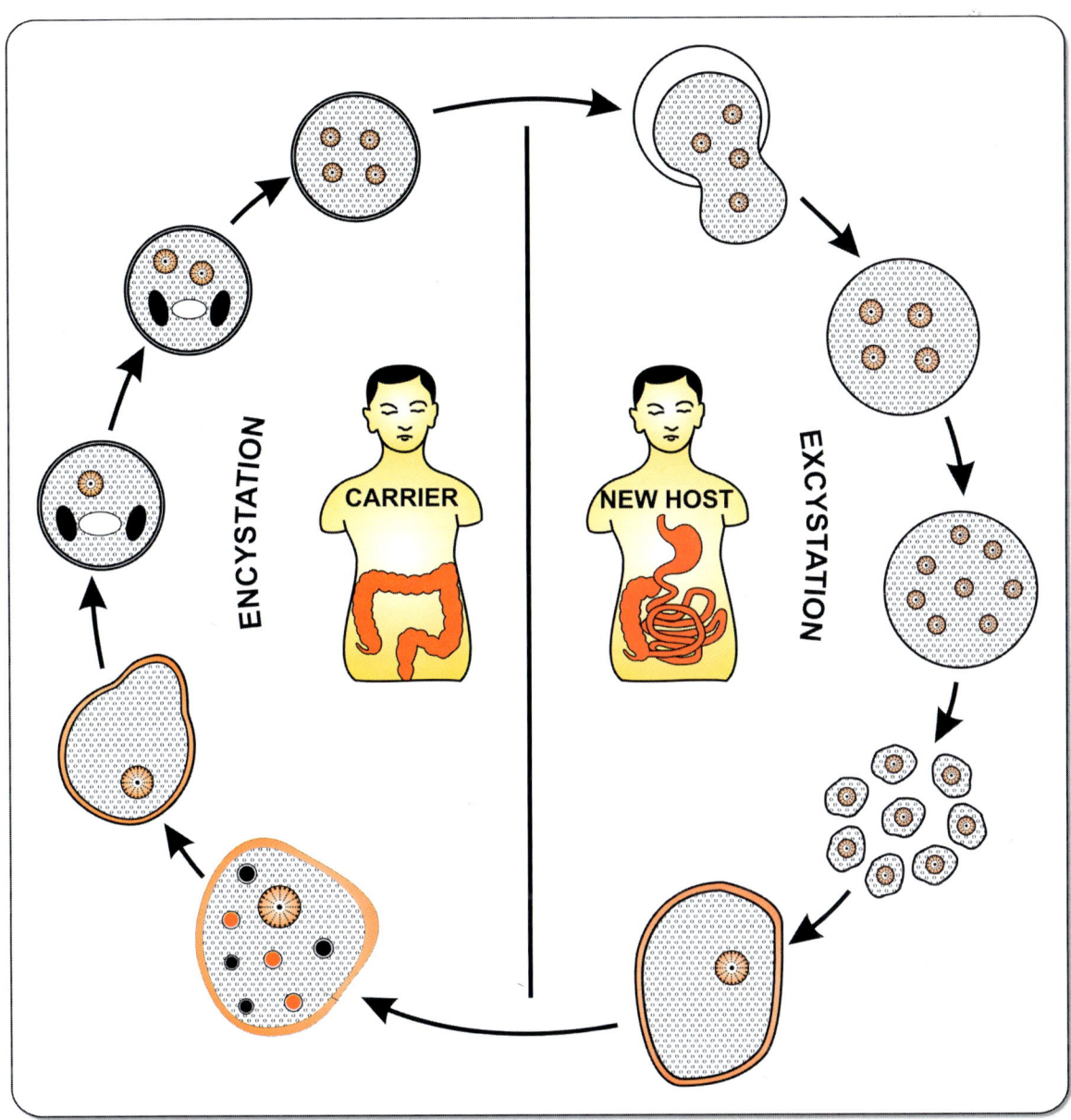

Fig. 56.2. Life cycle of *Entamoeba histolytica*.

During growth, *E. histolytica* secretes a **proteolytic enzyme of the nature of histolysin**, which brings about destruction and necrosis of tissue and produces flask-shaped ulcers (Fig. 56.3). The amoebae are mostly present at the periphery of the lesion. At this stage, a large number of trophozoites are excreted along with blood and mucus in the stool leading to amoebic dysentery. In a few cases, erosion of the large intestine may be so extensive that **trophozoites gain entrance into the radicals of portal vein** and are carried away to the liver where they multiply leading to amoebic hepatitis and amoebic liver abscess.

After some time, when the effect of the parasite on the host is toned down and patient has developed resistance, the lesions start healing and patient starts passing normal (formed) stools. The trophozoites, in the lumen of the large intestine, transform into precysts and then into mature quadrinucleate cysts. **These are the infective forms of the parasite.** This process is known as **encystation**. Cyst formation occurs only within the intestinal tract; once the stool has left the body, cyst formation does not occur.

Pathogenicity

E. histolytica causes intestinal and extraintestinal amoebiasis.

Intestinal amoebiasis

After an incubation period of 1–4 weeks, the amoebae invade the colonic mucosa, producing characteristic ulcerative lesions

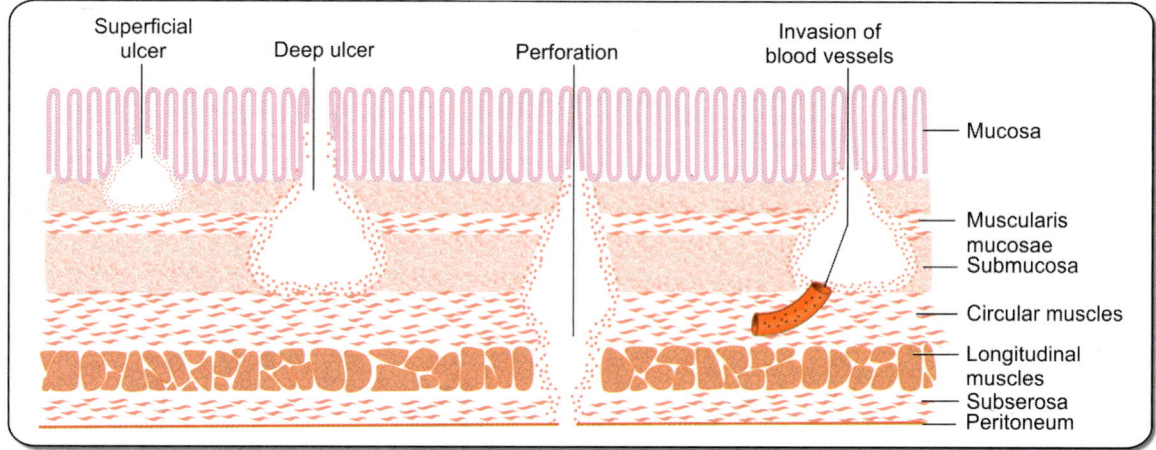

Fig. 56.3. Pathogenesis of intestinal amoebiasis.

and a profuse bloody diarrhoea (**amoebic dysentery**). The ulcers may be generalized involving the whole length of the large intestine or they may be localized in the ileocaecal (caecum, ascending colon, ileocaecal valve and appendix) or sigmoidorectal (sigmoid colon and rectum) region. Ulcers are discrete with intervening normal mucosa. They vary in size from pin-head size to more than 2.5 cm in diameter. They may be deep or superficial. Base of the deep ulcers is generally formed by muscular coat. However, superficial ulcers do not extend beyond muscularis mucosae (Fig. 56.3).

Extraintestinal amoebiasis

About 5% individuals with intestinal amoebiasis, 1–3 months after the disappearance of the dysenteric attack, develop hepatic amoebiasis. Trophozoites of *E. histolytica* are carried as emboli by the radicles of the portal vein from the base of the amoebic ulcer in the large intestine (Fig. 56.3). The capillary system of the liver acts as an excellent filter and holds these parasites. They multiply in the liver and lead to cytolytic action. The amoebae cause obstruction of the portal venules resulting in anaemic necrosis of hepatic cells. The destruction starts here and continues in concentric layers. Necrosis is followed by cytolysis. Small miliary abscesses coalesce to form big liver abscess.

Amoebic liver abscess

It varies greatly in size. It has been reported in patients of all ages, but predominate in adults between 20–60 years. It has a marked preference for the right lobe of the liver and it is at least three times more frequent in males than in females. The wall of the abscess cavity is ragged with shreds of connective tissue running across the abscess cavity. A section through the margin of the liver abscess can be differentiated into three zones:

1. A necrotic centre filled with thick pus with no amoebae.
2. An intermediate zone consisting of degenerated liver cells, a few red blood cells, leucocytes and occasional tropho-zoites of *E. histolytica*.

3. An outer zone of nearly normal hepatic tissue just being invaded by amoebae.

Pus of liver abscess

The centre of an amoebic liver abscess contains a viscous red-brown (anchovy sauce appearance) or grey-yellow fluid consisting of cytolysed liver cells, red blood cells and leucocytes. It is referred to as 'pus' but contains very few pus cells. Since the amoebae actively multiply in the walls of the abscess, the last few drops of pus obtained from the lesion are most likely to yield recognizable trophozoites of the parasite.

From the liver, *E. histolytica* may enter into general circulation involving other organs of the body like lungs, brain, spleen, skin, etc. Both faecal and sigmoidoscopic examinations for the parasite are negative in approximately half of the patients in extraintestinal disease.

Laboratory diagnosis

I. Intestinal amoebiasis

1. Stool examination

In acute amoebiasis, stool or colonic scrapings from ulcerated areas are examined by macroscopic and microscopic examination. It should be carefully differentiated from bacillary dysentery (Table 56.2). For microscopic examination stool is picked up with a matchstick or a platinum loop and emulsified in a drop of normal saline on a clean glass slide. A clean coverslip is placed over it and examined under microscope, first under low power and then under high power. This method is specially useful for the demonstration of the actively motile trophozoites of *E. histolytica*.

For the demonstration of cysts or dead trophozoites, stained preparation may be required for the study of the nuclear character. For this purpose iodine stained preparation is commonly employed. Stool is emulsified in a drop of five times diluted solution of Lugol's iodine, covered with a clean

Table 56.2. Differences between amoebic and bacillary dysentery

Character	Amoebic dysentery	Bacillary dysentery
Macroscopic		
Number	6–8 motions a day	Over 10 motions a day
Amount	Copious	Small
Odour	Offensive	Odourless
Colour	Dark red	Bright red
Reaction	Acidic	Alkaline
Consistency	Not adherent to the container	Adherent to the container
Microscopic		
RBCs	In clumps	Discrete, sometimes in clumps due to rouleaux formation
Pus cells	Few	Numerous
Macrophages	Few	Numerous, many of them contain RBCs; hence may be mistaken for *E. histolytica*
Eosinophils	Present	Scarce
Charcot-Leyden crystals	Present	Absent
Pyknotic bodies	Present	Absent
Ghost cells	Absent	Present
Parasites	Trophozoites of *E. histolytica*	Absent
Bacteria	Many motile bacteria	Few or absent

coverslip and examined under microscope. Both saline and iodine preparations may be prepared on the same slide. Since excretion of cysts in the stool is often intermittent, at least three consecutive specimens should be examined.

2. Blood examination

It shows moderate leucocytosis.

3. Serological tests

These are negative in early cases. However, in later stages of invasive intestinal amoebiasis antibodies appear and serological tests become positive. These tests include:

- indirect haemagglutination (IHA),
- indirect fluorescent antibody (IFA) test, and
- enzyme-linked immunosorbent assay (ELISA).

II. Hepatic amoebiasis

1. Diagnostic aspiration

Trophozoites of *E. histolytica* can be demonstrated by microscopy of the pus aspirated by exploratory puncture of amoebic liver abscess.

2. Liver biopsy

Trophozoites of *E. histolytica* can be demonstrated in the specimens of liver biopsy from cases of amoebic hepatitis or the wall of the liver abscess.

3. Blood examination

It shows leucocytosis with total leucocyte count of 15,000–30,000/µl, of which 70–75% are polymorphonuclear leucocytes.

4. Stool examination

In about 15% cases of amoebic hepatitis cysts of *E. histolytica* can be demonstrated in the stool. This indicates persistence of intestinal infection.

5. Serological tests

Serological tests like IHA, IFA and ELISA are of immense value in the diagnosis of hepatic amoebiasis. IHA and IFA tests have been reported positive with titres of $\geq 1 : 256$ and $\geq 1 : 200$ respectively, in almost 100% cases of amoebic liver abscess. ELISA is now replacing the IHA and is available commercially. Amoebic antibodies persist for months to years even after clinical cure.

Amoebic antigen can be detected in the patient serum by ELISA and a simple and economical slide agglutination test, the coagglutination test. It is present in serum only in active infection and disappears when the patient is cured of active amoebic disease.

6. Histology

A histological diagnosis of amoebiasis can be made when the trophozoites within the tissue are identified.

ENTAMOEBA COLI

It is a worldwide parasite. It lives freely in the lumen of large intestine of man and is non-pathogenic. Like *E. histolytica* it exists in three stages – trophozoite, precyst and cyst (Table 56.3). Life cycle of *E. coli* is similar to that of *E. histolytica*.

GIARDIA LAMBLIA

Trophozoite

It is pear-shaped with rounded anterior and pointed posterior end (Fig. 56.4). It measures 14 µm in length and 7 µm in maximum width. The dorsal surface is convex while on the ventral surface it has a shallow posteriorly notched concavity (sucking disc) that embraces anterior half of the organism. It acts as an organelle of attachment.

It is bilaterally symmetrical and has **one pair of nuclei**, one on each side of the midline, one pair of axostyles, one pair of parabasal bodies present on the axostyles and four pairs of flagella and probably four pairs of blepharoblasts, from which the flagella arise.

The **cytoplasm** is finely granular. The **nuclei** are rounded and possess a central karyosome. The nuclear membrane is

	Table 56.3. Trophozoites and cysts of *E. histolytica* and *E. coli*	
	E. histolytica	*E. coli*
Trophozoite		
Size	20–30 μm	20–50 μm
Motility	Active	Sluggish
Cytoplasm	Clearly defined into ectoplasm and endoplasm.	Not defined.
Cytoplasmic inclusions	Red blood cells, leucocytes and tissue debris but no bacteria.	Bacteria and cellular debris but never red blood cells.
Nucleus	Central karyosome, the nuclear membrane is delicate and is lined by fine chromatin granules. It is not visible in unstained preparations.	Eccentric karyosome, the nuclear membrane is thick and is lined by coarse chromatin granules. It is visible in unstained preparations.
Precyst	Oval with a blunt pseudopodium, 10–20 μm in diameter. Nucleus shows characteristics of that of its trophozoite.	20 μm in diameter, resembles in shape with that of *E. histolytica*. Nucleus shows characteristics of that of its trophozoite.
Cyst		
Size	Spherical, 10–15 μm in diameter.	Spherical, 15–20 μm in diameter.
Number of nuclei	1–4	1–8
Chromatoid bars	Rounded	Filamentous

delicate and is not lined by chromatin material. By rapid movement of flagella, the trophozoites move from place to place.

Cyst

Mature cyst is oval in shape and measures 12 × 7 μm in size. It has **two pairs of nuclei** which may remain clustered at one end or lie in pairs at opposite ends. The remains of the flagella and margins of the sucking disc may be seen inside the cytoplasm of the cyst (Fig. 56.4).

Life cycle

It passes its life cycle in one host. Mature cyst is the infective form of the parasite. **Man acquires infection by ingestion**

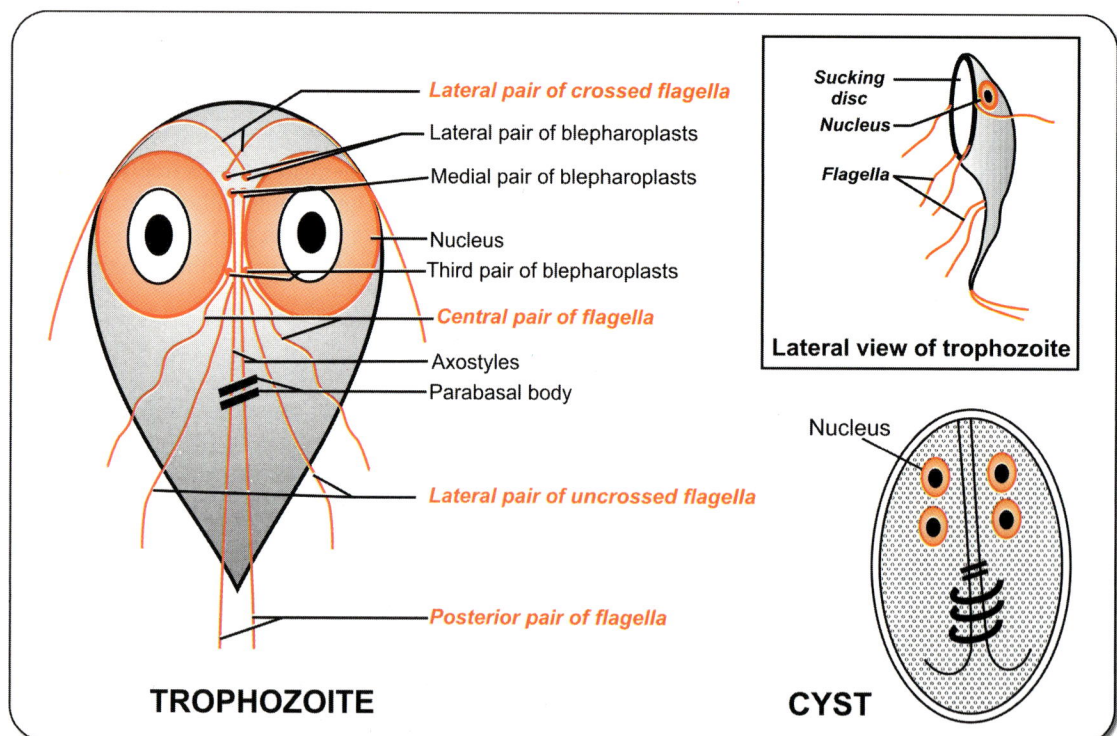

Fig. 56.4. Morphological forms of *Giardia lamblia*.

of water or food contaminated with the cysts. Infection may also be acquired by anal-oral sexual practices. Within 30 minutes of ingestion **excystation** occurs in the duodenum. The cyst hatches out two trophozoites, which then multiply to form enormous numbers and colonize in the duodenum and upper part of jejunum. To avoid acidity of duodenum, it may localize in biliary tract.

In frankly diarrhoeic stools, it is usual to find only the trophozoites. **Encystation** occurs commonly in transit down the colon where the intestinal contents lose moisture and patient starts passing formed stools. The trophozoites retract their flagella and secrete a thin, tough and hyaline cyst wall. As cyst matures, the internal structures are doubled, so that when **excystation** occurs, the cytoplasm divides, thus producing two trophozoites.

Pathogenicity

With the help of sucking disc the parasite attaches itself to the surface of the epithelial cells in the duodenum and jejunum and may cause duodenal and jejunal irritation leading to duodenitis and jejunitis. Patient may complain of dull epigastric pain, flatulence and **chronic diarrhoea of steatorrhoea type**. The stool is voluminous, foul smelling and contains large amount of mucus and fat but no blood. This is due to malabsorption since the parasites are coated on the mucosa, thus absorption suffers. Patient loses weight. When *Giardia* localizes in the biliary tract, it may lead to chronic cholecystitis and jaundice.

Laboratory diagnosis

Giardiasis can be diagnosed by identification of cysts of *G. lamblia* in the formed stools or the trophozoites of the parasite in diarrhoeal stools and bile aspirated from duodenum by intubation by normal saline and iodine preparation as in case of *E. histolytica*.

TRICHOMONAS

Genus *Trichomonas* contains three species which occur in humans:

1. *T. tenax*
2. *T. hominis*,
3. *T. vaginalis*

These flagellates exist **only in trophozoite stage**. Cystic stage is absent. They have four anterior flagella and one lateral flagellum, which is attached to the surface of the parasite to form undulating membrane. The undulating membrane is supported at the base by a rod-like structure known as costa. The axostyle runs down the middle of the body and ends in the pointed tail-like extremity. A round nucleus is located in the anterior portion.

TRICHOMONAS TENAX

It is a pyriform flagellate. It measures 5–12 µm in length and 5–10 µm in width (Fig. 56.5). It is a **harmless commensal of the human mouth**, living in the tartar around the teeth, in cavities of carious teeth, in necrotic mucosal cells in the gingival margins of gums and in pus pockets in tonsillar follicles. It is transmitted by kissing, salivary droplets and fomites.

Diagnosis can be made by demonstration of *T. tenax* in the tartar by microscopy. Better oral hygiene will rapidly eliminate the infection.

TRICHOMONAS HOMINIS

It is pyriform, measuring 5–14 µm in length and 7–10 µm in width (Fig. 56.5). **It inhabits the caecum of man and several other primate species** and feeds on enteric bacteria. It does not invade the intestinal mucosa. Though it has been occasionally found in the diarrhoeic stools, its pathogenicity is yet to be established.

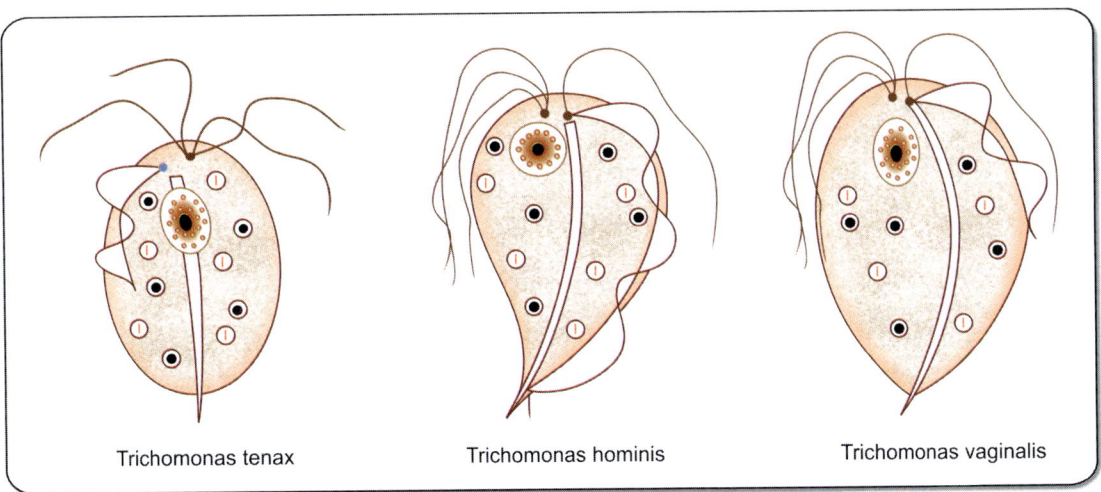

Trichomonas tenax Trichomonas hominis Trichomonas vaginalis

Fig. 56.5. Trophozoites of *Trichomonas* spp.

TRICHOMONAS VAGINALIS

Morphologically, it resembles *T. tenax* but it is larger than this. It measures 7–23 μm in length and 5–15 μm in width (Fig. 56.5). In a wet mount the trophozoite has a characteristic jerky motility. **The normal habitat of the parasite is the vagina and urethra of women and the urethra, seminal vesicles and prostate of man.** It may also be found in the Bartholin's glands and urinary bladder in female.

Pathogenicity

The parasite lives on the mucosa feeding on bacteria and leucocytes. *T. vaginalis* is an **obligate parasite**. It cannot live without close association with the vaginal, urethral or prostatic tissues.

The organism is responsible for a mild **vaginitis with discharge**. Vaginal discharge contains a large number of parasites and leucocytes and is liquid, greenish or yellow. Male patients usually have mild or asymptomatic infections. They may develop itching and discomfort inside penile urethra, especially during urination. The parasite is transmitted by sexual intercourse.

Laboratory diagnosis

The diagnosis can be made by demonstration of trophozoites of *T. vaginalis* in wet mounts of the sedimented urine, vaginal secretions or vaginal scrapings. In males it may be found in urine or prostatic secretions. Fixed smears may be stained with Papanicolaou (Fig. 56.6), Giemsa, Leishman and periodic acid-Schiff stain, and seen under light microscope.

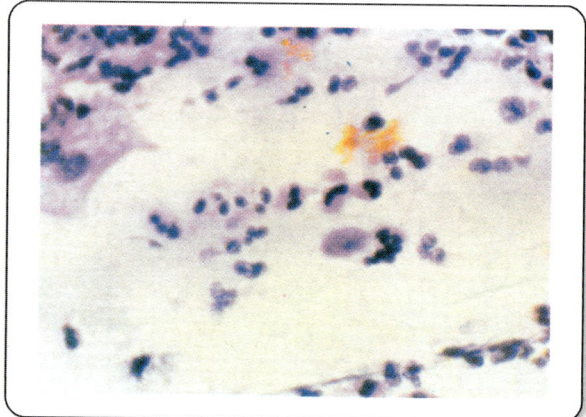

Fig. 56.6. Trophozoites of *Trichomonas vaginalis* in vaginal smear (Papanicolaou stain, ×400).

OLD WORLD LEISHMANIASIS

LEISHMANIA DONOVANI

Geographical distribution

L. donovani is endemic in Indian Subcontinent and East Africa.

Habitat

It is an **obligate intracellular parasite of reticuloendothelial cells**, predominantly of liver, spleen, bone marrow and lymph nodes of man and other vertebrate hosts (dog and hamster) where it occurs in amastigote form.

Morphology

The parasite exists in two morphological forms:

1. Amastigote
2. Promastigote.

Amastigote

In the amastigote form the parasite resides in the cells of reticuloendothelial system (macrophages, monocytes, polymorphonuclear leucocytes, or endothelial cells) of vertebrate hosts. It is non-motile, round or oval body measuring 2–4 μm in length along the longitudinal axis (Figs. 56.7 and 56.8). Cell membrane is delicate and can be demonstrated in fresh specimens only. Nucleus is round or oval, less than 1 μm in diameter. It is situated in the middle of the cell or along the side of the cell wall. Kinetoplast consists of parabasal body and blepharoplast, which are connected by one or more delicate fibrils. It lies tangentially or at right angle to the nucleus. The axoneme arises from the blepharoplast and extends to the margin of the body. It represents the intracellular portion of the flagellum. Alongside the axoneme lies a clear unstained space known as vacuole. In preparations stained with Giemsa or Wright stain, the cytoplasm appears pale blue, the nucleus red, parabasal body deep red and kinetoplast bright red.

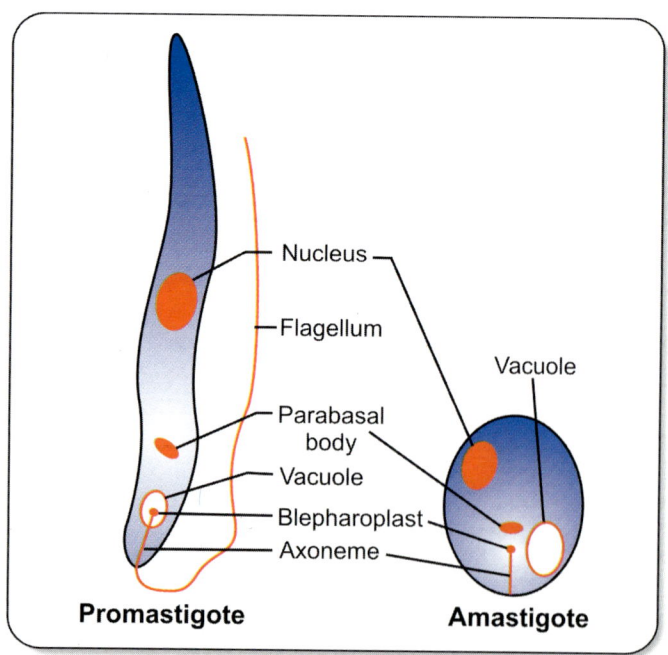

Promastigote   **Amastigote**

Fig. 56.7. Morphological forms of *Leishmania donovani*.

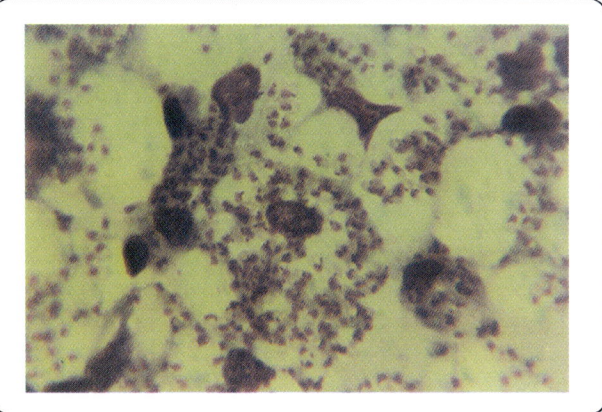

Fig. 56.8. Amastigote forms *of Leishmania donovani* in bone marrow (Giemsa stain, ×400).

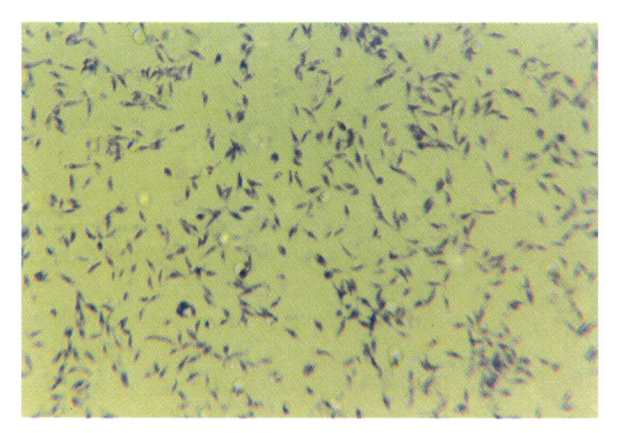

Fig. 56.9. Promastigote forms *of Leishmania donovani* in culture (Giemsa stain, ×400).

Promastigote

Promastigotes are found in **the digestive tract of insect vector (sandfly) and in the culture media**. These are elongated, motile, extracellular stage of the parasite. Fully developed promastigotes measure 15–25 μm in length and 1.5–3.5 μm in breadth. Nucleus is situated centrally. Kinetoplast lies transversely near the anterior end. In front of the kinetoplast lies a pale staining vacuole. From the blepharoplast arises the axoneme which projects from the anterior end of the parasite as free flagellum. Flagellum may be of the same length as the body of the parasite or longer. It does not curve round the body of the parasite, therefore, there is **no undulating membrane** (Fig. 56.7).

Cultivation

NNN medium

L. donovani can be cultured on N.N.N. medium which was first introduced by Novy and McNeal (1904), and later modified by Nicolle (1908). It consists of two parts of salt agar and one part of defibrinated rabbit blood. The tubed salt agar medium is melted and then cooled to 48° C. To each tube of medium one third of its volume of sterile defibrinated rabbit blood is added and mixed thoroughly by rotating the tubes. The tubes are slanted and allowed to cool preferably on ice, as more water of condensation is obtained.

Blood, aspirates, or small biopsy samples from spleen, liver, or bone marrow obtained aseptically are inoculated into water of condensation of the medium and incubated at 22°–25° C. The amastigote form changes into promastigote form which then multiplies rapidly by longitudinal fission to produce a large number of flagellates, particularly in the water of condensation at the bottom of the tube (Fig. 56.9).

Life cycle

L. donovani passes its life cycle in two hosts – man and also dog in some areas are the vertebrate hosts, and female sandfly of the genus *Phlebotomus* is the invertebrate host. Indian kala-azar is considered to be a non-zoonotic infection with man as the sole reservoir. Important sandfly hosts include *P. argentipes*, *P. orientalis* and *P. martini*. Of these *P. argentipes* is the Indian vector.

Cycle in sandfly

Amastigotes of the parasite are present in the blood stream of the patient, both free as well as phagocytosed by polymorphonuclear leucocytes and monocytes. These are taken up by the sandfly in a blood meal and reach midgut of the insect. Here the parasite transforms into promastigotes and multiplies producing enormous numbers. The parasites then proceed forwards to the pharynx and buccal cavity, which they block between the 6th and 9th day of its infective blood meal.

Cycle in man

Because of the blockage of pharynx and buccal cavity, the sandfly has difficulty in getting a blood meal, nevertheless, it pricks the skin of the victim and regurgitates the promastigotes in the wound caused by its proboscis. These are engulfed by nearby fixed macrophages and change into amastigotes within the cytoplasm of these host cells. Here the amastigotes multiply slowly and may remain more or less quiescent for weeks or months. Thereafter, parasitized macrophages are set free into the blood stream and are carried from the skin to spleen, liver, bone marrow, and other centres of reticuloendothelial activity. The amastigotes are now taken up by fixed macrophages such as Kupffer's cells in the liver, and multiply by simple binary fission till the cells become packed with the parasites (50–200 or more in the cytoplasm of the infected cell).

The infected cell ruptures and the parasites are liberated into the circulation. These are taken up by other reticuloendothelial cells followed by multiplication of the parasites and rupture of the cells. In this way the entire reticuloendothelial system becomes progressively infected. In the blood stream, some of the free amastigotes are phagocytosed by polymorphonuclear leucocytes and monocytes. A blood-sucking insect draws these free amastigotes, as well as those within the cells during its blood meal and the cycle is repeated.

Pathogenicity

L. donovani causes visceral leishmaniasis or kala-azar (*kala* meaning black and *azar* meaning disease), Dum Dum fever or tropical splenomegaly. In India, kala-azar has been known to occur in well defined areas in the eastern parts of the country mainly in Bihar, West Bengal, eastern districts of Uttar Pradesh, Assam, foothills of Sikkim, and to a lesser extent in Tamilnadu and Orissa.

Incubation period generally varies from 3–6 months, but it may be as short as 10 days or as long as 2 years. The parasite spreads from the site of inoculation to multiply in reticuloendothelial cells, especially in the spleen, liver, lymph nodes, and bone marrow. This leads to progressive enlargement of these organs. The host cellular and humoral defence mechanisms are stimulated. The former results in marked proliferation of macrophages. These cellular elements make up a large part of the bone marrow, compromising both the erythropoietic and granulocytic activity. The effect of this in the peripheral blood is leucopenia with granulocytopenia and relative monocytosis, anaemia (usually normocytic) and thrombocytopenia.

The spleen and liver become markedly enlarged, and hypersplenism contributes to the production of anaemia. It has been suggested that the erythrocytes adsorb immune complexes and become subject to enhanced phagocytosis by the macrophages of the liver and spleen. Lymphadenopathy is also produced. Production of globulin is greatly increased. This leads to reversal of the albumin: globulin ratio.

The disease is **reticuloendotheliosis** due to invasion of reticuloendothelial cells by *L. donovani*. Reticuloendothelial cells of various organs are proliferated and are packed with amastigote forms of the parasite. The disease manifests clinically with fever, malaise, headache, progressive enlargement of spleen, liver, and lymph nodes, anaemia, leucopenia and emaciation. Skin changes are often seen on the face, hands, feet, and abdomen, particularly in India, where patients acquire an earth-gray colour. If left untreated 75–95% patients die within 2 years. **Death in kala-azar is due to secondary infections.**

Visceral leishmaniasis and human immunodeficiency virus (HIV) together are synergistic infections because visceral leishmaniasis accelerates the development of acquired immunodeficiency syndrome (AIDS) and the presence of HIV infection enhances the spread of visceral disease. HIV may either activate subclinical leishmaniasis or make the patient susceptible to a new infection. *Visceral leishmaniasis has emerged as one of the most important opportunistic infections in HIV-infected patients.*

Immunity

In contrast to cutaneous leishmaniasis, cell-mediated immunity is impaired in active kala-azar patients, who consequently lack a delayed type hypersensitivity response, but this can be demonstrated after cure.

Laboratory diagnosis

Various tests which can be carried out for the laboratory diagnosis of kala-azar are given in Flowchart 56.1.

Flowchart 56.1. Laboratory diagnosis of Kala-azar

Non-specific tests
- Blood count- (pancytopenia mainly neutropenia and decreased erythrocyte count
- Haemoglobin estimation (anaemia)
- Estimation of serum proteins (raised serum proteins with reversal of albumin:globulin ratio due to greatly increased IgG level)

Parasitological diagnosis
- Peripheral blood film by thick film method (amastigote form)
- Blood culture in N.N.N. medium (promastigote form)
- Needle biopsy/aspiration

  Lymph node   Bone marrow   Liver   Spleen

- By touch preparation or smear stained with Giemsa stain (amastigote form)
- Culture in N.N.N. medium (promastigote form)
- Molecular methods
  – DNA probes
  – Polymerase chain reaction
- Animal inoculation

Immunological test

Non-specific tests
- Aldehyde test / Antimony test (Indicate greatly increased serum proteins)
- Complement fixation test with W.K.K. antigen

Specific tests
- Direct agglutination test
- Indirect haemagglutination test
- Indirect fluorescent antibody test
- Enzyme-linked immunosorbent assay
- Leishmanin or Montenegro skin test

Non-specific tests

These include:

1. **Blood count:** Total and differential leucocyte count reveals pancytopenia, mainly neutropenia and decreased erythrocyte count. The average total count of leucocytes is 3,000/μl of blood. During the course of the disease, the count may fall to 1,000/μl of blood or even below. Erythrocytes are also decreased in number.
2. **Haemoglobin estimation:** It reveals anaemia.
3. **Estimation of serum proteins:** It reveals raised serum proteins with reversal of the albumin: globulin ratio due to greatly raised IgG levels.

Parasitological diagnosis

Diagnosis of leishmaniasis can be confirmed by:

1. Peripheral blood film

Amastigote form of the parasite may be demonstrated inside circulating monocytes and less often in neutrophils, in the stained peripheral blood film by thick film method. Owing to the small number of *Leishmania* parasites present in the peripheral blood, an examination of a thin film is often negative.

2. Needle biopsy/aspiration

Deeper tissues, e.g., lymph node, bone marrow, liver and spleen may be sampled by needle biopsy/aspiration. Amastigote forms of the parasite can be demonstrated, within reticuloendothelial cells, in touch preparations or smears stained with Giemsa stain. Spleen aspirate is the most reliable material for demonstrating parasites in kala-azar. However, bleeding might continue from the puncture wound in the soft and enlarged spleen, resulting in death. Therefore, spleen puncture should not be performed in a patient with haemorrhagic diathesis and leukaemia.

3. Culture

Whatever material is collected (blood and biopsy/aspiration material from various organs), it should be inoculated into the water of condensation of NNN medium and incubated at 22°–25° C and examined microscopically twice a week for first 2 weeks and once a week thereafter for up to 4 weeks before they are reported as negative. Promastigote stages can be detected microscopically in wet mounts taken from centrifuged culture fluid. The material can also be stained with Giemsa stain to facilitate observation at a higher magnification.

4. Molecular methods

A number of molecular methods have been developed for species identification of the promastigotes, including the use of DNA probes and polymerase chain reaction.

5. Animal inoculation

Aspirate or biopsy material obtained from lymph node, spleen, liver, bone marrow, etc. is inoculated intraperitoneally in young hamster 2–4 months old. The infection in hamsters develops slowly and may take several months to produce detectable infection. Splenic aspirate is collected. Smear of splenic aspirate, and impression smear of spleen are stained with Giemsa stain and examined under microscope for amastigote forms of *Leishmania donovani*.

Immunological tests

These include non-specific and specific tests:

1. Non-specific tests

- Aldehyde test
- Antimony test
- Complement fixation test with W.K.K. antigen

1. **Aldehyde test:** A drop of full strength (40%) formalin is added to 1 ml of serum. A positive test is indicated by the rapid and complete coagulation of the serum. This serum test merely indicates greatly increased serum gamma globulin, and thus is non-specific. This test is not positive till the disease is of at least three months duration. This test has also been found to be positive in infections with *Schistosoma japonicum* and *Trypanosoma brucei gambiense*, multiple myeloma and cirrhosis liver.
2. **Antimony test:** This test also depends upon a rise of serum gamma globulin. When a 4% urea stibamine solution in distilled water is mixed with serum from a patient with kala-azar, it leads to the formation of a profuse flocculent precipitate. It is less reliable than aldehyde test.
3. **Complement fixation test with W.K.K. antigen:** Complement fixation test may be carried out for detection of serum antibodies in visceral leishmaniasis. The antigen originally used was prepared from human tubercle bacillus by Witebsky, Kleingenstein and Kuhn hence known as W.K.K. antigen. Since the antigen is not prepared from *L. donovani*, therefore, this test is non-specific.

2. Specific tests

Complement fixation test with W.K.K. antigen has been replaced with more specific tests such as indirect fluorescent antibody test (IFAT), indirect haemagglutination assay (IHA), and enzyme-linked immunosorbent assay (ELISA). These tests use the cultured promastigotes as antigen.

The direct agglutination test (DAT), using trypsin-treated Coomassie blue-stained promastigotes is a simple test for use in the diagnosis of kala-azar. This test detects specific IgM antibody at an early stage. It is useful in the detection of both clinical and subclinical infections.

Leishmanin or Montenegro test

It is a delayed hypersensitivity reaction to intradermal crude *Leishmania* antigen. It was first introduced in the South America by Montenegro. In this test, 0.2 ml of killed suspension of promastigotes of *L. donovani*, containing 6–10 million of the promastigotes per ml of 0.5% phenol saline, is injected intradermally. The test is read after 48–72 hours. A positive test shows an area of **erythema and induration 5 mm or more in diameter**. The test becomes positive 6–8 weeks after cure from kala-azar. Cell-mediated immunity is impaired in active kala-azar patients who consequently lack a delayed hypersensitivity response. Therefore, leishmanin test is negative in active cases of kala-azar. This test is of great value in epidemiological studies but is of little clinical use.

Diagnosis of visceral leishmaniasis in the presence of HIV infection is particularly difficult as the presentation may be very atypical and serological tests may be negative.

POST KALA-AZAR DERMAL LEISHMANIASIS

Post kala-azar dermal leishmaniasis (PKDL) was first described in patients with visceral leishmaniasis caused by *L. donovani* in India. It occurs in up to 20% of these patients. In India, skin lesions may appear 2–10 years after being partially treated, untreated or even those considered adequately treated for visceral leishmaniasis. In East Africa, lesions appear within a few months. It is caused by the reversal of *L. donovani* from viscerotropic to dermatotropic. It is not associated with *L. infantum* infection. PKDL is occasionally seen in patients with no history of visceral disease but only in places where *L. donovani* is transmitted, this is probably a sequel to subclinical infection.

Macules and papules usually appear first around the mouth and spread to the face and then to extensor surfaces of the arms, the trunk, and sometimes the legs. In the beginning they look like small hypopigmented patches; these then enlarge and may progress to nodules. The lesions are soft, painless, granulomatous of varying sizes and unless traumatized, do not ulcerate. When they are abundant, the clinical appearance may resemble that of lepromatous leprosy.

Laboratory diagnosis

Individuals with post kala-azar dermal leishmaniasis may be very important reservoirs for maintaining the infection in the population because of the high concentration of organisms in the skin.

Diagnosis of PKDL can be established by demonstration of amastigote form of *L. donovani* by a microscopical examination of Leishman-stained smear prepared from the biopsy material obtained from nodular lesions. Direct smear examination from the hypopigmented macules does not generally reveal any parasite.

LEISHMANIA TROPICA

Geographical distribution

The parasite is found in Central and Western Asia. In India, kala-azar is reported from eastern parts whereas *L. tropica* infection occurs in Central and Western India. It was first observed by Cunningham (1885) in Calcutta now Kolkata.

Habitat

It occurs inside reticuloendothelial cells (clasmatocytes) of the skin.

Morphology

The amastigote form occurs in man, whereas promastigote form is found in sandfly and in cultures. Morphologically, both these forms of *L. tropica* are indistinguishable from those of *L. donova*ni.

Cultivation

L. tropica, like *L. donovani*, can be cultured on N.N.N. medium.

Susceptible animal

As in case of *L. donovani*, hamster is susceptible to *L. tropica* infection.

Life cycle

The vertebrate host is man and invertebrate host is sandfly (*Phlebotomus sergenti*). The life cycle of *L. tropica*, in both vertebrate and invertebrate hosts, is similar to that of *L. donovani*, except that in man amastigote form of the former resides in the reticuloendothelial cells of skin and not in the viscera. One factor restricting the parasites causing cutaneous leishmaniasis to the skin may simply be temperature, to which some species of *Leishmania* are particularly sensitive.

Pathogenicity

L. tropica causes urban anthroponotic **cutaneous leishmaniasis** or **Oriental sore** or **Delhi boil**. Infection is transmitted to man either by direct inoculation of promastigotes of *L. tropica* through the bite of the sandfly or by crushing of the infected sandfly into the punctured wound caused by the bite. At the site of inoculation, promastigotes are phagocytosed by reticuloendothelial cells of the skin and are transformed into amastigotes.

A cutaneous lesion or **leishmanioma** develops at the site of infective sandfly bite. It is characterized by a chronic infective granuloma with fibrosis. In the early stage, the lesion is due to the proliferation of reticuloendothelial cells of skin that contain a large number of amastigotes. Later, round cell infiltration (lymphocytes and plasma cells) associated with a marked reduction in the number of parasites and development of a delayed hypersensitivity skin reaction (leishmanin reaction) occur.

Incubation period varies from a few weeks to 6 months and in some cases it may be 1–2 years. Clinically, the lesion begins as a raised papule about 2.5 cm in diameter. In majority of cases, it ulcerates. The ulcer has clean-cut margin with a raised indurated edge, surrounded by red areola. At this stage, the parasite is found along the red margin and not on the floor of the ulcer. The ulcer heals spontaneously, in about 6 months, leaving a depressed scar and a **solid immunity**.

There is a marked development of cell-mediated immunity but a weak antibody response, although specific antibodies can be detected. The cell-mediated immunity is responsible for a marked delayed type hypersensitivity response to leishmanin in active and cured cases. The sores are distributed on the exposed parts of the body, particularly on the face and extremities. The average number of sores is around two. **Oriental sore is not associated with systemic manifestations, although there may be enlargement of the draining lymph nodes.**

Laboratory diagnosis

Microscopy

Diagnosis of *L. tropica* infection is made by the microscopic examination of material obtained by puncture of the indurated edge of the sore and stained with Giemsa or Wright stain. Amastigote form of the parasite will be seen in large numbers inside the macrophages. Smears made by scraping the floor of the ulcer are often negative because amastigote-infected macrophages are destroyed in the presence of secondary bacterial infection. If smears are negative, biopsy from the margin of the ulcer at times provides specific proof of infection.

Culture

Isolation of promastigote of *L. tropica* may be made from the aspirates of the ulcer by culture in NNN medium. The specimen for culture is obtained by injecting a little volume of sterile physiological saline in the indurated margin of the ulcer and then aspirating it. A few drops of the aspirate are then inoculated into each medium.

Leishmanin skin test

Intradermal injection of leishmanin (killed promastigotes of *L. tropica* in 0.5% phenol saline) shows a marked delayed type hypersensitivity response.

NEW WORLD LEISHMANIASIS

LEISHMANIA BRAZILIENSIS COMPLEX AND LEISHMANIA MEXICANA COMPLEX

Geographical distribution

L. braziliensis complex and *L. mexicana* complex occur in tropical South America, and Central America respectively.

Habitat

These occur as intracellular parasites (amastigote form) inside the macrophages of the skin and mucous membrane of the nose and buccal cavity. These do not occur either in the internal organs or in the peripheral blood.

Morphology

These parasites are morphologically and culturally indistinguishable from other species of *Leishmania*.

Life cycle

The life cycle of *Leishmania* species causing the New World cutaneous and mucocutaneous leishmaniasis is similar to that of *L. donovani* and *L. tropica*, except that:

- amastigotes occur inside the macrophages of the skin and mucous membrane of the nose and buccal cavity but not in internal organs; and
- they are transmitted by sandflies of the genera *Lutzomyia* and *Psychodopygus*.

Pathogenicity

L. mexicana complex and *L. braziliensis* complex cause **chiclero's ulcer** and **espundia** respectively. These are zoonoses. The causative parasites are primarily those of wild animals. When the various sandfly vectors feed on humans these parasites may be transmitted. In this unnatural host they usually provoke an intense reaction and the eventual development of a skin lesion at the site of the bite. After about 7–10 days a tiny papule appears. In most cases it ulcerates, producing crater-like lesion with inflamed and elevated border.

The lesion may be single or multiple. The latter is due to the infected macrophages transporting the parasite to other parts of the body, thus establishing secondary lesion. *L. braziliensis* tends to produce such metastatic lesions in the nasal, pharyngeal and laryngeal mucosae. These lesions may appear within a few months of the original skin lesion, or years later when the patient appears to have been cured of his initial infection.

The pathology of skin lesion is similar to that of *L. tropica*. *L. mexicana* complex may also cause **'anergic diffuse cutaneous leishmaniasis' (ADCL)**. Histological examination of the skin and mucous lesion shows infiltration of lymphocytes, plasma cells and large mononuclear cells and necrosis of tissues. The parasites (amastigote forms) are found in large numbers inside the clasmatocytes and monocytes at the periphery of the lesion.

Laboratory diagnosis

Microscopy

The diagnosis is established by demonstration of amastigote forms of the parasites in the material obtained by puncture of the nodule or edge of the ulcer and stained with Giemsa or Wright stain.

Culture

L. mexicana complex and *L. braziliensis* complex can be isolated from clinical specimens by inoculation of NNN medium.

Animal inoculation

When inoculated into the skin of hamsters or mice *L. mexicana* complex causes large histiocytoma tumours containing abundant amastigotes, while *L. braziliensis* complex grows poorly in these animals.

Serology

- Antileishmanial antibodies may be detected in the patient serum by indirect fluorescent antibody (IFA) test using fixed amastigotes as antigens. It gives positive results in 89–95% of cases. IFA titre falls after successful chemotherapy.
- Enzyme-linked immunosorbent assay is also positive in 85% of cases.

Leishmanin or Montenegro skin test

This is positive in cutaneous and mucocutaneous leishmaniasis.

PLASMODIUM

Five species of *Plasmodium* are known to infect humans – *P. vivax*, *P. falciparum*, *P. malariae*, *P. ovale* and *P. knowlesi*. They cause the most important life-threatening protozoan disease called malaria.

Life cycle

Malaria parasites exhibit a complex life cycle (Figs. 56.10 and 56.11) involving alternating cycles of asexual division (schizogony) occurring in man (intermediate host) and sexual development (sporogony) occurring in female anopheles mosquito (definitive host). Therefore, **malaria parasites exhibit alternation of generations and alternation of hosts**.

Human cycle

The sporozoites are the infective form of the parasite. They are present in the salivary glands of female anopheles mosquito. Man gets infection by the bite of infected mosquito. The cycle in man comprises of following stages:

1. Primary exo-erythrocytic or pre-erythrocytic schizogony
2. Erythrocytic schizogony
3. Gametogony
4. Secondary exo-erythrocytic or dormant schizogony

1. Primary exo-erythrocytic or pre-erythrocytic schizogony

Within one hour all the **sporozoites** leave the blood stream and enter into liver parenchyma cells. The sporozoites which are elongated, spindle-shaped bodies become rounded inside the liver cells. They undergo a process of multiple nuclear division, followed by cytoplasmic division and develop into **schizont**. When primary exoerythrocytic schizogony is complete, the liver cell ruptures and releases merozoites into blood stream.

2. Erythrocytic schizogony

The **merozoites** liberated from primary exo-erythrocytic schizogony penetrate red blood cells where they multiply at the expense of the host cells. Here they pass through the stages of trophozoites, schizonts and merozoites (Table 56.4 and Figs. 56.10 and 56.11). Depending on the species about 6–24 nuclei are produced before cytoplasmic division occurs, and the red cell ruptures to release the individual merozoites, which then infect fresh red blood cells.

The parasitic multiplication during the erythrocytic phase is responsible for bringing on a clinical attack of malaria. Erythrocytic schizogony may be continued for a considerable period, but in the course of time the infection tends to die out. *P. falciparum* differs from the other forms of malaria parasites in that developing erythrocytic schizonts aggregate in the capillaries of the brain and other internal organs, so that only young ring forms are found in peripheral blood.

3. Gametogony

After malaria parasites have undergone erythrocytic schizogony for certain period, some merozoites develop within red cells into male and female gametocytes known as **microgametocytes** and **macrogametocytes**, respectively. They develop in the red blood cells of the capillaries of internal organs like spleen and bone marrow. Only mature gametocytes are found in the peripheral blood. They do not cause any febrile condition in human host. These are produced for the propagation and continuance of the species. The host carrying gametocytes is known as **carrier**. The microgametocytes of all the four species of *Plasmodium* are smaller in size, cytoplasm stains light blue and the nucleus (chromatin) is diffuse and large. On the other hand, the macrogametocytes are larger, the cytoplasm stains deep blue and the nucleus is compact and small (Table 56.4).

4. Secondary exo-erythrocytic or dormant schizogony

In case of *P. vivax* and *P. ovale*, some sporozoites on entering into hepatocytes enter into a resting (dormant) stage before undergoing asexual multiplication while others undergo multiplication without delay. The resting stage of the parasite is rounded, 4–6 μm in diameter, uninucleate and is known as **hypnozoite** or **sleeping form**. After a period of weeks, months or years (usually up to 2 years) hypnozoites are reactivated to become schizonts and release merozoites which infect red blood cells producing **relapse** of malaria. Hypnozoites are not formed in case of *P. falciparum* and *P. malariae*, therefore, relapses do not occur in disease caused by these species.

Mosquito (sexual) cycle

Sexual cycle actually starts in the human host itself by the formation of gametocytes which are present in the peripheral blood. Both asexual and sexual forms of the parasite are ingested by female anopheles mosquito during its blood meal from the patient. In the mosquito, only the mature sexual forms are capable of further development and rest die.

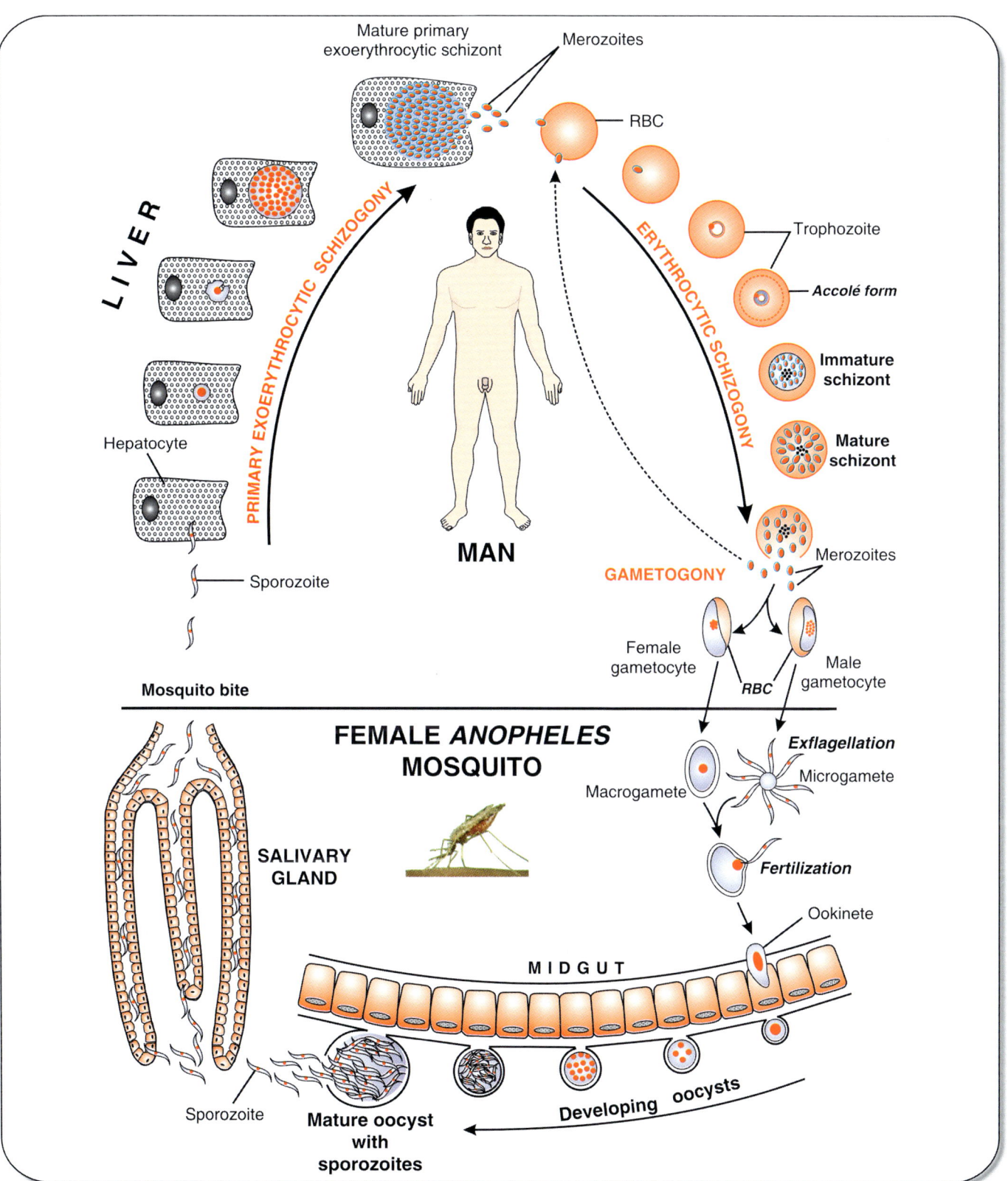

Fig. 56.10. Life cycle of malaria parasite.

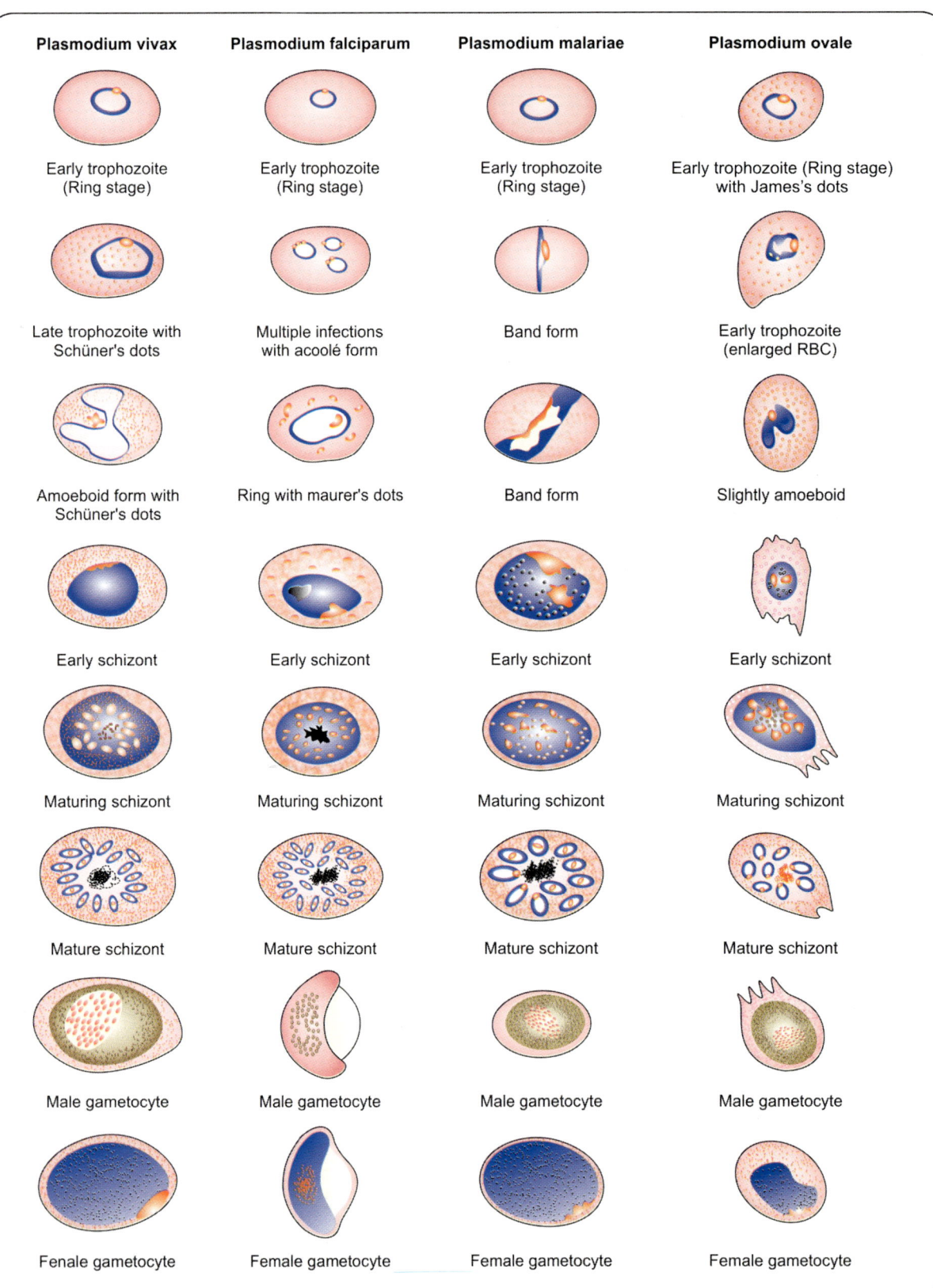

Fig. 56.11. Morphological forms of malaria parasites.

Table 56.4. Differential characters of erythrocytic phase of plasmodia of man

	P. vivax	P. falciparum	P. malariae	P. ovale
1. Forms in peripheral blood	Trophozoites, schizonts and gametocytes.	Rings and crescents (gametocytes).	Trophozoites, schizonts and gametocytes.	Trophozoites, schizonts and gametocytes.
2. Early trophozoite or ring stage	Large, 2.5 μm in diameter, usually one prominent chromatin dot, sometimes two, cytoplasm opposite the chromatin dot thicker, usually one and occasionally two rings in one red blood cell.	Small, delicate, 1.25–1.5 μm in diameter, often with two chromatin dots, two rings in one red blood cell are common. Some parasites lie along the red cell membrane. These are known as accolé forms.	Similar to that of P. vivax.	Similar to that of P. vivax.
3. Late trophozoite	Large, markedly amoeboid, prominent vacuole.	Medium-sized, compact and rounded.	Small, compact, band-shaped, slightly amoeboid, vacuole disappears early.	Slightly amoeboid.
4. Schizont	Large, 9–10 μm in diameter, almost fills an enlarged red cell.	Small, 4.5–5.0 μm in diameter, fills two-thirds of normal-sized red blood cell which is not enlarged.	Small, 6.5–7.0 μm in diameter, almost fills a normal-sized red blood cell.	Small, 6.2 μm in diameter, fills about three quarters of slightly enlarged red blood cell.
5. Number of merozoites	12–24.	14–32.	6–12.	6–12.
6. Microgametocytes	Spherical, 9–10 μm in diameter, compact, no vacuole, diffuse chromatin, cytoplasm stains light blue or reddish.	Crescent-shaped (banana-shaped), 8–10 μm × 2–3 μm, chromatin diffuse.	Similar to that of P. vivax but smaller.	Similar to that of P. vivax but smaller.
7. Macrogametocytes	Spherical, 10–12 μm in diameter, compact, larger than microgametocyte, compact chromatin, cytoplasm stains dark blue.	Crescent-shaped, longer and more slender, 10–12 μm × 2–3 μm, chromatin compact, cytoplasm stains dark blue.	Similar to that of P. vivax but smaller.	Similar to that of P. vivax but smaller.
8. Malaria pigment	Yellowish-brown; fine granules.	Dark brown; one or two solid blocks.	Dark brown coarse granules.	Dark yellowish-brown, coarser than those of P. vivax
9. Age of red blood cells invaded	Young.	All ages (young and old).	Old.	Young.
10. Alterations in infected red cell	Enlarged, pale and the portion of the cytoplasm not occupied by the parasite shows a dotted or stippled appearance, called Schüffner's dots. With Leishman stain they appear as fine pink granules.	Normal size and possesses 6–12 Maurer's dots which stain brick-red with Leishman stain.	Normal size and occasionally show fine stippling (Ziemann's dots) on prolonged staining.	Enlarged, pale, James's dots resembling Schüffner's dots appear early and infected cell may be oval.
11. Duration of erythrocytic schizogony	48 hours.	36–48 hours.	72 hours.	48 hours.
12. Presence of secondary exoerythrocytic cycle	Yes.	No.	No.	Yes.

In the stomach of the mosquito (Fig. 56.10) from one microgametocyte 5–8 thread-like filamentous structures called **microgametes** are formed by the process of exflagellation. The macrogametocyte does not show any exflagellation. It develops into a **macrogamete**, its nucleus shifts to the surface, where a projection is formed. **Fertilization** occurs when a microgamete penetrates this projection. The fertilized macrogamete is known as **zygote**. This occurs in 20 minutes to 2 hours. In next 24 hours, the zygote lengthens and matures into **ookinete**, a motile vermiculate stage. It penetrates the epithelial lining of the stomach of the mosquito and comes to lie between the external border of the epithelial cell and peritrophic membrane.

Here it develops into **oocyst**. It is rounded, 6–12 μm in diameter with a single vesicular nucleus. It increases in size from 6–60 μm in diameter. Inside this develop sporozoites. The number of sporozoites in each oocyst varies from a few hundreds to a few thousands and number of oocysts in the stomach wall varies from a few to more than a hundred. On about 10th day the oocyst is fully mature, ruptures and releases sporozoites in the body cavity of the mosquito. Through the body fluid the sporozoites are distributed to various organs of the body except the ovaries. They have special predilection for salivary glands and ultimately reach in maximum numbers in the salivary ducts. At this stage the mosquito is capable of transmitting infection to man.

Pathogenicity

Man develops infection by the bite of infected female anopheles mosquito. However, infection may also be transmitted by:

1. Transfusion of blood from a patient of malaria. This is known as **transfusion malaria**. Plasmodia can remain viable in refrigerated blood for up to 10 days.
2. Transmission of infection to foetus in utero through some placental defect. This is known as **congenital malaria**.
3. By the use of contaminated syringes particularly in drug addicts. This is known as **"mainline" malaria**.

The above conditions are also known as **trophozoite-induced malaria**. In this condition there is no primary and secondary exo-erythrocytic schizogony, incubation period is short and there is no relapse.

After an incubation period of 12 days for *P. falciparum*, 13–17 days for *P. vivax* and *P. ovale*, and 28–30 days for *P. malariae* patient develops malaria. The typical picture of malaria consists of febrile paroxysm, anaemia and splenomegaly.

Laboratory diagnosis

1. Microscopy

Diagnosis of malaria can be established by demonstration of malaria parasites in the blood. Thick and thin smears of the blood are prepared on the same or different slides. Blood is taken by pricking a finger or ear lobule before starting treatment with antimalarials. For preparation of thick smear take a large drop of blood on the slide. Spread it in an area of 1 cm square. Dehaemoglobinization of thick smear is done by keeping the slide in distilled water in Koplin's jar in vertical position for 5–10 minutes till the slide becomes white and then it is dried in air. Both thick and thin smears are stained with Leishman stain. The smears are then examined under oil-immersion lens.

The parasites are most abundant in peripheral blood late in the febrile paroxysm (a few hours after the height of paroxysm). Therefore, blood for smear should be collected at this period. All asexual erythrocytic stages, as well as gametocytes can be seen in peripheral blood in infection with *P. vivax*, *P. malariae* and *P. ovale*, but in *P. falciparum* infection, only the ring forms and crescent-shaped gametocytes can be seen. Late trophozoite and schizont stages of *P. falciparum* are usually confined to the internal organs and appear in peripheral blood only in severe or pernicious malaria.

The occurrence of **multiple rings** in an individual red blood cell with **accolé forms** is diagnostic of *P. falciparum* infection. Malaria pigments may be demonstrated inside the monocytes and polymorphonuclear leucocytes. The presence of malaria pigments only, in the absence of malaria parasites, suggests *P. falciparum* infection. Schüffner's dots, in the red blood cells, can be seen in case of *P. vivax* infection, while Maurer's dots, Ziemann's dots and James's dots are seen in case of *P. falciparum*, *P. malariae* and *P. ovale* infection, respectively. Red blood cells are enlarged in *P. vivax* infection.

Thin film is examined first and if parasites are found, there is no need for examining the thick film. If parasites are not seen in thin film in a few minutes the thick film should be examined. If parasites are seen in thick film but identity is not clear, the thin film is re-examined more thoroughly to determine the identity of the species. **The parasites are more along the upper and lower margins of the "tail" of the film.** Examination of thin film usually takes 15–20 minutes (≥ 300 oil-immersion fields), and examination of thick film usually requires 5–10 minutes (approximately 100 oil-immersion fields), before the smears are considered negative.

2. Other techniques

Malaria parasites in the peripheral blood may also be identified by quantitative buffy coat test, detection of antigens in lysed blood and polymerase chain reaction.

PLASMODIUM KNOWLESI

A fifth species, *P. knowlesi*, which normally infects long-tailed macaques (*Macaca fascicularis*) and pig-tailed macaques (*Macaca nemestrina*), is a significant cause of human malaria in Southeast Asia. It is transmitted by *Anopheles leucosphyrus* group of mosquitoes that reside in the upper canopy of the forests and has infrequent contact with humans. Similar to *P.*

falciparum, the erythrocyte invasion by *P. knowlesi* is not restricted to young or old RBCs which allows the development of high levels of parasitemia. It has a short life cycle of 24 hours (quotidian), and the development of the parasite in RBCs is not synchronous. *P. knowlesi* infection is usually misidentified as *P. falciparum* or *P. malariae* because its early trophozoites resemble the ring forms of *P. falciparum* and the later stages mimic those of *P. malariae*. In contrast to *P. falciparum*, *P. knowlesi* does not appear to sequester in the microvasculature, and the neurologic complications seen with *P. falciparum* infection have not been described.

RBCs infected with *P. knowlesi* exhibit a normal morphology, and all developmental stages may be seen in peripheral blood.

P. knowlesi, similar to *P. falciparum* and *P. malariae*, does not appear to produce hypnozoites in the liver. Relapses from the liver are not known to occur.

Human *P. knowlesi* infections have been described in high numbers only in Malaysia; however, because of reports of infection in the neighbouring countries of Thailand, Singapore, Brunei, Indonesia, Myanmar, Vietnam and the Philippines, it appears that *P. knowlesi* is a natural parasite of macaques throughout the Southeast Asia region.

TOXOPLASMA GONDII

Habitat

T. gondii is an obligate intracellular parasite, which is found inside the reticuloendothelial cells and many other nucleated cells.

Morphology

Tachyzoites (intracellular trophozoites or proliferative forms), tissue cysts and oocysts are important stages seen during the life cycle of the parasite (Figs. 56.12–56.14). All these stages are infectious to man.

Tachyzoite

It is crescent-shaped with a pointed anterior and a rounded posterior end. It measures 6 µm in length and 2 µm in breadth. The nucleus is spherical or rounded, and is usually situated towards the central area of the cell (Figs. 56.12 and 56.14).

Tachyzoite is the rapidly multiplying form seen during the acute stage of infection. It enters the host cell by active penetration of the host cell membrane. After entering the host cell the tachyzoite assumes an oval shape and becomes surrounded by a parasitophorous vacuole. It multiplies asexually within the host cell by repeated endodyogeny or internal budding, two daughter tachyzoites being formed within the parent cell. When the host cell becomes distended with the parasites it disintegrates releasing the trophozoites which infect other cells. Groups of proliferating tachyzoites within a host cell are known as **pseudocyst**.

Tissue cyst

Tissue cysts occur in chronic infection. These are formed when the parasites multiply and produce a wall within a host cell.

Oocyst

This stage is present in cat and other felines and not in humans. It is oval or spherical, 10–12 µm in diameter and contains a sporoblast.

Cultivation

T. gondii can be cultured in laboratory animals, chick embryos and cell cultures. Mice, hamsters, guinea pigs and rabbits are all susceptible, but mice are generally used as hosts because they are more susceptible. After intraperitoneal inoculation

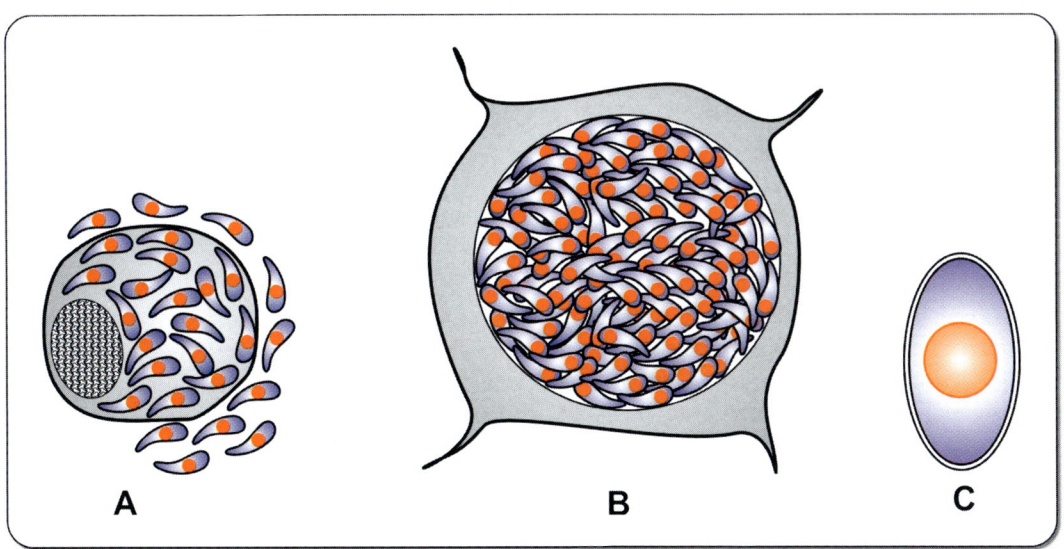

Fig. 56.12. Tachyzoites seen within and outside a cell (A), tissue cyst (B), and oocyst (C) of *Toxoplasma gondii*.

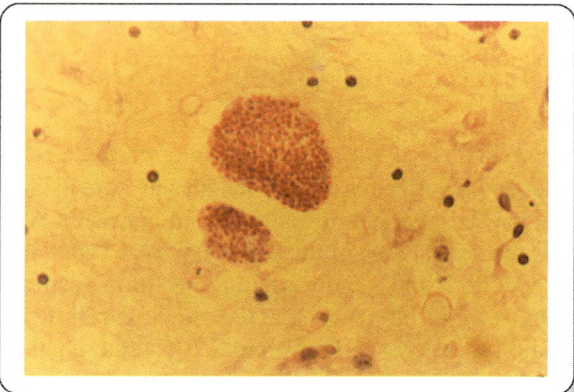

Fig. 56.13. Tissue cysts of *Toxoplasma gondii* in the brain (PAS stain, ×400).

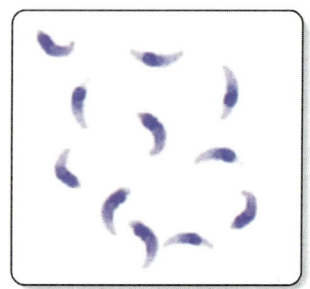

Fig. 56.14. *Toxoplasma gondii* tachyzoites, stained with Giemsa stain (×400), from a smear of peritoneal fluid obtained from a mouse inoculated with *T. gondii*.

of any of the three infectious stages, i.e., tachyzoites, bradyzoites and oocysts of *T. gondii*, some strains grow in the peritoneal cavity producing ascites, and tissue cysts are prominent in the brain after eight weeks. Virulent strains usually produce illness in mice and sometimes kill them within 1–2 weeks. *T. gondii* tachyzoites multiply in many cell lines in cell culture.

Life cycle

T. gondii has two types of life cycle (Fig. 56.15):

1. Enteric cycle.
2. Exoenteric cycle.

Enteric cycle

Enteric cycle occurs in domestic cat and other felines which are definitive hosts. It includes both asexual multiplication (schizogony) and sexual reproduction (gametogony) within the mucosal epithelial cells of the small intestine. Cat acquires infection by ingestion of any of the three infectious stages of *T. gondii*, i.e., tachyzoites and bradyzoites from tissue cysts in the flesh of other animals (mostly rodents), and sporozoites from oocysts in cat faeces. These invade mucosal cells of cat's small intestine in which they undergo several cycles of asexual generation before the sexual cycle begins with the

formation of male and female gametocytes which gives rise to male and female gametes respectively.

After sexual fusion (fertilization) of male and female gametes, oocysts develop, exit from host cell into the gut lumen, and pass out in the faeces. Freshly passed oocyst contains a sporoblast and is not infectious. It becomes infectious only after development in soil for 3–4 days. During this time, the sporoblast divides into two. These then become sporocysts by acquiring a cyst wall. Four sporozoites develop inside each sporocyst. The mature oocyst containing eight sporozoites is the infective form of the parasite. It can remain infective in the moist soil for about one year. When ingested, it can either repeat its cycle in a cat or if ingested by rodent or other mammal, including humans or certain birds, can establish an infection in which it reproduces asexually.

Exoenteric cycle

Exoenteric cycle occurs in humans, mice, rats, sheep, cattle, pigs, and certain birds, which are the intermediate hosts. Man acquires infection by:

- ingestion of food and drinks contaminated with cat's faeces containing sporulated oocysts, and
- ingestion of undercooked meat (mutton, pork and rarely beef) containing tissue cysts. In the duodenum the oocysts release sporozoites, and tissue cysts release bradyzoites.

These pass through the gut wall, circulate in the body, and invade various cells, especially macrophages, where they form tachyzoites, multiply, break out and spread the infection to other organs. Subsequently, they enter into the neural and muscular tissues, such as the brain, eye, and skeletal and cardiac muscles, where they multiply slowly (as bradyzoites) to form tissue cysts, initiating chronic stage of the disease. Tissue cysts may also develop in other organs such as lungs, liver and kidneys. Tissue cysts, when ingested by both definitive and intermediate hosts, are infective. Human infection may also be acquired by:

- organ transplantation or blood transfusion,
- transplacental transmission, and
- accidental inoculation of tachyzoites.

Maternal infection rate during the reproductive years is estimated to be between 3% and 5%.

Pathogenicity

T. gondii infection is widespread among humans and its prevalence varies from 16–80%. Most infections in humans are asymptomatic. However, fulminating fatal infections may develop in patients with congenital infections or in debilitated patients in whom underlying conditions may influence the final outcome of the infection. In immunocompromised patients, the infection most often involves the nervous system, with diffuse encephalopathy, meningoencephalitis, or cerebral mass lesions.

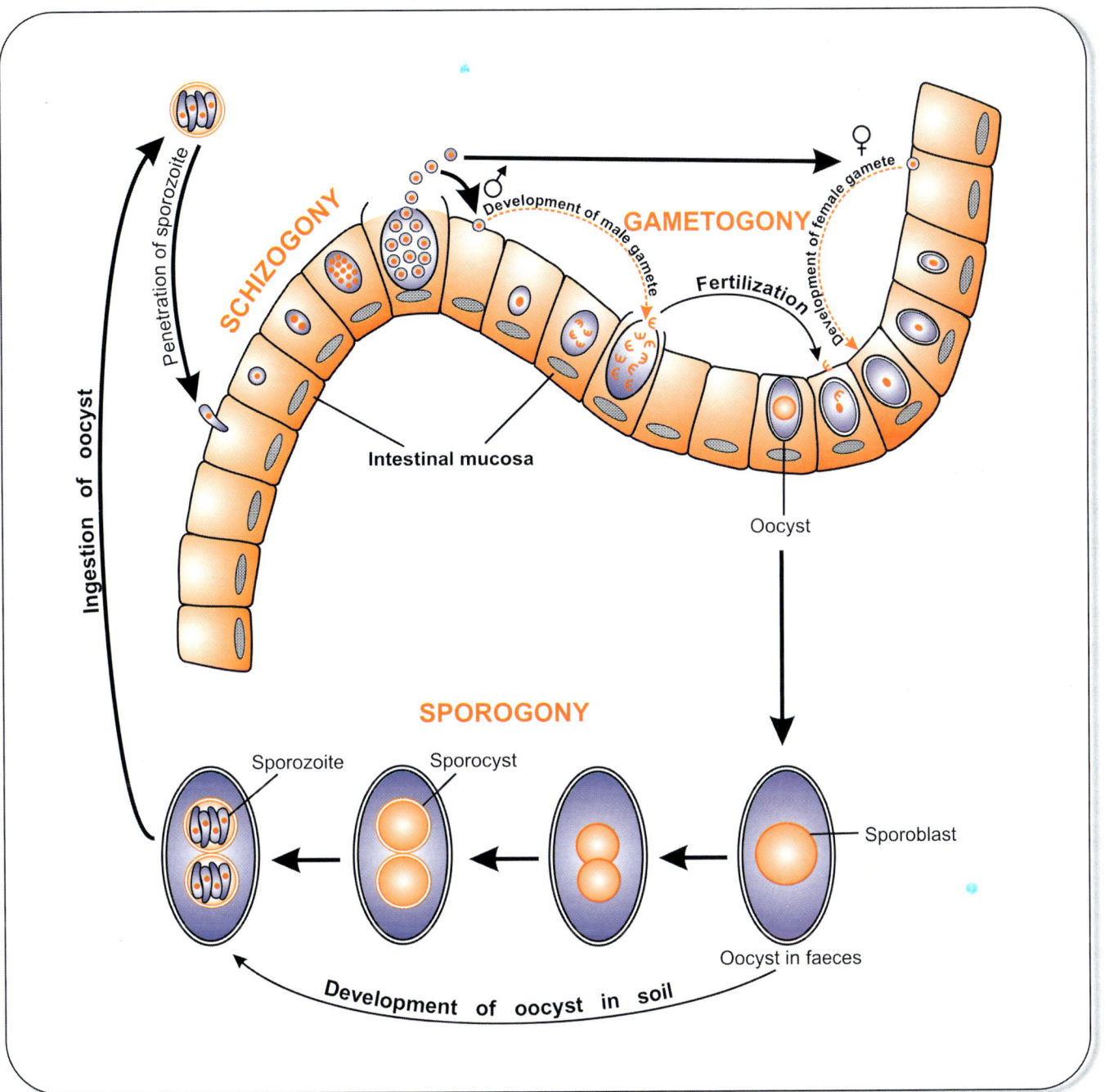

Fig. 56.15. Life cycle of *Toxoplasma gondii*.

Congenital infection

Congenital infection develops when mothers are infected during pregnancy. Although, the mother rarely has symptoms of infection, she does have a temporary parasitaemia. Focal lesions develop in the placenta and the foetus may become infected. In the foetus, there is generalized infection at first, but later it clears from visceral tissues and may localize in the central nervous system. Congenital infection leads to stillbirths, chorioretinitis, intracerebral calcification, psycho-

motor disturbances, and hydrocephaly or microcephaly. **Prenatal toxoplasmosis is a major cause of blindness and other congenital defects.**

Postnatally acquired infection

Postnatally acquired toxoplasmosis is much less severe than congenitally acquired disease. The commonest manifestation is lymphadenopathy. Although, any lymph node may be involved, the most frequently involved are the deep cervical lymph nodes. Lymphadenopathy may be associated with fever, malaise, headache, muscle pain, fatigue and sore throat. The illness is self-limited, though the lymphadenopathy may persist. Rarely there may be pneumonitis, myocarditis and meningoencephalitis, which may be fatal in some cases. Encephalitis is the most important manifestation of toxoplasmosis in immunosuppressed patients.

Laboratory diagnosis

Specimens

Blood (buffy coat of heparinized sample), sputum, bone marrow, cerebrospinal fluid and biopsy material from lymph node, spleen and brain.

Microscopic examination

Smears and sections stained with Giemsa or other special stains, such as periodic acid-Schiff may show the organisms. Tachyzoites of *T. gondii* in the smear are crescent-shaped and in sections round to oval (Figs. 56.12A, 56.13 and 56.14). Tissue cysts (Figs. 56.12B and 56.13) are usually spherical and lack septa, and the cyst wall stains with silver stains.

Animal inoculation

T. gondii can be isolated by intraperitoneal inoculation of body fluids or ground tissues into young laboratory mice that are free from infection. Peritoneal fluid and spleen smears may show the tachyzoites after 7–10 days.

Toxoplasma antigen detection

Toxoplasma antigen in blood or CSF may be demonstrated by ELISA.

Polymerase chain reaction (PCR)

Toxoplasmal DNA can be detected in the blood and CSF by PCR.

Serology

Serodiagnosis of toxoplasmosis is based primarily on detection of *Toxoplasma*-specific antibodies in the serum. Commonly used methods are as under:

1. **Sabin-Feldman dye test:** This test depends upon the appearance in 2–3 weeks of antibodies that render the membrane of laboratory-cultured living *T. gondii* impermeable to alkaline methylene blue, so that organisms are unstained in the presence of positive serum. Equal amounts (0.1 ml) of diluted patient serum (1 : 16, 1 : 64, 1 : 128 and 1 : 256 dilutions), live trophozoites of *T. gondii* obtained from the peritoneal exudates of infected mice and accessory factor (normal guinea pig serum as source of complement) are incubated for 1 hour at 37°C in a water bath. To each of the tubes is then added one drop of saturated alcoholic solution of methylene blue at pH 11. A drop of the mixture is then put on a slide, covered with a

cover slip and examined under high power lens of microscope. The number of tachyzoites with stained and unstained cytoplasm is counted. The highest dilution of the serum in which 50% or more of the tachyzoites have unstained cytoplasm is taken as the titre. It is one of the first methods used to diagnose toxoplasmosis. This highly sensitive and specific test is a complement-mediated neutralizing antigen-antibody reaction. It becomes positive within 1–2 weeks after infection. It remains positive at lower titres for years.

2. **Latex agglutination test:** It is a simple test. It shows 94.4% agreement with the dye test. The latex particles are coated with inactivated *T. gondii* soluble antigen. This test does not require heat inactivation of serum samples.

ISOSPORA BELLI

Morphology

Unsporulated oocysts of *I. belli* are ellipsoidal, measuring $20–33 \times 10–19$ μm (Fig. 56.16). Inside each oocyst develop two sporoblasts which later on convert into sporocysts. Each sporocyst is $9–14 \times 7–12$ μm and contains four crescent-shaped sporozoites. The oocyst is surrounded by a thin, smooth, two-layered cyst wall.

Life cycle

Man acquires infection by ingestion of food or water contaminated with sporulated oocysts from contaminated soil (Fig. 56.16). Eight sporozoites are released from two sporocysts in the upper small intestine and invade the epithelial cells of the distal duodenum and proximal jejunum and initiate schizogony. Upon rupture of the schizont, the merozoites are released, invade new epithelial cells, and continue the cycle of asexual multiplication. After a minimum of one week, the sexual stage (gametogony) begins with the development of micro- and macrogametes. Fertilization results in the development of oocysts that are excreted in the stool. Usually, the oocyst contains only one immature sporont, but two may be present. Continued development occurs in 3–4 days outside the body with the development of two mature sporocysts each containing four sporozoites. **The sporulated oocyst is the infective stage of the parasite.**

Pathogenicity

I. belli infects both immunocompetent and immunocompromised adults and children. Infection may be asymptomatic in immunocompetent individuals or it may lead to a mild, self-limiting diarrhoea lasting for 6 weeks to 6 months. Persistent non-bloody diarrhoea indistinguishable from that caused by microsporidia and *Cryptosporidium parvum*, is the major manifestation in immunocompromised individuals. Vomiting, headache, fever and malaise may also be present and dehydration follows when diarrhoea is severe. In AIDS patients, extra-intestinal infections can occur, though

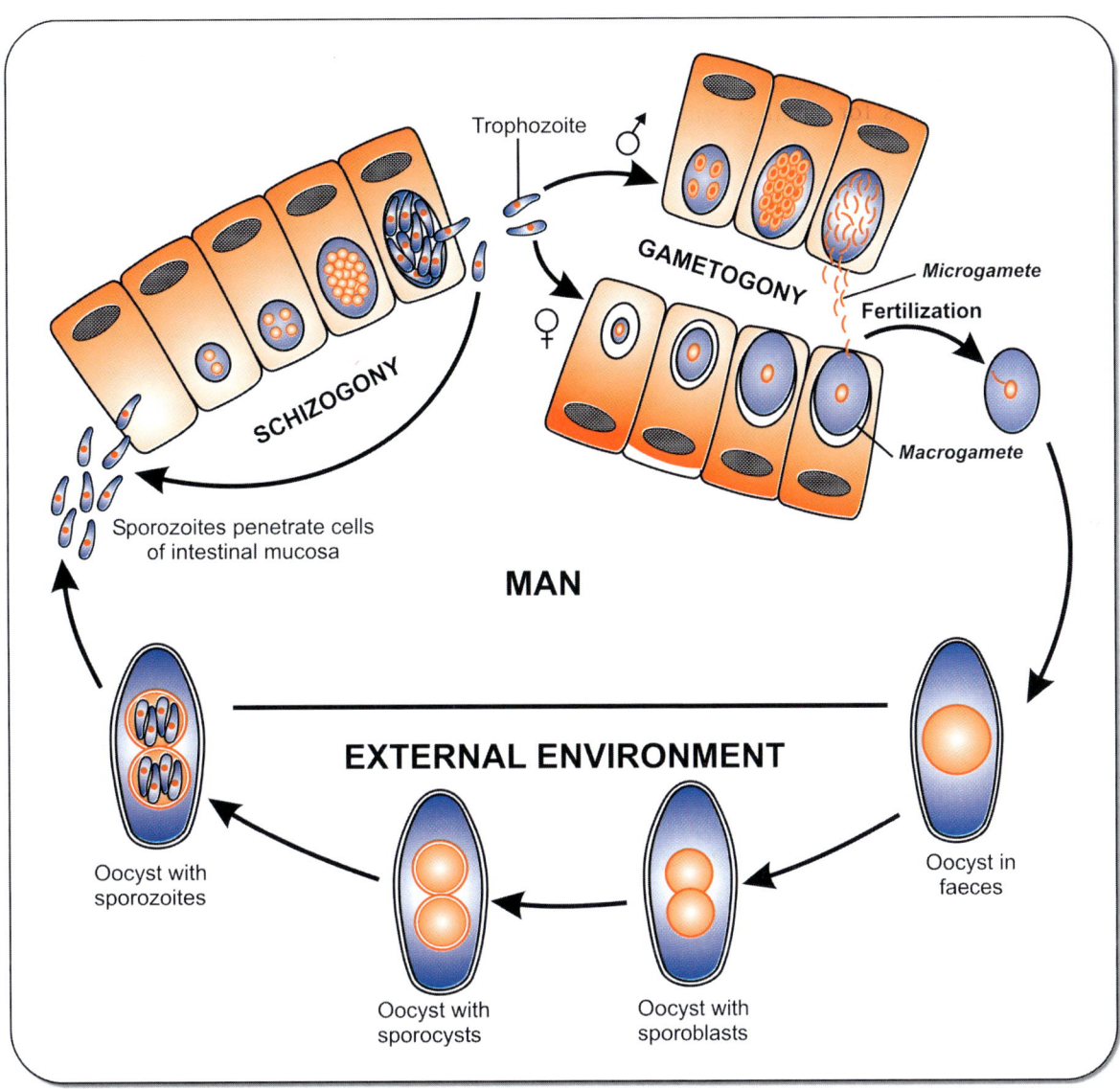

Fig. 56.16. Life cycle of *Isospora belli*.

they are rare. Necropsy, occasionally, reveals infection of mesenteric lymph nodes, liver, and spleen. Biliary disease has also been reported.

Laboratory diagnosis

Stool examination

Diagnosis can be established by:

- The demonstration of characteristic *I. belli* oocysts in the faeces by examination of unstained or iodine-stained direct smear preparations and by zinc sulphate centrifugal flotation as well as formalin-ether sedimentation methods.
- Oocysts can also be detected in faecal smears following acid-fast staining or staining with auramine-rhodamine. Oocysts tentatively identified by using auramine-rhodamine stains should be confirmed by wet smear examination or acid-fast stain, particularly if the stool contains other cells

or excess artifact material. With acid-fast stain oocysts appear red in colour.

Unstained oocysts are autofluorescent, appearing violet under ultraviolet light and green under green or blue-violet light.

Biopsy

- Various life cycle stages can be detected within the epithelial cells of intestinal mucosa obtained by biopsy. It is quite possible to have a positive biopsy specimen but not recover the oocysts in the stool because of the small number of organisms present. These organisms are acid-fast and can also be demonstrated by using auramine-rhodamine stains.
- Trophozoites of *I. belli* have also been reported to occur in tracheobronchial, mediastinal and mesenteric lymph nodes, gallbladder, liver and spleen in the AIDS patients.

Polymerase chain reaction (PCR)

A highly sensitive and specific method for diagnosis has employed PCR with primers for small-subunit rRNA sequences of *I. belli*.

CYCLOSPORA CAYETANENSIS

Morphology

Oocysts of *C. cayetanensis* are nonrefractile, spherical to oval, slightly wrinkled bodies (mulberry appearance) measuring 8–10 μm in diameter (almost twice the size of the oocysts of *Cryptosporidium* spp.). They contain two ovoid sporocysts, 4–6 μm in size. Each sporocyst contains two sporozoites. Thus, each sporulated oocyst contains four sporozoites.

Life cycle

Life cycle of *C. cayetanensis* is similar to that of *I. belli* in that oocysts are excreted unsporulated and require a period of time outside the host for maturation to occur. Man acquires infection by ingestion of food or water contaminated with sporulated oocysts from contaminated soil. In the intestine the oocyst releases sporozoites, which invade the enterocytes to form type I merozoites, and these form type II merozoites. The type II merozoites differentiate within the mucosal cells into sexual stages – the microgametes and macrogametes. The macrogamete is fertilized by the microgamete and produces a zygote. Unsporulated oocysts are then formed which are excreted in faeces. Sporulation occurs outside the body within approximately 7–13 days. The cycle is thus repeated.

Pathogenicity

It causes self-limiting diarrhoea, fever, fatigue, abdominal cramps lasting for 3–4 days and is associated with poor sanitation. As with other coccidian parasites, infection is more severe in immunocompromised patients, particularly with AIDS. In patients with AIDS, symptoms may persist for as long as 12 weeks. Biliary infection with accompanying symptoms has been observed in AIDS patients.

Laboratory diagnosis

Stool examination

Diagnosis can be made by microscopic detection of oocysts in stool:

- Oocysts may be detected by light microscopic examination of unstained faecal material (wet mount), where they appear as refractile, spherical to oval, slightly wrinkled bodies measuring 8–10 μm in diameter.
- Under ultraviolet illumination unstained oocysts of *C. cayetanensis* are autofluorescent, giving a rapid and inexpensive diagnostic method.
- Oocysts of *C. cayetanensis* are acid-fast and stain light pink to deep red in colour. Older cells may fail to stain.

- Oocysts stain orange red with safranin.
- They do not stain with iron-haematoxylin, Grocott-Gomori methenamine silver, iodine, or periodic acid-Schiff.
- *Cyclospora* oocysts may be excreted intermittently and in small numbers. Thus, a single negative specimen does not rule out the diagnosis. Three or more specimens at 2- or 3-day intervals may be required.
- Concentration procedures should be used to maximize recovery of oocysts. The method most familiar to laboratories is the formalin-ether sedimentation technique.

Jejunal biopsy

It reveals blunting of jejunal villi, villous atrophy, and crypt hyperplasia of varying degrees. Developmental stages resembling those of *I. belli* may be seen in jejunal enterocytes.

CRYPTOSPORIDIUM PARVUM

Morphology

The parasite released in the faeces is known as oocyst. It is colourless, spherical or oval and measures 4–5 μm in diameter. It contains four crescent-shaped naked or nonencysted sporozoites. Oocyst does not stain with iodine and is acid-fast (Fig. 56.17).

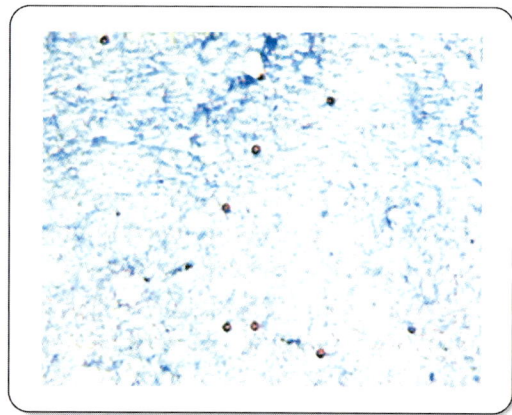

Fig. 56.17. Oocyst of *Cryptosporidium parvum* in faecal smear stained with modified acid-fast stain, ×400.

Life cycle

C. parvum undergoes both asexual (schizogony) and sexual (gametogony) multiplication in a single host (man, cattle, cat or dog). Man acquires infection by direct contact with infected animal or by ingestion of food or water contaminated with faeces containing oocysts of the parasite. After excysting from oocysts in the lumen of the intestine, sporozoites invade the epithelial cells, and undergo asexual and then sexual reproduction with the formation of oocysts (Fig. 56.18).

Pathogenicity

Humans become infected either from direct contact with

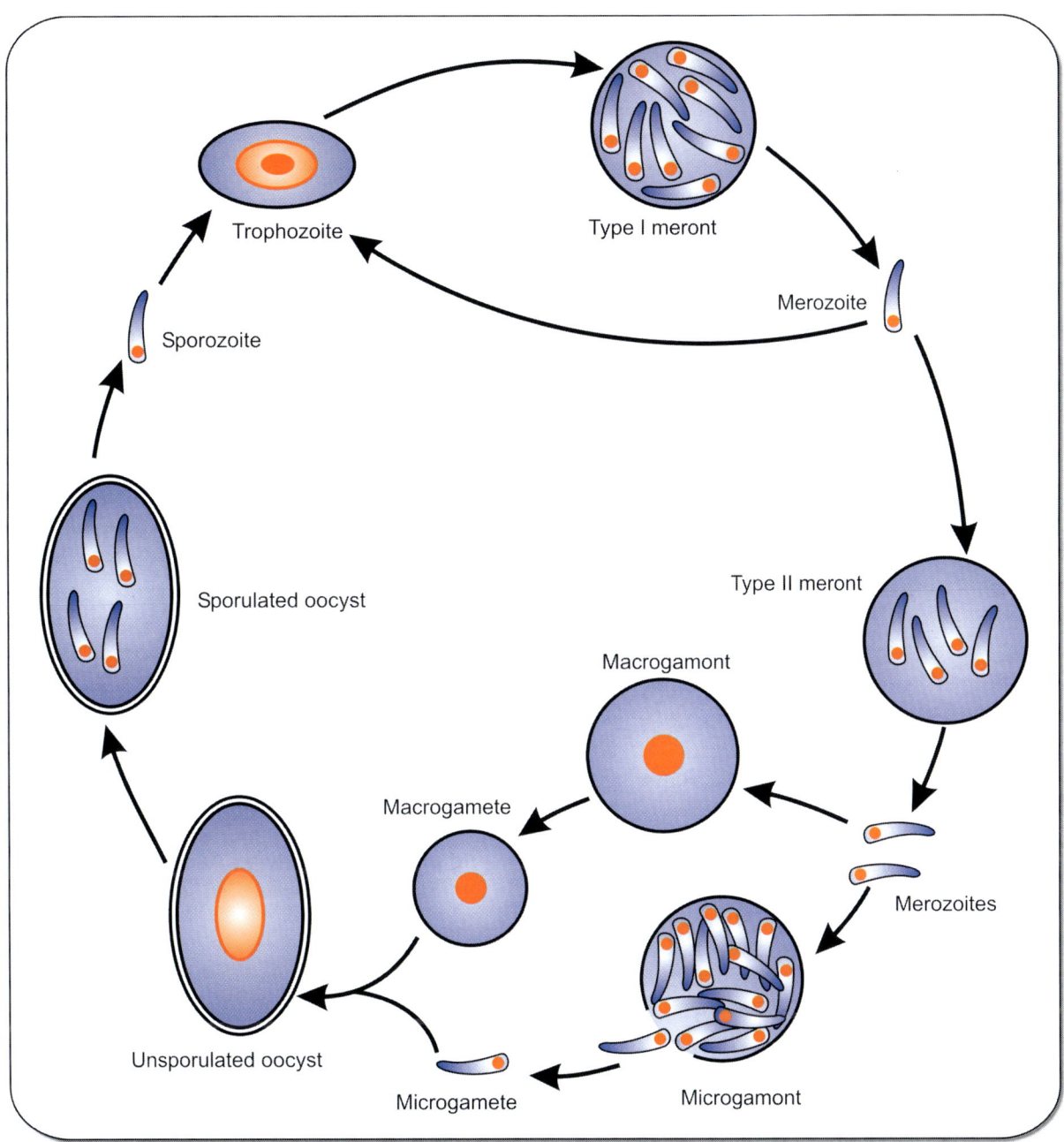

Fig. 56.18. Life cycle of *Cryptosporidium* spp.

infected animals or from ingestion of faecally contaminated food or water. People who are immunocompetent usually develop a short-term, self-limited diarrhoea lasting approximately 2 weeks. In contrast, those who are immunocompromised initially develop the same type of illness; however, it becomes more severe with time and results in a prolonged, life-threatening, cholera-like illness.

C. parvum infections are not always confined to the gastro-intestinal tract; additional symptoms (respiratory cryptosporidiosis, cholecystitis, hepatitis, and pancreatitis) have been associated with extraintestinal infections.

Laboratory diagnosis

Stool examination

For diagnosis, three consecutive specimens of stool should be examined. A direct wet mount of stool shows highly refractile, spherical or oval oocysts measuring 4–5 μm in diameter. Oocysts can be stained with modified acid-fast staining. By this method, oocysts appear bright red. Red stained oocysts can also be demonstrated in the sputum, bronchial washings and duodenal or jejunal aspirations by modified acid-fast staining methods.

Histopathological examination

Various life cycle stages of *C. parvum* can be detected in the microvillous region of intestinal mucosa obtained by biopsy. In haematoxylin and eosin-stained sections the parasites appear as small, spherical, basophilic bodies 1–3 μm in diameter. They are intracellular but extracytoplasmic and are found in parasitophorous vacuole in the microvillous region of epithelial cells of small intestine with jejunum being most heavily infected site.

Serodiagnosis

Antibodies specific to *C. parvum* can be detected by:

- IFA assays using endogenous stages of the parasite in tissue sections as antigens or intact oocysts as antigens.
- Specific anti-*Cryptosporidium* IgG or IgM or both may be detected by enzyme-linked immunosorbent assay using crude oocyst preparations as antigens.
- Cryptosporidial antigen in the faecal samples can be detected by ELISA.

Polymerase chain reaction (PCR)

PCR technology offers alternative to conventional diagnosis of *Cryptosporidium* in both clinical and environmental samples. Compared with microscopic examination by conventional acid-fast staining procedures, PCR is more sensitive and easier to interpret but requires more "hands on" time and expertise, as well as being more expensive. PCR has been used to detect *Cryptosporidium* DNA in fixed, paraffin-embedded tissue.

HELMINTHS

Medical helminthology deals with the study of helminths (parasitic worms). Most helminths are truly parasitic because they have no independent existence outside the host. Pathogenic manifestations of helminthic disease are due to the location of the worms, their size and life style. Helminths are divided into two major groups – nematodes or round worms and platyhelminths or flat worms. The latter are further divided into trematodes (flukes) and cestodes (tapeworms). Common helminths of man are given in Table 56.5.

ENTEROBIUS VERMICULARIS

Enterobius vermicularis infects children throughout the world. The adult worms live in caecum, vermiform appendix and adjacent portions of ascending colon.

Morphology

Adult worms

These are small, white, spindle-shaped and resemble short pieces of thread. At the anterior end, both male and female worms possess a pair of wing-like expansions, known as **cervical alae**. The male measures 2–4 mm in length and 0.1–

Table 56.5. Common helminths of man

Species	Common name
Nematodes	
• *Enterobius vermicularis*	Threadworm
• *Ascaris lumbricoides*	Common roundworm
• *Ancylostoma duodenale*	Old world hookworm
• *Necator americanus*	New world hookworm
• *Wuchereria bancrofti*	Bancroft's filaria
Cestodes	
• *Echinococcus granulosus*	Dog tapeworm
• *Taenia solium*	Pork tapeworm
• *Taenia saginata*	Beef tapeworm
Trematodes	
• *Schistosomes*	Blood flukes
• *Fasciola hepatica*	Sheep liver fluke
• *Fasciolopsis buski*	Large or giant intestinal fluke
• *Chlonorchis sinensis*	Chinese liver fluke
• *Paragonimus westermani*	Oriental lung fluke

0.2 mm in breadth. The posterior one third of the body is curved. The female is longer, 8–12 mm in length and 0.3–0.5 mm in width. Its posterior one third is straight and drawn out into a thin pointed pin-like tail (Fig. 56.19).

Eggs

The eggs are colourless, non-bile stained and flattened on one side (planoconvex). They measure 60 μm in length and 30 μm in width. They are surrounded by a transparent shell and usually contain fully developed larvae (Figs. 56.19 and 56.20). **They float in saturated solution of common salt.**

Life cycle

Of all the intestinal worms, it has the simplest life cycle (Fig. 56.19). It is completed in a **single host**. The adult worms live in caecum, appendix and adjacent portions of ascending colon. Male fertilizes female and dies, and is excreted in faeces. The gravid female migrates down the colon to the rectum. At night, when the host is in bed, it comes out of the anus. It then crawls on the perianal and perineal skin and deposits the eggs. Crawling of the gravid female worm leads to intense pruritis and the patient scratches the affected part.

Such patients have eggs of *E. vermicularis* on the fingers and under the nails. These individuals may develop auto-infection by direct anus-to-mouth transfer by finger contamination. Persons handling night clothes and bed linen of infected patients can also contract infection. Infection may also be acquired from contaminated objects like door knobs, table tops, etc. Airborne eggs that are dislodged from bed linens and clothes may get into mouth and swallowed.

The larvae, from embryonated eggs, hatch out in the small intestine. They then migrate to the caecum and vermiform appendix and develop into adult worms. Eggs laid on perianal

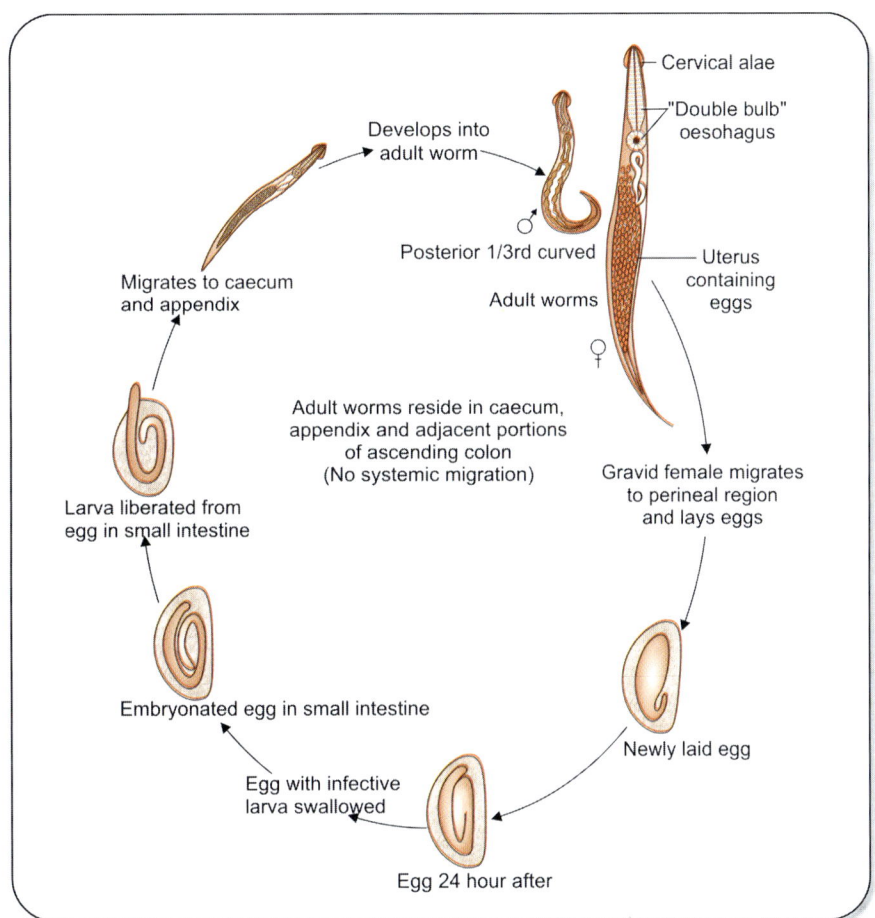

Fig. 56.19. Life cycle of *Enterobius vermicularis*.

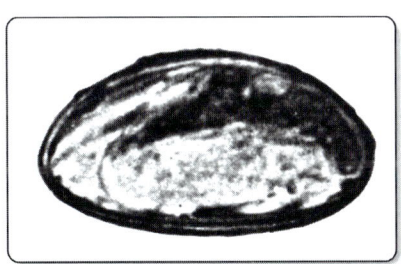

Fig. 56.20. Egg of *Enterobius vermicularis* (saline wet mount, ×400).

skin may immediately hatch into infective-stage larvae and may ascend through anus to develop into adolescent worms in the caecum and vermiform appendix.

After laying eggs on the perianal and perineal skin the worm may retreat into the anal canal and come out again to lay more eggs. The worm may also wander into the vulva, vagina, uterus, fallopian tubes and peritoneum.

Pathogenicity

It causes nocturnal perianal and perineal pruritis. It may also lead to appendicitis, vulvovaginitis and salpingitis.

Laboratory diagnosis

Detection of adult worms

The adult worms may be noticed by the patient or by the parents of the patient at the time of commencement of pruritis. They may be recovered in the stools after administration of a purgative or in the vermiform appendix during appendicectomy.

Demonstration of eggs

Since eggs are not discharged by the worm into faeces, therefore, faecal examination is not useful in the laboratory diagnosis of threadworm infection. However, in a small proportion of patients stool examination may show the presence of eggs of *E. vermicularis* (Fig. 56.20).

Eggs which are deposited in large numbers on the perianal and perineal skin at night can be demonstrated by scraping these areas with NIH (National Institute of Health) swab (Fig. 56.21) in the morning before the child goes to toilet and takes bath. NIH swab consists of a glass rod at one end of which a piece of transparent cellophane (with sticky surface out) is wrapped and held in place with a rubber band. The other end of the glass rod is fixed in a rubber stopper and kept in a test

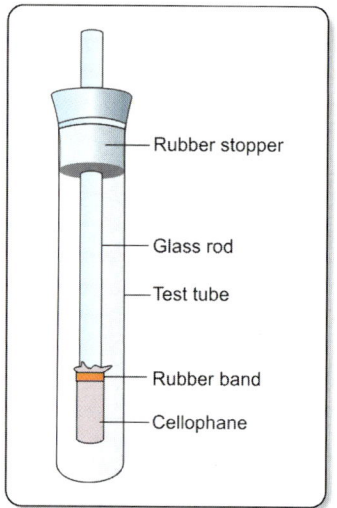

Fig. 56.21. NIH swab

tube. The cellophane part is used for swabbing by rolling over the perianal and perineal area. Then the cellophane is detached, spread over glass slide and examined microscopically. This procedure should be repeated on three successive days. Eggs may also be recovered from under the fingernails and the washings from garments.

ASCARIS LUMBRICOIDES

Morphology

Adult worm

It resembles an ordinary earthworm and is **the largest intestinal nematode parasitizing man**. It is elongated and cylindrical in shape with both ends tapering. The mouth opens at the anterior end. It possesses three finely toothed lips – one dorsal and two ventral. The digestive and respiratory organs of the worm float inside the body cavity possessing a **toxic fluid known as ascaron**. Allergic reactions seen in infected individuals are due to this toxin.

Male worm

It measures 15–30 cm in length and 3–4 mm in diameter. The posterior end is curved ventrally to form a hook. The ejaculatory duct along with the anus open into the cloaca from which arise a pair of copulatory spicules of equal size (Fig. 56.22).

Female worm

It is longer and stouter than the male worm and measure 25–40 cm in length and 5 mm in diameter. The tail is straight and conical. The anus is subterminal and opens on the ventral surface in the form of a transverse slit. The vulva opens at the junction of anterior and middle one third of the body on the midventral part of the worm. This part of the worm is narrow and is known as **vulvar waist** (Fig. 56.22). A mature female *A. lumbricoides* lays enormous number of eggs (nearly

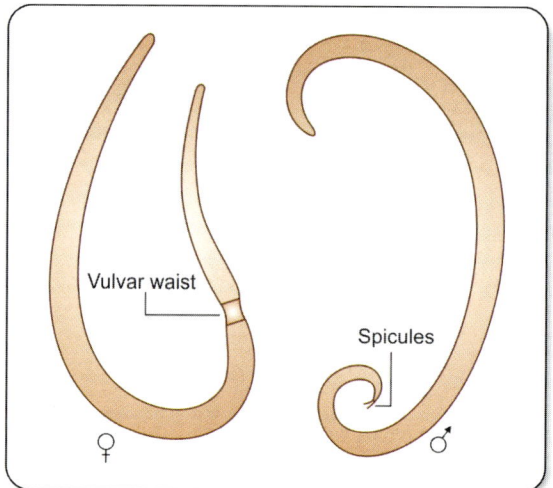

Fig. 56.22. Adult worms of *Ascaris lumbricoides*.

200,000 eggs daily) which are passed in the faeces. Eggs are of two types:

Fertilized eggs

The fertilized eggs are round or oval in shape and measure 60–75 µm in length and 40–50 µm in breadth (Fig. 56.23). They are bile-stained and brown in colour. They are surrounded by a thick, transparent shell, consisting of a relatively nonpermeable innermost lipoidal vitelline membrane, a thick transparent middle layer and an outermost coarsely mammillated albuminoid layer. Outer mammillated coat is sometimes lost. Such eggs are called **decorticated eggs**. They contain a large conspicuous unsegmented ovum with **a clear crescentic area at each pole. Fertilized eggs float in saturated solution of common salt.**

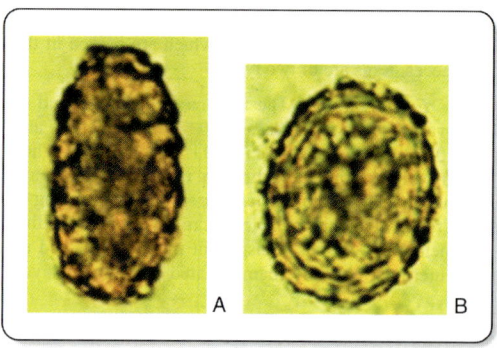

Fig. 56.23. Unfertilized (A) and fertilized (B) eggs of *Ascaris lumbricoides* (saline wet mount, ×400).

Unfertilized eggs

In the absence of a male worm, the female produces unfertilized (infertile) eggs. These are narrower and longer and measure 90 µm in length and 55 µm in breadth (Fig. 56.23). They are bile-stained and brown in colour. They have a small atrophied ovum and a thin shell within an irregular coating of albumin. The innermost lipoidal vitelline membrane of the shell is absent. The unfertilized eggs are heaviest of all the helminthic eggs, therefore, they **do not float in saturated solution of common salt**.

Life cycle (Fig. 56.24)

The life cycle of *A. lumbricoides* is passed **in only one host, man**. No intermediate host is required. Adult worms reside in the small intestine, particularly the jejunum of man. Fertilized eggs containing unsegmented ova are passed in the faeces. However, they are not immediately infective to man. They have to undergo a period of incubation in soil before acquiring infectivity. Depending on the temperature and humidity, a **rhabditiform larva** develops from the unsegmented ovum and undergoes first moulting within the egg shell in 10–40 days. The optimum temperature and humidity for the development of the larva within the egg shell is 20–40°C and more than 40%, respectively. **The embryonated eggs containing rhabditiform larvae are pathogenic to man.**

Man acquires infection by ingestion of food, water or raw vegetable contaminated with embryonated eggs. In the small intestine (duodenum) rhabditiform larvae are hatched out of the ingested eggs. These larvae then burrow their way through the mucous membrane of the small intestine and are carried by the portal circulation to the liver, where they reside for 3–4 days. They then pass via hepatic vein, inferior vena cava, right heart and pulmonary artery and reach the lungs. Here they grow in size and moult twice (first on 5th day and second on 10th day). The larvae then break through the capillary wall and reach the lung alveoli.

From the alveoli, the larvae migrate up the bronchi, trachea and larynx, crawl over the epiglottis to the pharynx and are swallowed. They pass down the oesophagus and stomach and

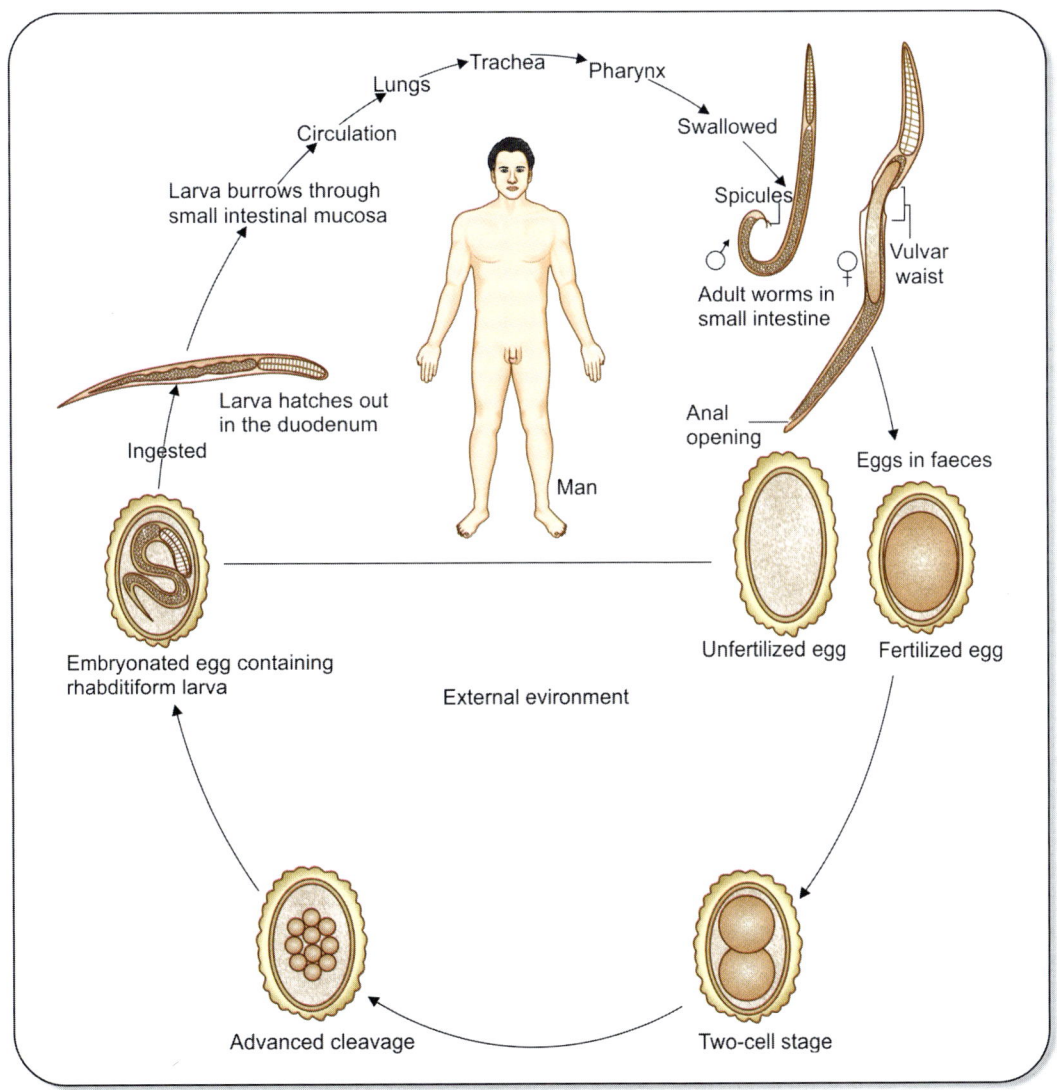

Fig. 56.24. Life cycle of *Ascaris lumbricoides*.

localize in the upper part of the small intestine, their normal abode. On twenty-fifth to twenty-ninth day of infection, the larvae undergo another moulting and transform into **adult worms**. In about 6–10 weeks they become sexually mature and by 12 weeks the gravid females begin to discharge eggs in the stool and the cycle is repeated.

Pathogenicity

Disease produced by *A. lumbricoides* is known as **ascariasis** and is caused by both adult worms and migrating larvae.

Pathogenicity of adult worms

1. By robbing the host of its nutrition, the adult worms affect the nutritional status of the host leading to **malnutrition and night blindness** due to vitamin A deficiency. The long-term effect of the malnutrition caused by ascariasis is **retardation of growth.**
2. The presence of adult worms in the intestine may also lead to intermittent colicky cramps and loss of appetite. In heavy infection, adult worms may cause **obstruction of the intestinal tract.**
3. **The worms are restless wanders.** They tend to probe and insinuate themselves into any aperture they find on the way. They may crawl out of mouth or may enter the nasal meatus via nasopharynx and pass out of a naris. From the oropharynx, the worm may enter a eustachian tube and penetrate to the middle ear and through the tympanic membrane to external auditory meatus. The worm may also enter into the trachea leading to **respiratory obstruction**. The worms may migrate downwards and lodge in appendix, bile duct and pancreatic duct leading to appendicitis, obstructive jaundice and acute haemorrhagic pancreatitis, respectively. They may perforate the intestinal wall weakened by ulcers or gangrene.
4. Release of toxic body fluid (ascaron) of the adult worm in the body of the patient may lead to various **allergic manifestations** such as fever, urticaria, angioneurotic oedema, wheezing and conjunctivitis.

Pathogenicity of migrating larvae

In persons repeatedly infected with *Ascaris* and sensitized to the parasite antigens, the migrating larvae may lead to inflammatory and hypersensitivity reactions in the lungs. There is formation of granuloma and eosinophilic infiltrates. It leads to fever, cough, dyspnoea, urticarial rash and eosinophilia. The sputum may be blood-tinged and may contain *Ascaris* larvae and Charcot-Leyden crystals. This condition is known as **Loeffler's syndrome.** Allergic inflammatory reaction to migrating larvae may involve other organs such as liver and kidneys.

Laboratory diagnosis

Parasitic diagnosis

Diagnosis of *A. lumbricoides* infection can be made by:

1. Demonstration of adult worms

Worm may be passed through anus, mouth, nose and rarely through ear. Barium meal may occasionally reveal the presence of adult worms in the small intestine.

2. Demonstration of larvae

Ascaris larvae may be detected in the sputum during the stage of migration.

3. Demonstration of both fertilized and unfertilized eggs

These may be detected by direct microscopy or concentration of the faeces by salt floatation or formol-ether sedimentation method. However, eggs may not be seen if only male worms are present.

ANCYLOSTOMA DUODENALE

Morphology

Adult worms

They are small, pinkish and fusiform in shape (Fig. 56.25). The anterior end is curved dorsally, hence the name hookworm. This curve is in the same direction as the general body curvature. The oral cavity is provided with four hook-like teeth on ventral surface and two knob-like teeth on dorsal surface (Fig. 56.26). The differences between male and female *A. duodenale* are given in Table 56.6. Owing to the position of genital openings of male and female worms they assume a Y-shaped figure during copulation.

Table 56.6. Differences between male and female *A. duodenale*

	Male	Female
Size	8 mm	12.5 mm
Posterior end	Expanded in an umbrella-like fashion. This is known as copulatory bursa.	Tapering
Genital opening	Opens posteriorly with cloaca.	Opens at the junction of posterior and middle third of the body.

Copulatory bursa

Copulatory bursa is present in the male worm for attachment with the female during copulation. This consists of three lobes. These lobes are supported by 13 chitinous rays, five each in lateral lobes and three in dorsal lobe (Fig. 56.26).

Eggs

Eggs are oval measuring 60 μm in length and 40 μm in width. They are colourless (not bile-stained) and are surrounded by a thin transparent hyaline shell. They possess a segmented ovum with usually four blastomeres. **There is a clear space between the segmented ovum and the egg shell** (Figs. 56.25 and 56.27). **The eggs float in saturated salt solution.**

Life cycle (Fig. 56.25)

Man is the only host. No intermediate host is required. Adult worms inhabit the small intestine of man attaching themselves to the mucous membrane by means of their mouthparts. The eggs containing segmented ova are passed out in the faeces of infected person. In the warm and moist soil, **rhabditiform larva** hatches out from the egg in 24–48 hours. The rhabditiform larva moults twice on the third and fifth day and develops into a **filariform larva**. This is capable of penetrating unbroken skin and is the **infective stage of the parasite**.

When a person walks barefooted on soil containing the filariform larvae they penetrate the skin, particularly the skin between the toes, the dorsum of the foot and the medial aspect of the sole. In farm workers the larvae may penetrate the skin of the hands. On reaching the subcutaneous tissue the larvae enter into the lymphatics or small venules and begin a migratory phase similar to that of *Ascaris*. Through lymph-vascular system they enter into venous circulation and are carried via the right heart into the pulmonary capillaries. Here they break through the capillary walls and enter into the alveolar spaces. From alveoli, the larvae migrate up the bronchi, trachea and larynx, crawl over the epiglottis to the pharynx and are swallowed.

During migration or on reaching oesophagus they undergo third moulting. Thereafter, they reach small intestine, undergo fourth moulting and develop into **adult worms**. They attach themselves to the mucous membrane of small intestine by means of their mouthparts. In about six weeks, from the time of infection, adult worms become sexually mature. Male fertilizes female and the latter lays eggs which are passed in faeces and the cycle is repeated.

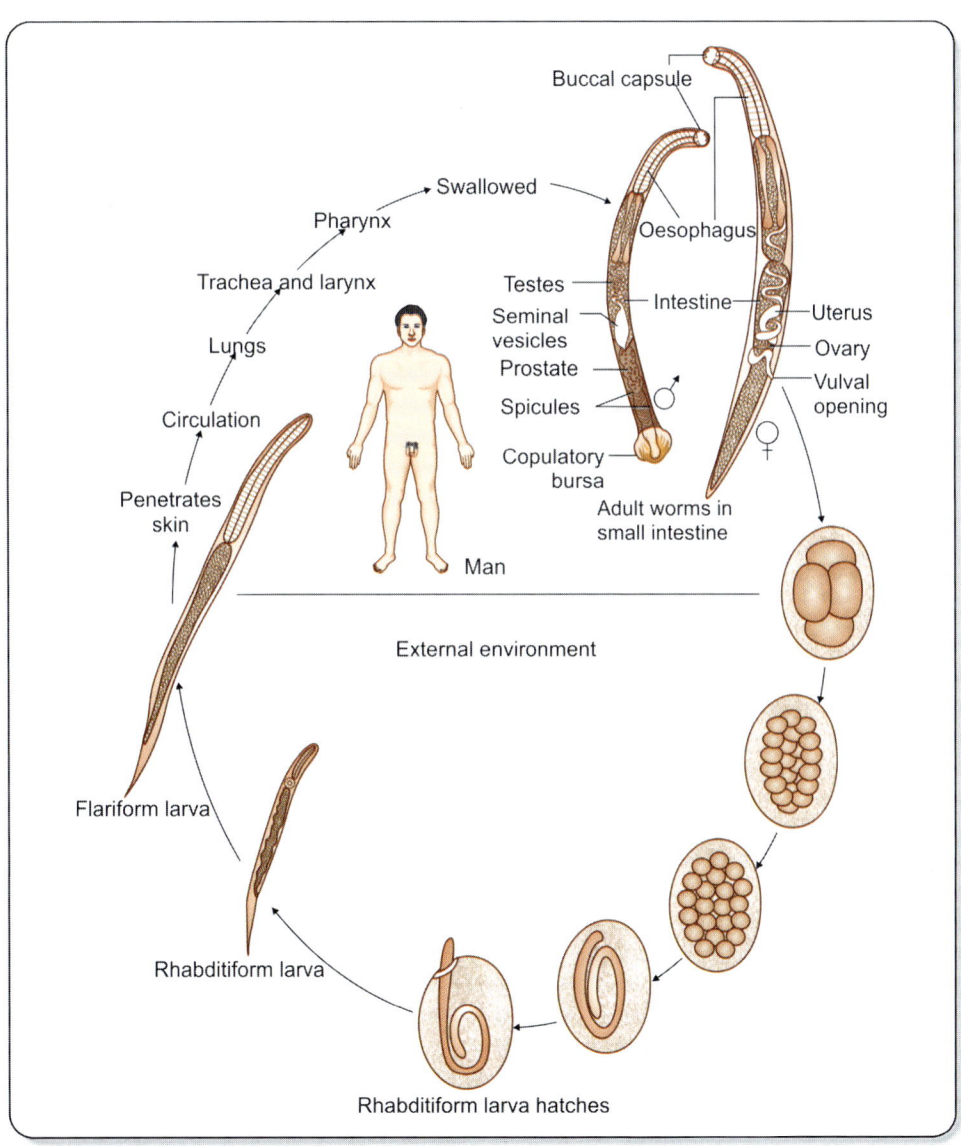

Fig. 56.25. Life cycle of *Ancylostoma duodenale*.

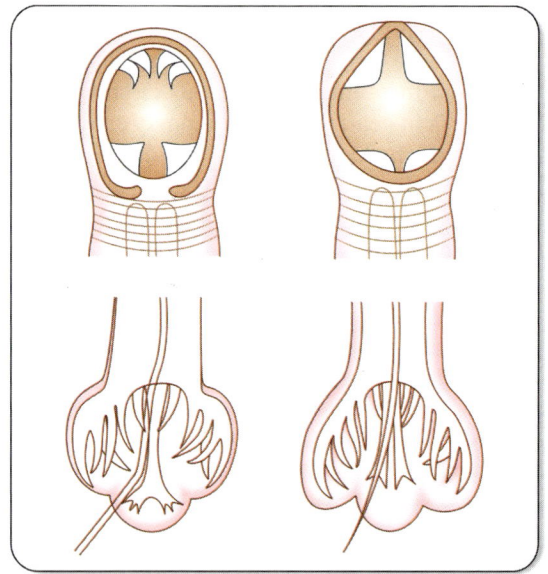

Fig. 56.26. Buccal capsule and copulatory bursa of (A) *Ancylostoma duodenale*, and (B) *Necator americanus*.

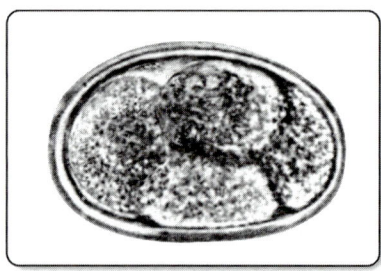

Fig. 56.27. Egg of *Ancylostoma duodenale* (saline wet mount, ×400).

Pathogenicity

Clinical disease in *A. duodenale* infection may be caused by the migrating larvae or adult worms.

Pathogenicity of migrating larvae

Migrating larvae of *A. duodenale* may cause two types of lesions:

1. Ancylostoma dermatitis or ground itch

When filariform larvae enter the skin they may lead to dermatitis. This causes intense itching and burning followed by erythema and oedema of the area which soon develops into papular and vesicular eruptions. This condition is more common with *N. americanus* than with *A. duodenale* infection. It disappears in 1–2 weeks.

2. Pulmonary lesions

When the filariform larvae break through the pulmonary capillaries and enter the alveoli, they may lead to bronchitis and bronchopneumonia. A **marked eosinophilia** occurs at this stage.

Pathogenicity of adult worms

The disease caused by adult worms is responsible for the syndrome commonly referred to as **hookworm disease**. The maturing and adult worms attach themselves to the mucosa of small intestine by means of their mouthparts. Hookworms ingest blood leading to microcytic, hypochromic type of iron deficiency anaemia. The degree of anaemia depends on the number of worms, body iron store and dietary iron. Patient develops epigastric pain, dyspepsia, vomiting and diarrhoea, the stool being reddish or black. Tongue, conjunctiva and skin become pale.

Laboratory diagnosis

Diagnosis of hookworm infection can be established by:

1. Direct methods

- Demonstration of characteristic eggs in the faeces by direct microscopy or by concentration methods.
- Adult worms may also be detected in the stool.
- Aspiration of duodenal contents by Ryle's tube may reveal eggs or the adult worms.

2. Indirect methods

- Blood examination may reveal microcytic, hypochromic anaemia and eosinophilia.
- In many cases of hookworm disease stool examination may show occult blood and Charcot-Leyden crystals.

NECATOR AMERICANUS

Necator americanus adult worms are slightly smaller and thinner than those of *A. duodenale*. The eggs of *N. americanus* are indistinguishable from those of *A. duodenale* and the life cycle, pathogenicity and diagnosis of the former is also similar to that of the latter.

WUCHERERIA BANCROFTI

Morphology

Adult worms

Adult worms (Fig. 56.28) are transparent, creamy white, long, hair-like structures. They are filiform in shape with both ends tapering. The male and female worms measure 2.5–4 cm × 0.1 mm and 8–10 cm × 0.2–0.3 mm, respectively. The posterior end of the female worm is straight, while that of the male is curved ventrally and contains two spicules of unequal length. Both male and female worms remain coiled together and it is difficult to separate them. The female is viviparous and liberates sheathed embryos (microfilariae) into lymph from where they find their way into blood.

Microfilaria

It is transparent and colourless with blunt head and pointed tail. It measures 290 × 6–7 µm in size and is covered by a hyaline sheath, which is much longer (359 µm) than the micro-

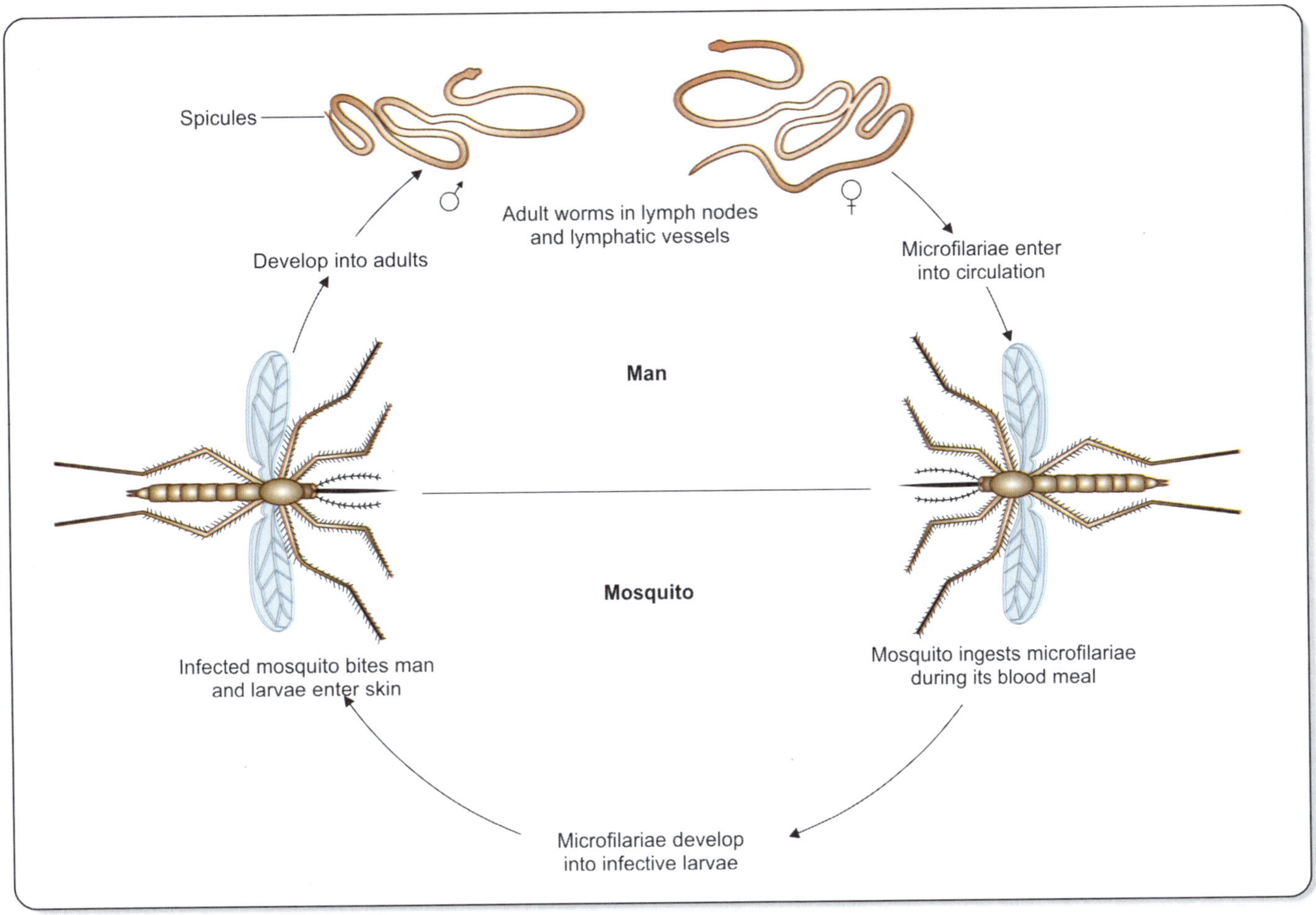

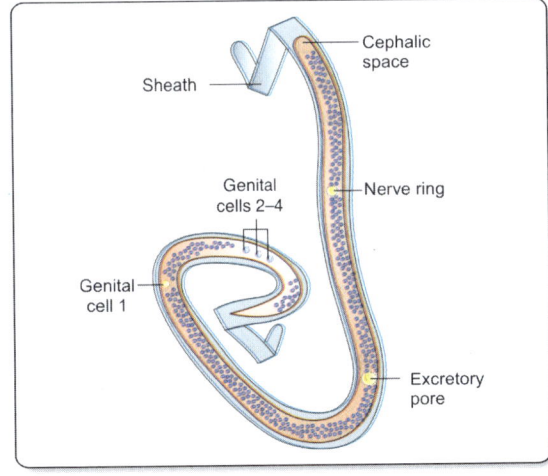

Fig. 56.28. Life cycle of *Wuchereria bancrofti*.

filaria. It can move forwards and backwards within the sheath. The somatic cells appear as granules in the central axis of the microfilaria. At places, these granules are absent. These form the landmarks for recognition of various microfilariae. The tail-tip is free from nuclei (Figs. 56.29 and 56.30).

Life cycle

W. bancrofti passes its life cycle in two hosts (Fig. 56.28). Man is the definitive host and the female mosquitoes belonging to the genera *Culex*, *Aedes* and *Anopheles* act as intermediate host. Adult worms reside in lymph nodes and lymphatics (usually inguinal, scrotal and abdominal) of man. The lymph provides nutrition to the adult worms. The male fertilizes female and the gravid female gives birth to microfilariae. Through lymphatics, they find their way into general circulation. The microfilariae appear in large numbers in peripheral blood at night, between 10 pm and 2 am. This correlates with the nocturnal biting habit of the insect vector.

Sheathed microfilariae are ingested by the mosquito during its blood-meal and reach the stomach of the mosquito. They cast off their sheaths, penetrate the stomach wall and reach thoracic muscles. Here they develop into infective stage of

Fig. 56.29. *Microfilaria bancrofti*.

the larvae. These larvae then migrate from thoracic muscles to the proboscis sheath of the mosquito. When the infected mosquito bites a human being, the larvae, in its proboscis, are deposited on the skin near the site of puncture. They then either enter through the puncture wound or penetrate through

10,000 eggs per day which are discharged in the faeces. The cycle is then repeated. Female worms can live for as long as 8 years.

Pathogenicity

Intimate contact of *T. trichiura* with the mucosa of large intestine leads to the inflammation of mucosa. Depending upon the intensity of infection, the inflammation may extend from the distal part of small intestine to the rectum. The mucosa may be oedematous and friable.

Prolonged massive infections lead to **iron deficiency anaemia**. This is due to the general malnutrition and **blood loss from the friable colon** and is not related to blood ingestion by the parasite.

Laboratory diagnosis

Specific diagnosis of trichuriasis can be made by the demonstration of the characteristic barrel-shaped eggs (Fig. 56.33) in the patient's faeces. Stool concentration methods such as simple salt floatation or formalin-ether sedimentation may be required to detect the light infection.

STRONGYLOIDES STERCORALIS

Habitat

Adult fertilized female lives buried under the mucosa of small intestine especially in the duodenum and jejunum.

Morphology

Adult worms

Strongyloides stercoralis is the **smallest nematode known to cause infection in man**. Parasitic females measure 2–3 mm in length and 30–50 μm in width (Fig. 56.34).

Eggs

The eggs measure 50–58 μm × 30–34 μm. They are thin-shelled, transparent and oval. They contain larvae ready to hatch. As soon as the eggs are laid, the rhabditiform larvae start hatching and bore their way out of the mucous membrane into the lumen from where they are passed in the faeces. As a result, it is the larvae which are excreted in faeces and the eggs are not routinely detected.

Life cycle

Adult female *S. stercoralis* lives buried under the mucosa of small intestine especially in the duodenum and jejunum (Fig. 56.34). As soon as the eggs are laid the rhabditiform larvae hatch and bore their way out of the mucous membrane into the lumen from where they are passed in the faeces. The rhabditiform larvae may metamorphose into filariform larvae during passage through the bowel. These may penetrate colonic mucosa or perianal skin without leaving the host and going through a soil phase again, thus providing a source of **autoinfection (hyperinfection)**.

Rhabditiform larvae may be voided with the faeces and may undergo two types of development in the moist, warm soil:

1. Direct development
2. Indirect development

Direct development

The rhabditiform larvae metamorphose, in 3–4 days, into filariform larvae. In this case each rhabditiform larva gives rise to one filariform larva.

Indirect development

The rhabditiform larvae develop into free-living adult males and females in the course of 24–30 hours. Male fertilizes female and the latter lays a second batch of rhabditiform larvae which are transformed into filariform larvae.

Filariform larvae, developed in the soil or faeces, are the infective form of the parasite. Man acquires infection by walking barefoot on the faecally contaminated soil. The filariform larvae penetrate the skin coming in contact with soil.

Once within the dermis, larvae invade the venous circulation and are carried by the blood stream to the right heart and then to the lungs, where they become trapped within capillaries and break through to the lung alveoli. They then migrate up the respiratory tree i.e. the bronchi, trachea, larynx, crawl over the epiglottis to the pharynx and are swallowed. They travel to the small intestine especially the duodenum and jejunum. Here they develop into adult parasitic females. The parasitic female then burrows into the mucous membrane and lays eggs. The rhabditiform larvae hatch out immediately and enter into lumen of the bowel. The cycle is then repeated.

Pathogenicity

Infection caused by *S. stercoralis* is known as **strongyloidiasis**. It is most frequently asymptomatic. In symptomatic cases the following lesions may be observed:

Skin lesions

On invading the skin, the filariform larvae produce petechial haemorrhage at each site of invasion, accompanied by intense pruritus.

Pulmonary lesions

When the larvae of *S. stercoralis* migrate through the lungs, they break out of the pulmonary capillaries into the alveoli leading to **haemorrhages in the lung alveoli and bronchopneumonia**.

Intestinal lesions

Patient develops intermittent abdominal pain, distension, bloating and diarrhoea alternating with constipation.

Laboratory diagnosis

The diagnosis of strongyloidiasis can be made by:

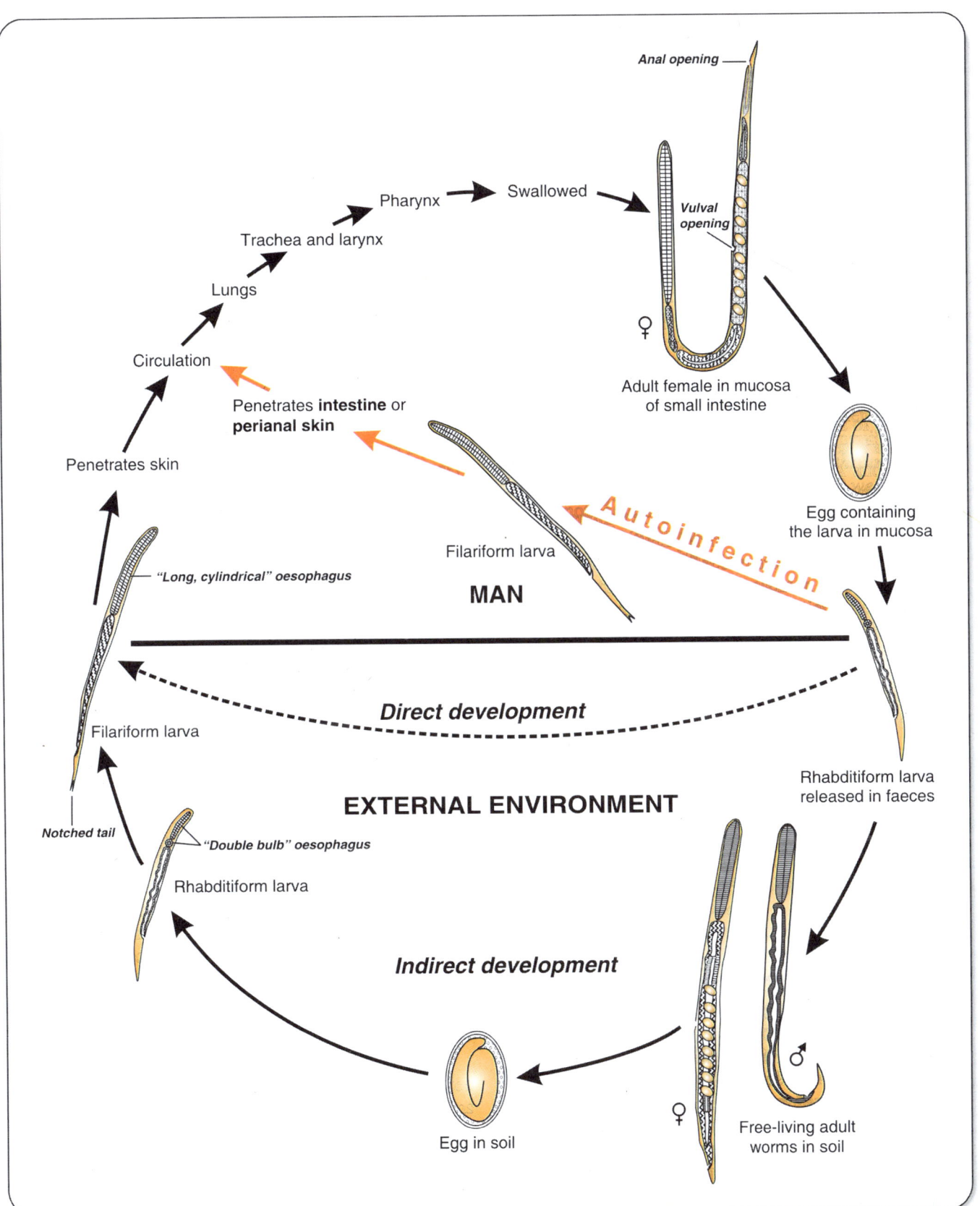

Fig. 56.34. Life cycle of *Strongyloides stercoralis*.

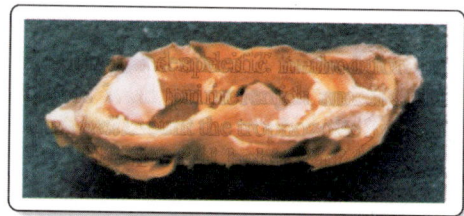

Fig. 56.37. Cysticerci (three in number) in tongue muscle.

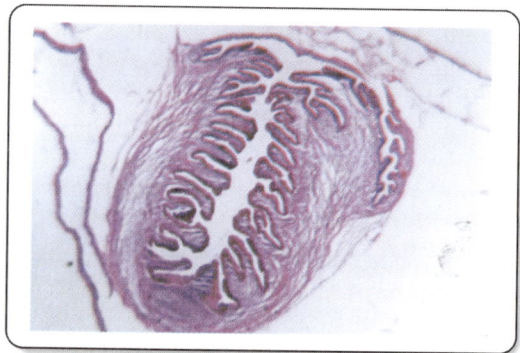

Fig. 56.38. Cysticercus cellulosae in tongue muscle (H&E stain ×100).

Gravid segments pass out with the faeces in chains of 5 or 6 and the cycle is repeated.

Cysticercus cellulosae can also develop in man as follows:

1. By ingesting the eggs with contaminated water and food.
2. A man harbouring adult worms may autoinfect oneself either by unhygienic personal habits or by reverse peristaltic movements of the intestine whereby the gravid segments are thrown into the stomach, equivalent to the swallowing of thousands of eggs. Further development to cysticercus cellulosae in man is similar to that in pig.

Pathogenicity

Adult worms in the small intestine usually produce no symptoms. But at times, they may cause vague abdominal discomfort, indigestion, persistent diarrhoea or diarrhoea alternating with constipation and loss of appetite.

Cysticercosis is a disease caused by larval stage of *T. solium*. Cysticercus cellulosae (larval form of *T. solium*) may develop in any organ and the effects produced depend on the location of cysticerci. They usually occur in large numbers, sometimes they may occur singly. They usually develop in the subcutaneous tissues and muscles forming visible nodules. It may also develop in brain leading to epileptic attacks, and in anterior and vitreous chamber of the eye.

Laboratory diagnosis

1. The diagnosis of *T. saginata* and *T. solium* adult worm infection can be carried out by:

- **Demonstration of characteristic eggs** in the stool by direct and concentration method by sedimentation technique (formol-ether sedimentation technique). **They do not float in saturated solution of common salt.**
2. The diagnosis of cysticercosis can be carried out by:
   - ***Biopsy of subcutaneous nodule:*** It may reveal cysticerci (Figs. 56.37 and 56.38).
   - ***Serological tests:*** Serological tests such as indirect haem-agglutination (IHA), indirect fluorescent antibody (IFA) and enzyme-linked immunosorbent assay (ELISA) can be used for demonstration of specific antibodies in the serum.

ECHINOCOCCUS GRANULOSUS

Morphology

Adult worm

It is a very small tapeworm measuring 3–6 mm in length. It consists of a scolex, neck and strobila (Fig. 56.39).

Scolex

It is piriform in shape and measures about 300 μm in diameter. It possesses four suckers and a protrusible rostellum with two circular rows of hooklets.

Neck

It is short and thick.

Strobila

It consists of three segments (occasionally four). The first segment is immature, the second is mature and the third (and the fourth when present) is gravid.

Eggs

These are indistinguishable from those of other *Taenia* species. These measure 31–43 μm in diameter and contain hexacanth embryos with three pairs of hooklets.

Larval form

This is found within the hydatid cyst which develops in the intermediate host (see pathogenicity).

Life cycle

E. granulosus passes its life cycle in two hosts (Fig. 56.39). The adult worm lives attached to the mucosa of small intestine of dog and other canine animals. The eggs are discharged in the faeces. These are swallowed by the intermediate hosts while grazing in the fields. Man acquires infection by a direct contact with infected dog or by allowing the dog to feed from the same dish or by ingesting water and food contaminated with dog's faeces containing eggs of *E. granulosus*.

In the duodenum the hexacanth embryos hatch out. These penetrate the intestinal wall and enter into the radicals of portal vein and are carried to the liver. The liver acts as the first

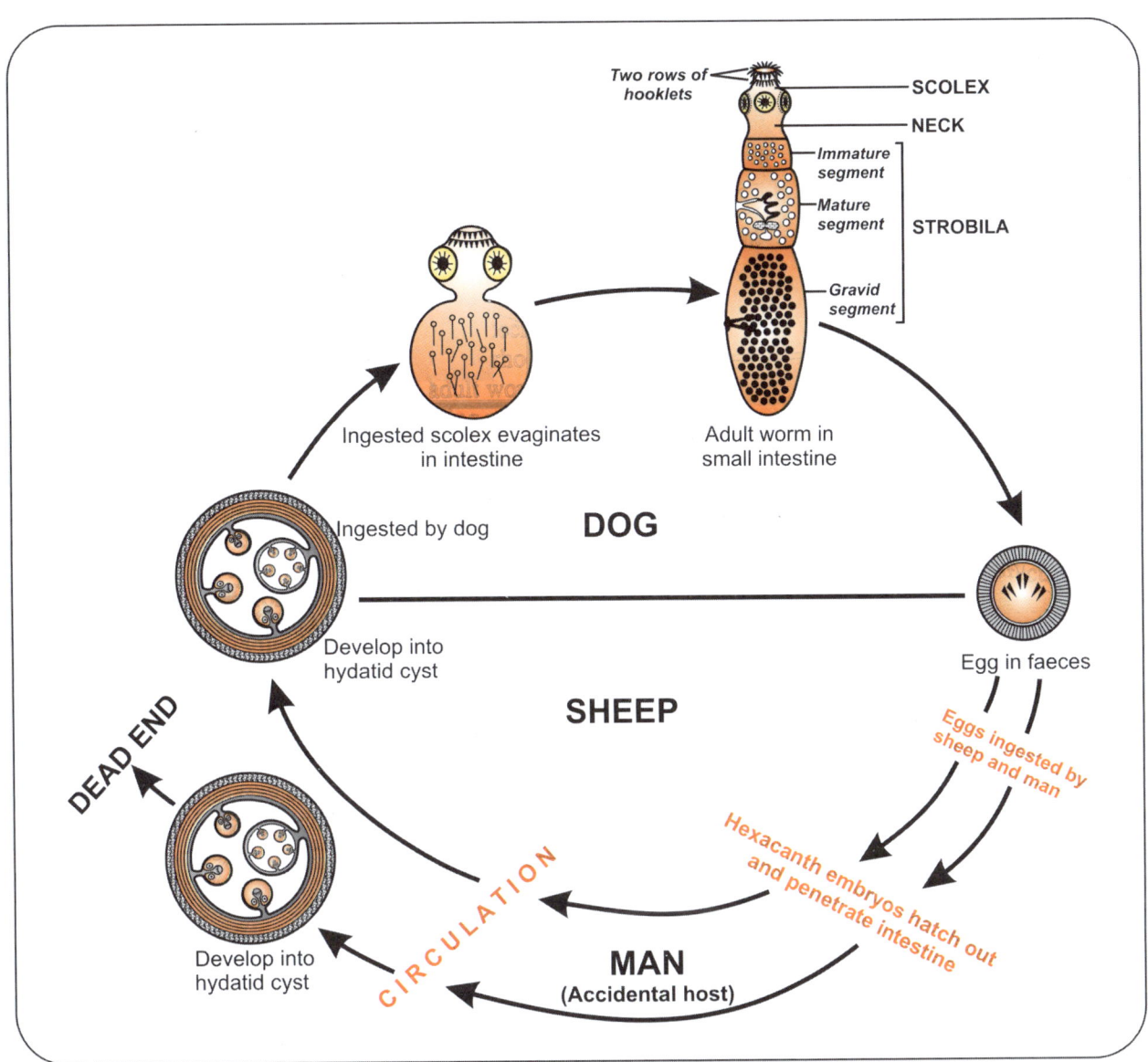

Fig. 56.39. Life cycle of *Echinococcus granulosus*.

filter where about 70% of human infections are located. Some embryos.may pass through the hepatic capillaries and enter the pulmonary circulation. Lungs act as the second filter. A few of these embryos may pass pulmonary circulation too and enter general circulation and may lodge in various organs and develop into hydatid cysts.

Wherever the embryos settle an active cellular reaction consisting of monocytes, giant cells and eosinophils takes place around the parasite. A large number of the parasites may, thus be destroyed by host defence mechanism. Some of the embryos, however, escape destruction and develop into hydatid cysts (Figs. 56.39–56.41). The cellular reaction in these cases gradually disappears, followed by appearance of fibroblasts and the formation of new blood vessels. Fibroblasts lay fibrous tissue, which envelops the growing embryo. This is known as **pericyst**. This merges with surrounding normal tissue. The parasite derives its nutrition through this layer. In old cysts the pericyst may become sclerosed or calcified and parasite within it may die.

Inside the pericyst, the embryo develops into a fluid-filled bladder known as **hydatid cyst**. From inner side of the cyst, **brood capsules** with a number of **scolices** are developed. The mature hydatid cyst when ingested by dog and other canine animals develop into a number of adult worms. These lay eggs which are passed in the faeces of infected animals and the cycle is repeated. Since dog has no access to the hydatid cysts developed in viscera of man, therefore, the life cycle of the parasite comes to a dead end.

Pathogenicity

E. granulosus causes **echinococcosis** or hydatid disease or **hydatid cyst** in man. It represents larval form of the parasite.

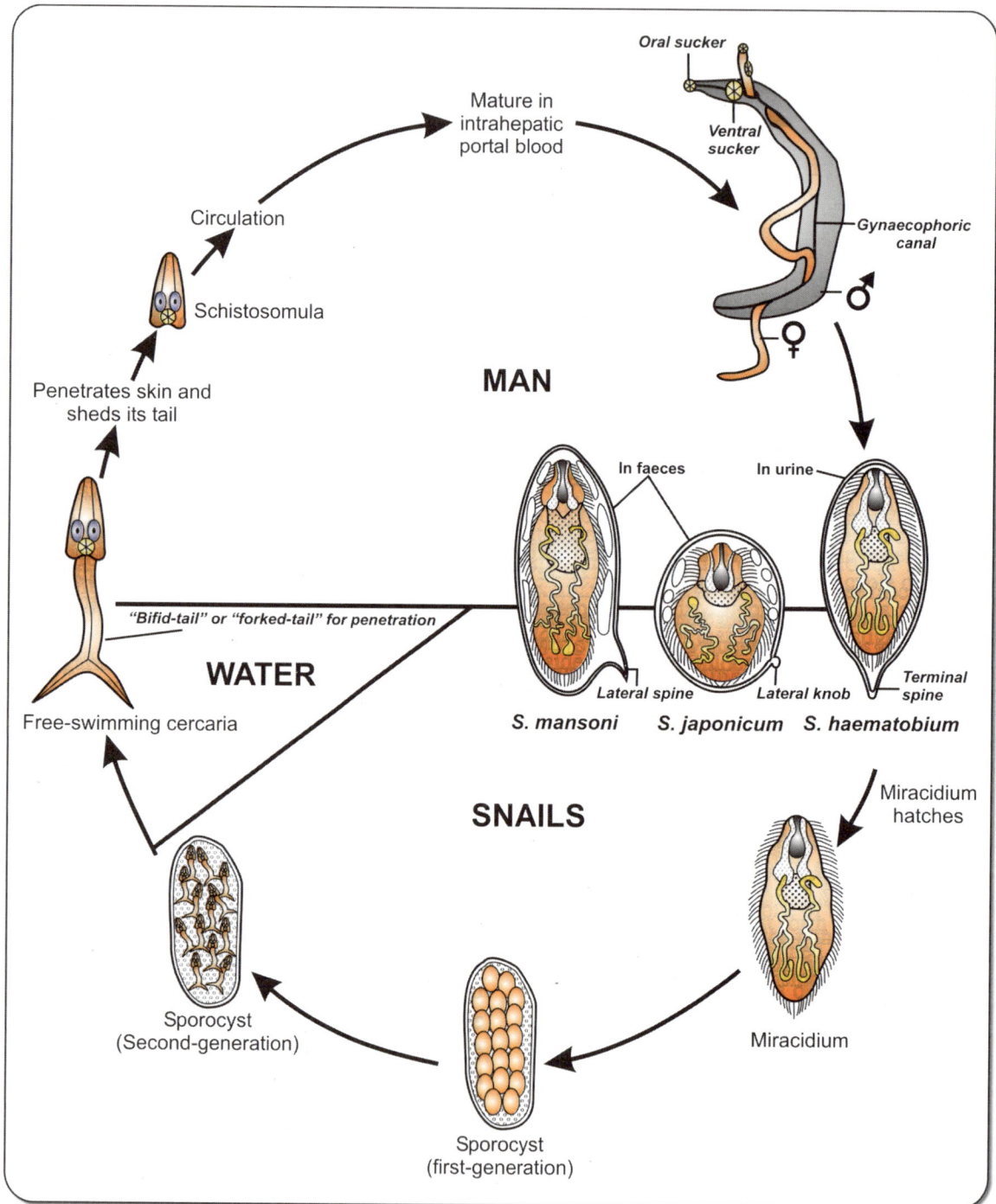

Fig. 56.42. Life cycle of *Schistosoma* species.

infective to man. The cercariae break off from the sporocysts and escape from the snail into water.

The free-swimming cercariae released from infected snails have the capability of directly penetrating the water-softened skin of human beings bathing or wading in this water. On entering the skin, the cercariae shed their tails and become **schistosomulae** which enter into peripheral venules. From here they are carried through the vena cava into the right heart,

the pulmonary circulation, the left heart and the systemic circulation. The majority of the schistosomulae, from the systemic circulation, are shunted in the abdominal aorta and gain access to the mesenteric artery, pass through capillary bed in the intestine and enter portal circulation and reach the liver.

In the intrahepatic portal veins the schistosomulae grow, pairing of worms take place on sexual maturation, and they

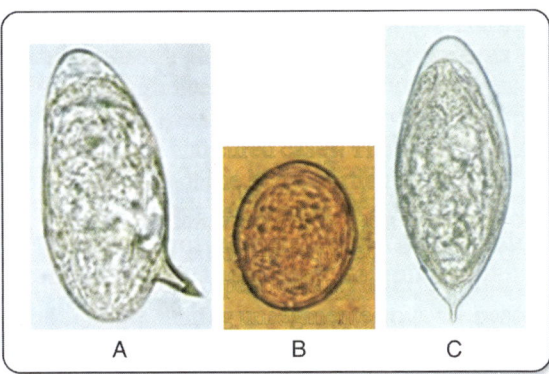

Fig. 56.43. Egg of *Schistosoma mansoni* (A) and *S. japonicum* (B) in stool, and that of *S. haematobium* in urine (C) (saline wet mount, ×400).

migrate against the blood current into the portal system venules, primarily those of the urinary bladder (*S. haematobium*), sigmoido-rectal region (*S. mansoni*) and ileo-caecal region (*S. japonicum*). Female worms lay the eggs which depending upon the species, are discharged in faeces or urine and the cycles are repeated.

Pathogenicity

Cercariae may induce **dermatitis** with itching and pruritic papular lesion in the skin within 24 hours of invasion by the cercariae. It disappears within a week. Migration of schistosomulae into lungs provoke cough and mild fever. In some patients anaemia may be observed.

Acute schistosomiasis or **Katayama fever** occurs in about a month after infection with *S. japonicum* and *S. mansoni* and rarely with *S. haematobium*. Characteristic symptoms include high fever, hepatosplenomegaly, lymphadenopathy, eosinophilia, and dysentery. This corresponds with the start of oviposition by mature female worms.

The International Agency for Research on Cancer (IARC) considers *S. haematobium* infection a definitive cause of urinary bladder cancer with an associated 5-fold risk.

Laboratory diagnosis

Specific diagnosis of schistosomiasis can be made by detection of the characteristic ova in the:

• Stool (*S. mansoni* and *S. japonicum*) or urine (*S. haematobium*) under microscopic examination (Fig. 56.43).

• Biopsy material obtained through the proctoscope (*S. mansoni* and *S. japonicum*) and cystoscope (*S. haematobium*) and examined microscopically after compression or sectioning.

Immunodiagnostic techniques such as immunofluorescent antibody test, ELISA, RIA and complement fixation test may be used as indirect methods for the diagnosis.

FASCIOLA HEPATICA

Common names

The sheep liver fluke; the common liver fluke.

Habitat

Adult worms reside in the biliary passages of the liver of sheep, goat, cattle and man.

Morphology

Adult worm

It is a large leaf-shaped fluke, measuring 30 mm × 13 mm and brown to pale grey in colour (Fig. 56.44). It is bilaterally symmetrical with three body layers, but has no true body cavity. At the anterior end there is a distinct conical projection. The posterior end is broadly pointed. The oral sucker measures 1 mm in diameter and is situated in the conical projection at the anterior end. The ventral sucker is 1.6 mm in diameter and is situated nearby in a line with two shoulders. The intestinal caeca, testes and vitelline follicles of the parasite are extensively branched. Life span of the adult worm is around 10 years.

Eggs

Eggs are large, elliptical to oval, operculate, **light yellowish-brown (bile-stained)** and measure 140 μm × 80 μm. The shell is thin with a smooth surface. Each egg contains a large unsegmented ovum in a mass of yolk cells (Figs. 56.44 and 56.45). It is excreted with the bile into the duodenum and then passed out along with the faeces. **It does not float in saturated solution of common salt.** Further development of the eggs takes place only in water.

Infective form

Metacercariae encysted on water plants that are ingested by humans.

Table 56.8. Morphology of eggs of *Schistosoma haematobium*, *S. mansoni* and *S. japonicum*		
S. haematobium	**S. mansoni**	**S. japonicum**
Elongated, 110–170 μm long and 40–70 μm wide; has a thin, smooth shell, a rounded anterior end and a characteristic terminal spine from the tapered posterior end.	Elongated, 115–180 μm long and 40–70 μm wide; has a thin, smooth shell with a prominent lateral spine near the more rounded posterior end; anterior end tends to be somewhat pointed and curved.	Oval or subspherical, 70–100 μm long and 55–65 μm wide; has a smooth, relatively thick shell; a small lateral knob may be seen; because it is often located in a depression in the shell, this is often difficult to see.

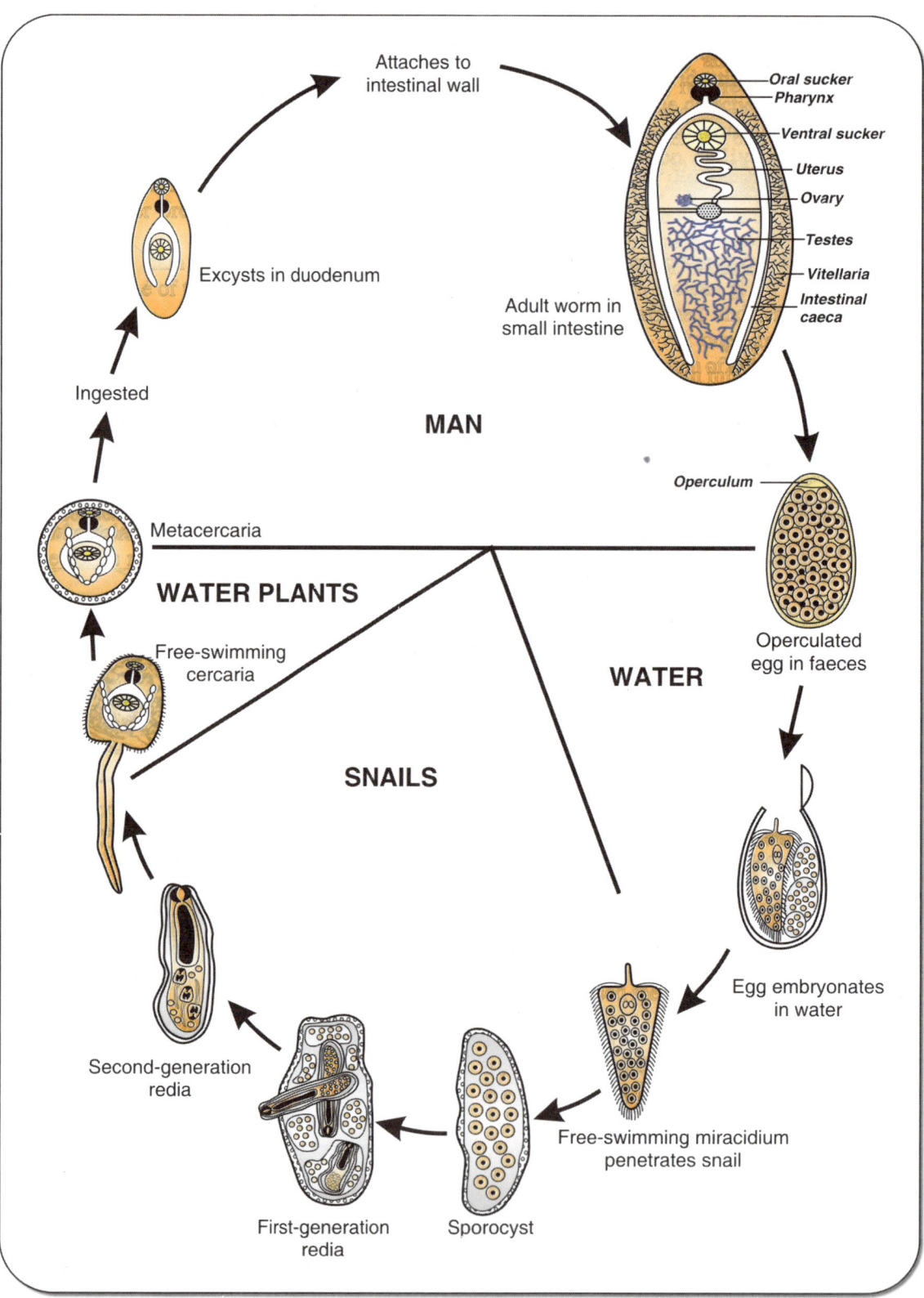

Fig. 56.46. Life cycle of *Fasciolopsis buski*.

Life cycle

Definitive hosts

Man and pig.

Intermediate hosts

- *First intermediate host:* Snails of the genera *Segmentina*, *Hippeutis* and *Polypylis*.
- *Second intermediate host:* Aquatic vegetations especially the seed pods of the water caltrop, the bulb of the water chestnut, and the roots of the lotus and water bamboo.

The life cycle of *F. buski* closely parallels that of *F. hepatica* (Fig. 56.46). The adult worms live attached to the mucosa of duodenum and jejunum of man and pig. The immature eggs are discharged in faeces and reach freshwater. The **miracidia** develop inside the eggs in 3–7 weeks at summer temperatures, after which they come out of the eggs and swim about in water. On contact with an appropriate snail, they burrow into the soft tissues and within a period of a few weeks **sporocysts, first- and second-generation rediae** and **cercariae** are produced in succession.

The cercariae, on coming out of the snail, encyst on the seed pods of the water caltrop, the bulb of the water chestnut and the roots of the lotus, water bamboo, and other aquatic vegetation becoming **metacercariae** or **infective forms**. Man acquires infection from peeling off the skin of these infested plants between the teeth and lips before swallowing the raw nut. The metacercariae excyst in the duodenum, become attached to the intestinal wall and develop into adult worms in about 3 months. Eggs are then liberated which exit in the faeces and the cycle is repeated.

Pathogenicity

Infection caused by *F. buski* is known as **fasciolopsiasis**. Patient complains of diarrhoea, initially alternating with constipation and persistent thereafter, abdominal pain, anorexia, nausea, vomiting, generalized toxic and allergic symptoms usually in the form of oedema particularly of the face, abdominal wall, and lower limbs. Ascites, anaemia, and asthenia are common and patient may die of profound toxaemia.

Laboratory diagnosis

Diagnosis of fasciolopsiasis can be made by:

- Detection of large, golden (**bile-stained**) operculated eggs in the faeces. The eggs of *F. buski* and *F. hepatica* are indistinguishable.
- Adult worms may be recovered and identified after a purgative or an anthelmintic.
- A marked eosinophilia and leucocytosis are commonly seen.

CLONORCHIS SINENSIS

Common names

The Chinese liver fluke; Oriental liver fluke.

Habitat

Adult worms are located in the biliary tract and occasionally in the pancreatic duct of man, dog, cat and rat.

Morphology

Adult worm

Clonorchis sinensis is narrow, oblong, flat worm with pointed anterior and somewhat rounded posterior end (Fig. 56.47). It measures 10–25 mm in length by 3–5 mm in breadth. The oral sucker is slightly larger than the ventral sucker. The latter is situated at the junction of the anterior and the middle third of the body just anterior to a loosely coiled uterus. The anterior sucker leads to an oesophagus, that branches into blind intestinal caeca, that extend laterally to the posterior end. It has two large deeply lobulated or branched testes. These are situated one behind the other in the posterior third of the body.

Eggs

The eggs are broadly ovoid, have a moderately thick, light **yellowish-brown shell** (**bile-stained**) and are provided with a distinct convex operculum resting on shoulders. A small knob is often seen at the posterior end. They measure 28–35 μm × 12–19 μm (average 29 μm × 16 μm). They contain ciliated embryos (**miracidia**) when discharged into the bile ducts (Figs. 56.47 and 56.48). They hatch only after ingestion by suitable molluscan hosts. **They do not float in saturated solution of common salt.**

Infective form

Metacercariae encysted in flesh of freshwater fish.

Life cycle

C. sinensis passes its life cycle in three hosts, one definitive host and two intermediate hosts (Fig. 56.47).

Definitive hosts

Man, pig, dog, cat and rat.

Intermediate hosts

- *First intermediate host:* Suitable species of operculate snails (*Bulimus, Parafossarulus, Semisulcospira, Alocinma*, and *Melanoides*).
- *Second intermediate host:* Freshwater fish of the family Cyprinidae.

Adult worms are located in the biliary tract and occasionally in the pancreatic duct of man, pig, dog, cat and rat. Eggs containing miracidia are discharged with the bile fluid into the faeces of definitive hosts and on entering into water, are ingested by the appropriate molluscan host. The **miracidium** hatches in the midgut of the snail, penetrates its intestinal wall and enters the vascular spaces where it passes through the stages of **sporocyst, first-generation rediae, second-generation rediae** and **finally cercariae.**

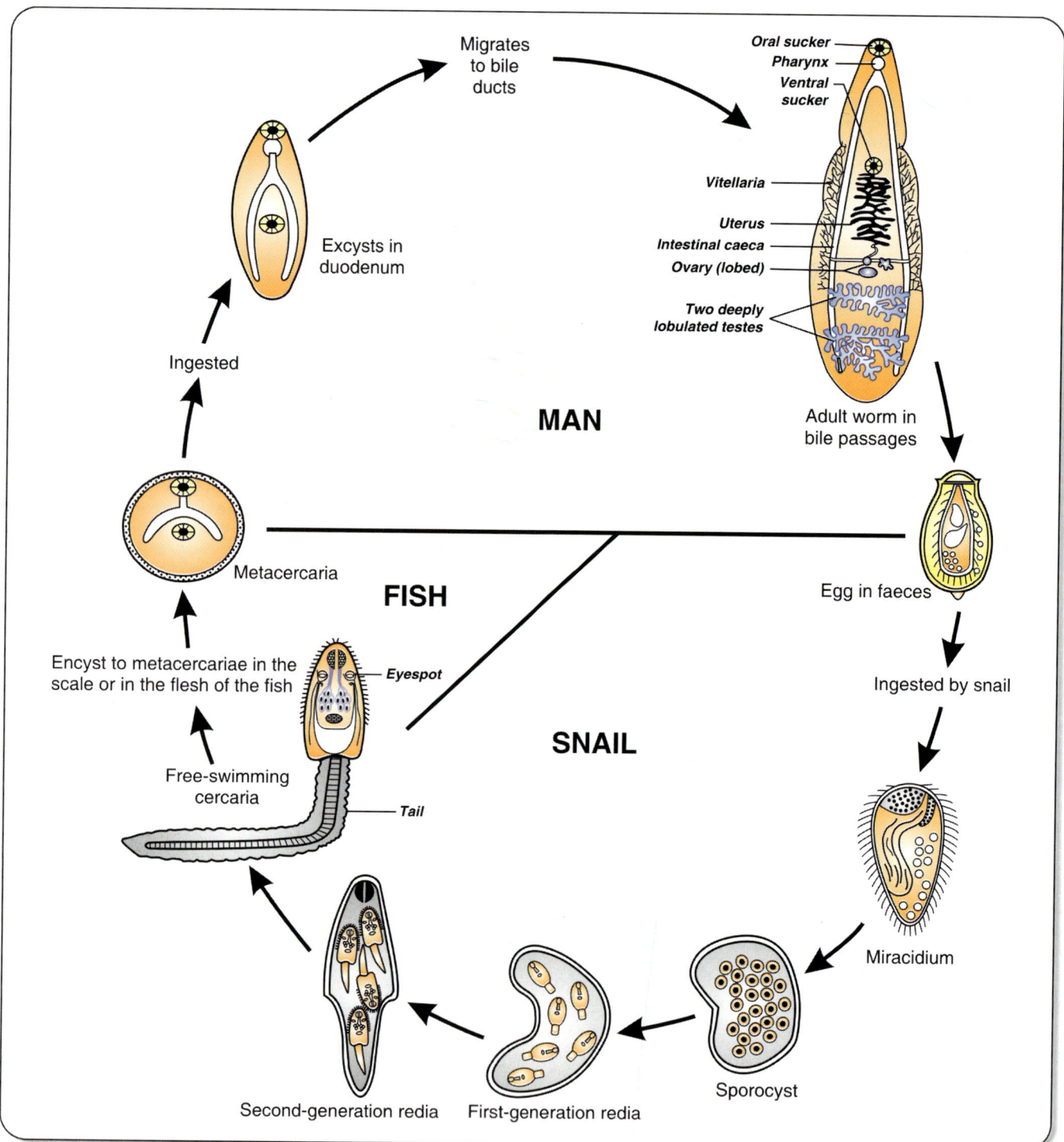

Fig. 56.47. Life cycle of *Clonorchis sinensis*.

The cercariae escape from the snail into water. After escape from the snail and a brief free-swimming existence, attack certain freshwater fish of the family Cyprinidae. The cercariae cast off their tails and encyst to metacercariae in the scale or in the flesh of the fish. The period of development in fish host, during summer, is 23 days.

Man acquires infection by eating raw, undercooked, salted or pickled freshwater fish harbouring metacercariae of *C. sinensis*. The metacercariae excyst in the duodenum, and usually enter the common bile duct through the ampulla of Vater and migrate to the distal bile capillaries, where they mature in about 1 month. Attachment and detachment of its

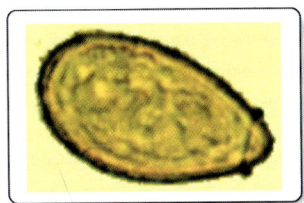

Fig. 56.48. Egg of *Clonorchis sinensis* (saline wet mount, ×400).

two suckers, together with a collar of spines on the immature worm, combined with extension and contraction of the body are presumably used, by *C. sinensis*, to migrate up the biliary tract, against the flow of bile. Mature worms probably move short distances within the ducts. Attachment is secured by the ventral sucker adhering to the biliary epithelium, leaving the oral sucker free for feeding. Adult worms produce an average of 10,000 eggs per day which exit the bile ducts and are excreted in the faeces. The cycle is then repeated.

Pathogenicity

C. sinensis causes proliferative and inflammatory reactions in the biliary epithelium of the bile ducts with which it makes contact. This is followed by encapsulating fibrosis of the ducts. Bile ducts are dilated particularly at the points where the flukes are attached to the inner lining, and biliary obstruction is rare except in extreme heavy infections. In most cases, the disease tends to remain low grade and chronic, with organisms persisting for three decades or more, producing only minor symptoms of abdominal distress, intermittent diarrhoea, and liver pain or tenderness.

C. sinensis has been linked to **cholangiocarcinoma**. *It is most frequently observed in areas where clonorchiasis is endemic. This cancer has a very poor prognosis, and few patients live longer than 6 months after diagnosis.*

Laboratory diagnosis

The diagnosis of clonorchiasis is based on:

- **Demonstration of eggs** by microscopical examination of faeces or aspirated bile by duodenal aspiration.
- **Differential leucocyte count** with eosinophilia (10–40%).
- Demonstration of antibodies against *C. sinensis* by ELISA, complement fixation test and indirect haemagglutination test.
- Skin test using extracts of adult *C. sinensis* as antigen.

PARAGONIMUS WESTERMANI

Common name

The Oriental lung fluke.

Habitat

The adult worms reside usually in pairs, in the parenchyma of lung, close to the bronchioles of man and other definitive hosts.

Morphology

Adult worm

It is thick, fleshy, oval-shaped and reddish-brown in colour with an integument covered with scale-like spines (Fig. 56.49). Its anterior end is slightly broader than the posterior end. It measures up to 16 mm in length, 8 mm in width and 5 mm in thickness. The ventral sucker is located towards the middle of the body and is of similar size to the oral sucker on the anterior end. The fluke possesses a large excretory bladder extending from the posterior extremity to the level of pharynx in the anterior region. The two blind intestinal caeca are unbranched and extend to the caudal region.

Life span of adult worm is about 6–7 years.

Eggs

The eggs of *P. westermani* are oval, **yellowish-brown**, measure 90 μm × 50 μm and have a prominent 'shouldered' operculum. The shoulder serves to distinguish the *Paragonimus* ova from those of *Diphyllobothrium latum*, the opercula of which are devoid of shoulders. *P. westermani* eggs also do not possess knoblike protrusion at the other end which is characteristic of *Diphyllobothrium* eggs. *P. westermani* eggs are unembryonated when laid.

Infective form

Metacercariae encysted in flesh of various crustaceans (cray-fish, crab).

Life cycle

Life cycle is passed in three hosts, one definitive host and two intermediate hosts (Fig. 56.49).

Definitive hosts

Man, wolf, fox, tiger, leopard, cat, dog and monkey.

Intermediate hosts

- *First intermediate host:* A freshwater snail of the genera *Semisulcospira* and *Brotia*.
- *Second intermediate host:* A freshwater crayfish or a crab (Crustacea).

The adult worms reside, usually in pairs, in the parenchyma of lung and lay eggs. Eggs escape into the bronchi and are coughed up and voided in sputum, or swallowed and passed in faeces. Freshwater bodies (lakes, canals, small ponds, rivers, flooded rice fields and other reservoirs of water) become contaminated with eggs from sputum and faeces. They develop and hatch in water after approximately 3 weeks, releasing a free-swimming **miracidium**, which burrows into the flesh of an appropriate snail.

Inside the snail, the miracidium passes through the stages of **sporocyst**, **first-generation rediae**, **second-generation rediae**, finally giving birth to **cercariae**. The mature cercariae

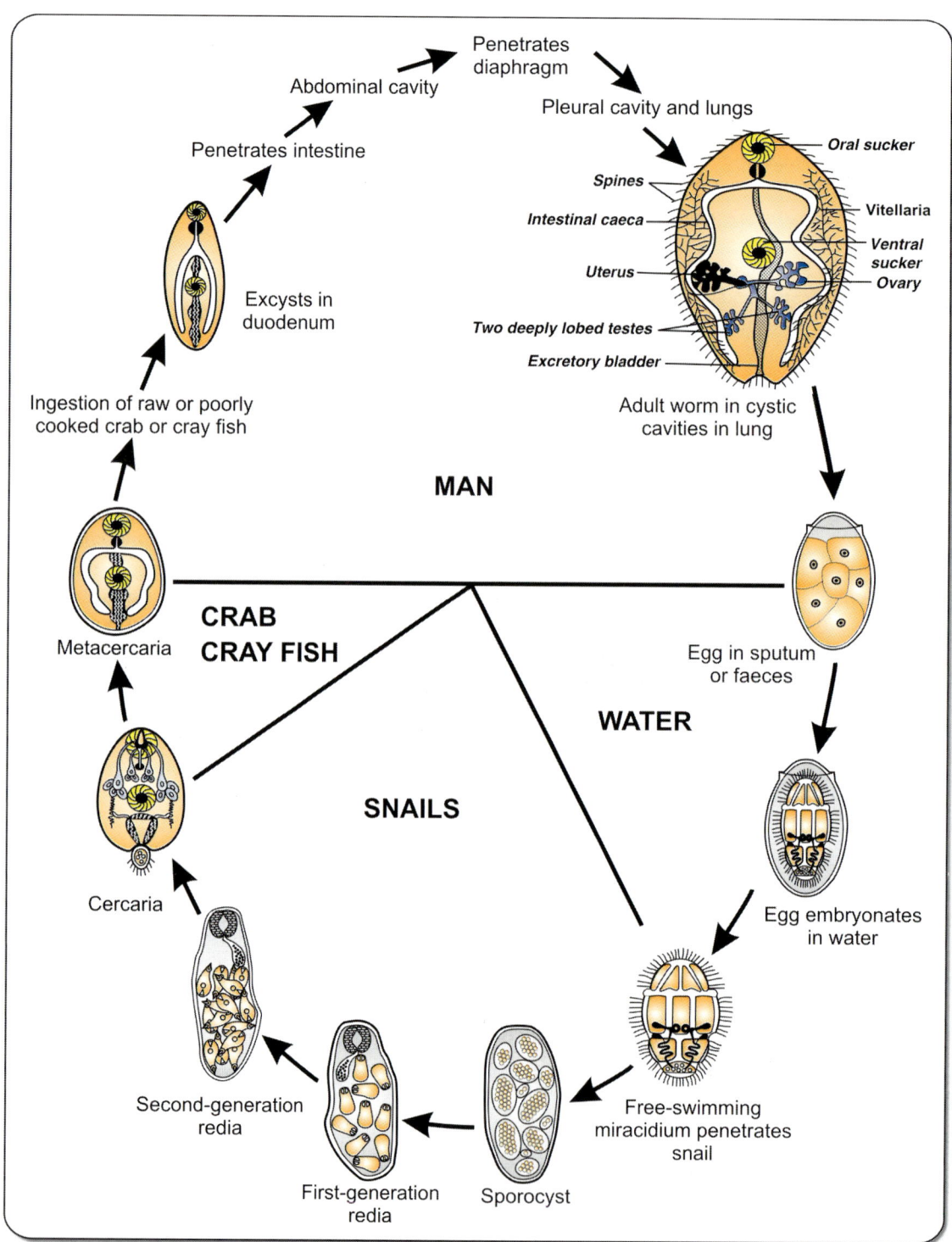

Fig. 56.49. Life cycle of *Paragonimus westermani*.

escape from the snail into water and penetrate gills and muscles of its second intermediate host, a freshwater crab or a crayfish. Crabs and crayfish can also become infected by eating the infected snail. Inside the crustacean host, the cercariae transform into **metacercariae** in the viscera, muscles and gills.

Humans become infected following ingestion of raw or poorly cooked or salted crab or crayfish, flesh of which contains encysted metacercariae. Ingested metacercariae excyst in the duodenum releasing larvae that attach to the duodenal mucosa. These larvae penetrate the intestine and enter into abdominal cavity. Then they migrate upwards, piercing through or around the diaphragm to the pleural cavity and lungs, finally arriving in the vicinity of the bronchioles, where they develop into adult worms usually in pairs encapsulated by host's inflammatory response and produce eggs. The time required for completion of their development in the definitive host is 65–90 days. Eggs are expelled in the sputum or may be dislodged by coughing, swallowed and excreted in faeces. The cycle is thus repeated.

Pathogenicity

During the migratory phase of *P. westermani* non-specific symptoms, e.g., chills, fever, marked eosinophilia, diarrhoea, abdominal and chest pain may be present. The adult worms in the lungs provoke granuloma formation consisting mainly of eosinophils and neutrophils, followed by development of a broad layer of fibrous tissue outside, thus producing a thick cystic encapsulation of the parasite. The cyst enlarges as the adult fluke grows, reaching up to 1.5–5 cm in diameter, and may break into an adjacent bronchiole.

Leakage of fluid into the bronchioles causes paroxysmal **coughing and haemoptysis**. Up to 50 ml of gelatinous, **rusty-brown sputum containing traces of blood and yellowish-brown parasite eggs** may be expectorated daily during paroxysmal coughing. It is often misdiagnosed as tuberculosis because of overlapping clinical manifestations including chest pain, cough and haemoptysis and confusing radiological findings in chest X-ray.

Laboratory diagnosis

Laboratory diagnosis of paragonimiasis can be made by:

1. Demonstration of eggs

Characteristic, **yellowish-brown, operculated eggs in the sputum**, aspirated pleural effusion or faeces. The sputum is blood-tinged and is peppered with rusty-brown flecks, consisting of clumps of yellowish-brown eggs.

2. Serological tests

A variety of serological tests, of which ELISA is sensitive and practical, are available.

3. Skin test

Skin test using extracts of adult *P. westermani* as antigen.

4. Biopsy

Parasite fragments and eggs can sometimes be seen in biopsy.

5. X-ray chest

It shows patchy foci of fibrotic change, with a characteristic 'ring shadow'.

57

Parasitic Diagnostic Procedures

Laboratory diagnosis of a parasitic infection can be carried out by detection and identification of the parasite or a stage in the life cycle of the parasite (trophozoite, cyst, egg, or larva) in various specimens (faeces, blood, bone marrow, urine, and biopsy material from spleen, liver, lymph nodes, etc.), cultivation of parasites, immunoassays, DNA probes and polymerase chain reaction.

EXAMINATION OF FAECES

COLLECTION OF THE SPECIMEN

Specimens should be collected in a wide-mouthed, clean, leak-proof container without contamination with urine, water or disinfectants because water may contain free-living organisms that can be mistaken for human parasites, and urine and disinfectants may destroy motile organisms. Faecal specimens, like other specimens received in the laboratory, must be handled with care to avoid acquiring infection from infectious parasites, bacteria, or viruses. Faeces may contain:

- **Infective forms of parasites** such as *Strongyloides stercoralis*, *Enterobius vermicularis*, *Taenia solium*, *Entamoeba histolytica*, *Giardia lamblia*, *Balantidium coli* and *Cryptosporidium parvum*.
- **Bacteria** such as *Shigella*, *Salmonella* and *Vibrio cholerae*.
- **Viruses** such as hepatitis A virus, hepatitis E virus and rotavirus.

Optimum time of specimen collection should ideally be as close to the onset of symptoms as possible, before initiation of antiparasitic therapy and first morning sample. Normally passed stool is preferable. Specimens obtained by purgation are generally less satisfactory. The specimen should be free of oil and other nonfaecal substances such as barium or bismuth. Patients who have received a barium enema may not excrete organisms in their stools for at least 1 week following barium enema, therefore, stool examination must be delayed for at least 1 week following the enema.

The amount of faeces requested may range from the whole stool, or series of stools over a specified period, to milligram amounts scraped from the gloved finger after rectal examination. The collection of three faecal specimens usually suffices to make the diagnosis of intestinal parasitic diseases, two obtained on successive days during normal bowel movement and a third after magnesium sulphate purge.

A total of six specimens, collected on successive days, may be required if intestinal amoebiasis or giardiasis is suspected. For obtaining scrapings of the ulcers in the rectum or the sigmoid colon, a proctoscope or a sigmoidoscope should be used. Every specimen should be identified with the following minimal information – patient's name and identification number, physician's name, and the date and time specimen was collected. The specimen should also be accompanied by a request form indicating which laboratory procedures are to be performed.

Because trophozoites disintegrate rapidly after defecation and do not encyst, liquid stool specimens should be examined within 30 minutes after collection (not 30 minutes after receipt in the laboratory) or semiformed stools within 60 minutes, to detect motile trophozoites, particularly in suspected infections with *Entamoeba histolytica* and *Giardia lamblia*. Formed stools, in which trophozoites are not expected, may be examined up to 24 hours after passage.

Preservation of stool

If there is delay from the time of collection of specimen and transport until examination in the laboratory, the use of stool preservatives should be considered. Several preservatives are available for permanent fixation of stool specimens that may be sent to reference laboratory for analysis. Preservation of stool helps in maintaining morphology of protozoan parasites and preventing further development of some helminth eggs

Table 57.1. Intestinal parasites found in faeces	
• *Entamoeba histolytica*	• *Giardia lamblia*
• *Dientamoeba fragilis*	• *Cryptosporidium parvum*
• *Isospora belli*	• *Cyclospora cayetanensis*
• *Balantidium coli*	• *Encephalitozoon intestinalis*
• *Enterocytozoon bieneusi*	• *Diphyllobothrium latum*
• *Taenia* species	• *Hymenolepis nana*
• *Hymenolepis diminuta*	• *Dipylidium caninum*
• *Schistosoma mansoni*	• *Schistosoma japonicum*
• *Fasciola hepatica*	• *Fasciolopsis buski*
• *Clonorchis sinensis*	• *Opisthorchis* species
• *Heterophyes heterophyes*	• *Metagonimus yokogawai*
• *Ascaris lumbricoides*	• *Ancylostoma duodenale*
• *Necator americanus*	• *Enterobius vermicularis*
• *Strongyloides stercoralis*	• *Trichuris trichiura*
• *Capillaria* species	

and larvae. Intestinal parasites which can be detected in faeces are given in Table 57.1.

Commonly used preservatives

Following are the commonly used preservatives:

Formalin solution

Faecal sample can be preserved in 10% formalin saline (100 ml formaldehyde in 900 ml 0.85% sodium chloride). Three parts of formalin preservative solution is thoroughly mixed with one part of stool specimen.

Advantages

- It is readily available, is easy to prepare, and serves as an all-purpose fixative.
- The prepared reagent has long shelf life.
- The morphology of helminth eggs, larvae, protozoan cysts, and coccidial forms are well preserved.
- Formalin preserved specimens are suitable for concentration procedures.

Disadvantages

- Formalin preserved specimens are not suitable for the preparation of trichrome-stained smears.
- Preservation is inadequate to maintain the morphology of protozoan trophozoites.
- Since the preservatives kill the parasites, therefore, characteristic motility of trophozoites cannot be seen.

Polyvinyl alcohol (PVA)

It preserves intestinal protozoa especially trophozoite stage. It is prepared by mixing 62.5 ml of 95% ethyl alcohol, 125 ml of saturated aqueous solution of mercuric chloride, 10 ml of glacial acetic acid, and 3 ml of glycerine in a 500 ml beaker. Then 10 gram of PVA powder is added, without stirring. The beaker is then covered and allowed to soak overnight. It is

then heated slowly to 75°C. When this temperature is reached, the mixture is removed from heat and it is stirred until a homogenous, slightly milky solution is obtained. For the preservation of stool, three parts of PVA is mixed with one part of the specimen.

Advantages

- The morphology of protozoan trophozoites and cysts is well preserved.
- Preserved samples remain stable for several months.
- Permanent slides can be prepared from PVA preserved stool specimens.

Disadvantages

- The morphology of helminth eggs and larvae, coccidian, and microsporidia are inadequately preserved.
- Unsuitable for acid-fast and safranin stains.
- The reagent is difficult to prepare in the laboratory.

Merthiolate-iodine-formalin (MIF) solution

MIF solution is prepared in two separate stock solutions to be mixed immediately before use:

- **Solution I** is prepared by mixing 250 ml of distilled water, 200 ml of thiomersal, 25 ml of formaldehyde, and 5 ml of glycerol.
- **Solution II** is Lugol's iodine (5% iodine in 10% potassium iodide solution in distilled water).

Before use, 9.4 ml (94 parts) of solution I is mixed with 0.6 ml (6 parts) of solution II. A small amount of the faecal specimen is added to this solution and mixed by stirring and shaking. It stains and fixes all microscopic parasite cysts, eggs, and larvae in the stool without any need for further staining by wet mounts. These are well preserved for 1 year or more.

Advantages

- The reagent components both fix and stain the parasitic forms.
- Preparation is easy and shelf life is long.
- Suitable for concentration procedures.

Disadvantages

- As with formalin preservative, it is not suitable for preparation of permanent trichrome smears.
- The morphology of protozoan trophozoites is poorly preserved.

Schaudinn's solution

It is prepared by mixing 45 gram of mercuric chloride, 310 ml of 95% ethyl alcohol, 50 ml of glacial acetic acid, 15 ml of glycerol and 625 ml of distilled water. In a 20 ml screw-capped vial, 1 ml of stool sample is mixed and stirred in 14 ml of Schaudinn's solution. The vial is then closed and shaken vigorously for 20–30 seconds. It fixes and preserves the specimen for 1 year or more.

Advantages

- Protozoan trophozoites and cysts are well preserved.
- Permanent stained smears are easily prepared.

Disadvantages

- The morphology of helminth eggs and larvae, coccidian oocysts and micrococcidian spores are poorly preserved.
- Less suitable than other preservatives for concentration procedures.
- Mercuric chloride is the main ingredient, making it difficult and expensive to dispose of the fixative.

METHODS OF EXAMINATION

Examination of stool consists of macroscopic and microscopic examination.

Macroscopic examination

Faeces should be examined for its consistency, colour, odour and presence of blood or mucus. Adult intestinal helminths, e.g., *Ascaris lumbricoides* and *Enterobius vermicularis* or segments of tapeworms may be seen in the stool specimen. Blood and mucus may be found in faeces from patients with amoebic dysentery, intestinal schistosomiasis, invasive balantidiasis, and in severe *Trichuris trichiura* infections. Fat-coloured and frothy specimens (containing fat) can be found in giardiasis.

Microscopic examination

Trophozoites of intestinal protozoa are usually found in liquid or soft and occasionally in semi-formed stools. These are not found in formed stools. Cysts are found in formed or semi-formed specimens. Coccidian oocysts and microsporidian spores can be found in any type of faecal specimen; in the case of coccidian oocysts, the more liquid the stool, the more oocysts that are found in the specimen. Helminth eggs may be found in any type of specimen, although the chances of finding of eggs in a liquid stool are reduced by the dilution factor.

Intestinal protozoa, and eggs and larvae of helminths can be detected and identified by microscopic examination of the stool. It includes saline wet mount, iodine wet mount, smear after concentration and permanent stained smear.

Saline wet mount

Saline wet mount is made by mixing a small quantity (about 2 mg) of faeces in a drop of saline placed on a clean glass slide. Remove any gross fibres or particles and cover with a coverslip. Avoid air bubbles by drawing one edge of coverslip slightly into the suspension and lowering it almost to the slide before letting it fall. The mount should be just thick enough that newspaper print can be read through the slide.

The smear is then examined under microscope. Begin at one corner of the smear and systematically examine successive adjacent swaths with the low power of the microscope. When a parasite-like object comes into view, it should be more closely examined and identified under high power. Saline wet mount is used for the detection of trophozoites and cysts of protozoa, and eggs and larvae of helminths. It is particularly useful for detection of live motile trophozoites of *E. histolytica*, *Giardia lamblia* and *Balantidium coli*.

Iodine wet mount

Stool is emulsified in a drop of five times diluted solution of Lugol's iodine on a clean glass slide covered with a clean coverslip and examined under microscope as above. Both saline and iodine wet mounts may be prepared on the same slide. For the preparation of Lugol's iodine, 10 gram of potassium iodide is dissolved in 100 ml distilled water and 5 gram of iodine crystals are then added slowly. *Potassium iodide renders the elemental iodine soluble in water through the formation of triiodide*. The solution is filtered and kept in a stoppered bottle of amber colour. It should be prepared every two weeks.

Iodine wet mount is used for the study of the nuclear character of cysts and trophozoites for the identification of the species. However, iodine immobilizes trophozoites. Iodine stained cysts of *E. histolytica* show pale refractile nuclei, yellowish cytoplasm and brown glycogen mass. The chromidial bars do not stain with iodine. Helminth eggs and larvae are readily identified without stain, but the iodine stain can be used advantageously in the examination of larvae as it immobilizes and kills them and stains some parts differentially.

Permanent stained smear

Permanent stained smears are essential for cytological details for accurate diagnosis. The detection and identification of *Entamoeba histolytica*, *Giardia lamblia* and other protozoan infections can be greatly enhanced. These can be prepared with both fresh and PVA preserved stool specimens. Iron-haematoxylin, trichrome and modified acid-fast stain are commonly used methods.

1. Iron-haematoxylin stain

A thin smear of faeces is made on a clean glass slide. It is fixed by keeping it in Schaudinn's solution for 15 minutes or longer. The smear is then immersed successively in 70% alcohol, 70% alcohol to which enough iodine has been added to give it a yellow colour, 70% alcohol, and 50% alcohol, 2–5 minutes in each.

It is washed in running tap water for 2–10 minutes and immersed in 2% aqueous ferric ammonium sulphate solution for 5–15 minutes followed by washing in running water for 3–5 minutes. It is then stained in 0.5% aqueous haematoxylin for 5–15 minutes and washed in running water for 2–5 minutes. Then it is differentiated in saturated aqueous solution of picric acid for 10–15 minutes and dehydrated by immersion for 2–5 minutes each in 50%, 70%, 80% and 95% alcohol and 5 minutes each in two changes of absolute alcohol. Stained smear is then cleared in two changes of xylol for 3–5 minutes each, mounted in Canada balsam and covered with coverslip.

2. Trichrome stain

The trichrome stain contains chromotrope 2 R, 0.6 gram; light green SF, 0.3 gram; and phosphotungstic acid, 0.7 gram. These dry components are mixed with 1.0 ml of glacial acetic acid and allowed to stand for 30 minutes, then diluted with 100 ml of distilled water. Faecal smear is prepared and fixed as in case of iron-haematoxylin staining. It is washed in 70% alcohol and in 70% alcohol containing enough iodine, to give it a yellow colour, for 1–5 minutes each. Then it is stained with trichrome solution for 10 minutes and differentiated in acid alcohol (99 parts 90% alcohol: 1 part glacial acetic acid) for 2–3 seconds. It is rinsed in absolute alcohol several times and dehydrated in two changes of absolute alcohol for 2–5 minutes each. Stained smear is then cleared in two changes of xylol for 2–5 minutes each, mounted in Canada balsam and covered with coverslip.

3. Modified acid-fast stain

Modified acid-fast stain is used for detection and identification of *Cryptosporidium parvum*, *Isospora belli* and *Cyclospora cayetanensis*. The staining solution contains:

1. *Carbol fuchsin*: 4 gram basic fuchsin is dissolved in 20 ml 95% ethanol. To this mixture, 100 ml distilled water is added slowly while shaking. Phenol is melted in a water bath at 56°C and 8 ml of this is added to above solution.
2. *Decolouriser*: It is 5% sulphuric acid.
3. *Counter stain*: It is 0.3% methylene blue in distilled water.

A thin smear of faeces is made on a clean glass slide. It is fixed by heat at 70°C for 10 minutes. It is kept on the staining rack and flooded with carbol fuchsin. The slide is heated till carbol fuchsin starts steaming. More carbol fuchsin is added to prevent slide from drying. The slide is allowed to stain for 9 minutes and washed with tap water. It is then decolourised with 5% aqueous sulphuric acid for 30 seconds, followed by washing with tap water and counter staining it with methylene blue for 1 minute. Finally, it is washed with tap water, dried, mounted in Canada balsam and covered with coverslip.

Oocysts of *Cryptosporidium parvum*, *Isospora belli* and *Cyclospora cayetanensis* stain red with carbol fuchsin and non-acid-fast background stains blue.

CONCENTRATION METHODS

Eggs, cysts, and trophozoites are often in such low numbers in faecal material that they are difficult to be detected in direct smears or mounts, therefore, concentration procedures should also be performed. Two commonly used methods are:

1. Floatation techniques
2. Sedimentation techniques

Both these methods are designed to separate intestinal protozoa and helminthic eggs from excess faecal debris.

Floatation techniques

Floatation involves suspending the specimen in a medium of greater density than that of the helminth eggs and protozoan cysts. The eggs and cysts float to the top and are collected by placing a glass slide on the surface of the meniscus at the top of the tube. Following floatation techniques can be used:

Saturated salt floatation technique

- About 1 gram of faeces is placed in a flat-bottomed vial (50 mm tall and 20 mm wide) and a few drops of saturated salt solution (specific gravity 1.200) are added.
- It is then stirred with a glass rod to make an even emulsion.
- More salt solution is added, so that the container is nearly full, stirring the solution throughout.
- Any coarse matter, which floats up, is removed. At this stage the container is placed on a level surface.
- The final filling of container is carried out by means of a dropper, until a convex meniscus is formed.
- A glass slide 7.5 cm × 5 cm is carefully laid on the top of the container, so that the centre is in contact with the fluid.
- The preparation is allowed to stand for 20–30 minutes, after which the glass slide is quickly lifted, turned over smoothly so as to avoid spilling of the liquid, and examined under the microscope. A coverslip may not be placed over the fluid.

It has been observed that all the helminth eggs float in the saturated salt solution except unfertilized eggs of *A. lumbricoides*, eggs of *Taenia solium*, *T. saginata* and all intestinal flukes. The *Strongyloides stercoralis* larvae also do not float in salt solution.

Zinc sulphate centrifugal floatation technique

- About 1 gram of faeces is thoroughly mixed in 10 ml of lukewarm distilled water. The coarse particles are removed by straining through gauze.
- The filtrate is poured into a 15 ml conical centrifuge tube and centrifuged at 2,500 revolutions per minute (rpm) for 1 minute.
- The supernatant fluid is poured off and distilled water is added to the sediment. It is shaken well, centrifuged and the process is repeated 2 or 3 times till the supernatant fluid is clear.
- The clear supernatant is poured off and 3–4 ml of 33% zinc sulphate (specific gravity 1.800) is added to the sediment and more zinc sulphate solution is added to fill the tube up to the top and centrifuged again at 2,500 rpm for 1 minute.
- With a platinum wire loop sample is taken from the surface, onto a clean glass slide, a coverslip is put on and examined under microscope.
- For protozoal cysts, one drop of iodine solution is added before the coverslip is put on.

Zinc sulphate centrifugal floatation technique effectively concentrates cysts of protozoa, eggs of nematodes, and small tapeworms. This method is not suitable for unfertilized eggs of *A. lumbricoides* and eggs of most trematodes and large tapeworms. However, the eggs of *Clonorchis sinensis* and *Opisthorchis* spp. are satisfactorily concentrated by this method. High concentration of the zinc sulphate suspension causes the opercula to pop open, fill with fluid, and sink to the bottom of the tube. Therefore, both the surface sample and the bottom sediment should be examined microscopically.

Sedimentation techniques

Concentration of intestinal parasites by sedimentation techniques, using either gravity or centrifugation, leads to a good recovery of cysts of protozoa and eggs of helminths. Cysts and eggs of parasites settle and are concentrated at the bottom because they have greater density than the suspending medium. Following are the commonly used sedimentation techniques:

Simple sedimentation

A sufficient amount of faeces is thoroughly mixed with ten to twenty times its volume of tap water and allowed to settle in a cone-shaped flask for an hour or two. This process is repeated several times till the supernatant fluid is clear. The clear supernatant fluid is discarded and the sediment at the bottom is examined for the eggs. This method is not suitable for protozoal cysts.

Formalin-ether sedimentation

- Half teaspoon of faeces is thoroughly mixed in 10 ml of water and strained through two layers of gauze in a funnel.
- The filtrate is centrifuged at 2,000 rpm for 2 minutes.
- The supernatant is discarded and the sediment is resuspended in 10 ml of physiological saline.
- It is again centrifuged and the supernatant is discarded.
- The sediment is resuspended in 7 ml of formalin saline and allowed to stand for 10 minutes or longer for fixation.
- To this is added 3 ml of ether.
- The tube is stoppered and shaken vigorously to mix.
- Then the stopper is removed and the tube is centrifuged at 2,000 rpm for 2 minutes.
- The tube is allowed to rest in a stand. Four layers become visible, the top layer consists of ether, second is a plug of debris, third is a clear layer of formalin saline and the fourth is sediment.
- The plug of debris is detached from the side of the tube with the aid of a glass rod, and the liquid is poured off leaving a small amount of formalin saline for suspension of the sediment.
- It is poured on a clean glass slide, covered with coverslip and examined under microscope.
- The sediment may also be mixed with a drop of iodine and examined.

Ether dissolves faecal fats and formalin fixes the parasites and removes faecal odour. Risk of laboratory acquired infection from faecal organism is minimized because organisms are killed by formalin solution.

QUANTIFICATION OF WORM BURDEN

For quantitative estimation of worm burden, two methods are commonly used:

- Direct smear egg count
- Stoll's method

Direct smear egg count

- Two mg of faeces is mixed in a small drop of saline on a slide and a coverslip is applied avoiding formation of air bubbles.
- The entire preparation is examined under low power of the microscope and the number of eggs (in 2 mg faeces) is counted and then the number of eggs per gram of faeces is calculated.

Stoll's method

This is commonly used method for determining the number of helminth eggs in faeces.

- Four gram of faeces is thoroughly mixed with 56 ml of N/10 NaOH in a flask to make a uniform suspension. This is facilitated by adding a few glass beads and closing the mouth with a rubber stopper and then shaking vigorously.
- 0.15 ml of the emulsion is removed with measuring pipette and is placed on a glass slide, a coverslip is put over it and all the eggs in the preparation are counted under low power of the microscope.
- The number of eggs per gram of faeces is calculated by multiplying the count with 100.
- The total egg production per day can then be calculated by multiplying the number of eggs/gram with a 24 hour faecal sample.
- Considering the consistency of faecal specimen, a correction factor (C.F.) is employed to convert the estimate to formed stool. For mushy-formed stool C.F. is 1.5, for mushy stool C.F. is 2, for mushy-diarrhoeic stool C.F. is 3, for frankly diarrhoeic stool C.F. is 4 and for watery stool C.F. is 5.

ANAL SCRAPINGS AND SWABS

- Amoebiasis cutis of the perianal area may be diagnosed by demonstrating motile trophozoites of *E. histolytica* in material scraped from ulcers and examined in saline suspension on a slide under a coverslip.
- *E. vermicularis* infection is usually diagnosed by demonstrating the presence of eggs on the perianal and perineal skin. This can be done by following methods:

1. Scotch cellulose adhesive tape method
2. NIH swab

Scotch cellulose adhesive tape method

Hold clear (not frosted) cellophane tape approximately 10 cm long between thumbs and forefingers with sticky surface facing outward. Before the patient has arisen from the bed in the morning (preferably while the child is still asleep), press the sticky side of the tape against the skin across the anal opening with even, thorough pressure. Gently, place the sticky side of the tape down against the surface of a clear glass slide for examination. A drop of toluene may be placed between the tape and slide. The toluene clears essentially everything except eggs and hair. Eggs of other helminths may also be seen in this preparation.

NIH swab

See Chapter 56.

ENTEROTEST

This is a simple and convenient method of sampling duodenal contents that eliminates the need for duodenal intubation. This device consists of nylon string weighted and coiled inside a gelatin capsule (Fig. 57.1).

The string protrudes through one end of capsule. This end of the string is taped to the side of the patient's face. The patient is then asked to swallow the capsule with water. In the stomach, gelatin capsule is dissolved and the weighted string is carried by peristalsis into the duodenum. The string is attached to the weight by a slipping mechanism. It is released and passed out in stool.

The string is recovered after 4 hours. After wearing the gloves bile-stained mucus clinging to the string can be removed by pulling the string between thumb and finger and collected in a small petri dish. The specimen should be examined immediately as a wet mount for motile organisms

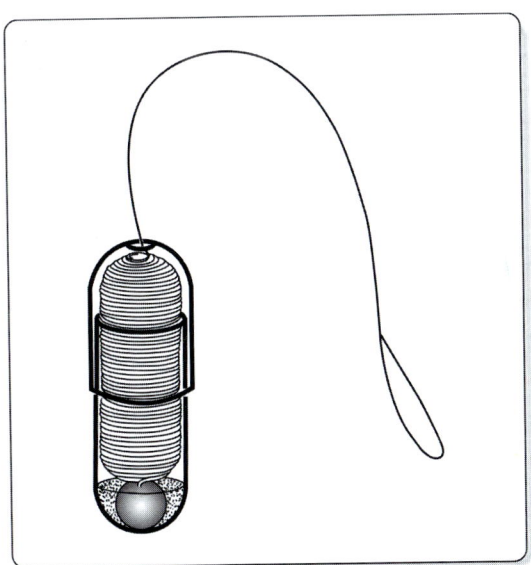

Fig. 57.1. Enterotest capsule for sampling duodenal contents.

(trophozoites of *Giardia lamblia* and larvae of *Strongyloides stercoralis*). Iodine may be added later to facilitate the identification of any organism present.

OBJECTS RESEMBLING ENTERIC PARASITES

A large variety of objects that closely resemble various parasite life cycle stages may be seen in faeces. White blood cells, macrophages, and squamous and columnar epithelial cells may resemble amoebae; yeasts and starch granules may resemble protozoal cysts; pollen and fungal conidia may resemble helminth eggs; plant fibres may resemble nematode larvae; and pieces of vegetables or vegetable skin may resemble adult worms or proglottids. Careful differentiation of these objects from real parasites is necessary to prevent inappropriate or unnecessary treatment.

EXAMINATION OF URINE

- *Trichomonas vaginalis* may be recovered in urine sediment from both male and female patients suffering from trichomoniasis.
- Eggs of *Schistosoma haematobium* and *Dioctophyma renale* may also be detected in the sediment of the urine. Samples of large volume should be allowed to settle for 1 or 2 hours. About 50 ml is then taken from the bottom sediment for centrifugation. A drop of sediment is placed on the glass slide covered with coverslip and examined under microscope.
- In case of *Wuchereria bancrofti* and occasionally in case of other filarial worm infections, the microfilariae may be discharged in the urine (chyluria). These may be detected in the centrifuged specimens. Rarely, *S. stercoralis* larvae may also be detected in the urine.

EXAMINATION OF SPUTUM

Sputum is commonly examined for the demonstration of:

- Eggs of *Paragonimus westermani* and *Capillaria aerophila* which reside in the respiratory tract of man.
- In pleuropulmonary amoebiasis, the rupture of the amoebic abscess into a bronchus results in coughing up the contents containing blood, necrotic tissue, and trophozoites of *E. histolytica*.
- Rupture of a pulmonary hydatid cyst is followed by discharge of its contents in which there are fragments of the laminated membrane and usually free scolices of *Echinococcus granulosus*.
- During migratory phase, larvae of *A. lumbricoides*, *Ancylostoma duodenale*, *Necator americanus* and *S. stercoralis* along with eosinophils and Charcot-Leyden crystals may be demonstrated in the sputum.

The sputum is spread in a petri dish and material suspected of bearing eggs (brown streaks) or pus and Charcot-Leyden crystals (opaque white or tan bronchial casts) is placed on a glass slide, covered with a coverslip and examined under microscope. Highly mucoid and gelatinous sputum is examined after the treatment with an equal volume of 3% sodium hydroxide.

EXAMINATION OF ASPIRATES

- The examination of aspirates from the liver is useful in the diagnosis of amoebic liver abscess and hydatid cyst. In amoebic liver abscess, trophozoites of *E. histolytica* are more likely to be found in material aspirated from the wall of the abscess than from the necrotic centre.
- Proctoscopic aspirates and scrapings are useful for the diagnosis of amoebic ulcers in the lower sigmoid colon and rectum.
- Duodenal aspirates may reveal trophozoites of *G. lamblia*, larvae of *S. stercoralis* and parasites in the gall bladder or biliary tract.
- Examination of aspirates (direct and Giemsa stained smears) from lymph nodes, spleen, liver, bone marrow, and spinal fluid is useful for the diagnosis of African trypanosomiasis, visceral leishmaniasis, Chagas' disease, and toxoplasmosis.
- The parasites may also be cultured from the aspirated material.
- The diagnosis of *Leishmania tropica* infection (oriental sore) is made by the microscopic examination of material obtained by puncture of the indurated edge of the sore and stained with Giemsa or Wright stain.

EXAMINATION OF CEREBROSPINAL FLUID

Examination of cerebrospinal fluid by direct microscopic examination of unstained and stained films is useful for the demonstration of:

- *Naegleria fowleri,*
- *Acanthamoeba* spp.,
- *Balamuthia* spp.,
- *Trypanosoma brucei gambiense*, and
- *T. b. rhodesiense.*

EXAMINATION OF BIOPSY MATERIAL

Biopsy is frequently useful, convenient and at times the only method for the diagnosis of a parasitic infection.

Skin biopsy

Skin biopsy can be used to demonstrate *E. histolytica*, *Leishmania* spp., and microfilariae of *Onchocerca volvulus*, *Mansonella streptocerca* and *M. ozzardi*, and encysted procercoid larvae of *Spirometra*.

Lymph node biopsy

Biopsy of an enlarged superficial lymph node may show *T. b. gambiense*, *T. b. rhodesiense*, *T. cruzi*, *Toxoplasma gondii*, *W. bancrofti*, *Brugia malayi* and *B. timori*.

Muscle biopsy

A muscle biopsy may reveal cysticerci of *T. solium*, larvae of *Trichinella spiralis* and *Toxocara*, and sarcocysts of *Sarcocystis lindemanni*.

Gastric biopsy

Gastric biopsy may reveal *Anisakis simplex*.

Small intestinal biopsy

Various life cycle stages of *Cryptosporidium parvum*, *Isospora belli* and *Cyclospora cayetanensis* may be seen in the epithelial cells of the mucosa of small intestine.

Colon and rectum biopsy

Biopsy of colon and rectum may demonstrate the eggs of *S. mansoni* and *S. japonicum*, and the trophozoites of *E. histolytica* and *B. coli*.

Brain biopsy

Brain biopsy may reveal trophozoites of *E. histolytica* and *N. fowleri*, trophozoites and cysts of *Acanthamoeba* spp. and *Balamuthia mandrillaris*, cysticercus cellulosae caused by *T. solium*, hydatid cyst caused by *E. granulosus* and coenurus caused by *Multiceps multiceps*.

Corneal scrapings

Corneal scrapings are helpful in making the diagnosis in cases of suspected *Acanthamoeba* keratitis. Wet mount preparation shows motile trophozoites. Cysts can be seen in stained preparations.

Liver biopsy

Liver biopsy may demonstrate *E. histolytica*, *L. donovani*, *E. granulosus*, *E. multilocularis* and *E. vogeli*.

Lung biopsy

Lung biopsy may demonstrate *E. histolytica*, *E. granulosus*, *P. westermani* and *C. aerophila*.

EXAMINATION OF BLOOD

Next to faeces, the blood provides the most common medium for recovery of various stages of animal parasites, e.g., *Plasmodium* spp., *Babesia* spp., *Leishmania* spp., *T. b. gambiense*, *T. b. rhodesiense*, *T. cruzi*, and microfilariae of *W. bancrofti*, *B. malayi*, *B. timori*, *Loa loa* and *M. ozzardi*. Whenever possible, specimens should be collected before treatment is initiated. When malaria and babesiosis are suspected, blood smears should be obtained and examined without delay. Since the parasitaemia may fluctuate, multiple smears might be needed. These can be taken at 8–12 hours intervals for 2–3 days. Microfilariae exhibit a marked periodicity depending on the species involved, therefore, the time of specimen collection is critical. If a filarial infection is suspected, the optimum collection time for demonstrating microfilariae is:

Loa loa	10 am to 2 pm
Wuchereria bancrofti and	
Brugia malayi	10 pm to 2 am
Mansonella	Any time
Onchocerca	Any time

Following methods can be used for the examination of parasites in the blood:

Wet preparation

A drop of anticoagulated blood can be placed on a clean glass slide, a coverslip put in place and examined microscopically for large, often motile, exoerythrocytic parasites, such as trypanosomes and microfilariae. **Use a suitable anticoagulant, e.g., sodium citrate for microfilariae, and EDTA for malaria parasites and trypanosomes.** Mix the blood well but gently with the anticoagulant. The blood must be examined within 1 hour of collection to avoid morphological changes in the appearance of parasites.

Permanent stained blood smear

Permanent stained blood smear is essential for accurate identification of blood parasites. Two types of blood films are used:

- Thin blood film
- Thick blood film
- Combined thick and thin films on the same slide

Thin blood film

Thin blood film is used primarily for the definitive species identification of plasmodia and other intraerythrocytic parasites. The pulp of a finger or lobe of an ear is wiped with spirit and allowed to dry. Thereafter, it is pricked with surgical cutting needle under aseptic condition. A drop of blood, about the size of pin head, is taken on a grease-free clean glass slide at about 2 cm from the right end. The drop of blood is touched with the edge of another slide. It is held at an angle of 30 degrees and pushed gently to the left, till the blood is exhausted. As the blood is exhausted, the film begins to form "tails" which end near about the centre of the slide. The film is allowed to dry. The thin film ideally is one cell thick, with erythrocytes lying flat on the glass surface. If the stain to be used is in an aqueous solution, e.g., Giemsa stain, the film must be fixed by covering it with absolute methyl or ethyl alcohol for 2–3 minutes to prevent dehaemoglobinization. For alcohol stains, e.g., Leishman stain, this treatment is not required.

Thick blood film

Thick blood film, many cells thick, contains 6–20 times as much blood per unit area as a thin film. A thick drop of blood is taken on a slide and spread with a needle or with the corner of another slide to form an area of about 12 mm square. It may also be prepared by taking 4 small drops of blood and joining the corners of the drops with a needle. The blood is continuously stirred for about 30 seconds to prevent formation of fibrin clots. If anticoagulated blood is used, stirring is not necessary because fibrin strands do not form. Potassium EDTA is the anticoagulant of choice. The film is allowed to air-dry in a dust-free area. The thickness of the film should be such as to allow a newsprint to be read or the hands of a wrist-watch to be seen through the dry preparation.

Once the film is dry, it should be dehaemoglobinized by placing the film in distilled water in a vertical position in a glass cylinder for 5–10 minutes. When the film becomes white, it is taken out and allowed to dry in an upright position. The disruption of the erythrocytes and the loss of their haemoglobin from the slide permits the remaining structures, including blood parasites, to be seen microscopically even when lying deep in the film. Dehaemoglobinization should be done as promptly as possible to assure total dehaemoglobinization. Thick blood films are especially useful in detecting malaria parasites in light infections.

Combined thick and thin films on the same slide

This method is of special value in survey work. Two drops of blood are taken; one, 1 cm and another, 2.5 cm from the right end of the slide. The former is made into a thick film and the latter into a thin film.

Staining blood film

Both thin and thick smears can be stained by Leishman and Giemsa stains. In addition, thick smear can be stained by Field stain.

Examination of thick smear

Since the erythrocytes (RBCs) have been lysed and the parasites are more concentrated, the thick smear is useful for screening of parasites and for detection of mixed infections.

- First screen the entire smear at low magnification (10× or 20× objective), to detect large parasites such as microfilaria.
- Then examine the smear using the 100× oil-immersion objective lens.
- If you see malaria parasites, make a tentative species determination on the thick smear and then examine thin smear to determine the species.
- NCCLS standards recommend examination of 100 fields using the 100× oil-immersion objective. It takes 5–10 minutes.

Examination of thin smears

Thin smears are useful for species identification of parasites already detected on thick smear, screening of parasites if thick smears are not available, and a rapid screen while thick smear is still drying.

- Screen at low magnification (10× or 20× objective lens) if this has not been done on the thick smears.
- Carefully examine the smear using the 100× oil-immersion objective lens. NCCLS standards recommend examination of at least 300 fields using the 100× oil-immersion objective. It takes 15–20 minutes.

Quantifying parasites

Malaria parasites can be quantified against blood elements such as RBCs or WBCs.

To quantify malaria parasites against RBCs: Count the parasitized RBCs among 500–2,000 RBCs on the thin smear and express the results as % parasitemia.

$$\% \text{ Parasitemia} = \frac{\text{Parasitized RBCs}}{\text{Total RBCs}} \times 100$$

If parasitemia is high (e.g., > 10%) examine 500 RBCs; if it is low examine 2,000 or more RBCs. Count asexual blood stage parasites and gametocytes separately. Only the former are clinically important. Gametocytes of *P. falciparum* can persist after elimination of asexual stages by drug treatment.

To quantify malaria parasites against WBCs: On the thick smear, tally the parasites against WBCs until you have counted 500 parasites or 1,000 WBCs, whichever comes first. Express the results as parasites per microlitre of blood using the WBC count, if known, or otherwise assuming 8,000 WBCs per microlitre of blood.

$$\begin{array}{c}\text{Parasites per}\\\text{microlitre of}\\\text{blood}\end{array} = \frac{\text{Parasites}}{\text{WBCs}} \times \begin{array}{c}\text{WBC count}\\\text{per microlitre}\\\text{(or 8,000)}\end{array}$$

Identification of blood parasites using fluorescent dyes

Fluorescent dyes that stain nucleic acids have been used for the detection of blood parasites. In the Kawamoto technique, blood smears on a slide are stained with acridine orange and examined under fluorescence microscope. This results in a differential staining of nuclear DNA in green and cytoplasmic RNA in red, which allows recognition of parasites. This method has been applied to malaria parasites (and to a lesser extent to African trypanosomes).

Leishman stain

Leishman stain is prepared by dissolving 0.15 gram of Leishman dry powder in 100 ml of absolute methyl alcohol in a bottle. The bottle is shaken until the powder is dissolved and allowed to stand for 48 hours with frequent shaking in between.

The smear is covered with 5–10 drops of stain. After 2 minutes, the stain is diluted by adding twice as many drops of buffered distilled water. The diluted stain is allowed to remain on the slide for 15–20 minutes for staining. The slide is washed with buffered distilled water, dried in air and examined under oil-immersion lens.

Giemsa stain

0.75 gram of Giemsa stain powder is placed in a mortar and 25 ml of glycerol is added to it and is grinded with a pestle until a paste is formed. To this is added 75 ml of methanol and stirred to make a solution. It is then poured in a dark coloured bottle and incubated at 37°C for 24 hours. This is used mainly for staining malaria parasites, trypanosomes, leishmanial parasites, and microfilariae.

The film is fixed by covering it with absolute methyl alcohol for 2–3 minutes. The slide is allowed to dry and immersed in 1:10 dilution of Giemsa stain in buffered distilled water for 30 minutes. It is then washed in buffered distilled water to remove excess stain and allowed to drain by keeping in the upright position and dried in air. The stained film is examined under oil-immersion lens.

Staining of thick and thin films on the same slide

For staining thick and thin films on the same slide, the thick film is first dehaemoglobinized and then stained along with the thin film. A line with a grease pencil is drawn between the films. The undiluted Leishman stain is poured over the thin film and after dilution the stain is flooded over the thick film. If the slide is to be stained with Giemsa stain then the thin part of the film is first fixed with methyl alcohol and after drying, the whole slide is flooded with dilute Giemsa stain and allowed to remain for half to two hours.

Field stain

This is a quick method of staining of malaria parasites in thick films (without fixation). This requires two solutions:

1. Solution A
2. Solution B

Solution A

Methylene blue	0.8 g
Azure I (or azure B)	0.5 g
Disodium hydrogen phosphate (anhydrous)	5.0 g
Potassium hydrogen phosphate (anhydrous)	6.25 g
Distilled water	500 ml

Solution B

Eosin	1.0 g
Disodium hydrogen phosphate (anhydrous)	5.0 g
Potassium hydrogen phosphate (anhydrous)	6.25 g
Distilled water	500 ml

The phosphate salts are first dissolved in water, then the stain is added. Solution of azure I or azure B is facilitated by grinding in a mortar with the phosphate solvent. The solutions are set aside for 24 hours and after filtration are ready for use.

Eosin solution should be renewed as soon as it becomes greenish.

- The thick film is placed in solution A for 1–2 seconds, or till the haemoglobin is removed and no trace of green colour is left.
- It is removed and immediately rinsed by waving gently in clean water for a few seconds until the stain ceases to flow from the film and the glass slide is free from stain.
- It is then placed in solution B for 1 second.
- It is removed and rinsed gently in clean water for 2–3 seconds. It is then allowed to stand upright to drain and dry.

Field stain is useful where large number of blood films have to be examined.

J.S.B. (Jaswant Singh, Bhattacharjee) stain

This is a rapid Romanowsky method of staining malaria parasites by water soluble stain. It consists of two solutions:

1. Solution I
2. Solution II

Solution I

This is prepared by dissolving methylene blue 0.5 gram in 500 ml distilled water in a narrow-mouthed flask. 1% sulphuric acid 3 ml and potassium dichromate 0.5 gram are added one after another, with the formation of a heavy deposit of amorphous purple coloured precipitate of methylene blue chromate. The solution is heated in a water-bath at boiling point for 2–3 hours. At the end of this period the solution turns blue. This indicates almost complete polychroming. The solution is allowed to cool at room temperature and the precipitate appears as steel-blue needle-like branched crystals. At this stage 10 ml of 1% potassium hydroxide is added, drop by drop, with the flask being shaken continuously. The liquid is filtered several times till the dye remaining on the filter paper is completely dissolved. The filtrate is blue having a violet iridescence and is a mixture of the azures with only a trace of methylene blue. It is left to mature at room temperature for 48 hours.

Solution II

This is prepared by dissolving 1 gram eosin in 500 ml distilled water.

Staining of thin film

Thin film is fixed with methyl alcohol for 3–5 minutes and allowed to dry. It is then immersed in solution I for 30 seconds, washed with acidulated tap water (pH 6.2–6.6), stained with solution II for 1 second, washed again with acidulated tap water for 4 seconds, immersed in solution I again for 30 seconds, washed again with acidulated water for 10 seconds, dried and examined under microscope.

Staining of thick film

The procedure for staining thick film is the same as for thin film except that the first step of fixation with methyl alcohol is omitted.

Smears from anticoagulated blood samples should be prepared as soon after collection as possible because the long exposure to the anticoagulant may compromise staining. Morphology of mature schizonts and gametocytes in particular may be altered. Sexual stages continue to develop during storage of blood sample in a warm laboratory environment, or following exposure of the blood sample to air. Gametocytes may exflagellate, releasing gametocytes into plasma. Merozoites, particularly those of *P. vivax*, may be released from mature schizonts and reinvade erythrocytes in which they may appear similar to the small accolé forms of *P. falciparum*.

BLOOD CONCENTRATION METHODS

Several concentration methods can be used for the detection of haemoparasites. These include:

1. Microhaematocrit centrifugation

Blood is collected aseptically by finger prick method in a microhaematocrit tube up to its two third of the volume. The end of the tube is sealed and centrifuged at 1,500 *g* for 7 minutes. The RBC-plasma interface is then examined under oil-immersion lens for **malaria parasites and trypanosomes**.

2. Triple centrifugation

9 ml of venous blood is mixed with 1 ml of 6% sodium citrate and centrifuged at 100 *g* for 10 minutes. The supernatant is collected and centrifuged at 250 *g* for 10 minutes. The supernatant is centrifuged again at 700 *g* for 10 minutes and the sediment is examined as a wet film or as stained smear. This method is useful for detection of **trypanosomes**.

3. Buffy coat concentration

5 ml of citrated or oxalated blood is centrifuged in a tube. Buffy coat present between the plasma and packed red cells is collected and stained for parasites. Trypanosomes, occasionally *Histoplasma capsulatum* (a fungus which appears as small oval yeast cells resembling those of *Leishmania* amastigote stage), and, in immunocompromised patients, *Leishmania* spp. (*L. infantum*, *L. chagasi* and *L. donovani*) are detected in the peripheral blood. These are found in the large mononuclear cells in the buffy coat. The nuclear material stains dark red-purple, and the cytoplasm stains light blue (*Leishmania* spp.). *H. capsulatum* appears as a large dot of nuclear material (dark red-purple) surrounded by a clear halo area. Trypanosomes in the peripheral blood also concentrate with buffy coat cells.

4. Knott concentration

2 ml of blood is thoroughly mixed with 10 ml of 2% solution of formalin and allowed to stand for 10 minutes or longer. It is then centrifuged at 200 g for 2 minutes and the sediment is examined microscopically for microfilariae.

5. Membrane filtration

1 ml of venous blood is drawn into a 10 ml syringe containing 0.1 ml of a 5% solution of sodium citrate. Then in the same syringe, 9 ml of 10% solution of Teepol in physiological saline is drawn and shaken gently for 1 minute. Needle of the syringe is removed and attached to a Swinney filter holder containing a 25 mm membrane filter of 5 mm porosity placed over a supporting filter paper pad of the same size, moistened with saline.

With gentle and steady pressure blood is forced through the filter. Filter is washed three times by passing 10 ml of physiological saline through it. Filter is removed and stained for 5 minutes in hot, but not boiling, Harris' haematoxylin, then it is briefly "blued" in running tap water. It is dried, covered with mounting medium and coverslip, and examined under microscope. This method is used for detection of microfilariae in the peripheral blood.

6. Gradient centrifugation

4 ml of Ficoll-Hypaque solution is mixed with an equal volume of heparinized blood. This is centrifuged at 150 g for 40 minutes. This shows three layers – white cell layer in the bottom, Ficoll-Hypaque layer in the middle and plasma layer on the top. Middle layer is examined for **microfilariae**.

CULTURE METHODS

The culture methods are frequently useful for accurate diagnosis of the organism, as a supplement to other methods or to provide positive diagnosis when routine methods have failed. These are also essential for preparation of antigen for immunodiagnosis of parasitic infections and for *in vitro* screening of drugs. Laboratory culture methods are available for many protozoan parasites. These include *E. histolytica*, *B. coli*, *N. fowleri*, *Acanthamoeba* spp., *B. mandrillaris*, *T. vaginalis*, *Leishmania* spp. and *Trypanosoma* spp. Brief methods for cultivation of these parasites are given in corresponding chapters.

SEROLOGIC DIAGNOSIS

The most reliable method for the diagnosis of a parasitic infection is by detection and identification of the infecting organism. However, the serologic approach to the evaluation of parasitic disease is most applicable when invasive techniques other than the routine examination of blood, faeces, or other body fluids are required to establish a diagnosis. For example, infective parasitic forms in toxoplasmosis, extra-intestinal amoebiasis, trichinosis, and cysticercosis are often lodged deep within tissues and organs and for the diagnosis either deep-needle or open surgical biopsies are needed. Various serologic tests and their clinical applications are given in Table 57.2.

Table 57.2. Serologic diagnosis of parasitic infections	
Test	**Disease**
Indirect haemagglutination test (IHA)	Amoebiasis, cysticercosis, echino-coccosis, filariasis, strongyloidiasis, fascioliasis, Chagas' disease
Fluorescent antibody test (FAT)	African trypanosomiasis
Indirect fluorescent anti-body test (IFAT)	Leishmaniasis, malaria, schisto-somiasis, toxoplasmosis
Enzyme-linked immuno-sorbent assay (ELISA)	Toxocariasis, toxoplasmosis, ascariasis
Complement fixation test (CFT)	Chagas' disease, paragonimiasis, leishmaniasis.
Latex agglutination	Echinococcosis
Bentonite flocculation	Trichinellosis, echinococcosis

MOLECULAR BIOLOGY

Molecular assays such as DNA probes and polymerase chain reaction (PCR) are available for the diagnosis of parasitic infections. DNA probe can be used for the diagnosis of malaria and filariasis and PCR can be used for the diagnosis of toxoplasmosis, leishmaniasis, Chagas' disease and oncho-cerciasis.

CONTROLLING MICROSCOPY

- Clean frequently the lenses of the eyepieces and objectives. The 40× objective can become easily contaminated when examining wet preparation.
- Use appropriate intensity of light for each objective and obtain adequate contrast by adjusting the condenser and iris diaphragm for the type of specimen and objective being used. When contrast is insufficient, parasites will be missed in unstained preparations, particularly trypanosomes in CSF, *T. vaginalis* in discharges, motile *E. histolytica*, *Giardia* trophozoites, and protozoal cysts and oocysts in faecal preparations. When light is insufficient for use with an oil-immersion objective, e.g., use of daylight with a binocular microscope, it will be practically difficult to identify malaria parasites in thick blood films.
- Use both 10× and 40× objectives to examine faecal preparations to avoid missing small parasites.
- Examine specimens for a sufficient length of time to avoid false negative reports and to ensure mixed *Plasmodium* infections, such as *P. falciparum* and *P. malariae*.

Index

A

Abnormal immunoglobulins, 67
ABO grouping, 105
Acid-fast bacteria, 7
Acid-fast cell wall, 7
Acinetobacter, 123, 126
Actinomyces, 207
Actinomyces israelii
   Actinomycosis showing a grain of, 208
   Colonies on blood agar medium, 208
Acute glomerulonephritis (AGN), 117
Acute rheumatic fever (ARF), 116
Adenoviruses, 244
   Morphology, 244
Aerobes, 19
Aerobic culture, 21
Agar-agar, 12
Agglutination reactions, 77
   Applications, 77
Albert's stain, 27
Alcohols, 38
Aldehydes, 38
Allergen, 95
Allergic asthma, 97
Allografts, 103
   Reaction, 103
      Mechanism of, 103
Amoebic and bacillary dysentery
   Differences, 297
Amoebic liver abscess, 296
Anaerobes, 20
Anaerobic culture, 21
   Methods, 21
Anaerobic jars, 21
Anaerobic media, 14
Anaphylaxis *in vitro* (Schultz-Dale
   phenomenon), 97
Ancylostoma duodenale, 322
   Differences between male and female, 322
   Egg, 324
   Life cycle, 323
Animal pathogenicity, 31

Annealing of primers, 46
Anthracoid bacilli, 133
Anthrax, 131
   Intestinal, 132
Antibiotic diffusion in agar
   Principle, 213
Antibiotic discs, 212
Antibodies, 63
   Production of, 90
Antibody paratopes of, 60
Antibody structure, 63
Antigens, 60
   Epitopes of, 60
   Fate in tissues, 90
Antigen-antibody reactions, 73
Antigen-presenting cells (APCs), 88
Antigenic specificity, 61
Antigenicity
   Determinants of, 60
Antiglobulin (Coombs') test, 78
Antimicrobial sensitivity testing, 212
Antisepsis, 33
Antonie van Leeuwenhoek, 3
Arthus reaction (local immune complex
   disease), 99
Ascaris lumbricoides, 320
   Adult worms, 320
   Eggs, 320
   Life cycle, 321
Ascoli's thermoprecipitin test, 132
Aspergillosis, 285
Aspergillus flavus, 286
Aspergillus fumigatus, 286
Aspergillus nidulans, 287
Aspergillus niger, 286
Aspergillus spp., 286
Aspergillus terreus, 287
Assimilation media for yeasts, 19
Atopic dermatitis (urticaria), 97
Atopy, 97
Atypical mycobacteria
   Diseases caused by, 146

Australian tick typhus (North Queensland
   tick typhus), 200
Autoclave, 36
Autografts, 103
Autoimmune diseases
   Classification of, 102
Autoimmunity, 101
   Mechanism of, 101
Automated ID and AST systems for bacteria
   and yeast, 222
Automated identification and antimicrobial
   susceptibility testing systems, 221
Automated specimen processing, 220
Automated system
   Comparison of currently available
      systems, 223
   Criteria for evaluation and selection, 224
   For identification of *Mycobacterium* spp.,
      223, 224
   of bacteria and yeasts
Automation in microbiology, 220
Autospecificity, 61
Autotrophs, 12
Auxanographic plate method, 19
Avian influenza (Bird flu), 253

B

B cell lymphoma, 242
B cells, 84, 85
B lymphocytes, 84, 86
Bacillary dysentery, 168
Bacillary lepromin, 149
Bacilli, 6
Bacillus anthracis, 131
Bacillus cereus, 133
Bacteria
   Environmental factors influencing growth,
      19
   Generation time, 11
   Identification of, 25
   L-forms, 10
   Microscopic morphology of, 25

Nutritional requirements for growth, 12
Shape of, 6
Size of, 5
Bacterial cell
Anatomy of, 6, 7
Wall, 6
Gram-negative, 7
Gram-positive, 7
Bacterial
Colonies
Appearance on solid media, 25
Flora in water, 215
Genetics, 42
Growth
Appearance in liquid media, 26
Growth curve, 11
Nucleus, 7
Nutrition, 12
Taxonomy, 31
Classification, 31
Identification, 32
Nomenclature, 31
Vaccines, 57
Bacteriocin (pyocin) typing, 178
Bacteriocin, bacteriophage and serotyping, 31
Bacteriological examination, 216
Bacteriological index (Ridley's scale), 147
Bacteriology
of air, 215, 218
of milk, 215, 217
of water, 215
Bacteriophage, 237
Bacteroides, 161
BactT/Alert 3D system, 222
Basal media, 13
Basic fungal morphology, 269
Basophils and mast cells, 88
BD Bactec system, 222
Biochemical reactions, 28
Biomedical waste (BMW), 40
Categories and their segregation, 40
Disposal of, 40
Bird seed agar or niger seed agar, 18
BK polyomavirus, 245
Black piedra, 272
Blastomyces dermatitidis, 281
Blastomycosis, 281
Blocking antibodies, 77
Blocking or non-agglutinating antibodies, 193
Blood culture by conventional and automated system, 221
Bone marrow, 84
Booster dose, 89
Bordetella, 186
Bordetella pertussis, 189
Borrelia, 152, 157
Borrelia burgdorferi, 158
Borrelia vincentii, 158
Boutonneuse fever, 200
Brain heart infusion (BHI) agar, 17

Brill-Zinsser disease (Recrudescent typhus), 199
Brucella, 191
Species and biotypes
Differential characteristics, 192
Bubonic plague, 174
Bubos, 205
Burkholderia, 175
Burkholderia cepacia, 180
Burkholderia mallei, 179
Burkholderia pseudomallei, 179
Burkitt's lymphoma, 242
Bursa-dependent areas, 85
'Bursa-dependent' or thymus-independent areas, 84
Bursa-independent areas, 85
Bursal lymphocytes, 84

C

CAMP test, 118
Reverse, 136
Campylobacter, 181
Differential characteristics of medically important species, 181
Candida albicans, 283
Blastoconidia and chlamydoconidia, 283
Germ tube and pseudohypha of, 284
Candidiasis, 282
Capsule, 7
Arrangement of, 8
Castaneda blood culture medium, 192
Castaneda method, 192
Catalase production, 30
Cell cultures in common use, 232
Cell-mediated immune responses, 91
Cell-mediated immunity (CMI), 83
Detection of, 92
Central dogma of molecular biology, 42
Chancre, 153
Chemiluminescence immunoassay (CLIA), 81
Chikungunya, 257
Chlamydia, 202
Chlamydia trachomatis
Inclusion body under fluorescence microscope, 206
Perinuclear inclusion body, 206
Chlamydiaceae
Classification, 202
Developmental cycle, 203
Chlamydiaceal infections of man, 204
Chlamydophila, 202
Cholera enterotoxin, 177
'Cholera red reaction', 176
Cholera toxin (CT), 177
Choleragen, 177
Christensen's medium, 30
Chromoblastomycosis, 277
Showing sclerotic bodies, 278
Cistron, 43
Citrate utilization, 29

Clonal selection theory of antibody production, 90
Clonorchis sinensis, 341
Egg, 343
Life cycle, 342
Clostridium, 134
Clostridium botulinum, 138
Clostridium difficile, 136
Clostridium perfringens (*Clostridium welchii*), 134
Typing of, 135
Clostridium species
Types of spores, 134
Clostridium tetani, 136
Coagglutination, 78, 111
Coagulase (tube coagulase) test, 111
Coagulase-negative staphylococci, 113
Cocci, 6
Coccidioides immitis, 282
Coccidioidomycosis, 282
Codon, 43
Cold agglutination, 77
Colicinogenic (col) factor, 46
Collection of water samples, 216
Commensals, 49
Common arthropods and diseases transmitted by them, 51
Common helminths of man, 318
Complement, 69
Biological effects of, 71
Activation
Alternative or properdin pathway, 70, 71
Classical pathway of, 69, 70
Fixation test (CFT), 78, 79
System, 69
Complete medium
Preparation of, 15
Blood agar, 16
Deoxycholate citrate agar (DCA), 16
Glycerol saline transport medium for enteric bacilli, 15
Heated blood agar ('chocolate agar'), 16
MacConkey agar, 16
Mueller Hinton agar, 16
Nutrient (meat extract) broth, 16
Nutrient agar, 16
Stuart's transport medium, 15
Thioglycollate broth, 15
Congenital malaria, 310
Conjugation, 45
Process of, 45
Constitutive enzymes, 43
Control strains, 212
Controlling microscopy, 356
Cornmeal agar, 17
Corynebacterium diphtheriae, 127
Differentiation of three biotypes, 128
Metachromatic granules, 127
Counterimmunoelectrophoresis, 76
Cryptococcus neoformans, 284
Cryptosporidium parvum, 316
Oocyst in faecal smear, 316

Cryptosporidium spp.
  Life cycle, 317
CSF container, 24
Culture in an atmosphere with added carbon dioxide, 21
Culture in microaerophilic atmosphere, 21
Culture media, 12
  For isolation of fungi, 17
  Preparation of, 14
    Alkaline peptone water, 14
    Cooked meat broth, 15
    Hiss's serum sugar media, 14
    Peptone infusion broth, 15
    Peptone water, 14
    Selenite F broth, 14
    Sugar fermentation media, 14
    Tetrathionate broth, 14
  Types of, 13, 14
    Anaerobic media, 14
    Basal media, 13
    Differential media, 13
    Enriched media, 13
    Enrichment media, 13
    holding media, 13
    Indicator media, 13
    Selective media, 13
    Storage media, 13
    Sugar media, 14
    Transport media, 13
Culture methods, 20, 356
Cutaneous anaphylaxis, 96
Cutaneous anthrax, 132
Cyclospora cayetanensis, 316
Cysticerci in tongue muscle, 332
Cysticercus cellulosae in tongue muscle, 332
Cytokines, 92
  Source and activity of, 93
Cytomegalovirus (CMV), 243
Cytoplasm, 7
Cytoplasmic membrane, 7

D

Dark-ground (dark-field) microscope, 5
Decarboxylase tests, 30
Deep infections, 283
Denaturation, 46
Dengue, 257, 258
Dermatophyte macroconidia
  Generic characteristics, 274
Dermatophytes
  Characteristics, 275
  Special types of hyphae, 274
Dermatophytosis, 273
Dick test, 115
Differential identification characteristics, 28
Differential media, 13
Diffusely adherent *E. coli* (DAEC), 163
Diplococci, 6
Disc contents of various antimicrobial agents, 213
Disinfectants
  Testing of, 39

Disinfection, 33
DNA
  Probes, 46
  Structure of, 42
  Viruses infecting humans, 233
  Watson and Crick model, 43
Donor, 103
Double diffusion in one dimension (Oakley-Fulthorpe procedure), 74
Double diffusion in two dimensions (Ouchterlony procedure), 75
Dry heat, 33
  Sterilization by, 34
Durham's tube, 29

E

Echinococcus granulosus, 332
  Life cycle, 333
Electroimmunodiffusion, 75
Electron microscope, 6
Elek's gel precipitation test, 130
Elek's test, 75, 130
ELISA (Enzyme-linked immunosorbent assay), 81
  Competitive, 81
  Indirect, 81
Embryonated hen's egg
  Cross-section, 231
Endemic (murine) typhus, 199
Endocarditis, 211
Endoflagella, 152
Endogenous infections, 50
Endometritis, 205
Endotoxins, 52
Enriched media, 13, 17
Enrichment media, 13
Entamoeba coli, 297
  Trophozoites and cysts, 298
Entamoeba histolytica, 293
  Life cycle, 295
  Morphological forms, 294
  Trophozoites and cysts, 298
Enteric fever, 170
Enteroaggregative *E. coli* (EAEC), 163
Enterobacter, 162, 165
Enterobius vermicularis, 318
  Egg of, 319
  Life cycle, 319
Enterococcus, 114, 118
Enteroinvasive *E. coli* (EIEC), 163
Enteropathogenic *E. coli* (EPEC), 163
Enterotest, 351
  Capsule for sampling duodenal contents, 351
Enterotoxigenic *E. coli* (ETEC), 163
Eosinophils, 56, 88
Epidemic (classical) typhus, 199
Epitopes, 60
Epstein-Barr virus (EBV), 242
Erysipeloid, 211
Erysipelothrix, 210

Erysipelothrix rhusiopathiae, 210
Escherichia, 162
Escherichia coli, 162
  Growth on MacConkey agar showing lactose fermenting colonies, 162
Ethylene oxide, 39
Eukaryotes, 5
Examination of
  Aspirates, 352
  Biopsy material, 352
  Blood, 352
  Cerebrospinal fluid, 352
  Faeces, 346
  Sputum, 351
  Urine, 351
Exogenous infections, 50
Exotoxins, 52
Exotoxins and endotoxins
  Differences, 53
Extrachromosomal genetic elements, 43
Extraintestinal amoebiasis, 296

F

Fasciola hepatica, 337
  Egg, 339
  Life cycle, 338
Fasciolopsis buski, 339
  Life cycle, 340
Fd piece, 64
Fertility (F) factor or F plasmid, 45
Filters
  Types of, 37
Fimbriae, 9
Flagella, 8
  Arrangement of, 8
  Structure of, 8
Floppy child syndrome, 138
Fluorescence microscope, 6
Food allergies, 97
Food-borne botulism, 138
Formaldehyde, 38
Formaldehyde gas, 39
Formalin solution, 347
Forssman antigen, 61
Fragment antigen binding (Fab), 63
Fragment crystallizable (Fc), 63
  Functions, 63
Friedlander's pneumonia, 165
Fungi
  Classification, 269
Fusobacterium, 161
Fusospirochaetosis, 158

G

Gardnerella, 210
Gardnerella vaginalis, 210
GasPak, 22
Gene, 43
  Acquisition of new genes, 43
Generation time, 11
GeneXpert system – XpertMTB/Rif test, 143

Index

Genotype, 43
Genotypic and phenotypic variations, 43
Ghon focus, 140
Giardia lamblia, 297
  Morphological forms, 298
Glutaraldehyde, 38
Gonorrhoea, 124
Graft, 103
  Types of, 103
Graft versus host reaction, 106
Gram stain, 26
  Mechanism of, 27
Group patterns, 6

H

H1N1 (Swine flu) virus, 253
Haemophilus, 186
Haemophilus ducreyi, 188
  Chancroid on the penis, 189
Haemophilus influenzae, 186
  Biotypes, 187
  Satellite growth, 187
Hair perforation test, 276
Halogens, 38
Hanging drop preparation, 26
Haverhill fever, 211
Hay fever (allergic rhinitis), 97
Heaf test, 140
Heat
  Types and principle, 33
Helicobacter, 181, 182
  Differential characteristics of medically
    important species, 181
Helicobacter cinaedi, 183
Helicobacter fennelliae, 183
Helicobacter pylori, 182
Helminths, 318
Hepatic amoebiasis, 297
Hepatitis A virus (HAV), 262
Hepatitis B carriers, 263
Hepatitis B infection
  Serological markers, 264
Hepatitis B virus (HBV), 262
Hepatitis C virus (HCV), 264
Hepatitis D virus (HDV), 264
Hepatitis E virus (HEV), 265
Hepatitis G virus (HGV), 265
Hepatitis viruses, 262
Herd immunity, 59
Herpes simplex virus (HSV), 240
  Multinucleated giant cells with
    intranuclear inclusion bodies, 241
Herpes zoster, 241
Herpesviruses, 239, 240
Heterogenetic (heterophile) specificity, 61
Heterophile agglutination, 77
  Test, 77
Heterotrophs, 12
Histamine, 95
Histocompatibility antigens, 61, 103
Histocompatibility testing, 105
Histoplasma capsulatum, 281

Histoplasmosis, 280
HIV infection
  Laboratory tests for the diagnosis, 261
HLA typing
  Uses, 105
Holding media, 13
Host, 293
Host-parasite relationships, 293
Hot air oven, 34
Human diploid cell (HDC) vaccine, 250
Human immunodeficiency viruses: AIDS,
  260
Human leucocyte antigen (HLA) complex,
  104
Humoral or antibody-mediated immunity
  (AMI), 83
Humoral response
  Primary, 89
  Secondary, 89
Hunterian chancre, 153
Hybridization, 46
Hydatid cyst, 334
Hydrogen peroxide fogging, 39
Hydrogen sulphide production, 30
Hypersensitivity, 95
  Delayed, 92
  Reactions
    Comparison of types I–IV, 100

I

ICRC bacillus, 147
Immune adherence, 72
Immune opsonization, 79
Immune responses, 83, 89
  Humoral or antibody-mediated, 89
  Primary cell-mediated, 91
  Secondary cell-mediated, 91
Immune system
  Architecture, 83
  Cells of, 85
Immunity, 54
  Acquired, 56
  Active, 56
    Artificial, 57
  Adoptive, 59
  Individual, 54
  Innate, 54
    Factors influencing, 54
    Mechanism of, 55
  Local, 59
  Passive, 58
    Artificial, 58
  Types, 57
Immunodiffusion (precipitation in gel), 74
  Tests, 75
    Types, 74
Immunoelectron microscopy, 82
Immunoelectrophoresis, 75, 76
Immunofluorescence (IF), 79, 80
  Direct, 80
  Indirect, 80

Immunogenicity, 60
Immunoglobulin
  A, 66
  Basic structure, 64
  Classes, 64
    Properties, 65
  D, 67
  Domains, 63
  E, 67
  G, 64
  M, 66
  Molecule
    Variable and constant domains, 65
Immunological memory, 57
Immunological tolerance, 93
Inclusion conjunctivitis, 204
Incomplete antigen or hapten, 60
Incubation, 22
Indicator media, 13
Indicator organisms, 215
Indole production, 28
Induced enzymes, 43
Infant botulism, 138
Infection, 49
  Endogenous, 50
  Exogenous, 50
  Modes of spread, 51
  Sources, 50
  Types, 49
Infectious mononucleosis (glandular fever),
  242
Infertility, 205
Influenza viruses, 251
  Inactivated vaccines, 252
  Live attenuated vaccines, 252
Inoculum, 212
Integral lepromin (Mitsuda lepromin), 149
Intestinal amoebiasis, 296
Intestinal parasites found in faeces, 347
Isografts, 103
Isospecificity, 61
Isospora belli, 314
  Life cycle, 315

J

Japanese encephalitis, 257, 258
JC polyomavirus, 245

K

Kala-azar
  Laboratory diagnosis, 302
Kauffmann-White scheme, 170
Keratomycosis, 289
Killer cells or K cells, 87
Kirby-Bauer disc diffusion method, 212
  Control strains, 212
  Interpretation chart of zone size, 214
Klebsiella, 162, 164
  Differentiation of species and subspecies,
    164

Koch's phenomenon, 140
Koch's postulates, 3, 4
Koplik's spots, 255
Koser's medium, 29
Kyasanur forest disease, 257, 258

L

Lawn culture, 20
Legionella pneumophila, 184
Legionnaires' disease, 184
Leishmania braziliensis complex, 305
Leishmania donovani, 300
   Amastigote forms in bone marrow, 301
   Morphological forms, 300
   Promastigote forms in culture, 301
Leishmania mexicana complex, 305
Leishmania tropica, 304
Lepromatous leprosy showing acid-fast
    bacilli in macrophages, 147
Lepromins, 149
   Test, 149
Leprosy
   Characteristics, 149
   Experimental animals used for
    experimental transmission, 148
Leptospira, 152
Leptospira interrogans, 159
Lichtheimia, 288
Light microscope, 5
Liquid culture, 21
Louis Pasteur, 3
Lyme disease, 159
Lymph nodes, 85
Lymphadenitis, 153
Lymphocytes, 85
Lymphogranuloma venereum, 205
Lymphoid organs
   Peripheral, 84
   Primary, 83
Lysis of target cell, 92
Lysogenic conversion, 44

M

Macroconidia in the three genera of
    dermatophytes, 274
Macroparasites, 49
"Mainline" malaria, 310
Major histocompatibility complex, 104
Malaria parasite
   Life cycle, 307
   Morphological forms, 308
Malassezia spp., 271
MALDI-TOF MS, 224
Mantoux test, 140
Mature HIV virion showing the localization
    of viral proteins, 260
McCartney bottle, 24
McCrady probability table, 217
McFadyean's reaction, 132
McIntosh-Fildes' anaerobic jar, 21
Measles virus, 255

Merthiolate-iodine-formalin (MIF) solution,
   347
Messenger RNA (mRNA), 43
Metallic salts, 38
Methicillin-resistant staphylococci (MRSA),
   112
Methyl red (MR) test, 28
MHC restriction, 88, 106
Microbial pathogenicity
   Factors predisposing, 52
Microbiology laboratory automation
   Current systems, 221
Microcapsule, 7
Microfilaria bancrofti, 325
   In peripheral blood, 326
Microorganisms likely to be present in milk,
   217
Microparasites, 49
Microphages, 56
Microscopy, 5
Migration inhibiting factor (MIF) test, 92
Minimum inhibitory and minimum
    bactericidal concentrations, 214
Minor histocompatibility antigens in man,
   106
Moist heat, 33
   Sterilization by, 35
Molecular biology, 356
Molluscum bodies, 240
Molluscum contagiosum, 240
   Multiple lesions in the pubic area, 240
Monoclonal antibodies, 90
   Applications of, 91
   Production of, 91
Moraxella, 123, 126
Moraxella (syn. *Branhamella*) *catarrhalis*,
   126
Morganella, 162, 166
Morphological forms of
   Entamoeba histolytica, 294
   Giardia lamblia, 298
   Leishmania donovani, 300
   Malaria parasites, 308
Morphology of T4 phage particle, 237
Mosquito (sexual) cycle, 306
Motility test, 30
Mucopurulent cervicitis, 205
Mucor, 288
Mucormycosis, 287
Mucosa-associated lymphoid tissues, 85
Mumps virus, 255
Mutation, 43
Mycetoma, 277
   Causative agents and colour of the grains,
    277
   Foot, 277
   Hand, 277
Mycobacterium avium, 145
Mycobacterium chelonae, 146
Mycobacterium fortuitum, 146
Mycobacterium gordonae, 145
Mycobacterium intracellulare, 145

Mycobacterium kansasii, 144
Mycobacterium malmoense, 145
Mycobacterium marinum, 145
Mycobacterium nonchromogenicum, 145
Mycobacterium phlei, 146
Mycobacterium scrofulaceum, 145
Mycobacterium simiae, 145
Mycobacterium smegmatis, 145
Mycobacterium szulgai, 145
Mycobacterium terrae, 145
Mycobacterium triviale, 145
Mycobacterium ulcerans, 145
Mycobacterium xenopi, 145
Mycobacteriosis, 144
Mycobacterium leprae, 147
Mycobacterium tuberculosis, 139
Mycolic acid, 7
Mycology, 269
Mycoplasma, 194
   Colonies showing 'fried egg' appearance,
    195
Mycoplasma genitalium, 196
Mycoplasma hominis, 196
Mycoplasma pneumoniae, 195
Mycoplasmas, 6
Mycoses
   Classification, 271
   Laboratory diagnosis, 269
   Opportunistic, 282
   Subcutaneous, 277
   Superficial, 271
   Systemic, 280
Mycotoxicosis, 290

N

Nagler's reaction, 135
Nasopharyngeal carcinoma, 242
Natural active immunity, 57
Natural killer (NK) cells, 55, 87
Natural passive immunity, 58
Necator americanus, 324
Negative staining, 28
Neisseria, 123
Neisseria gonorrhoeae (gonococcus), 124
Neisseria meningitidis (meningococcus), 123
   In CSF, 123
Nested PCR, 48
Neutralization tests, 79
Neutrophils, 88
New world leishmaniasis, 305
NIH swab, 320
Nine-banded armadillo (*Dasypus
    novemcinctus*), 148
Nitrate reduction, 29
Nocardia, 207, 208
Non-gonococcal urethritis (NGU), 205
Nontreponemal tests, 155
Nontuberculous mycobacteria, 144
   Classification, 144
   Differential characters, 146
Null cells, 87
Nutritionally deficient media, 17

O

Octads, 6
Old world leishmaniasis, 300
Ophthalmia neonatorum (inclusion blennorrhoea), 204
Opportunistic pathogens, 49
Opsonization, 72, 79, 80
Nonimmune, 79
Oral hairy leukoplakia, 242
Organ specificity, 61
Orientia, 198
Oropharyngitis (Vincent's angina), 158
Otomycosis, 289
Oxidase test, 30
Ozaena, 165

P

Papillomaviruses, 244, 245
Paracoccidioidomycosis, 281
Paragonimus westermani, 343
Life cycle, 344
Parainfluenza viruses, 254
Parasite, 49, 293
Classification of, 293
Parasitic infections
Diagnostic procedures, 346
Serologic diagnosis, 356
Paratope, 60
Paratyphoid fever, 170
Passive (indirect) agglutination, 78
Passive cutaneous anaphylaxis (PCA), 96
Passive immunization
Indications of, 59
Pathogenicity, 52
Pathogens, 49
Primary, 49
Paul-Bunnell test, 77
PCR
Applications in clinical laboratory, 48
Multiplex, 48
Real time, 48
Pelvic inflammatory disease, 205
Penicilliosis marneffei, 287, 288
Peptidoglycan, 7
Periappendicitis, 205
Perihepatitis, 205
Phaeohyphomycosis, 278
Phage assay, 238
Phage typing, 238
Phagocytic cells, 56
Phagocytosis
Events of, 56
Phase-contrast microscope, 5
Phenols, 38
Phenotype, 43
Phenylalanine deaminase test, 30
Piedra, 272
Black, 272
White, 272
Piedraia hortae, 273
Pili, 9

Pityriasis versicolor, 271
Plague, 173
Bubonic, 174
Pneumonic, 174
Septicaemic, 174
Plasma cells, 87
Plasmid, 43
Plasmodia of man
Differential characters of erythrocytic phase, 309
Plasmodium, 306
Plasmodium knowlesi, 310
Pneumococci in pus, 120
Pneumocystosis, 289
Pneumonic plague, 174
Polioviruses, 247
Polymerase chain reaction (PCR), 46, 47
Programming of cycles, 47
Polyoma viruses, 245
Polypeptide
Synthesis of, 42
Polyvinyl alcohol (PVA), 347
Post kala-azar dermal leishmaniasis, 304
Potassium cyanide test, 30
Pour-plate culture, 20
Poxviruses, 239
Prausnitz-Küstner (PK) reaction, 96
Precipitation and flocculation reactions
Applications, 73
Precipitation reactions, 73
Priming dose, 89
Principal protozoan pathogens of man, 294
Prions, 235
Prokaryotes, 5
Propionibacterium, 161
Proteomic based automated identification system, 224
Proteus, 162, 165
Proteus and *Morganella morganii*
Differentiation, 166
Protozoa, 293
Prozone phenomenon, 77, 193
Pseudomonas, 175
Pseudomonas aeruginosa, 178
Psittacosis, 205
Pulmonary anthrax, 132
Purified chick embryo cell (PCEC) vaccine, 250
Purified Vero cell (PVC) vaccine, 250
Pus cells, 109
Pus of liver abscess, 296

Q

Quantification of worm burden, 350
Quantifying parasites, 354
Quellung reaction, 8

R

RA factor, 78
Rabies vaccines, 249, 250

Rabies virus, 247, 248
Pathogenesis of, 248
Racial immunity, 54
Radioimmunoassay (RIA), 80
Reiter protein complement fixation test (RPCFT), 78
Relapsing fever, 157
Reservoir hosts, 50
Resistance plasmid or R plasmid or R factor, 46
Reversed passive agglutination, 78
Rhinoscleroma, 165
Rhinosporidiosis, 279
Rhinosporidium seeberi, 279
Rhizopus, 288
Ribosomal RNA (rRNA), 42
Rice-Tween 80 agar, 17
Rickettsia, 198
Rickettsiaceae, 198
Organisms causing human infections, 198
Rickettsial diseases of man, 199
Ritter's disease, 112
RNA
Structure of, 42
RNA viruses infecting humans, 234
Robert Koch, 3
Rocket electrophoresis, 76
Rocky Mountain spotted fever (RMSF), 200
Rotaviruses, 244, 246
RPR test, 156
RT-PCR, 48
Rubella, 257
Virus, 257

S

Sabouraud dextrose agar (SDA), 17
Emmons' modification of, 17
Sabouraud-cycloheximide-chloramphenicol agar, 17
Salmonella, 167, 169
Kauffmann-White classification, 170
Salmonella gastroenteritis, 172
Salmonella septicaemia, 172
Salmonellae
Antigenic structure, 169
Salpingitis, 205
Sandwich ELISA, 81
Saprophytes, 49
Satellitism, 186
Scalded skin syndrome, 112
Schaudinn's solution, 347
Schistosoma haematobium
Morphology of eggs, 337
Schistosoma japonicum
Morphology of eggs, 337
Schistosoma mansoni
Egg, 337
Morphology of eggs, 337
Schistosoma species
Life cycle, 336
Schistosomes or blood flukes, 335

Schultz-Charlton test, 115
Scrub typhus, 200
Selective and differential media, 18
Selective media, 13
Self-tolerance, 101
Sensitized individual, 95
Septicaemia, 211
Septicaemic plague, 174
Sereny test, 163
Serologic diagnosis, 356
Serratia, 162, 165
Serum sickness (systemic immune complex disease), 99
Sex pili, 9
Sexduction
    Process of, 45
Shigella, 167
    Differentiation of species, 167
Shigella boydii, 168
Shigella dysenteriae, 168
Shigella flexneri, 168
    Antigens of serotypes, 168
    Serotype 6 biotypes, 168
Shigella sonnei, 168
Siberian tick typhus (North Asian tick-borne spotted fever), 200
Silver impregnation method, 28
Simmons' citrate medium, 29
Single diffusion in one dimension (Oudin procedure), 74
Single diffusion in two dimensions (radial immunodiffusion), 74
Slide agglutination, 77
Slide coagulase test, 111
Slime layer, 7
Smallpox (variola), 239
Species immunity, 54
Species specificity, 61
Specimens
    Collection and transportation of, 23
        General rules, 23
    Criteria for rejection of, 23
Spirilla, 6
Spirochaetes, 6, 152
Spleen, 85
Sporangium, 9
Spore, 9
    Types of, 10
Sporothrix schenckii, 280
Sporotrichosis, 279
    Asteroid body in, 280
Sporulation, 9
    Morphological events in, 9
Spotted fevers, 200
Sputum container, 24
Sputum smear showing acid-fast tubercle bacilli, 139
Stab culture, 20
Staining techniques, 26
Standard tests for syphilis (STS), 155
Staphylococci, 109
Staphylococcus, 109

Staphylococcus aureus, 109
    Cell wall associated factors, 110
    Growth on blood agar showing haemolysis, 109
Steam sterilizer, 35
Sterilization, 33
    By radiation, 37
    Controls, 34, 36
Sterilization and disinfection
    Chemical agents, 38
    Physical agents, 33
Stool
    Examination methods, 348
Storage media, 13
Streak culture, 20
Streptobacillus, 210
Streptobacillus moniliformis, 211
Streptococci, 6
    Group B, 117
    Group D, 118
    In Gram-stained smear of pus, 114
Streptococcus, 114
Streptococcus MG, 119
Streptococcus MG agglutination, 77
Streptococcus pneumoniae (Pneumococcus), 120
Streptococcus pneumoniae and viridans streptococci, 121
Streptococcus pyogenes, 114
    Components of, 115
Stroke culture, 20
Strongyloides stercoralis, 328
    Life cycle, 329
Sugar fermentation, 29
Sugar media, 14
Superantigens, 62
Superficial infections, 283
Surface active disinfectants, 39
Syphilis
    Congenital, 154
    Laboratory diagnosis, 154
    Latent, 153
    Primary, 153
    Secondary, 153
    Tertiary, 154

T

T and B cells
    Development of, 84
T and B lymphocytes
    Differences, 87
T cells, 84, 85
    Differentiation, 86, 92
T lymphocytes, 84, 86
Taenia saginata, 330
    Life cycle, 331
Taenia solium, 330
    Life cycle, 331
Taenia saginata and *Taenia solium*
    Differentiating features, 330
Tetanolysin, 137

Tetanospasmin, 137
Tetanus toxins, 137
Tetrads, 6
Throat swabs, 24
Thymocytes, 86
Thymus, 83
'Thymus-dependent' regions, 84
Thymus-derived lymphocytes, 84
Tinea nigra, 272
Tissue typing (detection of MHC antigens), 105
Tolerance
    Mechanism of, 94
Tolerogens, 62
Toxin neutralization, 79
Toxoplasma gondii, 311
    Life cycle, 313
    Tachyzoites, 311, 312
    Tissue cysts in the brain, 312
Trachoma, 204
Transduction, 44
Transfer factor, 93
Transfer RNA (tRNA), 43
Transformation, 44
Transfusion malaria, 310
Transplant, 103
Transplantation immunology, 103
Transport media, 13
Transposon, 46
Treponema, 152
Treponema, *Borrelia* and *Leptospira*
    Differentiating features, 152
Treponema pallidum, 153
    Chancre on the penis, 154
    Chancre on the tongue, 154
    Nichol's strain, 153
Treponema phagedenis (*Reiter treponeme*), 153
Treponema refringens, 153
Treponemal tests, 156
Trichomonas, 299
Trichomonas hominis, 299
Trichomonas spp.
    Trophozoites of, 299
Trichomonas tenax, 299
Trichomonas vaginalis, 300
    Trophozoites in vaginal smear, 300
Trichuris trichiura, 326
    Egg, 327
    Life cycle, 327
Trophozoite-induced malaria, 310
Tube agglutination, 77
Tuberculosis
    Post-primary (secondary), 140
    Primary, 140
    Ziehl-Neelsen smear grading as per RNTCP recommendations, 141
Type I hypersensitivity
    Anaphylactic, 95
    Mechanism of, 95
Type II hypersensitivity: Cytotoxic, 97

Index

Type III hypersensitivity: Immune complex, 98

Type IV hypersensitivity: Cell-mediated or delayed, 99

Type V hypersensitivity: Stimulatory or antireceptor, 100

Typhoid fever, 170

Typhus fevers, 199

U

Ulcerative gingivostomatitis, 158

Unstained wet film, 26

Ureaplasma, 194

Ureaplasma urealyticum, 195

Urease test, 29

Urethritis, 205

Urine/stool container, 24

V

Vaccinia, 239

Vaccinia virion structure, 239

Vaginitis and vaginal discharge, 205

Vancomycin-resistant staphylococci, 113

Vapour-phase disinfectants, 39

Varicella, 241

Varicella zoster infection
    Vesicles on the left shoulder and neck, 242

Varicella-zoster virus (VZV), 241

VDRL test, 155

Verocytotoxigenic *E. coli* (VTEC), 163

Vibrio, 175

Vibrio cholerae, 175

Differences between classical and El Tor biotypes, 176

Vibrio cholerae non-O1, 178

Vibrio cholerae O1
    Phage types of strains of classical biotype, 177
    Phage types of strains of El Tor biotype, 177
    Subtypes, 176

Vibrios, 6

Viral infections
    Laboratory diagnosis, 235

Viral vaccines, 58

Viridans streptococci (oral streptococci), 114, 119

Viroids, 233

Virulence, 52
    Determinants of, 52

Virus isolation, 230

Virus neutralization tests, 79

Viruses
    Classification, 233
    General properties, 229
    Nomenclature, 233
    Replication, 230
    Shape, 230
    Structure, 229
    Symmetry of, 229

Voges-Proskauer (VP) test for acetoin production, 28

W

Wassermann reaction, 78

Waste segregation, 40

Water bacteriology
    Standard tests usually employed, 216

Water-borne pathogens, 215

Watson and Crick model of DNA, 43

Weil-Felix reaction, 77
    In rickettsial disease, 201

Weil's disease (infectious jaundice), 159

Western blotting, 82

White piedra, 272

Widal test, 77, 172
    Interpretation, 172

Woolsorter's disease, 132

Wound botulism, 138

Wuchereria bancrofti, 324
    In lymph node, 326
    Life cycle, 325

X

Xenografts, 103

Y

Yersinia pestis, 173
    Bipolar staining of, 173

Z

Ziehl-Neelsen stain, 27

Zone phenomenon, 73, 74

Zoonoses, 50

Zoonotic disease, 172, 173